CONTEMPORARY RESEARCH METHODS IN PHARMACY AND HEALTH SERVICES

VOLUME 2

CONTEMPORARY RESEARCH METHODS IN PHARMACY AND HEALTH SERVICES

VOLUME 2

Edited by

ALEDA M.H. CHEN
University of Arkansas for Medical Sciences, Little Rock, AR, United States

SHANE P. DESSELLE
Touro University, CA, United States

PARISA ASLANI
The University of Sydney, Sydney, NSW, Australia

FERNANDA STUMPF TONIN
University of Granada, Granada, Spain

TIMOTHY F. CHEN
The University of Sydney, Sydney, NSW, Australia

VICTORIA GARCÍA-CÁRDENAS
University of Granada, Granada, Spain

ELSEVIER

ACADEMIC PRESS
An imprint of Elsevier

Academic Press is an imprint of Elsevier
125 London Wall, London EC2Y 5AS, United Kingdom
50 Hampshire Street, 5th Floor, Cambridge, MA 02139, United States

For accessibility purposes, images in electronic versions of this book are accompanied by alt text descriptions independently provided by Elsevier, generated with the aid of AI. For more information, see https://www.elsevier.com/about/accessibility.

Books and Journals published by Elsevier comply with applicable product safety requirements. For any product safety concerns or queries, please contact our authorised representative, Elsevier B.V., at productsafety@elsevier.com.

Publisher's note: Elsevier takes a neutral position with respect to territorial disputes or jurisdictional claims in its published content, including in maps and institutional affiliations.

Notices
Knowledge and best practice in this field are constantly changing. As new research and experience broaden our understanding, changes in research methods, professional practices, or medical treatment may become necessary.

Practitioners and researchers must always rely on their own experience and knowledge in evaluating and using any information, methods, compounds, or experiments described herein. In using such information or methods they should be mindful of their own safety and the safety of others, including parties for whom they have a professional responsibility.

To the fullest extent of the law, neither the Publisher nor the authors, contributors, or editors, assume any liability for any injury and/or damage to persons or property as a matter of products liability, negligence or otherwise, or from any use or operation of any methods, products, instructions, or ideas contained in the material herein.

ISBN: 978-0-443-44607-8

For information on all Academic Press publications visit our website at https://www.elsevier.com/books-and-journals

Publisher: Andre Wolff
Editorial Project Manager: Pratishtha Gupta
Production Project Manager: Vijayaraj Purushothaman
Cover Designer: Raman Kumar

Typeset by Integra Software Services

Contents

IV
Technology advancing pharmacy research

Contributors

Nagham J. Ailabouni The University of Queensland, Brisbane, QLD, Australia

Anna Birna Almarsdóttir Department of Pharmacy, Faculty of Health and Medical Sciences, University of Copenhagen, Copenhagen, Denmark

Anneka Anderson University of Auckland, Te Kupenga Hauora Māori, Auckland, New Zealand

Lourdes Cantarero Arevalo Department of Pharmacy, Faculty of Health and Medical Sciences, University of Copenhagen, Copenhagen, Denmark

Isabelle Arnet medinform AG, Zurich, Switzerland

Mohsen Askar Department of Drug statistics, Norwegian Institute of Public Health, Oslo, Norway

Parisa Aslani Faculty of Medicine and Health, School of Pharmacy, The University of Sydney, Camperdown, NSW, Australia

Bethany Atkins School of Health Sciences, University of East Anglia, Norwich, Norfolk, United Kingdom

Adeola Bamgboje-Ayodele Discipline of Design, School of Architecture, Design and Planning, The University of Sydney, Camperdown, NSW, Australia

Carole Bandiera Sydney Pharmacy School, Faculty of Medicine and Health, University of Sydney, Sydney, NSW, Australia

Margaret Bermingham School of Pharmacy, University College Cork, Cork, Ireland

Debi Bhattacharya School of Health Sciences, University of East Anglia, Norwich, Norfolk, United Kingdom

Rachel Brown National Hauora Coalition, Auckland, New Zealand

Michael Bücker Münster School of Business - FH Münster, University of Applied Sciences, Münster, Germany

Caroline Buhl Department of Pharmacy, Faculty of Health and Medical Sciences, University of Copenhagen, Copenhagen, Denmark

Cathal Cadogan School of Pharmacy and Pharmaceutical Sciences, Trinity College Dublin, Dublin, Ireland

Rebecca Clarke Pharmacy Department, St James's Hospital, Dublin, Ireland

Michelle Cleary School of Nursing and Midwifery, Trinity College Dublin, Dublin, Ireland

Maeve Colleran Pharmacy Department, St James's Hospital, Dublin, Ireland

Jack C. Collins Faculty of Medicine and Health, School of Pharmacy, The University of Sydney, Camperdown, NSW, Australia

Jordan R. Covvey Duquesne University, School of Pharmacy, Pittsburgh, PA, United States

Robin Crunenberg Department of Pharmacy, ULiège, Liège, Belgium

Jacqueline Cumming Te Hikuwai Rangahau Hauora - Health Services Research Centre, Te Herenga Waka - Victoria University of Wellington, Wellington, New Zealand

Suelem Tavares da Silva Penteado Paraná State Department of Health, Curitiba, Brazil

Aline de Fátima Bonetti Pharmacy Department; Clinical Pharmacy Unit, Clinics Hospital Complex, Federal University of Paraná, Curitiba, Brazil

Alexandra L. Dima Avedis Donabedian Research Institute (FAD), Barcelona; Avaluació de tecnologies sanitàries en atenció primària i salut mental (PRISMA), Institut de Recerca Sant Joan de Déu (IRSJD), Esplugues de Llobregat; Universitat Autònoma de Barcelona (UAB), Barcelona; Consortium "Centro de Investigación Biomédica en Red" Epidemiology and Public Health (CIBERESP), Madrid, Spain

Carmel Doyle School of Nursing and Midwifery, Trinity College Dublin, Dublin, Ireland

Christiane Eickhoff Department of Medicine, Federal Union of German Associations of Pharmacists (ABDA), Berlin, Germany

Lynne Emmerton Curtin School of Diagnostic and Therapeutic Sciences, Curtin University, Perth, WA, Australia

Fernando Fernandez-Llimos Faculty of Pharmacy, Laboratory of Pharmacology, Department of Drug Sciences, University of Porto, Porto, Portugal

Michael R. Gionfriddo Geisinger College of Health Sciences, Scranton, PA, United States

Katri Hämeen-Anttila School of Pharmacy, Faculty of Health Sciences, University of Eastern Finland, Kuopio, Finland

Mark F. Harris International Centre for Future Health Systems, University of New South Wales, Sydney, NSW, Australia

Robert Haua Ngā Kaitiaki o Te Puna Rongoā o Aotearoa, Taupō, New Zealand

Joanna Hikaka Ngā Kaitiaki o Te Puna Rongoā o Aotearoa, Taupō; University of Auckland, Te Kupenga Hauora Māori, Auckland, New Zealand

Jun Ni Ho Quality Use of Medicines and Pharmacy Research Centre, School of Pharmacy and Biomedical Science, College of Health, Adelaide University, Adelaide, SA, Australia

Sara Sommer Holst Capital Region Pharmacy, Copenhagen University Hospital Bispebjerg, Copenhagen, Denmark

Kreshnik Hoti University of Pristina, Pristina, Serbia

Kimberly Illingworth Faculty Affairs and Pharmacy Practice, Purdue University, West Lafayette, IN, United States

Ramune Jacobsen Department of Pharmacy, Faculty of Health and Medical Sciences, University of Copenhagen, Copenhagen, Denmark

Dragana Jocic Faculty of Pharmacy, Novi Sad, Serbia

Suanne Kaae Department of Pharmacy, Faculty of Health and Medical Sciences, University of Copenhagen, Copenhagen, Denmark

Susanne Kaae Department of Pharmacy, Faculty of Health and Medical Sciences, University of Copenhagen, Copenhagen, Denmark

Melissa A. Kalarchian Duquesne University, School of Nursing, Pittsburgh, PA, United States

Renly Lim Quality Use of Medicines and Pharmacy Research Centre, School of Pharmacy and Biomedical Science, College of Health, Adelaide University, Adelaide, SA, Australia; Development and Innovation, Centre for Translational Research, Institute for Research, Development and Innovation, IMU University, Kuala Lumpur, Malaysia

Kate Lowrie Research Integrity and Ethics Administration, University of Sydney, Sydney, NSW, Australia

Cherie Lucas Faculty of Medicine and Health, University of NSW (UNSW) Sydney, Sydney, NSW, Australia

Valentina Marinkovic Faculty of Pharmacy, Belgrade, Serbia

Antonio Matoso Mendes Pharmacy Department; Clinical Pharmacy Unit, Clinics Hospital Complex - Federal University of Paraná, Curitiba, Brazil

Chyna McClendon Duquesne University, School of Pharmacy, Pittsburgh, PA, United States

Janet McDonald Te Hikuwai Rangahau Hauora - Health Services Research Centre, Te Herenga Waka - Victoria University of Wellington, Wellington, New Zealand

Brendon McIntosh Ngā Kaitiaki o Te Puna Rongoā o Aotearoa, Taupō, New Zealand

Gail Melanophy Pharmacy Department, St James's Hospital, Dublin, Ireland

Ardalan Mirzaei Faculty of Medicine and Health, School of Pharmacy, The University of Sydney, Sydney, NSW, Australia

Sabuj Kanti Mistry School of Population Health, University of New South Wales, Sydney, NSW, Australia

Christopher Mosch Pharmaceutical Biology and Clinical Pharmacy, Pharmacotherapy Research Group, Institute of Pharmacy, Paracelsus Medical University, Salzburg, Austria

Logan Thomas Murry Accreditation Council for Pharmacy Education, Continuing Pharmacy Education and Continuing Professional Development, Chicago, IL; Pharmacy Practice and Science, The University of Iowa College of Pharmacy, Iowa City, IA, United States

Jenny Leigh Newlon Birth Control Pharmacist, Oak Park, CA, United States

David A. Nolfi Duquesne University, Gumberg Library, Pittsburgh, PA, United States

Lotte Stig Nørgaard Department of Pharmacy, Faculty of Health and Medical Sciences, University of Copenhagen, Copenhagen, Denmark

Tara N. Officer Te Puna Hauora - School of Health, Te Herenga Waka - Victoria University of Wellington, Wellington, New Zealand

Ayomide Ogundipe Curtin School of Diagnostic and Therapeutic Sciences, Curtin University, Perth, WA, Australia

Ana Flávia Redolfi Oliota State University of Western Paraná, Cascavel, Brazil

Nora Parore Te Hikuwai Rangahau Hauora - Health Services Research Centre, Te Herenga Waka - Victoria University of Wellington, Wellington, New Zealand

L. Alison Phillips Department of Psychology, Iowa State University, Ames, IA, United States

Olaf Rose Department of Pharmaceutical Biology and Clinical Pharmacy, Institute of Pharmacy, Paracelsus Medical University, Salzburg, Austria

Elizabeth E. Roughead Quality Use of Medicines and Pharmacy Research Centre, School of Pharmacy and Biomedical Science, College of Health, Adelaide University, Adelaide, SA, Australia

Lynne Russell Te Hikuwai Rangahau Hauora - Health Services Research Centre, Te Herenga Waka - Victoria University of Wellington, Wellington, New Zealand

Cristín Ryan School of Pharmacy and Pharmaceutical Sciences, Trinity College Dublin, Dublin, Ireland

Marissa Ryan School of Pharmacy and Pharmaceutical Sciences, The University of Queensland; Pharmacy Department, Princess Alexandra Hospital, Brisbane, QLD, Australia

Leena Saastamoinen Research and Development Unit, Helsinki, Finland

Laura J. Sahm Pharmaceutical Care Research Group, School of Pharmacy, University College Cork; Pharmacy Department, Mercy University Hospital, Cork, Ireland

Carl Richard Schneider Faculty of Medicine and Health, School of Pharmacy, The University of Sydney, Sydney, NSW, Australia

Sion Scott School of Health Sciences, University of East Anglia, Norwich, Norfolk, United Kingdom

Tin Fei Sim Curtin School of Diagnostic and Therapeutic Sciences, Curtin University, Perth, WA, Australia

Kirsten Smiler Te Hikuwai Rangahau Hauora - Health Services Research Centre, Te Herenga Waka - Victoria University of Wellington, Wellington, New Zealand

Centaine L. Snoswell School of Pharmacy and Pharmaceutical Sciences, The University of Queensland, Brisbane, QLD, Australia

Nátalia Stollárová School of Pharmacy and Pharmaceutical Sciences, Trinity College Dublin, Dublin, Ireland; Department of Pharmacology and Toxicology, Faculty of Pharmacy, Comenius University Bratislava, Bratislava, Slovakia

Aimo Strömberg School of Pharmacy, Faculty of Health Sciences, University of Eastern Finland, Kuopio, Finland

Kristian Svendsen Department of Pharmacy, Faculty of Health Sciences, UiT-The Arctic University of Norway, Tromsø, Norway

Donna Thomas Sydney School of Health Sciences, Faculty of Medicine and Health, University of Sydney, Sydney, NSW, Australia

Fernanda S. Tonin Social and Legal Pharmacy Section, Pharmacy and Pharmaceutical Technology Department, University of Granada, Granada, Spain

Amaia Urionagüena Department of Pharmacy and Food Sciences, Faculty of Pharmacy, University of the Basque Country, UPV/EHU, Vitoria-Gasteiz, Spain

Jonathan Vella MCAST, Paola, Malta

Jouko Verho VATT Institute for Economic Research, Helsinki, Finland

Charlotte Vermehren Capital Region Pharmacy, Copenhagen University Hospital Bispebjerg; Department of Drug Design and Pharmacology, Faculty of Health and Medical Sciences, University of Copenhagen, Copenhagen, Denmark

Matthew Witry Department of Pharmacy Practice and Science, University of Iowa, Iowa City, IA, United States

Reginald Amin Yakob Faculty of Medicine and Health, School of Pharmacy, The University of Sydney, Camperdown, NSW, Australia

About the editors

Aleda M.H. Chen, PharmD, MS, PhD, FAPhA, is a Professor and Director of Assessment at the University of Arkansas for Medical Sciences College of Pharmacy. She is an Associate Editor at *Research in Social and Administrative Pharmacy* (RSAP) and coedits the major text *Pharmacy Management: Essentials for All Settings*. In 2024, she won the Lyman Award from the American Association of Colleges of Pharmacy (AACP) for the best educational research paper in the *American Journal of Pharmacy Education*, and in 2026, she received the AACP Distinguished Teaching Scholar Award. Her teaching and research interests focus on pharmacy assessment, competency-based education (CBE), implementation science, and behavior change, leading to over 125 published papers in peer-reviewed journals. Her work in CBE has led to her becoming a member of the International CBE Health Professions Collaborative and guest editing a collection of papers on the implementation of CBE for *Perspectives in Medical Education*.

Shane P. Desselle, RPh, PhD, FAPhA, is the Associate Dean for Research & Professional Affairs, Chair, and Professor at Touro University California. He is the founding Editor-in-Chief of *RSAP* and *Exploratory Research in Clinical and Social Pharmacy* (*ERCSP*). In addition, he coedits the major text *Pharmacy Management: Essentials for All Settings*, now in its sixth, worldwide edition. He has published over 170 papers in peer-reviewed journals. In 2020, he coauthored a paper winning the Wiederholt Prize for the best paper published in the *Journal of the American Pharmacists Association*, and in 2019, he won the AACP Sustained Contribution Award for his teaching, scholarship, and service in social/administrative pharmacy. His federally funded research focuses on organizational culture, quality of work life, and advancing the roles of various professionals within the medication use and education systems.

Parisa Aslani, BPharm(Hons), MSc, GradCertEdStud (Higher Ed), PhD, MRPharmS, FPS, FFIP, FANZCAP, is a Professor in Medicines Use Optimisation at The University of Sydney, Australia. She is known internationally for her research in the areas of consumer medicines information and adherence to therapy. Her research has impacted policy and education in the healthcare sector, and at the Australian Government level, and has led to a global initiative on developing medicine information strategies for implementation at national and local levels. Her research skills range from qualitative techniques to survey design and randomized control trials.

Fernanda Stumpf Tonin, PhD, is a Distinguished Professor at the Faculty of Pharmacy, University of Granada, Spain, and an Integrated Researcher at the Health & Technology Research Center, Instituto Politécnico de Lisboa, Portugal. She is also a senior researcher at the National Research Group in Health Technology Assessment (NATS/UFPR) in Brazil. She serves as Vice-Chair of the Pharmacy Practice Research Special Interest Group of the International Pharmaceutical Federation and as an associate editor of *ERCSP*. Her research focuses on health technology assessment, pharmacoeconomics, and health outcomes research, with more than 150 publications in international peer-reviewed journals. She has been ranked among the world's top 2% most-cited scientists by Stanford University. She also works as an HEOR and Market Access consultant in healthcare.

Timothy F. Chen, BPharm, DipHPharm, PhD, FFIP, FPS, FANZCAP, ARPharmS is a professor of Medication Management at The University of Sydney, Australia. Tim is nationally and internationally renowned for his research in medication review and strategies to reduce medication-related harm. He has published extensively in this and other areas of practice. Tim's research has informed significant practice change, through the implementation of the Australian Commonwealth Government funded Home Medicines Review program. Tim currently leads a large and productive postgraduate research team and is the recipient of university and national teaching awards.

Victoria García-Cárdenas, BPharm, MPharm, PhD, FFIP, is an associate professor at the University of Granada, Spain, where she serves as Vice-Dean for International Relations and Postgraduate Studies at the Faculty of Pharmacy. Her teaching and research focus on the development, evaluation, and implementation of professional pharmacy services, aiming to optimize the quality use of medicines and improve patient outcomes. Her work also addresses the advancement of patient-centered care and the integration of clinical pharmacy services within healthcare systems. She has authored over 90 peer-reviewed publications and has participated in several nationally and internationally funded research projects.

Preface

The first volume of the *Contemporary Research Methods in Pharmacy and Health Services* textbook outlined the historical underpinnings and growth of pharmacy and health services research. Following the positive reception of the first volume and the continued growth of this research area, the need for a second volume became readily apparent. This text offers another compendium of research methods, including new and emerging areas, to serve as an excellent resource for research programs to use as a complement to primary literature, providing examples, case studies, and discussion questions that can clarify best practices.

Further, this volume continues to represent global research efforts. Authors from around the world have contributed chapters, showcasing the breadth of research within pharmacy and health services and representing different resources and healthcare structures.

How the book is organized and its contents

For those familiar with the first volume, this volume follows a similar organization. Each chapter includes learning objectives, an overview of the methodology or analytical approach, questions for discussion, and application exercises. These components provide great opportunities for faculty and learners, at both the undergraduate and graduate levels, to engage in discussions, for example:

- Generating research ideas sparked by innovative methodologies or analytical approaches
- Debating which methodology or analytical approach to consider when beginning a project
- Comparing and contrasting the strengths and weaknesses of different approaches

Most of these chapters have been informed by various papers in the peer-reviewed journals, *Research in Social and Administrative Pharmacy,* and its newer counterpart, *Exploratory Research in Clinical and Social Pharmacy*. While every paper in those journals undergoes rigorous peer review, these chapters have been modified to focus on the methodology and analytical approaches, followed by more rounds of review. Thus, each chapter serves as a stand-alone resource and independent from other chapters; however, we have organized them into four sections, which are:

- Section I. Methodological Cornerstones of High-Quality Pharmacy and Health Services Research
- Section II. Designing and Evaluating Interventions in Pharmacy and Health Services Research
- Section III. Innovative Methods and Tools in Pharmacy and Health Services Research
- Section IV. Technology Advancing Pharmacy and Health Services Research

Notably, in this second volume, readers will see the juxtaposition of examining traditional and emerging methods. For example, several chapters focus on traditional research methodologies, where rigorous adherence may not be as common as desired. Conversely, several chapters on emerging technology and approaches examine the use of artificial intelligence in research methodology and analysis.

What we hope you will gain from this book

We hope that, much like the first volume, this will spark lots of research conversations among learners, mentors, and senior researchers, pushing them to ask: What are best practices? What are new approaches that I might consider? And how might I innovate and move research methodology in pharmacy and health services forward? Maybe it will even spark the papers that will comprise the next volume of this textbook!

To quote our previous preface, "we hope that the contents of the book will help the disciplines of social pharmacy and related health service research disciplines take another step forward in their respective scientific paradigms, help to enhance the quality of research undertaken, improve researchers' chances at getting funded and published, evoke new ideas to tackle age-old problems, and also provide a basis for provocative and edifying dialog between mentors and mentees in research." Thank you, and we are so excited to bring this second volume forward!

SECTION I

Methodological cornerstones of high quality pharmacy research

CHAPTER

1

How to validate self-reported questionnaires for pharmacy practice? Methodological recommendations with the 15-STARS as an illustrative example

Isabelle Arnet[a], *Alexandra L. Dima*[b,c,d,e], *Laura J. Sahm*[f,g], *and Christiane Eickhoff*[h]

[a]medinform AG, Zurich, Switzerland
[b]Avedis Donabedian Research Institute (FAD), Barcelona, Spain
[c]Avaluació de tecnologies sanitàries en atenció primària i salut mental (PRISMA), Institut de Recerca Sant Joan de Déu (IRSJD), Esplugues de Llobregat, Spain
[d]Universitat Autònoma de Barcelona (UAB), Barcelona, Spain
[e]Consortium "Centro de Investigación Biomédica en Red" Epidemiology and Public Health (CIBERESP), Madrid, Spain
[f]Pharmaceutical Care Research Group, School of Pharmacy, University College Cork, Cork, Ireland
[g]Pharmacy Department, Mercy University Hospital, Cork, Ireland
[h]Department of Medicine, Federal Union of German Associations of Pharmacists (ABDA), Berlin, Germany

CHAPTER OBJECTIVES

- To present the methodological, contextual, and practical challenges encountered during the validation procedure of questionnaires used as patient-reported outcome measures (PROMs).
- To use a novel self-reported questionnaire developed to screen for medication nonadherence as an example to discuss the standard validation requirements according to the COSMIN guideline.
- To explore and explain situations where adaptation of the standard validation requirements was needed in light of the questionnaire's purpose and content.

Contemporary Research Methods in Pharmacy and Health Services - Volume 2
https://doi.org/10.1016/B978-0-443-44607-8.00004-2

1 Introduction

The validation of questionnaires, which are used as patient-reported outcome measures (PROMs), is crucial to enable researchers and healthcare professionals to make an informed choice when selecting the most suitable tool for a given purpose or context of use. Validation procedures aim to ensure that an instrument is valid (i.e., it measures what it is intended to measure), reliable (i.e., the measure is consistent), relevant to clinical and practice use (i.e., actionable), and responsive (i.e., sensitive to clinical change over time) (Cook and Beckman, 2006). In addition to these methodological requirements, instruments should be practical (i.e., brief yet comprehensive) and adaptable across various cultures and languages. Standards have been developed over the last decades to help develop, report, and ultimately select the most appropriate questionnaire. COnsensus-based Standards for the selection of health Measurement INstruments (COSMIN) (Mokkink et al., 2024a, 2024b) has become the most recognized and widely used standard for validating PROMs due to its rigorous and systematic approach (Terwee et al., 2016; Churruca et al., 2021). Several measurement (or psychometric) properties have been adopted and categorized into three domains: for **validity**, 1.1. content validity, 1.2. face validity, 1.3. construct validity, 1.4. structural validity, 1.5. hypotheses testing, 1.6. cross-cultural validity, and 1.7. criterion validity; for **reliability**, 2.1. internal consistency and 2.2. test-retest; as well as 3.1. responsiveness and 3.2. interpretability and feasibility (Table 1.1). The performance of a questionnaire can thus be evaluated in each of these domains. To translate these abstract properties into concrete, measurable procedures and analyses that can be interpreted—i.e., to operationalize them—rigorous procedures are used, many of them involving statistical analyses (Table 1.1).

TABLE 1.1 Definitions of COSMIN properties with operationalization.

Definition	Operationalization
Domain 1: Validity	
1.1. Content validity	
• The items adequately reflect the concept (e.g., pain, quality of life, medication use) • The target population is clearly identified (age, condition, culture) • The items comprehensively cover all relevant aspects of the constructs being measured	• The target population and experts are involved in item generation • Cognitive interviews are conducted to confirm item relevance and understanding
1.2. Face validity [a]	
• The tool subjectively ("it looks like") covers the concept it is supposed to measure • The tool seems to be appropriate and understandable	• Feedback is collected upon the first questionnaire completion, often from users
1.3. Construct validity [b]	
• The items truly capture the underlying theoretical construct(s)	• The tool is compared to other validated instruments (not the gold standard) • Expected correlations and group differences have been reported
1.4. Structural validity	
• The item structure, whether as a single scale or divided into subscales, reflects the underlying conceptual model • The tool is unidimensional or multidimensional	• Exploratory/Confirmatory Factor Analysis (EFA/CFA) or Item Response Theory (IRT) analysis is conducted • Model fit indices are assessed
1.5. Hypothesis testing	
• The tool performs according to the theoretical assumptions	• Results are compared to predefined hypotheses
1.6. Cross-cultural validity	
• The tool performs equivalently across respondents with the same underlying trait, regardless of cultural, language, or demographic group	• Translation and back-translation are conducted for new language versions • Cross-cultural adaptation guidelines are used [e.g., ISPOR (Wild et al., 2005)] • Differential Item Functioning (DIF) is examined across groups
1.7. Criterion validity	
• The tool corresponds to a gold standard	•Expected correlation coefficient is reported

Definition	Operationalization
DOMAIN 2: Reliability	
2.1. Internal consistency	
• The items of a scale or subscale contribute to measuring the same underlying construct • There is consistency within subscales	• A measure of internal consistency is reported, depending on the type of scale tested [e.g., Cronbach's alpha or McDonald's omega; (Malkewitz et al., 2023)] • Expected item-total correlations are reported
2.2. Test-retest reliability	
• Stability of the tool's results over time under the same conditions for both tests (mode, settings, etc.)	• The questionnaire is administered twice, within a time interval during which the construct is expected to remain relatively stable, while also allowing the respondents to have less recollection of the first administration • The Intraclass Correlation Coefficient (ICC) is reported • Time interval is neither too short nor too long.
Domain 3: Responsiveness	
3.1. Responsiveness	
• The tool detects clinically meaningful changes over time	• Effect sizes (Cohen's d) or Standardized Response Means (SRMs) are reported • Minimal Clinically Important Difference (MCID) is defined
3.2. Interpretability and feasibility	
• A qualitative meaning can be assigned to the results	• The questionnaire displays key characteristics needed when applying the tool in real-world settings (understandability, appropriate length, acceptable completion time, and missing data rates)

[a]*COSMIN considers face validity as part of content validity, as a practical component.*
[b]*In the COSMIN guidelines, construct validity includes structural validity, hypothesis testing, and cross-cultural validity (Mokkink et al., 2010).*
Modified from Mokkink, L.B., Elsman, E.B.M., Terwee, C.B., 2024a. COSMIN guideline for systematic reviews of patient-reported outcome measures version 2.0. Qual. Life Res. 1573-2649. 33(11), 2929–2939. Available from: https://www.springer.com/journal/11136. doi:10.1007/s11136-024-03761-6.

In some cases, these psychometric requirements may need to be prioritized differently because applying them too strictly can be impractical or counterproductive in certain real-world contexts. Mainly, the COSMIN standard has been designed with research-level use in mind and is context-sensitive (Mokkink et al., 2024a, 2024b). Consequently, the need for maximizing construct validity or responsiveness may be lower for routine clinical use when weighed against other properties, such as feasibility, based on the instrument's purpose. Thus, matching the rigor of validation to the intended use of the questionnaire is often necessary, given the many constraints of data collection in some settings and the specificities of the measured constructs. An example is the length of a questionnaire. While many items are typically needed to ensure content validity by comprehensively covering all aspects of a construct, respondents are usually only willing to answer a limited number of questions. As a result, a trade-off between content validity and feasibility is often required. Thus, it might not be possible, nor necessary, to maximize all measurement properties simultaneously; instead, a balanced compromise is essential.

The 15-Screening Tool for AdheRence to medicineS (15-STARS) is a self-report questionnaire developed to address the need for a user-friendly tool that identifies difficulties with medication use (i.e., adherence) in everyday practice and serves as a basis for delivering support and tailored interventions. Items were identified through workshops, surveys, and meetings, and fall within two distinct conceptual domains used in the assessment of medication nonadherence: quantifying medicine use directly relative to a given time period and eliciting responses regarding medicine use behavior, as well as barriers to or beliefs about medicines that may influence medicine use behavior. The 15-STARS identifies modifiable factors of medication nonadherence (Arnet et al., 2024) with 15 single items. It detects different facets of nonadherent behavior and its determinants, such as handling difficulties, beliefs, reasons for not taking a medicine, frequency of missed doses, and the need for help from the pharmacy; i.e., it covers various aspects of one construct. The 15-STARS is a screening instrument designed to quickly identify potential issues and flag individuals who may need further evaluation. It was not designed to provide a definitive diagnosis or track changes over time. This focus on timely identification affects how strictly certain psychometric properties were applied. This chapter details the validation procedure of the 15-STARS against the COSMIN criteria as an illustrative example of the reasoning behind the selection of specific psychometric properties. Justification is provided in instances where some psychometric requirements were adapted, including a discussion of the need to adapt certain psychometric properties.

2 Methods

2.1 Content validity

Content validity is the most critical psychometric property, especially for self-reported instruments (US Food and Drug Administration, 2009). According to COSMIN, content validity is foundational and requires input from the target group and experts to ensure relevance, comprehensiveness, and comprehensibility. For a screening tool, the items must cover as many relevant domains as feasible, clearly and briefly.

For the 15-STARS development and validation, workshops were organized involving multiple stakeholders, including patients (target users), pharmacists (end users), and experts (content specialists). Qualitative, iterative development methods were used, with initial and revised items based on feedback. The workshops provided information about item generation, refinement, and face validity assessment with both patients and pharmacists.

Finding: The 15-STARS aligns well with COSMIN requirements and has a strong development process, which is acceptable for screening purposes.

2.2 Face validity

Face validity refers specifically to whether the items of a questionnaire appear to be appropriate and understandable to the target population. COSMIN does not treat face validity as a separate psychometric domain; rather, it considers face validity part of content validity as a practical and perceptual component (Mokkink et al., 2010). We present it separately here due to the special importance we give to this property and the distinct research tasks it requires.

Regarding the 15-STARS validation, face validity was assessed based on the clarity of the instrument for the target population (i.e., 144 German- and French-speaking patients). This assessment was based on missing data for each item, as well as written structured feedback from the patients. Items were revised as necessary. Respondents considered the 15-STARS to effectively measure behaviors and determinants relevant to medication adherence, which was also reflected in the high completion rates. There was less than 5% missing data.

Finding: The involvement of the target population and the low amount of missing data suggest that the items of the 15-STARS are generally understandable and acceptable to respondents. However, probing each item's understanding and interpretation by patients through cognitive interviews or "think-aloud" protocols was not performed. This might represent a gap relative to the COSMIN risk-of-bias checklist, which lists cognitive interviews to test for comprehensibility in a pilot study. Nevertheless, cognitive testing might be less critical for a screening instrument like the 15-STARS, which is designed primarily to initiate a subsequent conversation with a health-care professional.

2.3 Construct validity

Construct validity focuses on the theoretical relationships between the questionnaire and other instruments, as well as the differences in responses expected among different populations. However, a strong theoretical framework or well-developed theory explaining how the construct operates is often lacking for many questionnaires during the development process. In COSMIN, testing specific hypotheses about these relationships and differences is the recommended way to investigate construct validity, as no gold standards exist for PROMs (Mokkink et al., 2019). The property "hypothesis testing for construct validity" is divided into "convergent validity" for a comparison with other similar instruments and "discriminative or known-groups validity" for a comparison with different populations (Mokkink et al., 2019). In parallel with these two distinct requirements, the COSMIN taxonomy presents the property "construct validity" as including three distinct subcategories: "hypothesis testing", "structural validity", and "cross-cultural validity", with the same definition as "hypothesis testing" (Mokkink et al., 2010).

In contrast to COSMIN's recommendations, which consider construct validity as a general category encompassing a range of hypotheses to test convergent, discriminant, and known-groups validity (as well as structural and crosscultural validity), we prefer to present convergent and discriminant validity as the key criteria related to construct validity, bringing them into focus as the most commonly used and most relevant. Irrespective of the preferred classification, the same basic principles apply. For instruments measuring the same or similar construct (convergent validity), a high correlation is expected ($r > 0.5$). For instruments measuring unrelated constructs (discriminant validity), a low correlation is expected ($r < 0.3$).

Regarding the 15-STARS validation, construct validity was assessed by comparing two index questions as a proxy for medication adherence ["In the last 30 days, (1) Have you ever not taken at least one of your medicine(s)? and (2) If yes: on how many days did you miss at least one dose of any of your medicines?"] with item 12 ["Over the past 2 weeks, how often have you missed taking any of your medicines?"] and item 13 ["Over the past 6 months, have you ever decided to interrupt/stop taking any of your medicines?"]. The correlation between the averaged scores of the 15-STARS and the two external questions, based on the answers from 140 German- and French-speaking patients, was statistically significant and moderate ($r = 0.363$; $p < 0.001$; Arnet et al., 2024). This moderate convergent validity was indicative of construct validity of the 15-STARS for the two items addressing the dimension of self-report of missed doses. The low correlation factor is indicative of barriers to feasibility in terms of comprehension barriers: the different answer formats (yes/no versus frequency) may have weakened the correlation. In fact, the responses to the 15-STARS items and the index questions were skewed, with 56.4% and 65.7% of patients achieving the maximum score of 100% on the 15-STARS and the index questions, respectively.

Finding: The two index questions used as comparators are conceptually related to nonadherence and meet COSMIN expectations. However, none are true "gold standard" adherence measures, which, in this case, are electronic monitoring. Nevertheless, appropriate correlation analyses and group comparisons were used to examine the relationships between items and comparators, which are consistent with COSMIN standards. Given that the main focus of the 15-STARS development was to examine structural validity and other properties of the 15-STARS, the values obtained are acceptable (Arnet et al., 2024).

2.4 Structural validity

According to COSMIN, the analysis of dimensionality (i.e., factor structure) is examined using Exploratory Factor Analysis (EFA), Confirmatory Factor Analysis (CFA), or parametric or nonparametric Item Response Theory (IRT). Once the structure of the questionnaire is known, for example, from previous work on the construct, COSMIN prefers CFA for strong evidence, but EFA is acceptable in exploratory phases when the factor structure is not yet known. The recommended sample size ranges from a few responses for a short unidimensional questionnaire to thousands of responses for questionnaires with many items and dimensions. For a screening tool, structural validity is important but less critical, given that the goal is to identify several aspects that might be of concern in the shortest time. Thus, it might be less important to increase precision through the measurement of each aspect with a high number of items. Moreover, these aspects are selected based on their individual relevance to the behavior they aim to detect, and there are no theoretical constraints or expectations on their interrelationships. Nevertheless, exploring the structure provides useful information about how these aspects are related.

The 15-STARS does not measure a single unified construct. Instead, it is structured as a multidimensional screening tool, with single items or groups of items thematically grouped into four distinct aspects or reasons for nonadherence: practical barriers, beliefs, missed doses, and need for support.

Regarding the 15-STARS validation, nine items (five measuring practical barriers and four measuring beliefs) were included in an EFA with Varimax rotation to explore their structure. The remaining items, which are intended to measure distinct aspects of adherence (missed doses and need for support), were not used. Results differed between the French and German versions. In the French version, we identified a 4-factor solution, with three items loading on the first and second factors each (factor loadings 0.587–0.739 and 0.627–0.892, respectively, explaining 64.4% of the total variance), and the other items loading one on the third and two on the fourth factor (factor loadings 0.745 and 0.580–0.819, respectively). In the German version, we identified a 5-factor solution, with three items loading on the first factor (factor loadings 0.644–0.817), two items loading on the second and third factors each (factor loadings 0.646–0.851 and 0.855–0.867, respectively, explaining 69.0% of the total variance), and one other item loading on the fifth factor (factor loadings 0.840). One item ("because of the costs") was answered with "yes" by 98.4% of the respondents and was eliminated from the Varimax calculation. Only one item ("understand the instructions for my medicines") loaded onto a common factor for both versions.

Finding: The 15-STARS does not provide evidence for internal dimensionality but shows a multidimensional structure. This was expected according to the development of the tool, which incorporates various single aspects of adherence. However, the four-block structure was the result of conceptual development, not statistical analysis. Thus, applying CFA and IRT could be explored in future work to strengthen this initial evidence. Of note, this rating does not weaken the tool's usefulness.

2.5 Hypotheses testing

According to COSMIN, testing hypotheses about expected differences between relevant groups (i.e., known-groups hypothesis testing) consists of comparing groups' results with appropriate statistical tests (e.g., t-tests between groups). For screening tools, hypothesis testing is important to support construct validity but is not the most critical psychometric step.

Regarding the 15-STARS validation, no group differences were expected (e.g., between men and women, age groups, French and German); therefore, this property was not tested. Refer to 2.3. Construct validity with a correlation factor of 0.363.

Finding: The procedure of hypothesis testing for the 15-STARS was consistent with the general spirit of COSMIN, but it did not meet COSMIN's high methodological standards (i.e., several prespecified, explicit hypotheses with a positive/negative direction, an expected magnitude, and expected differences between known groups, with a large sample size). Thus, the quality of evidence relative to hypothesis testing is limited. Future studies might generate more hypotheses to test, such as comparing groups known to be more at risk of nonadherence based on previous research or contrasting the 15-STARS with other related constructs such as self-management, patient-provider relationships, health literacy, etc.

2.6 Crosscultural validity

According to COSMIN, cross-cultural validity must be assessed using quantitative testing of equivalence with multigroup analyses (e.g., multigroup CFA (MG-CFA) or differential item functioning (DIF) analysis). A sample size of ≥100–200 participants per group is preferred. For screening tools, cross-cultural validity is important for detecting issues equally well in all populations, independent of cultural context.

The 15-STARS questionnaire was developed in English and underwent validation in a bilingual context (French and German within Switzerland). Translation and adaptation procedures were followed according to the accepted guidelines from the International Society for Pharmacoeconomics and Outcomes Research (ISPOR) (Wild et al., 2005) including independent forward and backward translation, expert review, reconciliation, and cultural adaptation with a linguist. The qualitative approach of pretesting through cognitive interviews with target users enabled the identification and resolution of major issues. Separate analyses (e.g., internal consistency, test-retest reliability) were conducted for each language version and compared.

Finding: The full cross-cultural validation procedure per COSMIN standards (i.e., MG-CFA or DIF analysis) was not performed with the 15-STARS. Thus, it is theoretically unclear whether results can be meaningfully compared across populations. However, the 15-STARS underwent bilingual development and was tested in two linguistically and culturally distinct populations within Switzerland. The successful identification of similar adherence barriers across cultures indicates that the underlying concepts are transferable. This demonstrated early cross-linguistic transferability and sets a strong foundation, although the two language samples were analyzed together and equivalence across languages was not verified. Thus, the current validation status of the 15-STARS can still be considered acceptable. In addition, early-stage acceptability of the 15-STARS is justified because future cross-cultural translations and studies are planned, and the tool is currently used in exploratory research (Barbati et al., 2025) and not yet in clinical decision-making.

2.7 Criterion validity

COSMIN standards expect correlation with a gold standard, i.e., a trusted, established tool that measures the same construct. In the case of medication adherence, the gold standard consists of electronic monitoring data. If unavailable, an objective criterion can be used instead, for example, pharmacy dispensing/refill data. For subjective outcomes, construct validity is evaluated instead of criterion validity. For a screening tool, criterion validity should correspond with known indicators.

The 15-STARS questionnaire was not compared to a gold standard or to objective measures of adherence. Construct validity was evaluated instead using two validated single self-report questions that assess the frequency of missed medication (refer to 2.3. Construct validity).

Finding: Because self-report should not serve as a gold-standard comparator for a self-report tool, the interpretation of the criterion validity of the 15-STARS is ambiguous. Of note, this does not reflect poor quality of the 15-STARS but rather that COSMIN criterion validity requirements are not yet met. Nevertheless, the criterion validity is partially acceptable because the screening tool identifies adherence difficulties, which is sufficient for exploratory use. It is not yet robust enough for clinical decisions.

2.8 Internal consistency

COSMIN standards recommend Cronbach's alpha as the primary statistic for assessing internal consistency, provided that the unidimensionality of the scale has been confirmed. For multiple domains, alpha should be calculated separately for each subscale. A threshold of $\alpha \geq 0.70$ is desirable. For screening tools, internal consistency is of moderate importance because the items highlight different facets of the construct rather than a single construct.

Regarding the 15-STARS validation, Cronbach's alpha was calculated for the items that assess practical barriers and beliefs. These items reflect independent risk factors and are intentionally heterogeneous. Thus, they are not expected to correlate strongly, and a low Cronbach's alpha is anticipated. Values were acceptable for the French version ($\alpha = 0.61–0.72$) and low for the German version ($\alpha = 0.43–0.45$). Following these mixed results per COSMIN thresholds, the French version is marginally acceptable, while the German version is below standard, indicating issues with dimensionality or item functioning.

Finding: The 15-STARS was structured conceptually as various heterogeneous items grouped into four thematic blocks, but they were not tested as unidimensional subscales. Thus, the coherence of a unidimensional scale or of each block was unlikely, and a low Cronbach's alpha was expected. Therefore, the low internal consistency of the 15-STARS is of minor concern and not a critical flaw due to the contextual and conceptual screening purposes of the questionnaire.

2.9 Test-retest reliability

COSMIN standards recommend the use of the Intraclass Correlation Coefficient (ICC) or weighted Kappa to measure the degree of agreement between scores of the same respondents at two time points. A threshold of ICC or Kappa ≥ 0.70 is considered acceptable. Pearson's or Spearman's r are less preferred because they measure correlation rather than exact agreement. For a screening tool, test-retest reliability is desirable but not essential if it is used at only one time point. Because the 15-STARS does not produce a total score, correlation at the item-level was calculated (Zijlmans et al., 2018). Furthermore, as most items in the 15-STARS are binary responses, Pearson's correlations are more practical and provide an indication of temporal stability.

The 15-STARS questionnaire was administered twice, with a 2-week interval between the first and second administrations. Pearson's correlations between test and retest values were calculated for each item. All but one item reached an $r \geq 0.52$ (the item on forgetfulness in the French version, $r = 0.25$).

Finding: Because the total-score ICC was not possible to calculate, the test-retest reliability of the 15-STARS was not assessed following the COSMIN-recommended statistical methods. Poor stability of one item in one language was observed ($r = 0.25$) and may reflect an adherence determinant with less stability across the 2-week interval, which is common for adherence behavior (e.g., disruptions in routine). Nevertheless, the deviation from COSMIN standards is of minor concern due to the structure of the 15-STARS questionnaire and because it was not designed to monitor changes over time. Thus, precise test-retest agreement statistics are less critical.

2.10 Responsiveness

COSMIN standards view responsiveness as construct validity over time. As the changes should be meaningful and expected, prespecified hypotheses (with expected direction and magnitude of change) and clinical relevance (i.e., relationships with change in other measures) are crucial, not simply numerical change. Thus, effect size and standardized response mean, together with hypothesis testing, are expected to distinguish between pre and post values. Correlation with an external criterion may be an adequate analysis when a known gold standard of change is used.

Finding: The 15-STARS questionnaire did not include any evaluation of responsiveness in its validation study, which is acceptable in the early-stage development of the questionnaire. Thus, the ability of the 15-STARS questionnaire to detect change after an intervention remains unconfirmed and could be examined in future studies where the tool is used as part of an intervention targeting its determinants.

2.11 Interpretability and feasibility

Interpretability and feasibility of tools are crucial for their uptake. Unlike other psychometric properties, COSMIN standards treat interpretability and feasibility as qualitative attributes and process measures. Thus, no statistical tests are required, but analyses should be used to support interpretability and feasibility in clinical or research settings, such as time to complete, missing responses, respondent burden, administrative burden, mode of administration, and accessibility. For a screening tool, interpretability and feasibility are crucial, with quick and low-burden use being key.

The 15-STARS is concise (15 items), feasible for use in pharmacies, and demonstrated high acceptability with low missing data, below 5% per item. The low level of missing responses suggests the absence of floor or ceiling effects and alleviates concerns about clustering. No special training is required to use it; it can be utilized by untrained pharmacy staff during normal dispensing routines. Additionally, the tool appears to be feasible for use in other settings, such as hospitals or physicians' practices.

Finding: The 15-STARS fits well within COSMIN's requirements for interpretability and feasibility. Its practical strengths are demonstrated.

3 Discussion

COSMIN provides rigorous standards for evaluating the measurement properties of health-related questionnaires, i.e., reliability, validity, and responsiveness. These standards ensure the quality of the instruments and enable comparability between them. This should facilitate informed decision-making by researchers and healthcare practitioners when selecting an instrument. However, comprehensive standards for PROM development and validation can have disadvantages in practice and might even be unnecessary in many contexts, as not all PROMs are intended for the same purpose. A recent scoping review evaluated 40 existing guidelines on PROM development and validation and concluded that only 15 guidelines can be recommended, depending on the purpose of the PROMs to be developed (Jung et al., 2024). However, many of these guidelines were highly technical or exhaustive, and implementing every recommendation in full might be resource-intensive, time-consuming, or even unnecessary. For example, responsiveness testing is unnecessary for an assessment conducted at a single time point.

Thus, adapting the requirements during the questionnaire's development and validation might be appropriate. The strict application of the COSMIN requirements during the validation of the 15-STARS questionnaire was not always possible. Consequently, compared to COSMIN's rigorous psychometric criteria, the 15-STARS questionnaire falls short on several properties, such as structural validity and criterion validity, but still demonstrates strong content validity, acceptability, and feasibility, which are significant strengths. On the other hand, other standards exist, such as those defined by the International Society for Quality of Life Research (ISOQOL) in 2013 (Reeve et al., 2013). These standards include conceptual model, content validity, reliability (internal consistency/test–retest), construct validity (hypothesis testing), responsiveness, interpretability of scores, translation and cultural adaptation, and burden (feasibility and acceptability). The 15-STARS development and validation process aligns well with the ISOQOL minimum standard requirements.

However, and in a more relevant manner, PROM development and validation represent a process that takes place across multiple studies. Initial work may consist of several iterations of development and validation of some properties (e.g., content validity), based on which improved versions are proposed. Properties may be studied initially using exploratory methods, followed by confirmatory analyses (e.g., in structural validity and hypothesis testing). The timing of examining some properties might differ across questionnaires;, e.g., cross-cultural validity may be studied initially if a questionnaire is developed in multiple languages and cultures in parallel, or at a later stage for questionnaires developed in one language and translated to other settings after their validation in the original setting. The sequencing of the validation process also depends on access to the target population and the acceptability of different research design options (e.g., time available to participate, availability for repeated data collection). Thus, authors need to prioritize and sequence psychometric validation, balancing all these considerations in a research program rather than a single 'validation study'.

Based on the validation results of the 15-STARS, we recommend a validation process that balances scientific rigor and feasibility in the real-world setting by opting for statistical methods most adaptable to the purpose of the instrument. In addition, honest and transparent reporting should be mandatory, especially when deviating from standards, to enable users to understand what has been tested. Similarly, Jung et al. provided core principles of a pragmatic approach, such as prioritizing the essential steps and adapting the methods to the context (Jung et al., 2024).

In addition to applying the appropriate statistical tests for validity and reliability, two decisions must be made. Firstly, whether to use multivariate or bivariate statistics. Bivariate statistical tests are appropriate for examining certain measurement properties, such as construct validity and hypothesis testing. Pearson's or Spearman's correlations, Chi-square tests, t-tests, and ANOVA are easily executed in most statistical software packages; they are applicable to continuous or categorical variables, and their interpretation is relatively straightforward for nonstatisticians. As COSMIN recommends using the most appropriate statistical methods across all domains, bivariate statistics are not sufficient for full psychometric validation (Mokkink et al., 2024a, 2024b). Nevertheless, bivariate statistics can be recommended for exploring simple relationships between two variables, while multivariate statistics are needed for examining more complex relationships, such as causal relationships or controlling for confounders. This provides a good entry point for researchers with expertise in the topic or clinical area but limited statistical knowledge, as the primary focus of a questionnaire development and validation process is deepening the understanding of the construct being measured and determining how respondents can be supported to provide valid and reliable information through a respondent-friendly questionnaire response experience.

Secondly, the risk of false positive results when performing multiple tests on a relatively small dataset should be avoided. Three options exist to diminish this risk: (1) include a larger number of subjects (COSMIN judges fewer than 30 patients per group as inadequate and ≥100 as very good for comparing groups in construct validity testing); (2) measure only a few variables that are justified and specified in advance; or (3) interpret the results with caution. We opted for selected analyses and cautious interpretation for several reasons, mainly because a large sample size was impractical in the case of the 15-STARS validation due to high financial and resource burdens. In addition, it becomes unnecessary in the case of the 15-STARS, where the construct of the questionnaire is unambiguous and a clear pattern of results can be expected. Finally, a statistically significant but small correlation obtained with a large sample size might lack practical significance. It is therefore important to consider the clinical significance of the relationships examined in light of the construct the questionnaire aims to measure.

To conclude, we advocate for a pragmatic approach to the validation of health-related questionnaires, focusing on essential validation steps and applying standards after thorough consideration of the questionnaire's purpose, construct characteristics, use scenarios, and constraints of data collection in the target population, especially when real-world conditions make comprehensive validation impractical. Defining minimal acceptable criteria versus ideal standards, and viewing questionnaire development and validation as an ongoing process rather than a procedure limited in time, may offer a compromise that maintains both quality and usability. Moreover, one may flexibly "mix-and-match" the order and level of detail in examining each measurement property based on several considerations. As long as they are clearly justified and reported, scientific processes can move forward with research efforts, building on each other to reach higher levels of understanding of the constructs under study and the measures employed.

4 Questions for further discussion

- According to COSMIN, cognitive interviews with the target population are essential for evaluating a PROM's content validity. Which patient groups should be included? Are there any potential difficulties or limitations—for example, patients with low or no literacy?
- Mention has been made of the ISOQOL for the validation of health-related self-report instruments. Compared to COSMIN, ISOQOL's parameters appear less quantitative, providing a framework of good practice and general guidance in real-world use rather than methodological standards and detailed checklists. What are the specific differences between the two sets of recommendations? Which recommendation is most appropriate for a given health-related PROM or real-world context? Are the two recommendations complementary, and if so, in which contexts?
- Validation standards are likewise available for tests used in psychology, education, and the behavioral sciences. How do these standards align with COSMIN or ISOQOL? To what extent do their differences affect the overall quality assessment of the instrument?

5 Application exercise/scenario

Imagine your research team is developing an observational study to explore persistence with oral antibiotics and is embarking on using a published self-report questionnaire on adherence. After an intense literature search, several specific items from validated instruments are identified that would address your research question. However, your team is unsure about the validity of the selected items. What validation criteria will you check in the retrieved validation studies? What considerations will you use to determine whether your team can use the retrieved items or not?

References

Arnet, I., Sahm, L.J., Gregório, J., Tuula, A., Krüger, M., Wurmbach, V.S., Hoti, K., Schulz, M., Eickhoff, C., 2024. Development and validation of the 15-STARS—A novel self-report pharmacy-based questionnaire to screen for medication non-adherence. Res. Soc. Adm. Pharm. 1551-7411. 20 (3), 308–320. Available from: https://www.sciencedirect.com/science/journal/15517411. doi:10.1016/j.sapharm.2023.11.005.

Barbati, S., Stucki-Lickel, A., Rothen, J.-P., Allemann, S. S., Hruz, P., and Arnet, I. (2025). Usefulness of the Screening Tool for AdheRence to medicineS (15-STARS) in clinical practice: Subset-analysis of a multicentric study with inflammatory bowel disease (IBD) patients. Res. Soc. Admin. Pharm. 21 (11), 881–888. doi:10.1016/j.sapharm.2025.06.001.

Churruca, K., Pomare, C., Ellis, L.A., Long, J.C., Henderson, S.B., Murphy, L.E.D., Leahy, C.J., Braithwaite, J., 2021. Patient-reported outcome measures (PROMs): a review of generic and condition-specific measures and a discussion of trends and issues. Health Expect. 1369-7625. 24 (4), 1015–1024. Available from: http://onlinelibrary.wiley.com/journal/10.1111/(ISSN)1369-7625. doi:10.1111/hex.13254.

Cook, D.A., Beckman, T.J., 2006. Current concepts in validity and reliability for psychometric instruments: theory and application. Am. J. Med. 0002-9343. 119 (2), 166.e7. doi:10.1016/j.amjmed.2005.10.036.

Jung, A., Challoumas, D., Pagels, L., Armijo-Olivo, S., Braun, T., Luedtke, K., 2024. Guidelines for the development and validation of patient-reported outcome measures: a scoping review. BMJ Evid. Based Med. 2515-446X. 29 (6), 363–373. doi:10.1136/bmjebm-2023-112681.

Malkewitz, C.P., Schwall, P., Meesters, C., Hardt, J., 2023. Estimating reliability: a comparison of Cronbach's α, McDonald's ωt and the greatest lower bound. Soc. Sci. Humanit. Open. 2590-2911. 7 (1), 100368. doi:10.1016/j.ssaho.2022.100368.

Mokkink, L.B., Elsman, E.B.M., Terwee, C.B., 2024a. COSMIN guideline for systematic reviews of patient-reported outcome measures version 2.0. Qual. Life Res. 1573-2649. 33(11), 2929–2939. Available from: https://www.springer.com/journal/11136. doi:10.1007/s11136-024-03761-6.

Mokkink, L.B., Elsman, E.B.M., Terwee, C.B., 2024b. COSMIN Manual version 2.0—Conducting a systematic review of Patient-Reported Outcome Measures. Available from: www.cosmin.nl/wp-content/uploads/COSMIN-manual-V2_final.pdf.

Mokkink, L.B., Prinsen, D., Patrick, D., 2019. COSMIN study design checklist for patient-reported outcome measurement instruments. Available from: https://www.cosmin.nl/wp-content/uploads/COSMIN-study-designing-checklist_final.pdf.

Mokkink, L.B., Terwee, C.B., Patrick, D.L., Alonso, J., Stratford, P.W., Knol, D.L., Bouter, L.M., de Vet, H.C.W., 2010. The COSMIN study reached international consensus on taxonomy, terminology, and definitions of measurement properties for health-related patient-reported outcomes. J. Clin. Epidemiol. 0895-4356. 63 (7), 737–745. doi:10.1016/j.jclinepi.2010.02.006.

Reeve, B.B., Wyrwich, K.W., Wu, A.W., Velikova, G., Terwee, C.B., Snyder, C.F., Schwartz, C., Revicki, D.A., Moinpour, C.M., McLeod, L.D., Lyons, J.C., Lenderking, W.R., Hinds, P.S., Hays, R.D., Greenhalgh, J., Gershon, R., Feeny, D., Fayers, P.M., Cella, D., Brundage, M., Ahmed, S., Aaronson, N.K., Butt, Z., 2013. ISOQOL recommends minimum standards for patient-reported outcome measures used in patient-centered outcomes and comparative effectiveness research. Qual. Life Res. 0962-9343. 22 (8), 1889–1905. doi:10.1007/s11136-012-0344-y.

Terwee, C.B., Prinsen, C.A.C., Garotti, M.G.R., Suman, A., de Vet, H.C.W., Mokkink, L.B., 2016. The quality of systematic reviews of health-related outcome measurement instruments. Qual. Life Res. 1573-2649. 25 (4), 767–779. Available from: www.wkap.nl/journalhome.htm/0962-9343. doi:10.1007/s11136-015-1122-4.

US Food and Drug Administration, 2009. Guidance for industry—patient-reported outcome measures: use in medical product development to support labeling claims. Available from: www.fda.gov/downloads/Drugs/GuidanceComplianceRegulatoryInformation/Guidances/UCM193282.pdf.

Wild, D., Grove, A., Martin, M., Eremenco, S., McElroy, S., Verjee-Lorenz, A., Erikson, P., 2005. Principles of good practice for the translation and cultural adaptation process for patient-reported outcomes (PRO) measures: report of the ISPOR task force for translation and cultural adaptation. Value Health. 1098-3015. 8 (2), 94–104. doi:10.1111/j.1524-4733.2005.04054.x.

Zijlmans, E.A.O., van der Ark, L.A., Tijmstra, J., Sijtsma, K., 2018. Methods for estimating item-score reliability. Appl. Psychol. Meas. 1552-3497. 42 (7), 553–570. Available from: http://www.sagepub.com. doi:10.1177/0146621618758290.

CHAPTER

2

Hermeneutic phenomenology and member checking: Navigating tensions and advancing epistemological reflexivity philosophical critique, practical strategies, and reflective resources for qualitative research

Jonathan Vella
MCAST, Paola, Malta

CHAPTER OBJECTIVES

This chapter will:

- Examine the role and value of member checking within hermeneutic phenomenology, situating the practice within broader debates on interpretive inquiry.
- Explore the philosophical tensions between procedural validation logics and hermeneutic understandings of credibility, particularly in relation to interpretation, meaning, and researcher–participant dynamics.
- Present alternative strategies for enhancing trustworthiness in interpretive research, drawing on dialogical, reflexive, and analytic approaches aligned with the hermeneutic tradition.
- Discuss methodological adaptations appropriate for diverse, complex, or resource-constrained research contexts, with attention to feasibility, ethics, and interpretive coherence.
- Provide reflective prompts, scenarios, and resources to support critical engagement, enabling researchers, supervisors, and students to interrogate epistemological alignment and the rigor of their qualitative designs.

Contemporary Research Methods in Pharmacy and Health Services - Volume 2
https://doi.org/10.1016/B978-0-443-44607-8.00003-0

1 Introduction

1.1 Credibility, member checking, and the hermeneutic phenomenology debate

Qualitative research is grounded in exploring real-world contexts to understand how individuals interpret their experiences. It situates the researcher within naturalistic settings and uses diverse methods such as interviews, field notes, focus groups, and photographs to capture the depth and complexity of human experience (Tenny et al., 2022; Hadi and Closs, 2016). This approach prioritizes the meanings participants assign to phenomena over the pursuit of objectivity or generalizability (Anderson, 2010; Bush and Amechi, 2019). Rather than testing predefined hypotheses, qualitative research seeks to understand how and why particular experiences unfold, with an emphasis on meaning-making through dialogical and immersive engagement (Tong et al., 2007; Mays and Pope, 2000). Among the strategies used to establish credibility, member checking has long been prominent. However, as this chapter will show, its role is far from uncontested, particularly within hermeneutic phenomenology.

A defining characteristic of qualitative research is its embrace of subjectivity, acknowledging that knowledge is always shaped by the perspectives of those who produce it, and reflexivity, whereby researchers critically examine how their own assumptions and positions influence the research process (Denzin and Lincoln, 2000; Doyle, 2007). These commitments require methodological transparency by making the decisions and procedures that shape a study clear, and ethical sensitivity, which ensures respect, fairness, and care for participants at every stage (Lincoln and Guba, 2000, 1986). Flexibility is also valued, allowing studies to adapt to emerging insights and remain grounded in participants' lived realities (Lincoln and Guba, 1985; Moss, 2004). Ultimately, credibility in qualitative inquiry stems not from statistical validation but from the integrity and rigor of the interpretive process (Creswell and Miller, 2000; Hallett, 2013).

Within the diverse methodological traditions of qualitative research, such as narrative inquiry, ethnography, grounded theory, case study, and phenomenology, hermeneutic phenomenology offers a particularly nuanced lens. It emphasizes interpretation, contextuality, and the coconstruction of meaning, presenting both opportunities and challenges for how credibility is understood and achieved. It also prompts reflection on whether procedural strategies, such as member checking, can truly align with its philosophical foundations. The sections that follow (1.2–1.5) situate this issue within broader paradigm debates, unpack the hermeneutic lens in detail, and lay the groundwork for examining the divergence between member checking and hermeneutic phenomenology.

1.2 Research paradigms and trustworthiness in qualitative inquiry

Qualitative research is conducted within paradigmatic frameworks—overarching philosophical positions that shape how reality, knowledge, and meaning are understood. These paradigms, such as realist, constructivist, and social constructivist, carry distinct ontological and epistemological assumptions that influence how trustworthiness is defined and achieved (Stenfors et al., 2020). Realist paradigms assume an objective reality that can be discovered through systematic inquiry, with knowledge seen as a direct reflection of that reality and researcher neutrality emphasized. By contrast, constructivist and social constructivist paradigms view reality as multiple and contextually coconstructed. Constructivism highlights the individual's process of meaning-making, while social constructivism underscores the influence of language, power, and cultural interaction. In both perspectives, knowledge is cocreated, and the researcher is embedded within the interpretive process.

Within these interpretive paradigms, trustworthiness is understood less as confirming accuracy and more as demonstrating transparency, reflexivity, and engagement. It functions as the qualitative counterpart to internal validity, aiming to establish credibility while honoring the depth and contextuality of lived experience (Guba, 1981). Rigor is therefore achieved through practices such as reflexivity, triangulation, transparency in data analysis, and attention to outliers or atypical cases that complicate or test emerging interpretations, as well as participant engagement, often via member checking (Mays and Pope, 2000). These practices support the established criteria of credibility, transferability, dependability, and confirmability, but their use must always be sensitive to the paradigm in which the study is located.

Because of this diversity, quality in qualitative research cannot be judged by a single universal standard. Scholars increasingly argue that evaluative criteria must be aligned with specific epistemologies and disciplinary communities (Golafshani, 2003; Guba and Lincoln, 2005). This perspective contends that the multiplicity of research goals demands an equally diverse set of criteria, while also highlighting distinct emphases across traditions—for instance, narrative coherence in narrative inquiry, transcription accuracy in phenomenology, and systematic categorization in grounded theory (Bochner, 2000; Creswell, 2007). These tailored approaches are valuable but can be challenging for novices or interdisciplinary evaluators who may lack the paradigmatic fluency needed to apply them effectively (Lather, 2004).

This has led to a broader debate: can qualitative work be evaluated in a way that respects its paradigmatic foundations without collapsing into relativism or reimposing positivist standards? While some reject the very notion of cross-paradigmatic evaluation (Denzin and Lincoln, 2005), others, drawing on interpretive and poststructural traditions, advocate for flexible yet principled evaluative frameworks (Tracy, 2004; Richardson, 2000). This perspective reframes evaluation not as a search for universal criteria but as an effort to foster methodological transparency, ethical engagement, and resonance within a study's intended epistemological community.

Understanding these paradigmatic differences is essential for situating debates about credibility in qualitative research. Hermeneutic phenomenology offers a valuable case for exploring these issues because it adopts a strongly interpretive stance in which truth is understood as provisional, evolving, and inseparable from context. Within such a framework, meaning emerges through the dynamic interplay of researcher and participant rather than through verification against a fixed reality. This orientation sits uneasily alongside procedural strategies, such as member checking, which rest on the assumption that participants can confirm a singular, correct interpretation. The next section examines the philosophical foundations of hermeneutic phenomenology to illuminate why this tension arises and how it shapes the practice of establishing trustworthiness.

1.3 The hermeneutic lens and its implications for credibility in qualitative research

Hermeneutics, described as both a philosophy of interpretation and a science of understanding (Gadamer, 1975; Moules et al., 2015), moves beyond methodology to engage with foundational ontological and epistemological questions. Pioneered by Gadamer (1975) and Heidegger (1962), it examines how truth is understood, how meaning emerges, and how experiences are interpreted within their cultural, historical, and linguistic contexts. From this perspective, knowledge is conceived not as a static possession but as something continually in becoming—a dynamic unfolding through reflective dialog (Gadamer, 1975; Heidegger, 1962).

In qualitative research, especially when exploring lived experiences, a hermeneutic perspective invites researchers to embrace ambiguity, multiplicity, and the contextual nature of meaning (Moules et al., 2015; van Manen, 1990; Smith et al., 2009). Rather than seeking objective or generalizable truths, hermeneutic inquiry foregrounds understanding as evolving, situated, and interpretive. This orientation is particularly suited to studies of transition, identity, and meaning-making, where emotional, cultural, and institutional forces intersect. Interpretation extends beyond description to engage critically with the underlying dynamics of experience. Researchers are understood as self-interpreting beings who do not simply collect or decode data but coconstruct meaning through ongoing, dialogical interplay among context, phenomenon, and positionality (Lincoln et al., 2011; Schwandt, 2000). This embeddedness is not a bias to be eliminated but an essential condition for grasping situated truths.

A distinctive feature of hermeneutics is its focus on how meaning is shaped by language, temporality, and social embeddedness (Gillo, 2021; Crotty, 1998). Gadamer (1975) and Heidegger (1962) contend that all interpretation is historically and culturally situated, shaped by mood, disposition, and prior understanding. Understanding arises through a *fusion of horizons*—the merging and mutual transformation of researcher and participant perspectives. Because language mediates experience, it is through linguistic expression that meanings are articulated, shared, and reinterpreted. Hermeneutics also facilitates cross-contextual understanding, enabling researchers to locate individual accounts within broader institutional, cultural, and historical frameworks (Alsaigh and Coyne, 2021; Whitehead, 2004).

These distinctions can be further clarified through Table 2.1, which summarizes three broad orientations to validity, their philosophical underpinnings, and their implications for hermeneutic phenomenology.

As Table 2.1 indicates, hermeneutic phenomenology is most closely aligned with transformational and holistic approaches, both of which prioritize dialog, reflexivity, and evolving interpretations rather than fixed verification. This reinforces why procedural strategies, such as conventional member checking, may be difficult to reconcile with hermeneutic commitments.

TABLE 2.1 Validity orientations and their epistemological assumptions.

Validity orientation	Philosophical basis	Typical methods	Implications for hermeneutic phenomenology
Transactional validity	Postpositivist	Member checking for factual accuracy, triangulation	Risks imposing fixed 'truth' on fluid interpretation
Transformational validity	Constructivist/critical	Dialogic member checking, collaborative meaning-making	Aligns if designed as a dialogic and reflective process
Holistic validity	Interpretive/participatory	Integrated reflexivity, iterative feedback	Supports evolving, context-specific truths

Importantly, hermeneutics is not a prescriptive method but a philosophical orientation that provides guiding sensibilities rather than procedural rules. Researchers make deliberate, thoughtful choices about which aspects of the framework will guide inquiry. Truth, in this view, is not singular but plural and context-bound, emerging through reflective engagement rather than procedural verification. Rather than bracketing presuppositions, hermeneutics acknowledges that values, histories, and perspectives are integral to understanding (van Manen, 1990; Guba and Lincoln, 1994). This makes hermeneutic phenomenology particularly suited to studies seeking depth, nuance, and resonance over certainty or closure. It also bears directly on how credibility is established: procedural strategies such as member checking, which presume fixed meanings that participants can subsequently "verify," may sit uneasily with hermeneutic commitments to provisional, evolving, context-specific meaning (Moules et al., 2015; Laverty, 2003).

The next section examines this tension more closely and considers how rigor can be demonstrated without undermining hermeneutic foundations.

2 Examining member checking in context

2.1 Ensuring credibility in qualitative research: Strategies and paradigmatic fit

A central debate in qualitative research is how to establish the credibility and trustworthiness of findings, ensuring that results are meaningful and grounded in participants' perspectives (Hadi and Closs, 2016; Stenfors et al., 2020). Unlike quantitative research, which relies on statistical validation, qualitative inquiry enhances rigor through strategies such as triangulation, reflexivity, and member checking. Triangulation involves the use of multiple data sources, methods, or researchers to deepen interpretation, while reflexivity emphasizes the researcher's continuous self-examination of assumptions and positionality. Member checking, first articulated by Lincoln and Guba (Lincoln and Guba, 1985), entails presenting interpretations or thematic summaries to participants for feedback, enabling them to confirm, elaborate, or contest these accounts, and is often positioned as a hallmark of qualitative rigor (Morse et al., 2002; Birt et al., 2016).

The practice itself is referred to by a variety of terms, including member validation (Koelsch, 2013), respondent validation (Barbour, 2001), participant feedback (Curry et al., 2009), and member reflections (Tracy, 2010). These are more than semantic variations; they signal different epistemological assumptions. Labels such as validation imply the existence of a single objective truth to be confirmed, consistent with realist paradigms, while terms such as participant feedback or member reflections convey openness to multiple and evolving interpretations, more in line with constructivist and interpretivist traditions. Tracy (2010, p. 844), for example, deliberately avoided the term validation, preferring member reflections as an umbrella concept that accommodates paradigmatic diversity: "because the labels of member checks, validation, and verification suggest a single true reality, I instead offer the umbrella term member reflections" (Tracy, 2010).

In practice, member checking is often iterative and dialogical. Researchers may return transcripts, codes, or preliminary findings to participants, encouraging them to clarify, revise, or elaborate on emergent meanings (Lindheim, 2022; Zairul, 2021). This process positions participants as coconstructors of meaning and underscores a shared responsibility in representing lived experience (Thomas, 2017; Slettebø, 2021). Such dialogical use reflects interpretivist orientations that value evolving meaning over fixed confirmation.

However, strategies such as member checking cannot be assumed to apply universally across paradigms. What is taken as validation in one tradition may be philosophically incompatible with another. This reinforces the call for flexible evaluative criteria that are responsive to both methodological intent and epistemological alignment (Richardson, 2000; Tracy and Scott, 2006). From this perspective, credibility strategies should not be treated as procedural checklists but as principled choices that carry meaning only in relation to the paradigm in which they are deployed.

2.2 Validity, rigor, and the contested role of member checking

Validity in qualitative research refers to the process by which researchers provide evidence that their findings accurately represent the phenomenon under investigation (Guion et al., 2011; Jordan, 2018). It is often discussed alongside related concepts such as trustworthiness, credibility, and authenticity (Whittemore et al., 2001). While the concept of validity has been subject to critique and ongoing debate (Cho and Trent, 2006), it remains central to qualitative inquiry, particularly as a means of developing concepts and interpretations that may inform or complement other methodological approaches (Chesebro and Borisoff, 2007). Researchers describe several forms of validity in qualitative research, including:

- **Descriptive validity**: The factual accuracy of accounts, enhanced through strategies such as triangulation (Guion et al., 2011).
- **Interpretive validity**: The accurate representation of participants' perspectives, intentions, emotions, and experiences, often supported by verbatim quotations and member checking, which invites participants to engage directly with the researcher's interpretations (Sandelowski, 1993).

One key strategy for supporting interpretive validity is member checking, but this process can be undertaken in different ways and with different purposes. Scholars distinguish between two orientations that inform how it is used (Cho and Trent, 2006). A transactional orientation, often aligned with positivist assumptions, treats member checking as a procedural step to verify data accuracy, clarify misunderstandings, and correct factual errors (Varpio et al., 2017). A transformational orientation, aligned with constructivist and critical paradigms, views member checking as a dialogic and collaborative process that fosters shared meaning-making and participant empowerment (Brear, 2019). These orientations are not mutually exclusive; the choice depends on the study's purpose and epistemological stance (Cho and Trent, 2006).

These orientations reflect broader epistemological tensions. From a postpositivist perspective, member checking functions as a validation mechanism to ensure alignment between the researcher's account and the participant's intended meaning (Varpio et al., 2017). In contrast, constructivist and interpretivist paradigms reject the notion of a single, verifiable truth, positioning member checking as an opportunity to expand, challenge, or reinterpret meaning collaboratively (Sandelowski, 1993). This raises the question of whether its use always aligns with the philosophical foundations of a given study.

Within hermeneutic phenomenology, influenced by Heidegger's principles, truth is understood as contextual, historically situated, and shaped by the mood and disposition of both the researcher and the participant (Heidegger, 1962; Walsh, 1996). Meaning emerges through an evolving interpretive process rather than through post hoc validation. From this standpoint, member checking's underlying assumption—that participants can confirm a fixed interpretation—sits uneasily with a view that accepts multiple, shifting truths. Temporal distance between interviews and follow-ups can further complicate matters, as recollections evolve and second- or third-order interpretations may diverge significantly from initial accounts (Sandelowski, 1993; Mason, 1996).

Furthermore, beyond philosophical concerns, practical and ethical challenges persist. Member responses are often sparse or superficial, and outcomes are inconsistently reported (Goldblatt et al., 2011; Mero-Jaffe, 2011). When applied uncritically, the process can become a ritualistic exercise rather than a meaningful exchange (Koelsch, 2013), and additional feedback may dilute interpretive coherence or shift focus away from the original phenomenological moment (Varpio et al., 2017). Consequently, some quality appraisal frameworks, such as those developed by Hannes et al. (2010), omit member checking as a criterion altogether (Hannes et al., 2010). This omission reflects concerns that the practice may contribute little to rigor, is inconsistently documented in published studies, and can even risk distorting rather than strengthening interpretive analysis.

If retained in hermeneutic research, many scholars advocate reframing it not as a quest for accuracy or agreement but as an opportunity for participants to refine or re-narrate their experiences (Doyle, 2007; Koelsch, 2013). This constructivist and dialogical orientation is not merely a practical adjustment but a philosophical necessity if member checking is to remain consistent with hermeneutic commitments. It embraces evolving understandings but must be implemented with sensitivity to potential emotional and ethical risks (Goldblatt et al., 2011).

While these debates highlight the philosophical and practical complexities of member checking across qualitative traditions, the tensions become even more pronounced when examined within hermeneutic phenomenology. The following section focuses specifically on this paradigm, unpacking how its assumptions about truth, meaning, and interpretation both challenge and reshape the role of member checking.

3 Member checking and the question of validity in hermeneutic inquiry

The preceding discussion considered member checking's role in qualitative validity more broadly, including its philosophical alignment and practical application. This section narrows the focus to hermeneutic phenomenology, examining why its underlying assumptions about truth and meaning create particular tensions with procedural strategies such as member checking.

Hermeneutic phenomenology's emphasis on contextuality, interpretation, and reflexivity shapes not only how research is conducted but also how its credibility is evaluated. While member checking is often regarded as a gold standard for enhancing credibility in qualitative research, its compatibility with hermeneutic phenomenology is highly contested (Moules et al., 2015; Laverty, 2003). The tension stems from fundamental epistemological differences: member checking assumes that participants are the ultimate arbiters of their own "truths," confirming whether the researcher's interpretations align with their lived experience. In contrast, hermeneutic philosophy, particularly as informed by Heidegger and Gadamer, understands truth as emergent, provisional, and context-dependent (Heidegger, 1962; van Manen, 1990; Gadamer, 1975). Each recounting is thus a "snapshot in time," shaped by mood, context, and disposition, and revisiting participants for validation may alter the phenomenon itself rather than confirm it. In qualitative analysis, the development of second- and third-order constructs can progressively distance results from the original interview data, further complicating the notion of fixed validation (Sandelowski, 1993; Mason, 1996).

In hermeneutic inquiry, understanding is always situated and historically conditioned. Meanings evolve over time and may shift when revisited through new interpretive lenses. From this perspective, returning to participants for validation may undermine the phenomenological aim of capturing a particular horizon of meaning as it appeared in the original interpretive moment. Moreover, Gadamer's concept of a "fusion of horizons" underscores that understanding is coconstructed: interpretations arise through the dialogical interplay between the participant's narrative and the researcher's situated perspective. When participants are positioned merely as external validators rather than dialogical partners, this interpretive fusion is disrupted.

Livari (2018) illustrates how reconceived member checking can work differently: participants, invited to act as coinquirers, not only confirmed but also challenged and extended draft reports, enriching the interpretive process. This demonstrates the potential of member checking to deepen hermeneutic analysis when used dialogically, though such outcomes remain rare. As Lanzara (2016) describes, such encounters can generate "backtalk"—a process in which participants refine, resist, or reinterpret their earlier contributions, highlighting the dynamic and contested nature of interpretation. Evidence from other fields supports this concern: a review of psychology research articles using member checks found that studies often provided minimal information about their rationale, the process itself, and the impact of participant feedback on findings (Lanzara, 2016).

Ethical and methodological concerns add further complexity. Practical challenges include sparse or superficial responses, inconsistent reporting, and difficulties with follow-up in longitudinal or sensitive studies (Goldblatt et al., 2011; Mero-Jaffe, 2011). Requesting additional feedback may also dilute interpretive coherence or shift attention away from the original phenomenological moment (Varpio et al., 2017; Walsh, 1996). Power dynamics further shape how participants engage. Some may feel obliged to affirm the researcher's account, while others, particularly those in high-status roles, may seek to control how they are represented (Birt et al., 2016; Madill and Sullivan, 2017). In some institutional contexts, this can even extend to censorship, with senior figures attempting to sanitize or reshape findings for reputational protection (Bradshaw, 2001). Subtler effects, such as the "halo effect," can also emerge, with participants overemphasizing points they believe the researcher values. Finally, returning full transcripts to participants raises questions of ownership and control. While requests for deletion or revision can empower participants, they may also pressure researchers to make changes that compromise analytic coherence (Candela, 2019). These issues are summarized in Table 2.2.

Hermeneutics also challenges the assumption that participants can fully articulate their original intentions. Narratives are already interpretive by the time they are spoken, and researchers' subsequent engagement produces

TABLE 2.2 Challenges of member checking in hermeneutic inquiry.

Challenge	Description	References
Temporal and contextual shifts	Truth is emergent and shaped by time, mood, and context; repeated checking may alter, rather than confirm, the phenomenon	Heidegger (1962), Gadamer (1975), Mason (1996), Sandelowski (1993)
Risk to phenomenological moment	Follow-up contact can dilute or shift focus away from the original interpretive horizon	Walsh (1996), Varpio et al. (2017)
Sparse or inconsistent feedback	Responses are often minimal or inconsistently reported, which limits their methodological value	Goldblatt et al. (2011), Mero-Jaffe (2011)
Power dynamics	Participants may feel obliged to agree, or high-status individuals may control representation; halo effects can skew responses	Birt et al. (2016); Madill and Sullivan, 2018; Candela (2019)
Ownership and control of data	Requests for deletions or revisions empower participants but can compromise analytical coherence	Candela (2019)
Limited evidence of impact	Studies rarely document the rationale, process, or influence of feedback	Koelsch (2013); Livari (2018)

second-order interpretations—adding depth but also distance. This recursive nature of interpretation means that certainty is always partial, and misunderstanding is an inherent part of understanding (Walsh, 1996; Brogan, 2020; Zimmerman, 2015). Returning full transcripts to participants can, therefore, raise questions of ownership and control. While opportunities to refine or withdraw content may empower participants, they can also pressure researchers to make changes that compromise analytic coherence (Candela, 2019).

From a hermeneutic standpoint, the aim is not to validate the "correctness" of interpretations but to demonstrate rigor and transparency in the interpretive process. Some scholars argue that, if used at all in hermeneutic traditions, member checking should be reimagined as a dialogical space for exploring multiple truths rather than verifying a single account (Doyle, 2007; Koelsch, 2013). Participant engagement, in this view, is an invitation to expand interpretive horizons, not to authorize or correct the researcher's narrative. In practice-oriented studies, however—where outcomes may shape policy or services—it may still be important that participants recognize their experiences in the final account (Brear, 2019). Such engagement must nonetheless remain sensitive to hermeneutic commitments, avoiding recontact that pressures participants or undermines the temporal integrity of their accounts.

Given these challenges, practices such as prolonged engagement, iterative reflection, and transparent documentation of interpretive decisions provide more philosophically congruent approaches to establishing rigor. These strategies honor the fluid, coconstructed, and context-specific nature of meaning while supporting an ethically responsive understanding of lived experience.

The hermeneutic critique thus reveals that member checking, in its conventional form, rests on assumptions about truth, stability, and participant authority that are at odds with hermeneutic phenomenology. Yet many of the risks identified here—such as evolving narratives, participant burden, and power imbalances—also arise across other qualitative traditions. Recognizing these cross-cutting concerns is essential for deciding whether, when, and how member checking should be employed. The next section, therefore, turns to these broader ethical and epistemic considerations. Box 2.1 illustrates how evolving self-interpretation can transform the meaning of earlier accounts, exemplifying the temporal and dialogical movement that defines the hermeneutic inquiry.

4 Ethical and epistemic considerations in member checking

While hermeneutic phenomenology raises fundamental questions about the philosophical fit of member checking, ethical and epistemic challenges also arise in its practical application across qualitative traditions. These challenges concern how knowledge is produced, validated, and represented, and they often involve tensions between researcher authority and participant agency.

4.1 Epistemic concerns: Whose knowledge counts?

Participants' feedback is essential for fairness and representation, yet it is shaped by different forms of expertise. Researchers bring methodological and theoretical knowledge, while participants draw on lived experience. Because of this asymmetry, participants may lack the methodological grounding to fully critique analytic processes; their feedback may, therefore, focus more on content resonance than on methodological robustness.

BOX 2.1

Illustrative scenario 1: Evolving understanding over time

In a hermeneutic study exploring moral distress among clinical educators, participants initially expressed frustration and helplessness when confronting institutional constraints. Months later, when presented with the researcher's thematic synthesis, several resisted the framing of their experiences as "distress," preferring "moral alertness" or "ethical vigilance." The ensuing dialog revealed that their meanings had evolved as they discussed the study within their professional networks. Rather than invalidating the researcher's interpretation, this exchange illuminated Heidegger's notion that understanding is historically conditioned and always in motion. It exemplifies how member checking, when treated dialogically, can reveal temporal shifts in meaning and deepen reflexive awareness for both the researcher and participants.

This imbalance can create risks of epistemic injustice, where some voices or ways of knowing are marginalized in favor of the researcher's interpretive authority (Fricker, 2007; Jordan, 1997). At the same time, seeking consensus can oversimplify complex realities, obscuring dissenting perspectives or silencing tensions that are vital for interpretation (Doyle, 2007; Rolfe, 2006). Narratives themselves are not fixed: recollections evolve over time, and participants may reinterpret their experiences in ways that diverge from earlier accounts (Sandelowski, 1993). Such shifts can prompt disagreement, disconfirmation, or ambivalence (Birt et al., 2016; Madill and Sullivan, 2017; Caretta and Pérez, 2019), requiring researchers to reflect carefully on how to address competing interpretations without reducing complexity.

4.2 Ethical issues: Respect, consent, and emotional impact

Inviting participants to review data or interpretations can raise sensitive ethical issues. Some may request deletions or withdraw data—particularly if they feel misrepresented or emotionally overwhelmed (Buchbinder, 2011; Fahie, 2014). While such requests respect autonomy, they also raise questions about data ownership and the balance between participant agency and preserving analytic coherence. Re-engaging participants can also cause distress, especially when findings are abstract, theoretical, or disconnected from their self-perceptions (Birt et al., 2016). Although safeguards for emotional distress are often built into data collection, they are less common at the member-checking stage (Dickson-Swift et al., 2007).

It is also important to recognize that member checking may lead not only to individual emotional responses but also to tangible changes within organizations and the lives of participants. In studies seeking to influence practice or policy, enabling participants to recognize their experiences in final outcomes can be crucial for credibility and for the transferability of findings to wider communities. This potential impact should, therefore, be weighed carefully at the planning stage. Box 2.2 presents an illustrative scenario that highlights how these tensions can emerge in practice, showing how ethical responsibility extends beyond procedural consent to the ongoing care of participants' representation.

4.3 Practical challenges: Engagement and representation

Transcript-based member checking often yields low engagement and superficial feedback (Carlson, 2010). Participants may lack the time, interest, or capacity to engage with lengthy or linguistically complex material. While inviting participants to modify or redact content respects autonomy, especially with vulnerable groups (Candela, 2019), it may limit their understanding of how individual accounts are anonymized and integrated into broader analyses, potentially skewing feedback. Providing participants with relevant excerpts from final reports, including direct quotations, can help them assess how their contributions are represented and address concerns about anonymity or misinterpretation (Fahie, 2014; Pinto et al., 2022). Selectively sharing only the sections that pertain to each participant can also protect confidentiality while maintaining the participatory spirit of the process.

4.4 Balancing researcher authority and participant agency

Disagreements in member checking are inevitable. Researchers hold theoretical and methodological expertise (Morse, 2015), but dismissing participant feedback can undermine the participatory ethos of qualitative

> **BOX 2.2**
>
> **Illustrative scenario 2: Ethical tensions in representation**
>
> *In a project on interprofessional collaboration, a participant requested that her quotations be removed from the final report after recognizing that her wording could identify her within a small clinical team. The researcher faced a dilemma: preserving analytic coherence required keeping the account, yet ethical responsibility demanded respect for withdrawal. Following reflective dialog and consultation with supervisors, the excerpt was removed, and the thematic narrative reworked to preserve conceptual integrity without attribution. This scenario highlights that ethical responsibility in hermeneutic inquiry extends beyond procedural consent to an ongoing attentiveness to how representation, recognition, and power shape the participant's sense of ownership.*

research. Conversely, granting participants too much control over final interpretations may compromise analytic coherence. Navigating this balance requires ethical reflexivity, transparency, and awareness of the power dynamics that shape both the research relationship and the knowledge produced (Caretta and Pérez, 2019; Motulsky, 2021).

In sum, member checking is not inherently harmful. For some participants, the process can be validating or even therapeutic, particularly when they see their experiences accurately reflected or recognize shared struggles (Harper and Cole, 2012). For others, however, it may provoke confusion, discomfort, or distress—especially when faced with raw transcripts or unfamiliar interpretations (Mero-Jaffe, 2011). This variability underscores that it must be approached as a context-sensitive, dialogical process rather than a procedural requirement. These considerations highlight that member checking, if used at all, must be designed with attention to both epistemological alignment and ethical responsibility. The following section examines how member checking can be reframed to serve dialogical, reflexive, and transformative purposes, moving beyond verification to more collaborative forms of meaning-making. Box 2.3 illustrates how these asymmetries can manifest in practice, highlighting the importance of reflexivity and transparency in navigating divergent participant responses.

5 Practical and reflexive considerations in member checking

While philosophical and ethical debates highlight the complexities of member checking, its practical implementation also demands careful planning and reflexive awareness. To be meaningful, the process must be designed in alignment with the study's epistemology, the researcher's positionality, and the realities of the research context. This requires more than simply adding member checking as a procedural step; it involves embedding it into the overall methodological design so that it reflects the underlying philosophical stance of the study. In a realist design, the process may focus on verifying factual accuracy and ensuring alignment with participant intent. In a hermeneutic study, it may be oriented toward exploring alternative interpretations and examining how meanings evolve over time, while in a critical or participatory approach, it can be developed as a platform for coanalysis and coownership of findings. Regardless of the paradigm, researchers must have a comprehensive understanding of their philosophical position and ensure that member checking is conducted in a manner that is consistent with it, avoiding practices that inadvertently undermine interpretive integrity or credibility.

Because member checking is often scheduled late in the research cycle, it can be rushed or underresourced, resulting in low engagement, superficial feedback, or ethical oversights. To mitigate this, planning should begin before data collection and establish the purpose, scope, and format of the process in relation to the study's aims. Adequate time must be scheduled for participants to respond, especially if translation or additional support is required, and the nature of the process should be communicated early in the research relationship. Clear instructions should explain both the purpose of member checking and the epistemological stance of the study, clarifying how participant feedback will be used and ensuring that contributors understand its interpretive rather than confirmatory orientation.

Figure 2.1 guides researchers in determining whether member checking is epistemologically and contextually appropriate. The process begins with identifying the study's epistemology, clarifying the specific purpose of member

BOX 2.3

Illustrative scenario 3: Power dynamics and epistemic authority

A doctoral researcher studying leadership culture in a teaching hospital invited senior managers and junior nurses to review emerging interpretations. Senior participants provided extensive feedback, requesting changes that softened critical language, while junior staff offered minimal responses, fearing reprisal. Incorporating these revisions verbatim would have compromised the analytic integrity of the study, yet ignoring them risked dismissing participant voices. The researcher documented this tension in the reflexive journal and reported both sets of perspectives transparently. This case demonstrates how member checking can inadvertently reproduce hierarchical power relations, reinforcing the need for epistemic reflexivity—recognizing whose voices carry authority, how institutional power circulates, and how interpretive integrity can be preserved amid asymmetry.

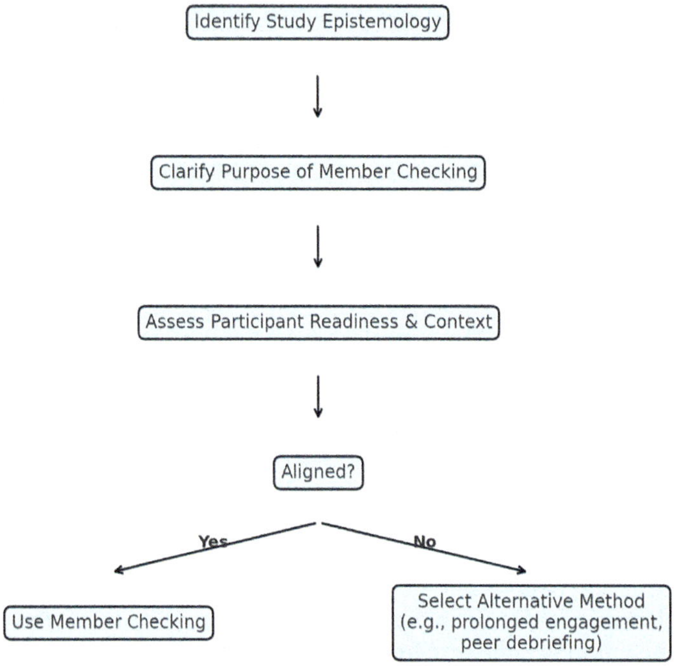

FIG. 2.1 Paradigm fit versus misfit decision tree. Decision-making flowchart for evaluating the appropriateness of member checking in qualitative research. The process emphasizes alignment with epistemology, study purpose, and participant readiness, guiding researchers either toward member checking or alternative strategies (e.g., prolonged engagement, peer debriefing).

checking, and assessing participant readiness and context. If the practice aligns with the study's philosophical stance and research conditions, member checking may be implemented. If not, researchers are advised to select alternative strategies, such as prolonged engagement or peer debriefing, that are more congruent with their epistemological commitments.

The researcher's role in member checking is inherently complex, particularly for those new to qualitative inquiry. Novice researchers may find themselves caught between acting as an expert who interprets and analyzes data and as a collaborator who invites participants into shaping those interpretations. Without careful reflexivity, there is a risk of repeatedly adjusting codes in response to feedback without critically examining how these changes align with the broader interpretive framework. This challenge is heightened for novice researchers, who must learn to balance these dual roles. Overreliance on participant preferences can result in superficial revisions, whereas developing the skill to calibrate responses to divergent perspectives strengthens both reflexivity and interpretive depth. Reflexivity here involves maintaining an ongoing record of decisions about when and how feedback is integrated, engaging in dialog with colleagues to surface potential biases, and distinguishing between changes that enhance coherence and those that dilute interpretive depth.

Disagreement between researchers and participants—or among participants themselves—is not only possible but expected. At times, participants may overemphasize certain points because they believe the researcher values them (the "halo effect"). In other cases, they may soften or withhold criticism to maintain face or avoid sensitive issues altogether due to organizational politics or personal considerations. Such dynamics require researchers to make careful decisions about when to adapt interpretations and when to preserve the original analysis. If feedback is not incorporated, the rationale should be documented and, where appropriate, communicated transparently in reporting. Nonparticipation in member checking should also be acknowledged, along with its implications for credibility, as some participants may decline involvement or offer superficial agreement out of politeness or convenience rather than genuine engagement. In some cases, retaining the original interpretation may be necessary despite disagreement—for example, to preserve analytic coherence when divergence stems from organizational politics, face-saving needs, or limited familiarity with the theoretical framework guiding the analysis.

Participants may also struggle to recognize their own narratives in findings that synthesize multiple accounts, particularly when these have been theoretically abstracted. This highlights the importance of

TABLE 2.3 Methodological do's and don'ts for member checking in hermeneutic or interpretive research.

Do's	Don'ts
Align with epistemology: Ensure procedures are consistent with the philosophical stance of the study. Avoid imposing verification logic on interpretive paradigms	**Don't treat it as a checklist**: Avoid including member checking merely to 'tick a box' for rigor
Plan early: Integrate member checking into the research design from the outset, ensuring clear objectives and effective participant communication	**Don't overburden participants**: Refrain from extensive reviews of raw transcripts unless clearly beneficial and consented to
Be transparent: Explain the purpose, potential impact, and epistemological assumptions to all participants	**Don't disregard power dynamics**: Remain attentive to how authority and relationships influence feedback, especially in hierarchical settings
Accommodate participants: Use formats and timings that respect participants' capacities, contexts, and preferences	**Don't dilute interpretive coherence**: Avoid changes that compromise analytic integrity solely to achieve consensus
Document the process: Record who participated, the nature of the feedback, and how it shaped the interpretation	

explaining how individual contributions have been anonymized and integrated into broader interpretations, and clarifying the type of feedback sought—whether it concerns factual accuracy, thematic resonance, or interpretive nuance. Offering relevant excerpts of the analysis rather than full datasets can make engagement more manageable, while examples of constructive feedback can help participants understand the role expected of them. Providing flexible modes of engagement—such as written responses, follow-up interviews, or group discussions—further accommodates participants' preferences and capacities, increasing the likelihood of meaningful participation.

Ultimately, effective member checking requires early design decisions grounded in epistemology, adequate allocation of time and resources, reflexive awareness of the researcher's role and influence, constructive engagement with disagreement, and transparent communication throughout the process. By treating member checking as a relational and context-sensitive activity rather than a fixed procedural requirement, researchers can ensure that it contributes meaningfully to both methodological rigor and ethical accountability. These practical considerations also provide a foundation for exploring the diversity of paradigms and innovative adaptations to member checking, which are discussed in the following section. To consolidate the philosophical, ethical, and practical insights outlined above, Table 2.3 summarizes key methodological do's and don'ts for researchers considering member checking in hermeneutic or interpretive qualitative inquiry.

The learning activity at the end of the chapter applies this decision logic to three contrasting research scenarios.

6 Paradigms, methods, and the lack of consensus

The diversity of ethical, epistemic, and methodological challenges outlined above helps explain why there is no clear consensus on what constitutes "good" member-checking practice. In response to these complexities, researchers have developed a range of innovative approaches designed to align the process with participants' needs, study contexts, and the epistemological commitments of the research.

While traditional approaches often rely on written or verbal feedback, alternative strategies include visual and arts-based techniques such as found poetry, diagrammatic elicitation, and card sorting (Harry et al., 2005; Sahakyan, 2023), as well as iterative, participatory models grounded in community engagement (Birt et al., 2016; Brear, 2019; Chase, 2017; Urry et al., 2024). These approaches reflect an evolving understanding of member checking as a family of practices shaped by methodological intent, participant capacity, and contextual realities. Scholars call for a flexible orientation—one that centers participants' agency and preferences while remaining sensitive to their priorities (Carlson, 2010; Erdmann and Potthoff, 2023).

Paradigmatic commitments also shape how member checking is conceptualized. Within critical or transformative frameworks, the aim extends beyond confirming accuracy to exploring how participation affects self-understanding, agency, and the redistribution of power (Doyle, 2007). In this view, validity is assessed not by correspondence with "truth" but by the potential to challenge dominant narratives, amplify marginalized voices,

TABLE 2.4 Alternatives to member checking for ensuring rigor.

Alternative method	Description	Suitability for hermeneutic phenomenology
Prolonged engagement	Extended researcher immersion in the participant context	High—builds trust and depth of interpretation
Peer debriefing	Critical dialogue with colleagues	High—surfaces researcher assumptions
Reflexive journaling	Ongoing documentation of reflections	High—strengthens transparency
Collaborative analysis	Joint interpretation with participants/peers	Moderate to high—needs careful facilitation

and promote social change (Brear, 2019; Motulsky, 2021). At the other end of the spectrum, some researchers adopt a pragmatic, hybrid approach, combining tools and philosophical orientations as needed to address the research question and context (Johnson and Onwuegbuzie, 2004). This middle ground reflects the growing diversity of qualitative inquiry and the need to tailor practices to real-world conditions rather than follow rigid methodological rules.

Whether arts-based, participatory, or hybrid, these innovations bring their own ethical and practical considerations. Participants may face barriers to engagement—technological, linguistic, emotional, or cognitive. Requests for additional time and interpretive labor require careful management, particularly in research with trauma-experienced or underresourced participants (Barbour, 2001; Motulsky, 2021). Researchers must, therefore, critically assess not only whether member checking is used, but also how, when, and why—and to what ethical and epistemic ends.

In resource-constrained contexts, member checking often requires further adaptation. Strategies include integrating validation discussions into scheduled data collection visits to minimize additional travel and costs (Birt et al., 2016), using low-bandwidth communication such as short message service (SMS), WhatsApp voice notes, or local radio announcements for remote communities (Chilisa, 2012), and working with community intermediaries or local research assistants when literacy or language barriers exist (Marshall and Rossman, 2016). Short, focused validation sessions using printed thematic summaries rather than full transcripts can also reduce participant burden while supporting interpretive dialog (Koelsch, 2013). These approaches must still preserve ethical standards, ensure voluntary participation, and remain congruent with the study's epistemological stance.

Taken together, this range of practices and paradigmatic positions underscores that there is no single "best" way to conduct member checking. Instead, its design must be responsive to epistemology, participant capacity, and the specific ethical and methodological aims of the research. Building on this diversity, the next section considers how member checking can be reframed to move beyond procedural verification toward more dialogical, ethically grounded, and transformative forms of engagement.

In light of these debates, it is important to recognize that member checking is not the only strategy available to enhance rigor. A range of alternative methods can be employed, many of which are particularly well-suited to hermeneutic phenomenology because they emphasize reflexivity, dialog, and sustained engagement rather than procedural verification. Table 2.4 summarizes several widely used alternatives and their relevance to hermeneutic research.

7 Reframing member checking: Practices, purposes, and transformative potential

Previous sections have outlined the philosophical tensions, ethical complexities, and methodological diversity that challenge a one-size-fits-all approach to member checking. This section shifts from critique to reconstruction, examining how the practice can be reimagined to align with interpretive and hermeneutic principles while remaining responsive to the practical realities of contemporary qualitative research.

7.1 From verification to dialogue

Rather than treating member checking as a procedural safeguard against error or misrepresentation, a reframed approach positions it as a dialogical process that can deepen understanding, enhance ethical engagement, and foster participant agency. Some scholars describe this orientation as *transformational validity*—a process that "involves a deeper, self-reflective, empathetic understanding of the researcher while working with the researched" (p. 322) (Cho and Trent, 2006). In this view, the goal is not to confirm a single correct account but to engage in mutual meaning-making that reshapes both participants' and researchers' perspectives.

Evidence of such transformation can be found in several studies. In one example, researchers used member checking not only to review interpretations but also to invite participants to reflect on personal changes over time (Koelsch, 2013). Another study reported that stepfathers experienced increased clarity and reduced emotional overwhelm after engaging with their own and others' narratives, suggesting that member checking can provide psychological benefits beyond its methodological aims (Harper and Cole, 2012). In community-based and program evaluation contexts, participant feedback has also functioned as a mechanism of ethical accountability, ensuring that detailed and personal accounts are represented fairly and that those represented have a voice in shaping the narrative (Rodríguez-Campos, 2012).

7.2 Hermeneutic and interpretive alignment

Within hermeneutic and other interpretive paradigms, reframed member checking can serve as an extension of the hermeneutic circle—a recursive process in which understanding emerges through ongoing dialog between parts and whole, researcher and participant (Klein and Myers, 1999). Designed as a collaborative encounter, it encourages participants to revisit, challenge, and extend interpretations rather than simply verify them.

Livari (2018) provides a compelling example: participants invited to interpret draft reports engaged in affirming, challenging, and reworking the texts, either collaboratively or individually. This process both refined the findings and acknowledged participants as coinquirers, disrupting the traditional researcher–participant hierarchy. Box 2.4 illustrates this process through a findings-based example, showing how shared reflection between researcher and participant can generate richer, more resonant understandings of lived experience.

7.3 Findings-based member checking: An operational model

One way to operationalize this reframed philosophy is through findings-based member checking. Rather than returning raw data, such as transcripts, which often elicit only minor factual corrections, this approach invites participants to engage directly with the interpretive products of the research, such as thematic summaries, representative quotations, or conceptual frameworks. This shift directs attention to how experiences are represented to others and how meaning is constructed in relation to other participants' accounts.

To support this process, a brief, structured protocol can be used once participants have reviewed the findings. Follow-up can be conducted through written feedback or short interviews (10–15 minutes) using questions such as:

- *After reading the findings, what are your general thoughts?*
- *How accurately do they capture your experiences or perspectives?*
- *What could be added to better reflect your viewpoint?*
- *Is there anything you would like removed, and why?*

BOX 2.4

Illustrative scenario 4: Findings-based, dialogical engagement

A hermeneutic study of mentoring relationships in nursing education employed findings-based member checking by sharing thematic summaries rather than transcripts. Participants discussed how the themes resonated with or diverged from their lived experiences. One mentor proposed reframing "knowledge transfer" as "mutual learning," emphasizing reciprocity rather than hierarchy. The researcher integrated this insight, resulting in a conceptual refinement that mirrored Gadamer's "fusion of horizons." The exercise not only enhanced interpretive depth but also modeled how participants can act as coinquirers, extending meaning through dialog rather than verifying accuracy.

These questions not only promote reflexivity and dialog but also provide participants with a mechanism to protect privacy or correct misrepresentations, which is particularly relevant in studies involving sensitive topics or marginalized groups (Fahie, 2014; Pinto et al., 2022).

7.4 Potential outcomes and benefits

When participants see their experiences situated alongside those of others, it can prompt reinterpretation of their own narratives and generate new insights (Koelsch, 2013; Harper and Cole, 2012). For researchers, such engagement can reveal unrecognized assumptions, expand analytic depth, and strengthen ethical transparency. Even if participant feedback does not lead to major revisions, documenting the process—who was invited, who responded, the nature of the feedback, and how it was handled—reinforces the collaborative and provisional nature of qualitative interpretation.

In sum, reframing member checking from a tool of verification to a vehicle for dialog, reflection, and transformation shifts the focus from accuracy to coconstruction. When aligned with the epistemological commitments of a study, such approaches not only strengthen methodological rigor and relational ethics but also open space for personal and collective transformation.

8 Conclusion and way forward

This chapter has explored the complex and often contested role of member checking in qualitative research, with particular attention to its philosophical alignment—or lack thereof—with hermeneutic phenomenology. Throughout the discussion, a central theme has emerged: member checking is neither inherently essential nor inherently flawed. Its value depends on how, when, and why it is used, as well as on whether it aligns with the epistemological, ethical, and relational foundations of the study.

From this analysis, several key principles can be distilled:

- Epistemological congruence is essential. The choice to use—or not to use—member checking must reflect the study's ontological and epistemological commitments, as well as the researcher's positionality.
- Planning and transparency are critical. Member checking should be considered from the outset, with clear goals, protocols, and communication about how feedback will be incorporated.
- Ethical sensitivity is required. This includes recognizing power imbalances, avoiding undue burden, and ensuring participant autonomy in how they engage.
- Reflexivity is nonnegotiable. Researchers must critically examine how their assumptions, theoretical frameworks, and interpretations shape both the process and the outcomes of member checking.

From a hermeneutic perspective, meaning is fluid, coconstructed, and situated. Conventional notions of "verification" risk oversimplifying this dynamic and may inadvertently distort the temporal and contextual integrity of lived experience. Yet, when reimagined as a dialogical and interpretive practice—such as in findings-based member checking—the process can enhance dialog, prompt reflection, and generate richer, more ethically grounded interpretations.

Future research should investigate how to optimize member checking for diverse contexts and populations, particularly those with varied levels of methodological or technological literacy. There is also scope for innovation in using asynchronous and digital platforms to broaden accessibility while preserving opportunities for meaningful engagement.

Ultimately, member checking should be regarded as one tool among many available to qualitative researchers. Its adoption must always be a deliberate, principled choice—grounded in research aims, respectful of participants, and committed to enhancing both methodological rigor and ethical integrity. Reframed in this way, member checking can contribute not as a universal standard but as a context-sensitive practice that supports credibility and resonance within interpretive inquiry.

To support researchers in translating these principles into practice, the following checklist and reflective prompts provide a practical guide for deciding whether, when, and how to incorporate member checking. Together, these tools highlight that member checking is best approached not as a procedural requirement but as a context-sensitive, dialogical choice that can enhance interpretive rigor when aligned with the philosophical commitments of a study.

Checklist—"Before You Member Check ... "

- Is member checking epistemologically aligned with my study?
- Will it enhance interpretation rather than force verification?
- Are participants willing and able to engage meaningfully?
- Do I have the resources and time to support the process?
- Have I planned how to integrate divergent feedback?

Reflective sidebar—How would member checking affect interpretative rigor in MContext?

Consider your own research setting:

- Would member checking enhance or constrain your ability to interpret lived experiences faithfully?
- How might participants' feedback shift your understanding of the phenomenon?
- In what ways could power dynamics influence the process and outcomes?
- How would you communicate the epistemological stance of your study to participants so that they can engage meaningfully?

Reflect on these questions as you consider whether and how to incorporate member-checking into your qualitative research design.

Learning activity: Making decisions about member checking

This activity supports readers in applying the methodological decision points illustrated in Fig. 2.1 to concrete research situations. Rather than assuming that member checking is universally required, the cases invite reflection on how epistemological alignment, the purpose of participant engagement, and contextual considerations shape decisions about whether, when, and how member checking may be appropriate.

The activity reinforces a central argument of the chapter: *methodological rigor in qualitative research emerges from epistemological alignment and reflexive judgment, rather than from the routine application of validation techniques.*

By engaging with these cases, readers are encouraged to make deliberate, philosophically informed decisions about the role of member checking within their own research designs, including when alternative strategies may be more congruent.

Case 1: Cointerpreting change in a professional development program

Research context and purpose

This study evaluates a year-long interprofessional professional development program aimed at improving collaborative decision-making among healthcare staff. The research is embedded within the program and adopts a critical–constructivist orientation, with an explicit commitment to dialog, reflexivity, and participant empowerment.

Aim

To explore how participants interpret changes in their professional roles, relationships, and sense of agency as a result of engaging in the program.

Methodology and epistemological stance

- **Design:** Qualitative interpretive study
- **Epistemology:** Constructivist/critical
- **Data collection:** Longitudinal semistructured interviews conducted at two time points (n = 15)
- **Analysis:** Iterative thematic analysis focused on meaning-making, contradictions, and transformation
- **Intended use of findings:** Program refinement and critical reflection on professional power relations

Participants are positioned as active contributors to knowledge production rather than as sources of data to be verified.

Consideration of member checking

The researcher is considering whether member checking is appropriate and, if so, what form it should take. The purpose would not be to verify accuracy but to create opportunities for participants to engage with emerging interpretations, particularly where these raise questions about power, role boundaries, or institutional norms. Participants are familiar with reflective dialog through the program and are accustomed to collective discussion.

Reflective prompts

- Which epistemological assumptions are shaping how credibility is understood in this study?
- What purpose would member checking serve here, if used at all?
- How does the research context and participant readiness influence whether dialogic engagement is appropriate?
- What ethical considerations arise when participants are invited to respond to potentially challenging interpretations?

Case 2: Understanding professional becoming in early-career academics

Research context and purpose

This study adopts a hermeneutic phenomenological approach to explore how early-career academics experience professional becoming within competitive university environments. The focus is on meaning, temporality, and the evolving nature of self-understanding.

Aim

To interpret how early-career academics make sense of belonging, legitimacy, and professional identity over time.

Methodology and epistemological stance

- **Design:** Hermeneutic phenomenology (Heidegger–Gadamer orientation)
- **Epistemology:** Interpretive
- **Data collection:** In-depth conversational interviews (n = 12)
- **Analysis:** Recursive interpretive analysis, producing second- and third-order themes
- **Researcher stance:** Explicitly reflexive; interpretation is acknowledged as historically and contextually situated

Findings are presented as a synthesized interpretive narrative rather than individualized accounts.

Consideration of member checking

The researcher is uncertain whether member checking should be undertaken. While participants are capable of engaging in reflective dialog, there is concern that revisiting accounts may alter the phenomenological moment or introduce expectations of verification. The researcher considers whether alternative strategies might better support rigor without re-contacting participants.

Reflective prompts

- How does the epistemological stance of this study shape expectations about participant involvement after analysis?
- What would be the purpose of member checking in this context, and is that purpose compatible with the study's aims?
- How do temporal distance and participant context affect the appropriateness of follow-up engagement?
- What approaches could be used to demonstrate rigor and transparency in ways aligned with the study's interpretive intent?

Case 3: Evaluating a medication safety intervention

Research context and purpose

This study is a qualitative service evaluation of a newly implemented medication reconciliation protocol in an acute hospital setting. The evaluation was commissioned to assess implementation processes and inform service improvement initiatives.

Aim

To explore healthcare professionals' experiences in implementing the medication reconciliation protocol and to identify operational barriers affecting adherence.

Methodology

- **Design:** Qualitative descriptive study
- **Data collection:** Semistructured interviews with pharmacists and nurses (n = 18)
- **Analysis:** Thematic analysis focused on accurately representing reported practices and workflow processes
- **Intended use of findings:** Policy refinement, staff training, and audit preparation

The study prioritizes clarity and accuracy in accounts of clinical practice to support organizational decision-making.

Consideration of member checking

The researcher is considering member checking primarily to ensure the factual accuracy of descriptions relating to workflow, timing, and professional responsibilities. Participants are accustomed to audit and feedback processes, and engagement would be brief and task-focused.

Reflective prompts

- What assumptions about knowledge and accuracy underpin this study design?
- What purpose would member-checking serve in this context?
- How does participant context and readiness shape the form that member checking might take?
- What risks might arise if participant confirmation is treated as validation of a fixed account?

Comparative reflection

Consider the following across all cases:

- How does identifying the study's epistemology shape subsequent decisions about credibility strategies?
- How does the *purpose* of engaging participants after analysis differ across cases?
- How do participant readiness and research context influence whether member checking is appropriate?
- In which cases does alignment lead toward member checking, and in which cases might alternative strategies be more congruent?

AI disclosure

During the preparation of this work, the author(s) used ChatGPT for sentence construction and paraphrasing. After using this tool/service, the author(s) reviewed and edited the content as needed and take(s) full responsibility for the content of the publication.

References

Alsaigh, R., Coyne, I., 2021. Doing a hermeneutic phenomenology research underpinned by Gadamer's philosophy: a framework to facilitate data analysis. Int. J. Qual. Methods 20, 16094069211047820. doi:10.1177/16094069211047820.

Anderson, C., 2010. Presenting and evaluating qualitative research. Am. J. Pharm. Educ. 74 (8), 141. doi:10.5688/aj740814.

Barbour, R.S., 2001. Checklists for improving rigour in qualitative research: a case of the tail wagging the dog?. BMJ 322 (7294), 1115–1117. doi:10.1136/bmj.322.7294.1115.

Birt, L., Scott, S., Cavers, D., Campbell, C., Walter, F., 2016. Member checking: a tool to enhance trustworthiness or merely a nod to validation?. Qual. Health Res. 26 (13), 1802–1811. doi:10.1177/1049732316654870.

Bochner, A.P., 2000. Criteria against ourselves. Qual. Inq. 6 (2), 266–272. doi:10.1177/107780040000600209.

Bradshaw, M., 2001. Contracts and member checks in qualitative research in human geography: reason for caution?. Area 33 (2), 202–211. doi:10.1111/1475-4762.00020.

Brear, M., 2019. Process and outcomes of a recursive, dialogic member checking approach: a project ethnography. Qual. Health Res. 29 (7), 944–957. doi:10.1177/1049732318812448.

Brogan, W., 2020. Basic concepts of hermeneutics: gadamer on tradition and community. Duquesne Stud. Phenomenol. 1 (1), 1–13.

Buchbinder, E., 2011. Beyond checking: experiences of the validation interview. Qual. Soc. Work. 10 (1), 106–122. doi:10.1177/1473325010370189.

Bush, A.A., Amechi, M.H., 2019. Conducting and presenting qualitative research in pharmacy education. Curr. Pharm. Teach. Learn. 11 (6), e1–e7. doi:10.1016/j.cptl.2019.02.030.

Candela, A., 2019. Exploring the function of member checking. Qual. Rep. 24 (3), 619–628. doi:10.46743/2160-3715/2019.3726.

Caretta, M.A., Pérez, M.A., 2019. When participants do not agree: member checking and challenges to epistemic authority in participatory research. Field Methods. 31 (4), 359–374. doi:10.1177/1525822X19866578.

Carlson, J.A., 2010. Avoiding traps in member checking. Qual. Rep. 15 (5), 1102–1113.

Chase, E., 2017. Enhanced member checks: reflections and insights from a participant-researcher collaboration. Qual. Rep. 22 (10), 2689–2703. doi:10.46743/2160-3715/2017.2957.

Chesebro, J.W., Borisoff, D.J., 2007. What makes qualitative research qualitative?. Qual. Res. Rep. Commun. 8 (1), 3–14. doi:10.1080/17459430701617846.

Chilisa, B., 2012. Indigenous Research Methodologies. Sage Publications, Thousand Oaks, CA.

Cho, J., Trent, A., 2006. Validity in qualitative research. Qual. Res. 6 (3), 319–340. doi:10.1177/1468794106065006.

Creswell, J.W., 2007, Qualitative Inquiry and Research Design: Choosing among Five Approaches, 2nd. Sage Publications, Thousand Oaks, CA.

Creswell, J.W., Miller, D.L., 2000. Getting good qualitative data to improve educational practice. Theory Pract. 39 (3), 124–130. doi:10.1207/s15430421tip3903_2.

Crotty, M., 1998. The Foundations of Social Research: Meaning and Perspective in the Research Process. Sage Publications, London, UK.

Curry, L.A., Nembhard, I.M., Bradley, E.H., 2009. Qualitative and mixed methods provide unique contributions to outcomes research. Circulation 119 (10), 1442–1452. doi:10.1161/CIRCULATIONAHA.107.742775.

Denzin, N.K., Lincoln, Y.S., 2000. Introduction: the discipline and practice of qualitative research. In: Denzin, N.K., Lincoln, Y.S. (Eds.). Handbook of Qualitative Research, 2nd. Sage Publications, Thousand Oaks, CA, pp. 1–29.

Denzin, N.K., Lincoln, Y.S., 2005. Introduction: the discipline and practice of qualitative research. In: Denzin, N.K., Lincoln, Y.S. (Eds.). The Sage Handbook of Qualitative Research, 3rd. Sage Publications, Thousand Oaks, CA, pp. 1–32.

Dickson-Swift, V., James, E.L., Kippen, S., Liamputtong, P., 2007. Doing sensitive research: what challenges do qualitative researchers face?. Qual Res. 7 (3), 327–353. doi:10.1177/1468794107078515.

Doyle, S., 2007. Member checking with older women: a framework for negotiating meaning. Health Care Women Int. 28 (10), 888–908. doi:10.1080/07399330701615325.

Erdmann, A., Potthoff, S., 2023. Decision criteria for the ethically reflected choice of a member check method in qualitative research: a proposal for discussion. Int. J. Qual. Methods 22 (1), 16094069231177664. doi:10.1177/16094069231177664.

Fahie, D., 2014. Doing sensitive research sensitively: ethical and methodological issues in researching workplace bullying. Int. J. Qual. Methods 13 (1), 19–36. doi:10.1177/160940691401300108.

Fricker, M., 2007. Epistemic Injustice: Power and the Ethics of Knowing. Oxford University Press, Oxford, UK.
Gadamer, H.G., 1975. Truth and Method (Barden G, Cumming J, trans.). Seabury Press, New York, NY.
Gillo, M.D., 2021. Fundamentals of hermeneutics as a qualitative research theoretical framework. Eur. J. Educ. Pedagogy 2 (3), 42–45. doi:10.24018/ejedu.2021.2.3.77.
Golafshani, N., 2003. Understanding reliability and validity in qualitative research. Qual. Rep. 8 (4), 597–606. doi:10.46743/2160-3715/2003.1870.
Goldblatt, H., Karnieli-Miller, O., Neumann, M., 2011. Sharing qualitative research findings with participants: study experiences of methodological and ethical dilemmas. Patient Educ. Couns. 82 (3), 389–395. doi:10.1016/j.pec.2010.12.016.
Guba, E.G., 1981. Criteria for assessing the trustworthiness of naturalistic inquiries. Educ. Technol. Res. Dev. 29 (2), 75–91. doi:10.1007/BF02766777.
Guba, E.G., Lincoln, Y.S., 1994. Competing paradigms in qualitative research. In: Denzin, N.K., Lincoln, Y.S. Eds., Handbook of Qualitative Research. Sage Publications, Thousand Oaks, CA, Accessed August 29, 2025 http://www.uncg.edu/hdf/facultystaff/Tudge/Guba%20&%20Lincoln%201994.pdf.
Guba, E.G., Lincoln, Y.S., 2005. Paradigmatic controversies, contradictions, and emerging confluences. In: Denzin, N.K., Lincoln, Y.S. (Eds.). The Sage Handbook of Qualitative Research, third ed. Sage Publications, Thousand Oaks, CA, pp. 191–216.
Guion, L.A., Diehl, D.C., McDonald, D., 2011. Triangulation: establishing the validity of qualitative studies. EDIS 2011 (3), 1–3. doi:10.32473/edis-fy394-2011.
Hadi, M.A., Closs, S.J., 2016. Ensuring rigour and trustworthiness of qualitative research in clinical pharmacy. Int. J. Clin. Pharm. 38 (3), 641–646. doi:10.1007/s11096-015-0237-6.
Hallett, R.E., 2013. Dangers of member checking. In: Midgley, W., Danaher, P.A., Baguley, M., Eds., The Role of Participants in Education Research: Ethics, Epistemologies, and Methods. Routledge, New York, NY, pp. 29–39.
Hannes, K., Lockwood, C., Pearson, A., 2010. A comparative analysis of three online appraisal instruments' ability to assess validity in qualitative research. Qual. Health Res. 20 (12), 1736–1743. doi:10.1177/1049732310378656.
Harper, M., Cole, P., 2012. Member checking: can benefits be gained similar to group therapy?. Qual. Rep. 17 (2), 510–517. doi:10.46743/2160-3715/2012.2139.
Harry, B., Sturges, K.M., Klingner, J.K., 2005. Mapping the process: an exemplar of process and challenge in grounded theory analysis. Educ. Res. 34 (2), 3–13. doi:10.3102/0013189X034002003.
Heidegger, M., 1962. Being and Time. SCM Press, London, UK.
Johnson, R.B., Onwuegbuzie, A.J., 2004. Mixed methods research: a research paradigm whose time has come. Educ. Res. 33 (7), 14–26. doi:10.3102/0013189X033007014.
Jordan, A., 2018. Approaches to validity in qualitative research. Int. J. Qual. Methods 17, 1–6. doi:10.1177/1609406918788237.
Jordan, S., 1997. Embodying the generic? A comparison of interpretive methodologies. Int. J. Qual. Stud. Educ. 10 (4), 449–463. doi:10.1080/095183997237124.
Klein, H.K., Myers, M.D., 1999. A set of principles for conducting and evaluating interpretive field studies in information systems. MIS Q. 23 (1), 67–93. doi:10.2307/249410.
Koelsch, L., 2013. Reconceptualizing the member check interview. Int. J. Qual. Methods 12 (1), 168–179. doi:10.1177/160940691301200105.
Lanzara, G.F., 2016. Shifting Practices: Reflections on Technology, Practice, and Innovation. MIT Press, Cambridge, MA.
Lather, P., 2004. Scientific research in education: a critical perspective. Br. Educ. Res. J. 30 (6), 759–772. doi:10.1080/0141192042000279490.
Laverty, S.M., 2003. Hermeneutic phenomenology and phenomenology: a comparison of historical and methodological considerations. Int. J. Qual. Methods 2 (3), 21–35. doi:10.1177/160940690300200303.
Lincoln, Y.S., Guba, E.A., 1985. Naturalistic Inquiry. Sage Publications, Beverly Hills, CA.
Lincoln, Y.S., Guba, E.G., 1985. Naturalistic Inquiry. Sage Publications, Newbury Park, CA.
Lincoln, Y.S., Guba, E.G., 1986. But is it rigorous? Trustworthiness and authenticity in naturalistic evaluation. New Dir. Program Eval. 1986 (30), 73–84. doi:10.1002/ev.1427.
Lincoln, Y.S., Guba, E.G., 2000. Paradigmatic controversies: contradictions and emerging confluences. In: Denzin, N.K., Lincoln, Y.S. (Eds.). Handbook of Qualitative Research, 2nd. Sage Publications, Thousand Oaks, CA, pp. 163–188.
Lincoln, Y.S., Lynham, S.A., Guba, E.G., 2011. Paradigmatic controversies, contradictions, and emerging confluences, revisited. In: Denzin, N.K., Lincoln, Y.S. (Eds.). The Sage Handbook of Qualitative Research, 4th. Sage Publications, Thousand Oaks, CA, pp. 97–128.
Lindheim, Ø., 2022. Member checking in qualitative research: reflections for researchers. Qual. Rep. 27 (11), 2525–2535. doi:10.46743/2160-3715/2022.5826.
Livari, N., 2018. Using member checking in interpretive research practice: a hermeneutic analysis of informants' interpretation of their organizational realities. Inf. Technol. People. 31 (1), 111–133. doi:10.1108/ITP-07-2016-0168.
Madill, A., Sullivan, P., 2017. Mirrors, portraits, and member checking: managing difficult moments of knowledge exchange in the social sciences. Qual. Psychol. 4 (2), 214–229. doi:10.1037/qup0000069.
Madill, A., Sullivan, P., 2018. Mirrors, portraits, and member checking: Managing difficult moments of knowledge exchange in the social sciences. Qual. Psychol. 5 (3), 321–339. doi:10.1037/qup0000089.
Marshall, C., Rossman, G.B., 2016, Designing Qualitative Research, sixth ed. Sage Publications, Thousand Oaks, CA.
Mason, J., 1996. Qualitative Researching. Sage Publications, London, UK.
Mays, N., Pope, C., 2000. Qualitative research in health care. Assessing quality in qualitative research. BMJ 320 (7226), 50–52. doi:10.1136/bmj.320.7226.50.
Mero-Jaffe, I., 2011. "Is that what I said?" interview transcript approval by participants: an aspect of ethics in qualitative research. Int. J. Qual. Methods 10 (3), 231–247. doi:10.1177/160940691101000304.
Morse, J.M., 2015. Critical analysis of strategies for determining rigor in qualitative inquiry. Qual. Health Res. 25 (9), 1212–1222. doi:10.1177/1049732315588501.
Morse, J.M., Barrett, M., Mayan, M., Olson, K., Spiers, J., 2002. Verification strategies for establishing reliability and validity in qualitative research. Int. J. Qual. Methods 1 (2), 13–22. doi:10.1177/160940690200100202.
Moss, G., 2004. Provisions of trustworthiness in critical narrative research: bridging intersubjectivity and fidelity. Qual. Rep. 9 (2), 359–374.

Motulsky, S.L., 2021. Is member checking the gold standard of quality in qualitative research?. Qual. Psychol. 8 (3), 389–400. doi:10.1037/qup0000181.

Moules, N.J., McCaffrey, G., Field, J.C., Laing, C.M., 2015. Conducting Hermeneutic Research: From Philosophy to Practice. Peter Lang, New York, NY.

Pinto, A., Rodriguez, A., Smith, J., 2022. Research sensitive topics in healthcare. Evid. Based Nurs. 25 (2), 41–43. doi:10.1136/ebnurs-2021-103501.

Richardson, L., 2000. Evaluating ethnography. Qual. Inq. 6 (2), 253–256. doi:10.1177/107780040000600208.

Rodríguez-Campos, L., 2012. Stakeholder involvement in evaluation: three decades of the American Journal of Evaluation. J. Multidiscip. Eval. 8 (17), 57–79.

Rolfe, G., 2006. Validity, trustworthiness and rigour: quality and the idea of qualitative research. J. Adv. Nurs. 53 (3), 304–310. doi:10.1111/j.1365-2648.2006.03727.x.

Sahakyan, T., 2023. Member checking through diagrammatic elicitation: constructing meaning with participants. TESOL Q. 57 (2), 686–701. doi:10.1002/tesq.3210.

Sandelowski, M., 1993. Rigor or rigor mortis: the problem of rigor in qualitative research revisited. Adv. Nurs. Sci. 16 (2), 1–8. doi:10.1097/00012272-199312000-00002.

Schwandt, T.A., 2000. Three epistemological stances for qualitative inquiry: interpretivism, hermeneutics, and social constructionism. In: Denzin, N.K., Lincoln, Y.S. (Eds.). Handbook of Qualitative Research, 2nd. Sage Publications, Thousand Oaks, CA, pp. 189–214.

Slettebø, T., 2021. Participant validation: exploring a contested tool in qualitative research. Qual. Soc. Work. 20 (5), 1223–1238. doi:10.1177/1473325020968189.

Smith, J.A., Flowers, P., Larkin, M., 2009. Interpretative Phenomenological Analysis: Theory, Method and Research. Sage Publications, London, UK.

Stenfors, T., Kajamaa, A., Bennett, D., 2020. How to assess the quality of qualitative research. Clin. Teach. 17 (6), 596–599. doi:10.1111/tct.13242.

Tenny, S., Brannan, J.M., Brannan, G.D., 2022. Qualitative study. StatPearls [Internet]. StatPearls Publishing, Treasure Island, FL. Accessed August 29, 2025 https://www.ncbi.nlm.nih.gov/books/NBK470395/.

Thomas, D.R., 2017. Feedback from research participants: are member checks useful in qualitative research?. Qual. Res. Psychol. 14 (1), 23–41. doi:10.1080/14780887.2016.1219435.

Tong, A., Sainsbury, P., Craig, J., 2007. Consolidated criteria for reporting qualitative research (COREQ): a 32-item checklist for interviews and focus groups. Int. J. Qual. Health Care. 19 (6), 349–357. doi:10.1093/intqhc/mzm042.

Tracy, S.J., 2004. The construction of correctional officers: layers of emotionality behind bars. Qual. Inq. 10 (4), 509–533. doi:10.1177/1077800403259716.

Tracy, S.J., 2010. Qualitative quality: eight "big-tent" criteria for excellent qualitative research. Qual. Inq. 16 (10), 837–851. doi:10.1177/1077800410383121.

Tracy, S.J., Scott, C., 2006. Sexuality, masculinity and taint management among firefighters and correctional officers: getting down and dirty with "America's heroes" and the "scum of law enforcement. Manag. Commun. Q. 20 (1), 6–38. doi:10.1177/0893318906287898.

Urry, J., Law, J., Mol, A., 2024. Rethinking participation: dialogical models for qualitative research. Qual. Inq. 30 (2), 145–162. doi:10.1177/10778004231123456.

van Manen, M., 1990. Researching Lived Experience: Human Science for an Action Sensitive Pedagogy. SUNY Press, Albany.

Varpio, L., Ajjawi, R., Monrouxe, L.V., O'Brien, B.C., Rees, C.E., 2017. Shedding the cobra effect: problematising thematic emergence, triangulation, saturation and member checking. Med. Educ. 51 (1), 40–50. doi:10.1111/medu.13124.

Walsh, K., 1996. Philosophical hermeneutics and the project of Hans-Georg Gadamer: implications for nursing research. Nurs. Inq. 3 (4), 231–237. doi:10.1111/j.1440-1800.1996.tb00050.x.

Whitehead, L., 2004. Enhancing the quality of hermeneutic research: decision trail. J. Adv. Nurs. 45 (5), 512–518. doi:10.1046/j.1365-2648.2003.02934.x.

Whittemore, R., Chase, S.K., Mandle, C.L., 2001. Validity in qualitative research. Qual. Health Res. 11 (4), 522–537. doi:10.1177/104973201129119299.

Zairul, M., 2021. Can member check be verified in real time? Introducing ARC (asking, record, confirm) for member checking validation strategy in qualitative research. Eng. J. 25 (1), 245–251. doi:10.4186/ej.2021.25.1.245.

Zimmerman, J., 2015. Hermeneutics: A Very Short Introduction. Oxford University Press, Oxford, UK.

CHAPTER

3

Scientific visibility and medical subject heading terms: The case of 'pharmaceutical sciences'

Fernanda S. Tonin[a] *and Fernando Fernandez-Llimos*[b]

[a]Social and Legal Pharmacy Section, Pharmacy and Pharmaceutical Technology Department, University of Granada, Granada, Spain

[b]Faculty of Pharmacy, Laboratory of Pharmacology, Department of Drug Sciences, University of Porto, Porto, Portugal

CHAPTER OBJECTIVES

This chapter aims to:

- Provide a better understanding of the role of Medical Subject Headings (MeSH) descriptors in the retrieval and visibility of scientific literature
- Identify the gaps in the representation of pharmacy within biomedical indexing systems
- Highlight the limitations of the current indexing process and propose practical strategies to improve its accuracy, consistency, and overall effectiveness
- Enhance the visibility and accessibility of pharmacy practice publications

1 Introduction

1.1 Concepts and relevancy of medical subject headings thesaurus

Medical Subject Headings (MeSH) thesaurus is the controlled vocabulary developed by the U.S. National Library of Medicine (NLM) to index, catalog, and search for biomedical and health-related literature, including scientific articles, books, and other research sources. Initially created in the 1960s, MeSH was composed of around 4000 terms derived from subject headings used in card catalogs from libraries. In 2025, the number of descriptors appearing in MEDLINE (a primary bibliographic database of life sciences and biomedical literature that forms PubMed and houses over 31 million records) reached 30,000. The terms are annually updated in the English language to reflect changes in terminology and account for variations in language, synonyms, and alternate spellings (National Library of Medicine, 2025b).

Different types of terms exist within the MeSH thesaurus. The descriptors, or main headings, represent the primary subjects of indexed content, organized into 19 categories (e.g., category A for anatomic terms, category B

https://doi.org/10.1016/B978-0-443-44607-8.00007-8

for organisms, category C for diseases, etc.). Each category is further divided into subcategories where descriptors are arranged both alphabetically and hierarchically to reflect broader (i.e., upper in the tree structure) and narrower (i.e., descendant in the tree structure) concepts. This allows users to retrieve not only the selected MeSH term but also all its specific subordinate terms automatically—a process known as 'automatic exploding' or 'extended search'. Moreover, most descriptors are accompanied by a short description or definition, cross-references to related descriptors, and a list of synonyms or very similar terms (known as 'entry terms') that enhance searchability by accommodating variations in terminology. Descriptors may be further supplemented by qualifiers—topical subheadings that refine meaning by specifying certain aspects of a subject, such as diagnosis, therapeutic use, or drug effects. In addition, MeSH includes publication types that describe the methodological design of a resource (e.g., clinical trials, reviews) and geographic descriptors to tag regional context. Supplementary concept records further extend the thesaurus by covering entities not included as main descriptors, such as chemicals, rare diseases, organisms, and population groups (National Library of Medicine, 2025c; National Library of Medicine, 2025a). Although these supplementary records are not part of the hierarchical tree, they are mapped to related descriptors to maintain semantic coherence (Baumann, 2016). An overview of MeSH components is summarized in Table 3.1.

TABLE 3.1 Core components of the MeSH thesaurus.

Elements	Definitions
Class 1 descriptor: Main headings	Core terms representing concepts in biomedical literature are used to index citations in NLM's MEDLINE database for cataloging publications and other databases, and they are searchable in PubMed as Main Headings "[MH]". These terms are organized hierarchically, ranging from broad to specific topics, and are usually updated on an annual basis.
Class 2 descriptors: Publication characteristics (publication type)	Describe the type or format of a publication (e.g., charts, editorial, clinical trial). They function as metadata rather than being about the content. These records are searchable in PubMed as Publication Type "[PT]".
Class 3 descriptors: Check tags	This class of descriptors is used for tagging (i.e., filtering and statistical purposes) citations that contain certain categories of information. They do not appear in the MeSH tree. Currently, only two Class 3 descriptors remain: "Male" and "Female."
Class 4: descriptors Geographics	Descriptors include continents, regions, countries, states, and other geographic subdivisions. They are not used to characterize subject content but rather to indicate physical location. These descriptors are listed in category Z of the MeSH Tree Structures.
Tree numbers	Alphanumeric codes are assigned to descriptors, indicating their position in the hierarchy (e.g., A01.111 for a specific anatomical structure).
Hierarchy levels	The tree is structured with broader terms at higher levels and narrower terms as descendants, allowing for specificity in indexing and searching. Example of the hierarchical structure of the MeSH 'pharmaceutical services': *Pharmaceutical services* • *Community pharmacy services* • *Drug information services* • *Adverse drug reaction reporting systems* • *Clinical pharmacy information systems* • *Prescription drug monitoring programs* • *Medication therapy management* • *Pharmaceutical services, online* • *Pharmacy services, hospital* • *Prescriptions* • *Drug prescriptions* • *Drug substitution* • *Electronic prescribing* • *Non-medical prescribing*
Entry terms (synonyms)	Alternative names or synonyms are linked to descriptors, helping users find relevant terms even when they use different terminology.
Qualifiers (subheadings)	There are 78 topical terms used for indexing and cataloging in conjunction with Descriptors. They indicate a specific aspect of a subject (e.g., diagnosis, therapy) and are searchable in PubMed as MeSH Subheadings "[SH]".
Supplementary concept records	These terms are used to index chemicals, drugs, and other concepts, such as rare diseases, for MEDLINE and are searchable by Substance Name "[NM]" in PubMed. They are not organized in a tree hierarchy. Five classes exist: chemicals, protocols, diseases, organisms, and population groups.

Until 2011, the assignment of MeSH terms was performed entirely manually by trained NLM staff or subcontracted catalogers, following the structured framework of the MeSH vocabulary. Shortly thereafter, the NLM implemented the Medical Text Indexer (MTI), an algorithm designed to assist in the indexing process while maintaining human oversight (data curation) for quality control. Since April 2022, MEDLINE indexing has transitioned fully to an automated system [MTI-Auto (MTIA)], although selected citations (e.g., those involving genes and proteins, ambiguous terms with multiple meanings, clinical trials) and random sets of citations continue to undergo human review. Although the use of full-text indexing has been considered, the MTIA currently relies only on titles, abstracts, and MeSH terms from related PubMed records to generate a final list of MeSH descriptors, supplementary concepts, and publication types (Fernandez-Llimos et al., 2024; Mork et al., 2017; Chen et al., 2023).

The most significant contribution of MeSH to the research community is its role in enhancing the efficiency and precision of literature searches, minimizing the inclusion of irrelevant records. Unlike free-text keywords provided by authors—which often vary in terminology, spelling, and specificity—MeSH terms offer a standardized and hierarchically structured vocabulary that ensures consistent indexing across biomedical literature. Free-text keywords (i.e., search terms that are entered in natural language without being restricted to a predefined list, category, or structured vocabulary) are especially problematic when dealing with synonymous or closely related concepts, as they can impair the identification of relevant publications. Moreover, appropriate MeSH terms can significantly increase the visibility and discoverability of articles, thereby improving citation potential (Jenuwine and Floyd, 2004; Chang et al., 2006; Doig and Simpson, 2003). Articles that lack MeSH terms (either because authors do not incorporate them into abstracts and titles or because journals do not require their use) may be less easily retrieved in bibliographic searches, reducing their chances of being cited. This has a dual impact: authors may receive less recognition for their work, and journals may experience a lower citation count, ultimately affecting impact metrics (Yang and Lee, 2018). To support accurate MeSH term identification and consistent use, researchers may rely on three main approaches: the MeSH Browser, which allows for structured exploration of the descriptors; the MeSH terms listed under relevant PubMed articles; and the MeSH on Demand tool, which uses natural language processing to suggest appropriate MeSH terms based on free-text input (Baumann, 2016; Jimeno-Yepes et al., 2013).

2 MeSH in pharmacy: Differences between practice and representation

Despite the extensive scope of the MeSH thesaurus in covering biomedical disciplines, it contains fewer and often less specific terms compared to Emtree, the controlled vocabulary used by Scopus—another relevant database. Moreover, several studies have highlighted insufficient coverage of certain specialized fields in MeSH, as well as inconsistencies and inaccuracies in the assignment of terms by NLM indexers—whether performed manually or via the MTIA system. These pitfalls can introduce significant bias in literature retrieval and citation patterns (Portaluppi, 2007; Richter and Austin, 2012; Tonin et al., 2022; Minguet et al., 2015, 2014; Rotta et al., 2017; Fernandez-Llimos, 2025).

Yet, pharmacy is not a core area of interest for the NLM, a limitation that has been highlighted in several research studies on the underrepresentation of pharmacy journals in both PubMed and MEDLINE (Mendes et al., 2019). The number of pharmacy-related MeSH terms in the thesaurus remains lower than those assigned to other similar health professions, despite recent efforts to incorporate newly proposed terms. As of 2014, only 26 pharmacy-specific MeSH terms were available, compared to 94 in nursing and 145 in dentistry. Although at least 16 new pharmacy-related terms have since been proposed, only five have been adopted by the NLM (Minguet et al., 2014; Fernandez-Llimos et al., 2017; Salgado and Fernandez-Llimos, 2019). Furthermore, pharmacy journals often face longer delays in MeSH indexing compared to general medical journals, further limiting their visibility and impact (Rodriguez, 2014). As of August 2025, around 40 MeSH terms relevant to pharmacy are available (including pharmacy-specific terms and pharmacy-adjacent terms); Table 3.2 provides an overview of the pharmacy-specific terms, primary definitions, and year of introduction in MEDLINE.

This lack of comprehensive and timely indexing is concerning, given the evolving scope of contemporary pharmacy and how it is (or is not) captured in major biomedical indexing systems. Pharmacists are increasingly involved in clinical decision-making, patient education, interprofessional healthcare teams, public health initiatives, and pharmacoeconomic analysis—roles that extend the traditional dispensing functions. However, these broader responsibilities are not adequately represented in indexing vocabularies, which tend to focus more heavily on pharmacological agents and drug-related effects rather than professional services, patient-centered care, or health systems integration. This mismatch, often caused by professional domains advancing faster than the terminological frameworks, limits the retrieval of relevant literature, reduces the visibility of pharmacy-related research, and distorts bibliometric analyses by underrepresenting the profession's full impact on healthcare (Raza et al., 2022; Marriott, 2018; Gernant et al., 2020).

TABLE 3.2 Main pharmacy-related MeSH terms.

Pharmacy-related MeSH	Definition	Year introduced[a]
Behind-the-counter drugs	Medicines that are stocked behind the counter of a pharmacy require the attention or advice of a pharmacist before being dispensed or handed over to a consumer or patient	2010
Clinical pharmacy information systems	Information systems, usually computer-assisted, are designed to store, manipulate, and retrieve information for planning, organizing, directing, and controlling administrative activities associated with the provision and utilization of clinical pharmacy services	1991
Community pharmacy services	Total pharmaceutical services are provided to the public through community pharmacies	1968
Dictionaries, pharmaceutic as topic	Works about specialized reference lists and descriptions of drugs and related concepts	2018 (1966)
Drug compounding	The preparation, mixing, and assembly of a drug	2017
Drug information services	Services providing pharmaceutical and therapeutic drug information and consultation	1981(1977)
Economics, pharmaceutical	Economic aspects of the fields of pharmacy and pharmacology apply to the development and study of medical economics in rational drug therapy and the impact of pharmaceuticals on the cost of medical care. Pharmaceutical economics also includes the economic considerations of the pharmaceutical care delivery system and drug prescribing, particularly regarding cost-benefit values.	1994
Education, pharmacy	Formal instruction, learning, or training in the preparation, dispensing, and proper utilization of drugs in the field of medicine	1999
Education, pharmacy, continuing	Educational programs are designed to inform graduate pharmacists about recent advances in their field	1968
Education, pharmacy, graduate	Educational programs for pharmacists who have a bachelor's degree or a Doctor of Pharmacy degree are designed for those entering a specific field of pharmacy, and they may lead to an advanced degree	1968
Ethics, pharmacy	The principles of proper professional conduct concern the rights and duties of the pharmacist, relations with patients and fellow practitioners, as well as the actions of the pharmacist in health care and interpersonal relations with patients' families	1968
Evidence-based pharmacy practice	The practice of pharmacy involves the pharmacist making decisions while taking into account the best available current research evidence, the pharmacist's expertise, and the needs and preferences of the patient	2020
Faculty, pharmacy	Teaching and administrative staff with academic rank in a pharmacy school or department	2017
Fees, pharmaceutical	Amounts charged to the patient or third-party payer for medication include the pharmacist's professional fee and the cost of ingredients, containers, etc.	1968
History of pharmacy	Study of the origins and development of the field of pharmacy	2019
Insurance, pharmaceutical services	Insurance provides for the payment of services rendered by the pharmacist. These services include the preparation and distribution of medical products	1968
Legislation, pharmacy	Laws and regulations pertaining to the field of pharmacy, proposed for enactment or enacted by a legislative body	1968
Licensure, pharmacy	The granting of a license to practice pharmacy	1968
Medication adherence	Voluntary cooperation of the patient in taking drugs or medicines as prescribed includes timing, dosage, and frequency	2009
Nonprescription drugs	Medicines that can be sold legally without a 'drug prescription'	2009(1973)
Non-medical prescribing	Prescribing by a healthcare professional other than a doctor or dentist	2024
Nuclear pharmacy	An application of pharmacy involving the preparation and dispensing of radioactive materials for use in medications	2017
Pharmaceutical preparations	Drugs intended for human or veterinary use, presented in their finished dosage form. Included here are materials used in the preparation or formulation of the finished dosage form.	1998(1963)
Pharmaceutical services	Total pharmaceutical services are provided by qualified pharmacists. In addition to the preparation and distribution of medical products, these services may include consultative support offered to agencies and institutions that do not have a qualified pharmacist.	1968

Pharmacy-related MeSH	Definition	Year introduced[a]
Pharmaceutical services, online	Pharmacy services accessed via electronic means	2012
Pharmacies	Facilities for the preparation and dispensing of drugs	1968-1978
Pharmacists	Those individuals legally qualified by education and training to engage in the practice of pharmacy	1968
Pharmacy	The practice of compounding and dispensing medicinal preparations	1999
Pharmacy administration	The business and managerial aspects of pharmacy in their broadest sense	1968
Pharmacy and therapeutics committee	An advisory group composed primarily of staff physicians and a pharmacist, which serves as the communication link between the medical staff and the pharmacy department	1968
Pharmacy research	Research activity focused on pharmacy	2017
Pharmacy residencies	Advanced programs of training are designed to meet specific professional requirements in the practice of compounding and dispensing medicinal preparations	2014
Pharmacy Service, Hospital	Hospital department responsible for receiving, storing, and distributing pharmaceutical supplies	1978
Pharmacy technicians—previous pharmacists' aides (1971–2016)	Persons who perform certain functions under the supervision of a pharmacist	2017
Pharmacovigilance	The detection of long and short-term side effects of conventional and traditional medicines through research, data mining, monitoring, and evaluation of healthcare information obtained from healthcare providers and patients	2012
Practice patterns, pharmacists'	Patterns of practice related to how pharmacists prepare or compound prescription drugs are especially influenced by the cost of the service requested and provided	2021
Schools, pharmacy	Educational institutions for individuals specializing in the field of pharmacy	1968
Societies, pharmaceutical	Societies whose memberships are limited to pharmacists	1968
Students, pharmacy	Individuals enrolled in a school of pharmacy or a formal educational program leading to a degree in pharmacy are pursuing specialized training in the field of pharmaceutical sciences	1968
Technology, pharmaceutical	The application of scientific knowledge or technology to pharmacy and the pharmaceutical industry includes methods, techniques, and instrumentation in the manufacture, preparation, compounding, dispensing, packaging, and storing of drugs and other preparations used in diagnostic and determinative procedures, as well as in the treatment of patients	1968

[a] *Year in which the term was introduced; some had their definitions refined (year in parentheses).*

However, simply expanding the number of MeSH terms is not sufficient to ensure proper representation of the pharmacy field. Existing MeSH descriptors must also be appropriately and consistently assigned to articles—either by NLM staff or through automated systems. Previous work has demonstrated that the quality of MeSH term assignment in pharmacy literature is suboptimal, with over half of the articles indexed without a single pharmacy-specific MeSH (Minguet et al., 2015). Yet, an important barrier to both the proposal of new MeSH terms and the precise indexing of articles is the inconsistent use of terminology within the pharmacy community itself—including authors, researchers, peer-reviewers, and editors (Salgado and Fernandez-Llimos, 2019; Gernant et al., 2020; Fernandez-Llimos and Salgado, 2021). This issue is evident in the terminology used to describe 'pharmaceutical services', which varies widely and includes overlapping or loosely defined terms such as 'clinical pharmacy', 'pharmaceutical care', 'medication therapy management', and 'comprehensive medication management'. To address these challenges, the International Collaboration of Pharmacy Journal Editors (ICPJE) has identified the promotion of pharmacy and pharmacy journals within NLM databases—including the MeSH thesaurus—as one of its key objectives (Alves da Costa et al., 2025; Fernandez-Llimos et al., 2023). Achieving this goal requires robust, well-designed research studies on the gaps in coverage and indexing, as well as increased commitment from pharmacy researchers to use standardized terminology that can be adopted into MeSH.

The following section presents a case study on the use of one of the most common MeSH terms in the pharmacy domain, aiming to illustrate key pitfalls and challenges that still hinder the scientific visibility of the pharmacy practice field (Tonin et al., 2022).

3 Methods: Case study

3.1 Study design and data collection

This case study presents findings from a published meta-research study that, through a multistep process, assessed how the MeSH descriptor 'pharmaceutical services' (Unique ID: D010593) and related terms are assigned to articles on pharmacists' interventions (Tonin et al., 2022; Harpe, 2021). 'Pharmaceutical services' was introduced by the NLM in 1968, encompassing a broad range of pharmacy-related activities. Currently, it includes 14 descendant MeSH terms across three generations (see Table 3.1—Hierarchy Levels). According to the NLM's official definition, it refers to the "total pharmaceutical services provided by qualified PHARMACISTS", including preparation, distribution, and consultative functions.

For this study, the initial dataset was built upon a previously published systematic review by Bonetti et al. (2020, 2022), which was updated to identify all meta-analyses evaluating the impact of pharmacist-delivered services on economic, humanistic, clinical, or process outcomes. Literature searches were conducted in PubMed, Scopus, and Web of Science (up to January 2022) and supplemented by manual searches of references. Eligible studies included meta-analyses of interventional or observational studies comparing pharmacist-led interventions to standard care or other professionals' care. Non-meta-analytic reviews, outdated analyses, or those lacking focus on pharmacists were excluded. From the final set of meta-analyses, all the primary studies were identified. Duplicates were removed, and only those indexed in PubMed with assigned PubMed Identifiers were selected for analysis. This process followed international recommendations on the conduct and reporting of systematic reviews and meta-analyses from the Cochrane Collaboration and Preferred Reporting Items for Systematic Reviews and Metaanalyses guidelines (Higgins et al., 2024; Page et al., 2021).

3.2 MeSH terms extraction and classification

MeSH terms for each included primary article were systematically extracted from PubMed (date of extraction: March 2022) using the 'save into PubMed' format feature to create a .txt file, which was further imported into an Excel (Microsoft, Redmond, WA) data sheet. Particular attention was given to the assignment of:

- 'Pharmaceutical services' MeSH term and its descendants *(Note: the term 'nonmedical prescribing' was excluded from this analysis, as it was only recently introduced in 2024 and has not yet generated a sufficient number of indexed articles.)*
- 26 additional pharmacy-related MeSH terms, previously described in the literature and potentially related to pharmaceutical services (Minguet et al., 2015, 2014)

The analysis also differentiated between all assigned MeSH descriptors and those designated as 'Major MeSH' in the database (which denote the article's primary focus and are marked with an asterisk). Data extraction and organization were performed using Excel (Microsoft, Redmond, WA) and EndNote X21 (Clarivate, Philadelphia, PA).

3.3 Data analysis

The study combined descriptive statistics to summarize MeSH use. A Spearman test was used for nonparametric correlations on the number and percentage of MeSH terms and Major MeSH terms with the year of publication. Sensitivity analyses were also conducted on articles explicitly mentioning 'pharmacy' or 'pharmacist' in their objectives/goals to reduce the influence of multidisciplinary studies. Analyses were performed in IBM SPSS (Statistical Package for the Social Sciences) v. 24.0 (IBM Corp., Armonk, NY), and p-values below 5% were considered statistically significant.

Additionally, social network analysis using Gephi's ForceAtlas2 model (Bastian et al., 2009) was performed to visualize the cooccurrence of MeSH terms, highlighting the structural links between pharmacy-specific descriptors and those related to 'pharmaceutical services'.

3.4 Key findings

The study revealed significant terminological dispersion. Among the 2012 primary studies on pharmacists' interventions analyzed, a total of 1893 different MeSH terms were identified (median number of 15 [IQR - interquartil range 12–18] MeSH terms per article), with over one-third of them (37.6%) appearing only once across the dataset. In the sensitivity analysis, limited to more pharmacy-specific articles (n = 1099), results were similar (1312 different MeSH terms, with 520 [39.3%] of them appearing in only one article). A slightly positive time trend regarding the number of MeSH terms assigned per article was observed (Spearman rho = 0.193; $p < 0.001$). Figure 3.1 depicts the

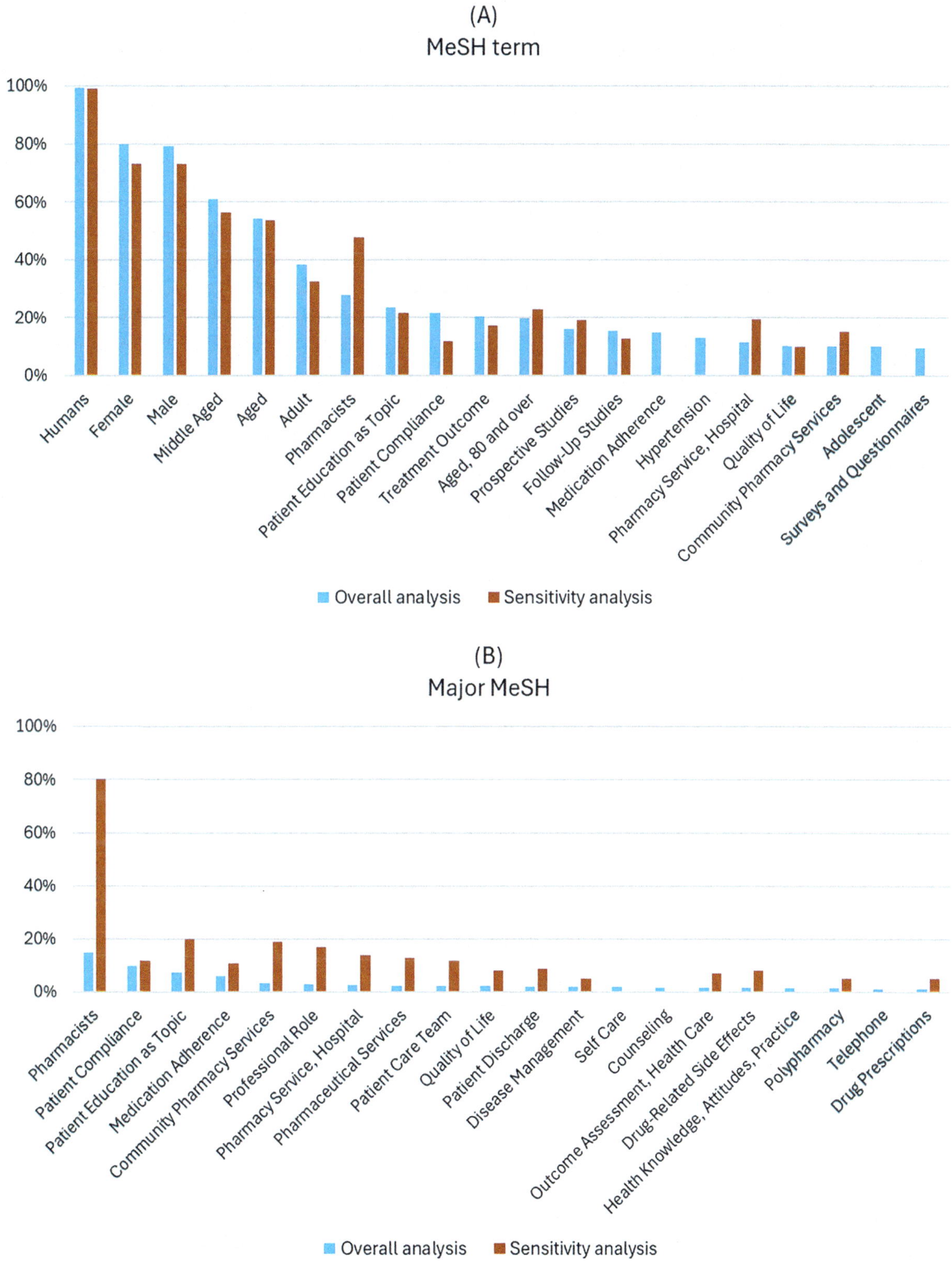

FIG. 3.1 Top terms most frequently assigned to pharmacists' intervention articles as (A) MeSH terms and (B) Major MeSH terms. Overall analysis: terms assigned to the 2012 articles. Sensitivity analysis: terms assigned to the 1099 articles presenting the words 'pharmacist' or 'pharmacy' in the objective.

top 20 most frequently reported terms in the included articles—most of which are not directly related to pharmacy (e.g., humans, adult, middle-aged, prospective studies), revealing a fragmented use of descriptors.

Among pharmacy-related terms, broad descriptors such as 'pharmacists', "pharmacy service, hospital," and 'community pharmacy services' were the most frequently assigned, though their overall use remained low—around 30%, 12%, and 10%, respectively, in the overall analysis. These rates showed a slight increase in the sensitivity analysis of pharmacy-focused articles, reaching 48%, 20%, and 15%, respectively. With the exception of 'pharmacists'—designated as a Major MeSH in 15% of cases in the overall analysis and 80% in the sensitivity analysis—the assignment of other pharmacy-related terms as primary indexing descriptors was even less frequent, remaining below 5% overall and increasing to 10%–20% in the sensitivity analysis.

A notably poor utilization of relevant descriptors within the 'pharmaceutical services' branch was also identified. Only 36.6% of all 2012 articles were indexed with any term from this category. Even in the more pharmacy-specific articles (n = 1099), this proportion increased modestly to around 58%. Furthermore, when such terms were used, they were scarcely prioritized: only 11.5% of the indexed articles had a 'pharmaceutical services' term marked as a Major MeSH, suggesting these descriptors were not considered central to the studies' focus. Other specific MeSH terms were rarely employed, appearing in less than 1% of the studies. See Tables 3.3 and 3.4.

The social network analysis (depicted in Fig. 3.2) confirmed weak structural connections between 'pharmaceutical services' terms and other pharmacy-specific descriptors. The only notable cooccurrence was with the term 'Pharmacists', and even that was limited to a few related MeSH terms.

TABLE 3.3 Frequency of other pharmacy-specific MeSH terms assigned to pharmacists' intervention studies.

MeSH term	Overall analysis[a] (n = 2,012)		Sensitivity analysis[b] (n = 1,099)	
	N	%	N	%
Behind-the-counter drugs	0	0.0	0	0
Dictionaries, pharmaceutical	0	0.0	0	0
Drug compounding	1	0.0	0	0
Education, Pharmacy	8	0.4	6	0.55
Education, pharmacy, continuing	4	0.2	4	0.36
Education, pharmacy, graduate	0	0.0	0	0
Ethics, pharmacy	0	0.0	0	0
Evidence-based pharmacy practice	0	0.0	0	0
Faculty, pharmacy	0	0.0	0	0
Fees, pharmaceutical	1	0.0	1	0.09
History of pharmacy	0	0.0	0	0
Insurance, pharmaceutical services	11	0.5	6	0.55
Legislation, pharmacy	4	0.2	4	0.36
Licensure, pharmacy	0	0.0	0	0
Pharmacies	55	2.7	48	4.37
Pharmacists	560	27.8	524	47.68
Pharmacists' aides	0	0.0	0	0
Pharmacy	7	0.3	5	0.45
Pharmacy administration	2	0.1	2	0.18
Pharmacy research	0	0.0	0	0
Pharmacy and therapeutics committee	2	0.1	2	0.18
Practice patterns, pharmacists'	0	0.0	0	0
Schools, pharmacy	1	0.0	1	0.09
Societies, pharmaceutical	0	0.0	0	0
Students, pharmacy	2	0.1	2	0.18
Technology, pharmaceutical	0	0.0	0	0

[a]*Terms assigned to the 2012 articles.*
[b]*Terms assigned to the 1099 articles presenting the words 'pharmacist' or 'pharmacy' in the objective.*

TABLE 3.4 Frequency of 'pharmaceutical service' terms assigned to pharmacists' intervention studies.

MeSH term	Overall analysis[a] (n = 2,012)		Sensitivity analysis[b] (n = 1,099)	
	N	%	N	%
Pharmaceutical services	181	9.00	168	15.29
Community pharmacy services	205	10.19	192	17.47
Drug Information services	9	0.45	8	0.73
Adverse drug reaction reporting systems	11	0.55	7	0.64
Clinical pharmacy information systems	18	0.89	13	1.18
Prescription drug monitoring programs	0	0	0	0
Medication therapy management	68	3.38	46	4.19
Pharmaceutical services, online	0	0	0	0
Pharmacy service, hospital	232	11.53	215	19.56
Prescriptions	5	0.25	4	0.36
Drug prescriptions	108	5.37	78	7.10
Drug substitution	4	0.19	2	0.18
Electronic prescribing	9	0.45	1	0.09
Non-medical prescribing[c]	–	–	–	–
Pharmaceutical services	50	2.49	47	4.28
Community pharmacy services	68	3.38	67	6.10
Drug Information services	2	0.10	2	0.18
Adverse drug reaction reporting systems	4	0.20	3	0.27
Clinical pharmacy information systems	9	0.45	5	0.45
Prescription drug monitoring programs	0	0	0	0
Medication therapy management	21	1.04	15	1.36
Pharmaceutical services, online	0	0	0	0
Pharmacy service, hospital	53	2.63	50	4.55
Prescriptions	1	0.05	0	0
Drug Prescriptions	1	0.05	18	1.64
Drug Substitution	27	1.34	1	0.09
Electronic Prescribing	1	0.05	0	0
Non-Medical Prescribing[d]	–	–	–	–

[a]*Terms assigned to the 2012 articles.*
[b]*Terms assigned to the 1099 articles presenting the words 'pharmacist' or 'pharmacy' in the objective.*
[c]*Not evaluated (term introduced in 2024).*
[d]*Not evaluated (term introduced in 2024).*

4 Discussion

Given the growing relevance of pharmacy-based interventions in healthcare systems worldwide, one would expect high visibility and consistent indexing of related descriptors in scientific literature—which is not observed in practice. The metaresearch case study highlights a persistent and consequential issue in pharmacy literature: the underutilization and inconsistent assignment of standardized indexing terms, despite the existence of pharmacy-specific descriptors—many of which are organized under the 'pharmaceutical services' branch. This underrepresentation reduces the field's visibility and undermines bibliometric evaluations that are paramount for academic recognition, research funding, and policy impact in healthcare. Considering that the main goal of a bibliographic database, such as MEDLINE, should be to facilitate the retrieval of scientific literature, having a robust search engine, like PubMed, may not always be sufficient. Controlled vocabularies of subject headings, such as the MeSH thesaurus, were created to standardize terms, index and catalog scientific articles, and thus avoid terminology variations among researchers (Fatehi et al., 2014; Sivarajkumar et al., 2024).

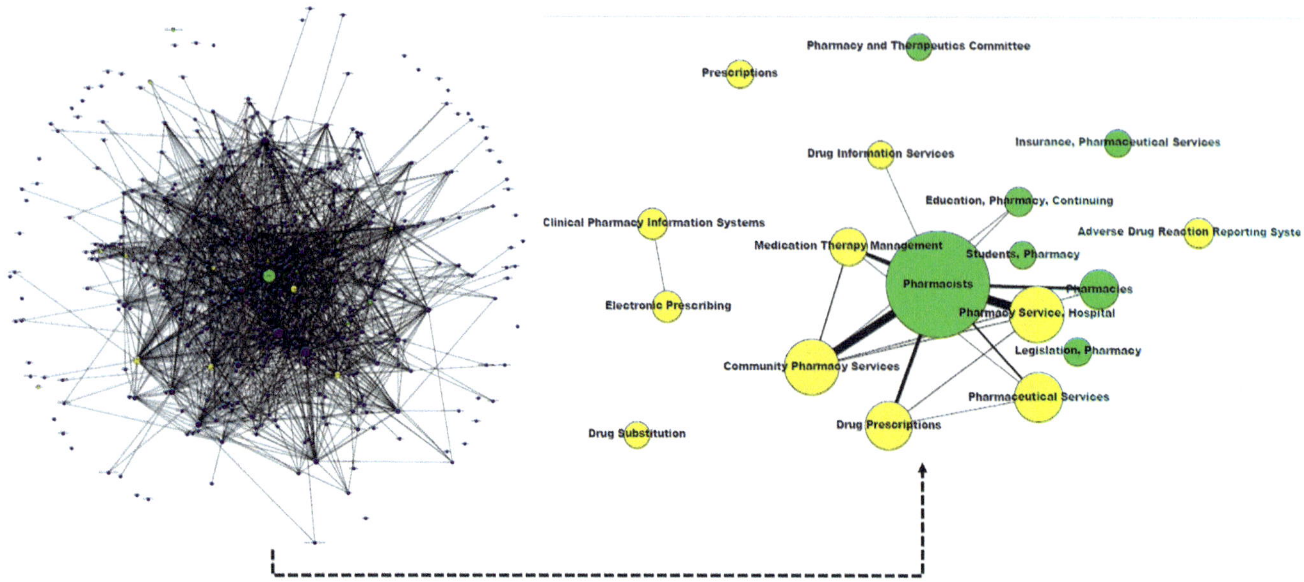

FIG. 3.2 Social network analyses of the cooccurrence of MeSH terms. Yellow nodes represent the MeSH terms from the 'pharmaceutical services' branch. Green nodes represent pharmacy-specific MeSH terms. Blue nodes represent the remaining nonpharmacy-specific MeSH terms.

At its core, this challenge is shaped by language. The terminology used by authors—whether standardized or ad hoc, often created to defend a research group's so-called "innovation"—directly influences whether studies can be effectively retrieved through database searches. This inconsistent use not only reduces search sensitivity but also weakens the request for new pharmacy-related MeSH terms. According to NLM policy, the introduction of new descriptors relies on consistent use of the term in the literature (Salgado and Fernandez-Llimos, 2019). However, this consistency is often lacking in pharmacy due to author oversight: many researchers assume indexers will identify appropriate descriptors and, therefore, do not prioritize precise terminology in their own articles. This issue is exacerbated by journal submission systems that provide limited guidance or flexibility in MeSH term selection. At a broader level, systemic limitations in indexing systems like MEDLINE—which became fully automated in 2022 and relies only on titles and abstracts—compromise indexing accuracy in the absence of standardized language (Chen et al., 2023; Jimeno-Yepes et al., 2013).

Additional barriers stem from structural issues in the MeSH hierarchy itself. In contrast to other health professions, for instance, where relationships such as 'nurse–patient relations' or 'dentist–patient relations' exist as distinct MeSH terms, the pharmacy equivalent was not formally created. Instead, the NLM embedded it as a subordinate concept within the broader taxonomy 'professional–patient relations' MeSH. The issue is further compounded by the dispersion of pharmacy research across more than 500 journals, many of which are not pharmacy-specific. While interdisciplinary publishing may broaden exposure and citation, it often decreases visibility within the pharmacy field and reduces the likelihood of accurate MeSH assignment. This journal scattering also undermines peer-level editorial feedback, which could otherwise help refine both the manuscript and its terminological precision (Fernandez-Llimos et al., 2023).

4.1 Lessons learned and recommendations

Improving indexing in pharmacy requires a collective, global effort as advocated by the ICPJE (https://www.icpje.org/). Standardizing terminology, refining editorial practices, and engaging with indexing authorities are all essential steps toward a more visible, connected, and scientifically credible field. The findings from this case-study offer several lessons and point to tangible strategies for improvement:

- **Language matters:** Standardizing terminology across pharmacy research is paramount to improving the visibility and recognition of the field
- **Indexing systems are not neutral:** They reflect institutional priorities and may perpetuate historical gaps unless actively challenged and updated
- **Collaborative advocacy is needed:** Pharmacy researchers, editors, and associations must engage with national libraries (e.g., NLM) to propose and support revisions or additions to the MeSH vocabulary. Health sciences

librarians and information specialists should also be more integrated into the research and publication process to guide the appropriate use of terminology
- **Education and awareness:** Authors must be encouraged and trained to select accurate descriptors, and journal editors and reviewers should prioritize descriptor quality during the peer review process

5 Questions for further discussion

- Why are pharmacy-related concepts often underrepresented in biomedical indexing systems?
- What impact does this underrepresentation have on research visibility and accessibility?
- What other methods and approaches could be explored to improve MeSH selection and ensure consistent use?
- What role should journals and editors play in selecting or promoting MeSH terms?

5.1 Considerations for future application

To address the persistent underrepresentation of pharmacy-related concepts in biomedical indexing systems, future efforts should also explore the integration of artificial intelligence (AI) and text-mining tools. These technologies can assist in identifying inconsistencies and gaps within the MeSH hierarchy, particularly where terms relevant to pharmaceutical services, policy, or practice remain underused or absent. For instance, recent work has demonstrated the potential of hybrid approaches that combine vector space models and description logics to improve biomedical document indexing by enabling approximate matching and filtering of irrelevant concepts through the structured knowledge in MeSH (Boukhari and Omri, 2020). Moreover, AI techniques that use weak supervision have proven useful in enhancing semantic indexing by allowing for more detailed identification of concepts. One example involves training systems to recognize specific terms that frequently appear in articles about certain diseases. This strategy leads to more precise tagging of topics, going beyond the general categories provided by standard MeSH descriptors (Nentidis et al., 2020; You et al., 2021; Tang et al., 2023). Integrating these strategies could significantly enhance the visibility of pharmacy-related research, ensuring its appropriate representation in biomedical databases and improving its discoverability by clinicians, researchers, and policymakers.

Additionally, building international coalitions of researchers and professional bodies can lend strength and legitimacy to advocacy aimed at reshaping-controlled vocabularies like MeSH or Emtree. Collective action is essential not only for proposing new terms but also for promoting transparency and inclusivity in the curation of indexing systems. Equally important is the incorporation of discussions on metadata, indexing practices, and controlled vocabularies into graduate and postgraduate research training (Kipnis and Childs, 2004; Maggio et al., 2009). Educating emerging scholars on the implications of terminology and classification equips them to participate actively in shaping how their disciplines are represented and accessed (Bass et al., 2022). Another emerging policy avenue in this context involves integrating MeSH term selection directly into the editorial processes of scientific journals, thereby reinforcing the role of editors and peer reviewers in the appropriate allocation of indexing terms. For instance, journals could include in their author guidelines a curated list of preferred MeSH terms aligned with the journal's scope, encouraging authors to use these terms in the titles and abstracts of their submissions (Fernandez-Llimos, 2025).

5.2 Final remarks

The way scientific knowledge is categorized has far-reaching consequences—not only for the visibility of individual articles but also for the broader recognition of academic fields. In the case of pharmacy, the limited presence and inconsistent use of key MeSH terms, such as those from the 'pharmaceutical services' branch, underscore the need for greater critical engagement with indexing processes. More than a technical issue, this also raises concerns about how knowledge from certain fields is recognized and valued. Researchers in pharmacy and related disciplines must recognize that controlled vocabularies are not neutral—they reflect and reinforce hierarchies within science. Engaging with them strategically is essential for advancing both the visibility and the integrity of the field.

6 Application exercise/scenario

6.1 Practical activity

Read the following two versions of a hypothetical abstract available on PubMed regarding patient adherence to treatment, and compare them carefully (Table 3.5). The first version lacks appropriate MeSH terminology, whereas the second has been revised to incorporate relevant indexing terms (highlighted in the text) for improved scientific visibility.

Questions for reflection and discussion:

- What are the main differences in terminology between the two titles and abstracts?
- Which version do you think is more likely to be indexed and cited in scientific databases?
- Using PubMed or another scientific database, search for articles on "medication adherence" and note how MeSH terms are used in highly cited articles.

TABLE 3.5 Comparison of abstracts on the use of MeSH terms.

Version 1—Without standardized terminology	Version 2—With standardized terminology
Compliance with medication in chronic diseases: a cross-sectional study from the perspective of pharmaceutical professionals	Medication adherence in chronic diseases: a cross-sectional study from the perspective of pharmacists
Background: adherence to medication remains a critical factor in the management of chronic diseases, directly affecting treatment efficacy and healthcare outcomes. Healthcare professionals play a central role in identifying barriers and promoting strategies to improve patient adherence.	Background: adherence to medication remains a critical factor in the management of chronic diseases, directly affecting treatment efficacy and healthcare outcomes. Pharmacists, particularly those engaged in community pharmacy services and hospital settings, play a central role in identifying barriers and promoting strategies to improve patient compliance with therapy.
Methods: a cross-sectional survey was conducted between January and March 2025, involving 250 community and hospital-based pharmacists across five major urban centers in southern Spain. Participants responded to a structured questionnaire assessing their perceptions of patient adherence, observed barriers, and strategies implemented to support adherence. Quantitative data were analyzed using descriptive statistics and logistic regression.	Methods: a cross-sectional survey was conducted between January and March 2025, involving 250 community pharmacies and hospital-based professionals across five major urban centers in southern Spain. Pharmacists responded to a structured questionnaire assessing their perceptions of patient compliance, observed barriers, and strategies implemented to support adherence. Quantitative data were analyzed using descriptive statistics and logistic regression.
Results: participants estimated that only 75% of patients with chronic conditions consistently adhered to their prescribed regimens. The most frequently reported barriers were forgetfulness (80%), misunderstanding of treatment instructions (65%), and lack of perceived need for the medication, including over-the-counter therapies (52%). Only 22% of respondents indicated that patients regularly returned for follow-up counseling. Pharmacists working in community settings were more likely to report implementing adherence-promoting strategies, such as reminder systems (45%) and educational interventions (40%), compared to those in hospital settings (27% and 15%, respectively; $p < 0.05$). Lack of time (72%) and insufficient patient engagement (65%) were the most cited professional challenges.	Results: pharmacists estimated that only 75% of patients with chronic conditions consistently adhered to their prescribed regimens. The most frequently reported barriers were forgetfulness (80%), misunderstanding of treatment instructions (65%), and lack of perceived need for the medication, including nonprescription drugs such as behind-the-counter drugs (52%). Only 22% of respondents indicated that patients regularly returned for follow-up counseling. Pharmacists working in community settings were more likely to report implementing adherence-promoting strategies, such as reminder systems (45%) and educational interventions (40%), compared to those in hospital settings (27% and 15%, respectively; $p < 0.05$). Lack of time (72%) and insufficient patient engagement (65%) were the most cited professional challenges.
Conclusions: professionals perceive suboptimal medication compliance among patients with chronic diseases and identify multiple behavioral and systemic barriers. There is a clear need for structural support, training, and policy integration to enhance the impact of pharmacy services on chronic disease management.	Conclusions: pharmacists perceive suboptimal medication adherence among patients with chronic diseases and identify multiple behavioral and systemic barriers. There is a clear need for pharmacy research on structural support, training, and policy integration to enhance the impact of pharmaceutical services on chronic disease management.

References

Alves da Costa, F., Fernandez-Llimos, F., Desselle, S., Arnet, I., Babar, Z., Bond, C., Cordina, M., Cardenas, V.G., Hajj, M.S.E., Jacobsen, R., Law, A.V., Nørgaard, L.S., Polidori, C., Shcherbakova, N., Stewart, D., Tonin, F.S., Weidmann, A.E., 2025. The international collaboration of pharmacy journal editors (ICPJE) formally constituted to foster quality around clinical and social pharmacy practice research publications. Curr. Pharm. Teach. Learn.. 1877-1300. 17 (4), 102317. doi:10.1016/j.cptl.2025.102317.

Bass, M.B., Molina, R.L., Reardon, E.E., Porcello, L., Goldberg, J., Nickum, A., Lipke, L., Zeigen, L., Eldredge, J.D., Wallerstein, N.B., 2022. Trends in … controlled vocabulary and health equity. Med. Ref. Serv. Q. 1540-9597. 41 (2), 185–201. Available from: http://www.tandfonline.com/toc/wmrs20/current. doi:10.1080/02763869.2022.2060638.

Bastian, M., Heymann, S., Jacomy, M., 2009. Gephi: an open source software for exploring and manipulating networks. In: International AAAI Conference on Weblogs and Social Media.

Baumann, N., 2016. How to use the medical subject headings (Me SH). Int. J. Clin. Pract.. 1368-5031. 70 (2), 171–174. doi:10.1111/ijcp.12767.

Bonetti, A.F., Rocca, A.M.D., Lucchetta, R.C., Tonin, F.S., Fernandez-Llimos, F., Pontarolo, R., 2020. Mapping the characteristics of meta-analyses of pharmacy services: a systematic review. Int. J. Clin. Pharm.. 2210-7711. 42 (5), 1252–1260. Available from: http://springerlink.metapress.com/content/2210-7703/. doi:10.1007/s11096-020-01058-5.

Bonetti, A.F., Tonin, F.S., Lucchetta, R.C., Pontarolo, R., Fernandez-Llimos, F., 2022. Methodological standards for conducting and reporting meta-analyses: ensuring the replicability of meta-analyses of pharmacist-led medication review. Res. Social Adm. Pharm. 1551-7411. 18 (2), 2259–2268. Available from: http://www.journals.elsevierhealth.com/periodicals/rsap. doi:10.1016/j.sapharm.2021.06.002.

Boukhari, K., Omri, M.N., 2020. Approximate matching-based unsupervised document indexing approach: application to biomedical domain. Scientometrics. 1588-2861. 124 (2), 903–924. Available from: http://www.springerlink.com/content/0138-9130. doi:10.1007/s11192-020-03474-w.

Chang, A.A., Heskett, K.M., Davidson, T.M., 2006. Searching the literature using medical subject headings versus text word with PubMed. Laryngoscope. 0023-852X. 116 (2), 336–340. doi:10.1097/01.mlg.0000195371.72887.a2.

Chen, Y.Y., Bullard, J., Giustini, D., 2023. Automated indexing using NLM's medical text indexer (MTI) compared to human indexing in medline: a pilot study. J. Med. Libr. Assoc.. 1558-9439. 111 (3), 684–695. doi:10.5195/jmla.2023.1588.

Doig, G.S., Simpson, F., 2003. Efficient literature searching: a core skill for the practice of evidence-based medicine. Intensive Care Med. 29 (12), 2119–2127. doi:10.1007/s00134-003-1942-5.

Fatehi, F., Gray, L.C., Wootton, R., 2014. How to improve your PubMed/MEDLINE searches: 3. advanced searching, MeSH and my NCBI. J. Telemed. Telecare. 1758-1109. 20 (2), 102–112. doi:10.1177/1357633X13519036.

Fernandez-Llimos, F., 2025. Consistency of medical subject headings assignment: a test-retest reliability analysis. Res. Social Adm. Pharm. 1551-7411. doi:10.1016/j.sapharm.2025.05.008

Fernandez-Llimos, F., Desselle, S., Stewart, D., Garcia-Cardenas, V., Babar, Z.U.D., Bond, C., Dago, A., Jacobsen, R., Nørgaard, L.S., Polidori, C., Sanchez-Polo, M., Santos-Ramos, B., Shcherbakova, N., Tonin, F.S., 2023. Improving the quality of publications in and advancing the paradigms of clinical and social pharmacy practice research: the Granada statements. Pharm. Educ. 1477-2701. 23 (1), 109–117. Available from: https://pharmacyeducation.fip.org/pharmacyeducation/article/view/2111/1458. doi:10.46542/pe.2023.231.109117.

Fernandez-Llimos, F., Minguet, F., Salgado, T.M., 2017. New pharmacy-specific medical subject headings included in the 2017 database. Am. J. Health-Syst. Pharm.. 1535-2900. 74 (15), 1128–1129. Available from: http://www.ajhp.org/content/ajhp/74/15/1128.full.pdf. doi:10.2146/ajhp170046.

Fernandez-Llimos, F., Negrao, L.G., Bond, C., Stewart, D., 2024. Medical subject headings (MeSH) selection for pharmacy practice journals. Res. Social Adm. Pharm. 20 (9), 911-917. doi:10.1016/j.sapharm.2024.06.003.

Fernandez-Llimos, F., Salgado, T.M., 2021. Standardization of pharmacy practice terminology and the Medical Subject Headings (MeSH).. Res. Social Adm. Pharm. 17 (4), 819-820. doi:10.1016/j.sapharm.2020.07.005.

Gernant, S.A., Bacci, J.L., Upton, C., Ferreri, S.P., McGrath, S., Chui, M.A., Rickles, N.M., Smith, M., 2020. Three opportunities for standardization: a literature review of the variation among pharmacists' patient care services terminology. Res. Social Adm. Pharm.. 1551-7411. 16 (6), 766–775. Available from: http://www.journals.elsevierhealth.com/periodicals/rsap. doi:10.1016/j.sapharm.2019.08.034.

Harpe, S.E., 2021. Meta-research in pharmacy: time for a look in the mirror. Res. Social Adm. Pharm.. 1551-7411. 17 (12), 2028–2035. Available from: http://www.journals.elsevierhealth.com/periodicals/rsap. doi:10.1016/j.sapharm.2021.04.006.

Higgins, J.P., Thomas, J., Chandler, J., Cumpston, M., Li, T., Page, M.J., Welch, V.A., 2024. Cochrane Handbook for Systematic Reviews of Interventions Version 6.5 (Chichester (UK): John Wiley & Sons).

Jenuwine, E.S., Floyd, J.A., 2004. Comparison of medical subject headings and text-word searches in MEDLINE to retrieve studies on sleep in healthy individuals. J. Med. Libr. Assoc.. 1536-5050. 92 (3), 349–353. Available from: http://www.pubmedcentral.nih.gov/picrender.fcgi?artid=442177&blobtype=pdf.

Jimeno-Yepes, A.J., Plaza, L., Mork, J.G., Aronson, A.R., Diaz, A., 2013. MeSH indexing based on automatically generated summaries. BMC Bioinform. 14 (208). doi:10.1186/1471-2105-14-208.

Kipnis, D.G., Childs, G.M., 2004. Educating Generation X and Generation Y: teaching tips for librarians. Med. Ref. Serv. Q 23 (4), 25–33. doi:10.1300/J115v23n04_03.

Maggio, L.A., Bresnahan, M., Flynn, D.B., Harzbecker, J., Blanchard, M., Ginn, D., 2009. A case study: using social tagging to engage students in learning medical subject headings. J. Med. Libr. Assoc.. 1558-9439. 97 (2), 77–83. Available from: http://www.pubmedcentral.nih.gov/picrender.fcgi?artid=2670207&blobtype=pdf. doi:10.3163/1536-5050.97.2.003.

Marriott, J.L., 2018. What can be done to help the pharmacy profession advance globally? Am. J. Pharm. Educ.. 0002-9459. 82 (8), 7040. doi:10.5688/ajpe7040.

Mendes, M., Tonin, F.S., Buzzi, M.F., Pontarolo, R., Fernandez-Llimos, F., 2019. A lexicographic analysis. Res. Social Adm. Pharm. 15, 1464–1467.

Minguet, F., Boogerd, L.V.D., Salgado, T.M., Correr, C.J., Fernandez-Llimos, F., 2014. Characterization of the medical subject headings thesaurus for pharmacy. Am. J. Health-Syst. Pharm.. 1535-2900. 71 (22), 1965–1972. Available from: http://www.ajhp.org/content/71/22/1965.full.pdf+html. doi:10.2146/ajhp140073.

Minguet, F., Salgado, T.M., van den Boogerd, L., Fernandez-Llimos, F., 2015. Quality of pharmacy-specific medical subject headings (MeSH) assignment in pharmacy journals indexed in MEDLINE. Res. Social Adm. Pharm.. 1551-7411. 11 (5), 686–695. Available from: http://www.journals.elsevierhealth.com/periodicals/rsap. doi:10.1016/j.sapharm.2014.11.004.

Mork, J., Aronson, A., Demner-Fushman, D., 2017. 12 Years on—Is the NLM medical text indexer still useful and relevant? J. Biomed. Semantics 12 (1), 8.

National Library of Medicine, 2025a. Concept Structure in MeSH https://www.nlm.nih.gov/mesh/concept_structure.html

National Library of Medicine, 2025b. History of MeSH https://www.nlm.nih.gov/mesh/intro_preface.html#pref_hist

National Library of Medicine, 2025c. Frequently Asked Questions about Indexing https://www.nlm.nih.gov/bsd/indexfaq.html#produced

Nentidis, A., Krithara, A., Tsoumakas, G., Paliouras, G., 2020. Beyond MeSH: fine-grained semantic indexing of biomedical literature based on weak supervision. Inf. Process. Manag.. 0306-4573. 57 (5), 102282. doi:10.1016/j.ipm.2020.102282.

Page, M.J., McKenzie, J.E., Bossuyt, P.M., Boutron, I., Hoffmann, T.C., Mulrow, C.D., Shamseer, L., Tetzlaff, J.M., Akl, E.A., Brennan, S.E., Chou, R., Glanville, J., Grimshaw, J.M., Hróbjartsson, A., Lalu, M.M., Tianjing, L., Loder, E.W., Mayo-Wilson, E., McDonald, S., McGuinness, L.A., Stewart, L.A., Thomas, J., Tricco, A.C., Welch, V.A., Whiting, P., Moher, D., 2021. The PRISMA 2020 statement: an updated guideline for reporting systematic reviews. BMJ (Clin. Res. Ed.) 372. doi:10.1136/bmj.n71

Portaluppi, F., 2007. Consistency and accuracy of the medical subject Headings® thesaurus for electronic indexing and retrieval of chronobiologic references. Chronobiol. Int.. 1525-6073. 24 (6), 1213–1229. doi:10.1080/07420520701791570.

Raza, M.A., Aziz, S., Noree, M., Anjum, I., Raza, S.M., 2022. A portrait of the pharmacy profession globally: pharmacist universal professional identity and establishment of global pharmacy council. Innov. Pharm.. 2155-0417. 13 (1), 4. doi:10.24926/iip.v13i1.4502.

Richter, R.R., Austin, T.M., 2012. Using MeSH (Medical Subject Headings) to enhance PubMed search strategies for evidence-based practice in physical therapy. Phys. Ther.. 1538-6724. 92 (1), 124–132. Available from: http://ptjournal.apta.org/content/92/1/124.full.pdf+html. doi:10.2522/ptj.20100178.

Rodriguez, R.W., 2014. Delay in indexing articles published in major pharmacy practice journals. Am. J. Health-Syst. Pharm.. 1535-2900. 71 (4), 321–324. Available from: http://www.ajhp.org/content/71/4/321.full.pdf+html. doi:10.2146/ajhp130421.

Rotta, I., Souza, T.T., Salgado, T.M., Correr, C.J., Fernandez-Llimos, F., 2017. Characterization of published randomized controlled trials assessing clinical pharmacy services around the world. Res. Social Adm. Pharm. 1551-7411. 13 (1), 201–208. Available from: http://www.journals.elsevierhealth.com/periodicals/rsap. doi:10.1016/j.sapharm.2016.01.003.

Salgado, T., Fernandez-Llimos, F., 2019. Medical subject headings (MeSH) terms: problems and solutions. Res. Social Adm. Pharm. 15, 1189-1190 .

Sivarajkumar, S., Mohammad, H.A., Oniani, D., Roberts, K., Hersh, W., Liu, H., He, D., Visweswaran, S., Wang, Y., 2024. Clinical information retrieval: a literature review. J. Healthc. Inform. Res. 2509-498X. 8 (2), 313–352. Available from: https://www.springer.com/journal/41666. doi:10.1007/s41666-024-00159-4.

Tang, W., Klang, M., Medved, D., Nugues, P., Nilsson, J. 2023 Automatic annotation of PubMed articles with MeSH qualifiers. Proceedings of the Annual International Conference of the IEEE Engineering in Medicine and Biology Society, EMBS. 9798350324471 Institute of Electrical and Electronics Engineers Inc., Sweden doi:10.1109/EMBC40787.2023.10340998

Tonin, F.S., Gmunder, V., Bonetti, A.F., Mendes, A., Fernandez-Llimos, F., 2022. Pharmaceutical services' medical subject headings (MeSH) in articles assessing pharmacists' interventions. Explor. Res. Clin. Soc. Pharm. 7, p. 1. doi:10.1016/j.rcsop.2022.100172 .

Yang, H., Lee, H.J., 2018. Research trend visualization by MeSH terms from PubMed. Int. J. Environ. Res. Public Health. 1660-4601. 15 (6). Available from: http://www.mdpi.com/1660-4601/15/6/1113/pdf. doi:10.3390/ijerph15061113.

You, R., Liu, Y., Mamitsuka, H., Zhu, S., 2021. BERTMeSH: deep contextual representation learning for large-scale high-performance MeSH indexing with full text. Bioinformatics. 1460-2059. 37 (5), 684–692. Available from: http://bioinformatics.oxfordjournals.org/. doi:10.1093/bioinformatics/btaa837.

CHAPTER

4

Lexicographic analysis as a methodological tool for mapping healthcare integration

Amaia Urionagüena[a] *and Fernando Fernandez-Llimos*[b]

[a]Department of Pharmacy and Food Sciences, Faculty of Pharmacy, University of the Basque Country, UPV/EHU, Vitoria-Gasteiz, Spain

[b]Department of Drug Sciences, Laboratory of Pharmacology, Faculty of Pharmacy, University of Porto, Porto, Portugal

CHAPTER OBJECTIVES

This chapter aims to:

- Introduce lexicographic analysis as an effective methodological approach for mapping and organizing complex concepts in scientific literature, with a focus on healthcare integration
- Demonstrate how this technique facilitates the identification and classification of key terms and emerging themes related to healthcare integration, enabling a more structured understanding of the field
- Illustrate the practical use of lexicographic analysis research, using empirical results to support its application

1 Introduction

1.1 Contemporary challenges in healthcare systems

The Constitution of the World Health Organization (WHO) affirms that *"the enjoyment of the highest attainable standard of health is one of the fundamental rights of every human being without distinction of race, religion, political belief, economic or social condition"* (World Health Organization, 1948). To uphold this right, countries have established healthcare systems as essential instruments for promoting, maintaining, and restoring health. However, in recent decades, health systems worldwide have encountered increasingly complex and multifaceted challenges that threaten their sustainability, equity, and efficiency.

Among the most pressing concerns is the growing burden of chronic conditions, which demands long-term and coordinated care. This trend, coupled with demographic shifts such as population aging, has significantly increased

Contemporary Research Methods in Pharmacy and Health Services - Volume 2
https://doi.org/10.1016/B978-0-443-44607-8.00019-4

the demand for health services. Simultaneously, advancements in medical technology, pharmaceuticals, and diagnostic tools, though undeniably beneficial, have also escalated healthcare costs (Lucero-Prisno et al., 2025), exerting financial pressure on both public budgets and out-of-pocket spending by patients.

A particularly critical and persistent issue in patient care is the fragmentation of healthcare delivery (World Health Organization, 2016a; Gröne and Garcia-Barbero, 2001). Patients frequently experience care as a disjointed series of encounters across various levels and sectors, including primary, secondary, and tertiary care, as well as between public and private providers. This lack of integration undermines the continuity of care, compromises patient safety and outcomes, and leads to inefficiencies such as duplication of services and poor resource allocation (Lalani et al., 2023).

The COVID-19 pandemic has further exposed and intensified structural weaknesses within health systems (Cutler, 2023). It highlighted significant disparities in access to care and underscored the urgency of developing stronger, more flexible, and more inclusive health infrastructures capable of responding to both routine and emergent public health challenges.

In addressing these pressures, there is a clear imperative to enhance the responsiveness and adaptability of health systems. Meeting this demand requires systemic reforms that promote coordination, sustainability, and equity across all levels of care (Tichenor and Sridhar, 2017). Increasingly, policymakers and researchers are turning their attention to organizational models that foster collaboration, continuity, and patient-centeredness. Among these, the concept of "*healthcare integration*" has emerged as a promising direction, one that warrants closer examination.

1.2 Integration as a strategic response

Healthcare integration represents a deliberate and systemic response to the fragmentation and inefficiencies that characterize many contemporary health systems. Rather than functioning as isolated units, integrated systems aim to coordinate services across all levels of care, primary, secondary, tertiary, and social, creating cohesive and patient-centered care pathways.

Integration encompasses a broad spectrum of coordinated activities. These include the alignment of services and tasks involved in patient care, the formulation of policies that promote the integration of multidisciplinary teams, the evaluation and monitoring of care delivery and patient follow-up, and the strengthening of collaboration between health and social sectors (World Health Organization, 2016a; Zonneveld et al., 2018). It also involves establishing shared values and a unified organizational culture, improving access to shared information systems, and fostering the decentralization and empowerment of local services (Zonneveld et al., 2018).

Beyond optimizing the allocation of resources and streamlining service delivery, integration contributes significantly to enhancing equity and improving the quality of care (World Health Organization, 2025). By facilitating more equitable access to services and reducing variation in care standards, integration addresses systemic inefficiencies and social determinants that contribute to disparities in health outcomes (World Health Organization, 2025; Graham and White, 2016). The movement towards integration reflects a necessary adaptation to a rapidly changing global health environment, characterized by demographic shifts, epidemiological transitions, and evolving patient expectations.

Healthcare integration models are underpinned by core principles such as collaboration among multidisciplinary teams, the use of interoperable and patient-centered information systems, and the alignment of financial incentives to support coordinated service provision (Suter et al., 2009; Simoens and Scott, 2005; Nolte and McKee, 2008). These models aim to dismantle traditional silos within health systems, encouraging synergy between stakeholders to collectively address the broad spectrum of patient needs, whether biomedical, psychological, or social (Suter et al., 2009).

The WHO strongly advocates for Integrated, People-Centered Health Services (IPCHS) (World Health Organization, 2016b), which emphasize organizing health systems around the comprehensive needs and preferences of individuals, rather than around isolated diseases or institutional hierarchies. Achieving this vision requires a rethinking of conventional healthcare models and the adoption of innovative strategies that prioritize integration across all levels of care. This shift represents not only a technical reform but a profound cultural transformation toward more inclusive, collaborative, and sustainable health systems.

1.2.1 Primary care

Primary care constitutes the key element of any effective and equitable healthcare system. As the first point of contact for individuals within the public health system, it plays a pivotal role in delivering accessible, comprehensive, and continuous care that addresses the vast majority of health needs throughout the life course (Starfield et al., 2005; Rotenstein and Gitomer, 2023). Beyond direct clinical care, primary care also encompasses essential functions in health promotion, disease prevention, early diagnosis, and the coordination of services across other levels of the system (World Health Organization, 2022).

Due to its foundational role, primary care serves as the central axis around which the broader health system is organized. It acts as a gatekeeper, guiding patients through complex care pathways and ensuring that services are used appropriately and efficiently. Moreover, robust primary care is strongly associated with improved health outcomes, reduced health disparities, and more cost-effective care delivery (Sawicki et al., 2021; Hudon et al., 2019; Hughes et al., 2022).

However, in many countries, primary care is currently under significant strain (Andueza, 2022; Mahtani and Abrams, 2025; Allen et al., 2025; Matthews et al., 2025). The rising demand for health services, driven by demographic changes, epidemiological transitions, and growing patient expectations, has overwhelmed the capacity of many primary care systems. Compounding this issue is a critical shortage of health professionals. In search of better working conditions and professional opportunities, many health workers migrate to regions or sectors that offer more favorable environments (Matthews et al., 2025). This human resource imbalance exacerbates service gaps, particularly in underserved or rural areas, placing additional pressure on already limited resources.

These challenges underscore the urgent need to rethink and restructure the delivery of primary care services (Martín et al., 2023). Strengthening this level of care must be a policy priority for governments and health authorities. Strategies should include targeted investments in the professional development and retention of primary care workers, improvements in work environments, and the provision of adequate infrastructure and technological support (De Vries et al., 2023).

Importantly, the process of healthcare integration should begin at the primary care level. It is at this level that patient needs are first identified and addressed, making it the ideal starting point for coordinated care pathways that extend upward through secondary and tertiary care. Effective integration efforts must therefore prioritize the strengthening of primary care as both a structural and functional prerequisite for broader system transformation.

1.2.2 The emerging role of community pharmacy in integration

Historically, pharmacists have been recognized primarily as professionals responsible for the compounding and dispensing of medications. However, over the past few decades, the role of the pharmacist has undergone a transformation. This evolution reflects a growing recognition of pharmacists as clinical care providers, capable of assuming a more proactive and patient-centered role within the broader health system. Key milestones, such as the 1985 Hilton Head Conference (Hepler, 1985) that declared pharmacy a clinical profession and the seminal 1990 article by Hepler and Strand (Hepler and Strand, 1990), signaled a paradigm shift toward pharmaceutical care as a core component of the practice of pharmacy.

As community pharmacy has moved toward a more clinical and patient-focused model, its function within the health system has expanded significantly. Pharmacists' proximity to the population, frequent patient interactions, and growing involvement in health promotion and disease prevention position them uniquely within integrated care frameworks (World Health Organization, 2016a).

The COVID-19 pandemic further underscored the critical value of community pharmacies as accessible and trusted healthcare resources (DiPietro Mager and Bright, 2023). During the crisis, pharmacies served as essential contact points for health advice, medication access, and public health information, often in settings where other health services were limited or disrupted. This experience highlighted the untapped potential of community pharmacies to act as frontline healthcare providers, particularly in support of overstretched primary care systems.

Recognizing this, there is growing interest in formally incorporating community pharmacies into healthcare system strategies for integration and resilience. Community pharmacists have the expertise to optimize therapeutic outcomes through effective medication management, adherence support, and chronic disease monitoring (World Health Organization, 2016a, 2018). Their integration into multidisciplinary care teams can improve patient safety, reduce hospital readmissions, and contribute to better population health outcomes (World Health Organization, 2016a, 2018). Furthermore, by managing minor ailments, delivering preventive services, administering vaccines, and supporting health education initiatives, pharmacists can help reduce the burden on general practitioners and emergency services.

To realize this potential, however, systemic changes are required. These include policy reforms that acknowledge and support the clinical role of pharmacists, interprofessional collaboration mechanisms, and sustained investment in pharmacy infrastructure and workforce development. Equally important is the need to shift perceptions, within both the health system and the public, about the capabilities and responsibilities of pharmacists in delivering integrated care.

In this context, integrating community pharmacies into primary healthcare seems necessary. Primary care represents the front line of healthcare access, and the widespread network of community pharmacies offers a valuable, yet underutilized, resource to strengthen this level of care. The integration of pharmacists into primary care must be understood not as an ancillary measure, but as a strategic imperative to enhance care coordination, increase system efficiency, and ensure continuity across the care continuum.

Therefore, the role of community pharmacy should be reconceptualized within the health system integration agenda, as a critical enabler of accessible, patient-centered, and collaborative health services capable of addressing current and future health system challenges. But for that, it is necessary to understand what is meant by the concept of "integration".

1.3 The concept of integration

The term "integration" is a complex and multifaceted concept that has been widely debated over time (Leutz, 1999; Armitage et al., 2009; Singer et al., 2011).

The idea of integration is deeply rooted in both systems theory (Johansen, 1993) and organizational theory (Lawrence and Lorsch, 1986). Systems theory emphasizes the importance of analyzing systems as "wholes" rather than merely as collections of isolated parts. Historically, scientific inquiry often relied on a reductionist approach, breaking down phenomena into individual components to study them independently. While this method can yield valuable insights, it falls short when dealing with complex systems, where elements are interdependent and continuously interact with one another and with their environment (Johansen, 1993). In healthcare systems, a reductionist perspective might examine hospitals, clinics, and care providers as separate entities. However, true understanding and effective functioning of the system require viewing these components as interconnected parts of a single, dynamic whole. Integration, in this sense, means fostering meaningful interactions between different units so that they operate in a coordinated way toward shared goals, such as improving health outcomes and enhancing patients' quality of life.

Organizational theory complements this view by addressing how organizations respond to external demands. According to this perspective, organizations often divide into specialized units, each tasked with managing specific aspects of their external environment. This segmentation reflects the same reductionist logic found in systems theory. Yet, to function cohesively, these separate units must also be able to work together. Here, the concept of integration becomes essential; it refers to the capacity of an organization to coordinate and align its various parts to respond effectively to the broader environment (Lawrence and Lorsch, 1986). A classic formulation of this concept is offered by Lawrence and Lorsch (1986), who defined integration as *"the quality of the state of collaboration that exists among departments that are required to achieve unity of efforts by the demands of the environment"*. This highlights that integration is not simply structural—it is relational and strategic, aimed at harmonizing the internal diversity of an organization to achieve common objectives.

Over time, the concept of integration has expanded and gained complexity, especially in fields like healthcare. It now goes beyond linking different units; it includes the coordination of processes, resource sharing, and alignment of various services across the entire system (World Health Organization, 2016a; Suter et al., 2009). Moreover, it encompasses the involvement of diverse stakeholders, not only healthcare providers but also patients, communities, administrators, and broader social and environmental actors. This evolving perspective sees integration as a dynamic, inclusive, and continuous process, essential for building responsive and resilient systems (Evans et al., 2014).

However, the concept of integration remains multifaceted and often ambiguous, leading to varied interpretations and implementations across different health systems. Understanding the nuances of integration is crucial for developing coherent policies and practices that truly benefit patients and healthcare providers alike.

1.3.1 *Integration as an ambiguous and polysemic concept*

This conceptual complexity is compounded by terminological inconsistencies. The term "integration" is often used interchangeably with related concepts, such as collaborative practice, coordination, cooperation, interprofessional work, and integrated care. This overlap in terminology has led to significant conceptual ambiguity, making it difficult to establish a clear and shared understanding of what integration actually entails in practice.

A particularly notable point of confusion arises between the concepts of "integration" and "integrated care". Although "integration" and "integrated care" are different concepts, some authors use the older, direct definition of integration to define integrated care. For instance, Valentijn et al. (2013) describe integrated care as the effort to link healthcare systems with other social services to improve outcomes, borrowing almost word-for-word from an earlier definition of integration by Leutz (1999) (Table 4.1). This conflation exemplifies how terms are often repurposed without sufficient conceptual clarification, deepening the overall lack of terminological precision in the field.

Moreover, definitions of integration differ widely depending on disciplinary focus and contextual application. Some emphasize structural and administrative alignment, while others focus on relational processes and shared governance among independent actors. For example, Kodner and Spreeuwenberg (2002) describe integration as a structured set of methods across multiple levels—financial, organizational, and clinical—aimed at fostering coordination within and between health and care sectors. In contrast, Contandriopoulos' et al. (2003) define integration as a long-term process

TABLE 4.1 Comparison of "integration" (Leutz) vs. "integrated care" (Valentijn) definitions.

Definitions
Leutz (1999): "Integration is defined, for the purposes of this paper, as the search to connect the health care system (acute, primary medical, and skilled) with other human service systems (e.g., long-term care, education, and vocational and housing services) in order to improve outcomes (clinical, satisfaction, and efficiency)" (Leutz, 1999).
Valentijn et al. (2013): Integrated care: "The search to connect the healthcare system (acute, primary medical and skilled) with other human service systems (e.g., long-term care, education and vocational and housing services) to improve outcomes (clinical, satisfaction and efficiency)" (Valentijn et al., 2013).

of creating common frameworks to manage interdependence among autonomous stakeholders. Still others view integration more as a unification of services or entities, as in the case of Maslin-Prothero and Bennion (2010), who associated integration with reducing service fragmentation for the benefit of users, particularly those with complex needs.

These diverse definitions reflect the multifaceted nature of integration. Its meaning shifts depending on the goals, contexts, and stakeholders involved. While this flexibility can be useful, it also introduces challenges for evaluation and implementation exercises. The broad and often vague use of the term risks undermining its utility as an analytical or strategic tool.

Importantly, achieving integration does not necessarily imply the physical or organizational merging of all entities involved (Shortell et al., 1994). Rather, integration can be achieved through a variety of arrangements, including formal partnerships, contractual agreements, or strategic alliances. The optimal level of integration may vary across services and units, depending on the nature of their functions and the specific outcomes they aim to achieve. What is essential is not uniformity, but coherence and alignment in service of common goals. Identifying and implementing the right degree of integration for each context is, therefore, key to maximizing system performance and improving patient outcomes.

1.3.2 *Integration as a process with different stages*

Integration in healthcare is widely recognized not as a static goal but as an evolving process, characterized by distinct stages that help organizations respond to the complex demands of implementation. This process-oriented understanding allows for the exploration of multiple dimensions and approaches, tailored to the particularities of each context.

Various academics have proposed stage-based models to conceptualize the development of integration. Notable contributions came from Leutz (1999), Ahgren and Axelsson (2005), and Bradley et al. (2012), each of whom offered a different trajectory. For instance, Leutz outlines a linear progression from linkage to coordination and eventually full integration. Ahgren and Axelsson expand this model, adding intermediate steps such as segregation, linkage, coordination in networks, cooperation, and full integration. Bradley and colleagues—following Armitage's collaborative theory (Armitage, 1983)—present a progression from isolation and initial encounters to communication, collaboration between two agents, and ultimately collaboration throughout the organization.

Although no unified framework or definitive roadmap to achieving integration exists, the evidence in the literature consistently points to a series of commonly observed stages. The process typically begins with a phase of initial contact among healthcare providers, where informal interactions and early discussions set the foundations. These early stages are generally characterized by limited coordination and low levels of shared activity.

As relationships strengthen, more structured forms of coordination begin to emerge. These may involve agreed-upon communication protocols, joint planning activities, or aligned service delivery procedures. Over time, these efforts pave the way for true collaboration, where actors begin to share not only information but also resources, goals, and responsibilities. Ultimately, the process may conclude in a stage of full integration, where the health system functions as a cohesive network, responding collectively to patient and population needs.

This progressive structure suggests that integration is inherently a multifaceted and adaptive endeavor. The pace and nature of its evolution depend on numerous factors, including organizational readiness, policy environments, stakeholder commitment, and the specific health challenges being addressed. Crucially, integration is not a one-size-fits-all solution, but must be flexible and context-sensitive, with strategies tailored to each system's unique configuration.

1.3.3 *Types of integration: Breadth, enablers, types by system levels and intensity*

The concept of integration within health systems is multifaceted and challenging to operationalize. To move beyond simple definitions and provide a more robust framework for analysis, particularly for understanding the complexity involved in integrating new actors like community pharmacy, a comprehensive classification model seemed essential.

The following framework, derived from a narrative review of the integration literature, was adopted to structure our analysis. This model organizes the different types of integration into four key dimensions: breadth of integration; integration enablers (effective integration occurs supported by a range of enablers that facilitate its implementation and sustainability); types of integration classified by system levels (integration occurs across three levels of the health system); and intensity of integration (higher intensity implies stronger interdependencies and more robust integration) (Urionagüena et al., 2023) (Table 4.2).

This classifying model underscores that integration is a dynamic process, not a fixed state. It requires structural, cultural, relational and contextual alignment. Understanding these dimensions is essential for designing flexible strategies, particularly when integrating community pharmacy into primary care, where ownership models (public versus private), policy environments, and professional roles often diverge. While the model is a valuable tool for conceptualizing integration, it must be complemented by practical factors that make it work in practice.

1.3.4 Components of integration

As part of a scoping review of theories, models, and frameworks for health systems integration, eleven core components that are consistently addressed across the literature were identified (Piquer-Martinez et al., 2024a). These factors interact dynamically and their intensity can vary across the health system.

1. Stakeholder management: Active participation and alignment of all involved parties, from policymakers to patients.

TABLE 4.2 Summary of the classification framework for different types of integration.

Framework for Classifying Integration Types		
Breath of integration		
Type of integration	Definition	
Vertical integration	Unifies services and actors from different hierarchical levels (e.g., hospitals and primary care centers) under a single management.	
Horizontal integration	Connects services at the same level (e.g., community pharmacies and general practitioners) relying on collaborative practices, mutual agreements, and shared objectives, instead of hierarchical oversight.	
Integration enablers		
Type of integration	Definition	
Functional integration	Coordination of support functions/activities across units	
Normative integration	Shared goals and improvement plans	
Financial integration	Shared fiscal and clinical responsibility	
Contextual integration	Organizational capacity to allocate resources for complex interventions	
Informational integration	Use of IT systems for data sharing and analysis	
Cultural integration	Alignment of values and practices	
Structural integration	Formal links between teams and organizations	
Types of integration classified by system levels		
Level	Definition	Type(s) of integration
Macro level	Focus on governance, regulation, and policy coordination	System integration
Meso level	Address how different healthcare professionals and institutions collaborate and align their operations	Professional integration and organizational integration
Micro level	Involves the daily coordination of patient care across providers and settings	Clinical integration and Service integration
Intensity of Integration		
Constructs	Definition	
Consensus	Shared objectives and joint decision making	
Connectivity	Technological and informational linkages	
Communication	Structured, bidirectional information flow	
Trust	Mutual recognition and respect	

2. Adequate funding: Financial resources, incentives, and strategic allocation are essential for sustainable integration efforts.
3. Technological connectivity: Shared IT systems and data platforms are fundamental for communication, enhance clinical decision-making, reduce duplication, and improve continuity and coordination of care.
4. Roles: Clear and well-defined roles are necessary to improve coordination, respect, trust, and mutual understanding.
5. Governance: Strong leadership and shared decision-making structures guide the integration process and ensure accountability, alignment with strategic goals, and coordination.
6. Communication: Consistent and transparent communication, both formal and informal, builds trust and ensures efficient information flow.
7. Shared vision, values, and goals: A common purpose unifies efforts and ensures all actors work toward shared outcomes.
8. Context: Integration strategies must be adapted to specific political, economic, organizational, and cultural conditions.
9. Culture: Promoting a culture of collaboration, learning, and shared identity facilitates system-wide engagement and transformation.
10. Community engagement: Involving patients and communities in the integration processes ensures that services are people-centered and responsive to local needs.
11. Colocation: Physical proximity of services can facilitate communication, trust-building, and coordination, but it must be complemented by integrative processes.

These components form a comprehensive foundation for creating more responsive, effective, and sustainable integrated care systems.

1.4 The need for terminological clarification and conceptual mapping

Beyond the multiplicity of existing definitions surrounding the concept of integration, the real issue on the integration of community pharmacy and primary care is the absence of a coherent conceptual framework capable of organizing and distinguishing the various terms, analytical levels, and theoretical perspectives used across the literature (Evans et al., 2014; Contandriopoulos' et al., 2003; Urionagüena et al., 2023, 2024a; Piquer-Martinez et al., 2024b). This lack of terminological precision hinders interdisciplinary dialogue and impairs the development of analytical tools that can be applied consistently across different contexts.

Integration, whether understood as a process, an outcome, or even as a normative supreme, is frequently blended with a wide range of related concepts, which are often used without clear boundaries or critical reflection. The task, therefore, is not only to define individual terms but to understand their interrelationships, overlaps, and distinctions based on context, stakeholder perspectives, and intended goals. Conceptual mapping becomes useful by providing a structured way to organize this complex semantic field, uncovering conceptual gaps, highlighting persistent ambiguities, and building bridges across theoretical traditions (Gray et al., 2018; de Ries et al., 2022).

Conceptual mapping involves identifying and organizing the various dimensions, attributes, and relationships associated with integration. This process can uncover underlying assumptions, highlight areas of consensus and divergence, and reveal gaps in knowledge. By elucidating the conceptual landscape of integration, researchers and practitioners can develop more precise and effective models of care, tailored to specific contexts and populations. Such clarity is essential for evaluating the impact of integration efforts and for scaling successful initiatives across different healthcare settings.

From a methodological standpoint, conceptual mapping helps delineate the scope of inquiry, guides the selection of relevant indicators, facilitates model comparison, and promotes coherence between theoretical, operational, and evaluative dimensions (de Ries et al., 2022). It also enables researchers and practitioners to uncover implicit assumptions embedded in terminology and to critically examine how language not only describes but also shapes our understanding of reality.

Terminological clarification is particularly crucial in practical settings, where conceptual confusion can lead to poorly aligned strategies, miscommunication among stakeholders, and unclear accountability. While a common language cannot by itself ensure successful implementation, it lays the groundwork for more effective cross-sector collaboration, clearer policy formulation, and more accurate evaluation of health integration initiatives.

Moving toward meaningful integration in health systems demands more than structural changes or technical solutions. It requires a deliberate effort to construct shared conceptual foundations. Conceptual mapping and terminological clarification thus emerge as key methodological strategies, useful not only for enhancing the clarity and coherence of academic discourse but also for supporting informed, coordinated, and context-sensitive action in complex healthcare environments.

1.5 Lexicographic analysis as a methodological tool

As part of the broader effort to establish shared conceptual foundations for healthcare integration, lexicographic analysis emerges as a valuable methodological strategy for addressing the complex and often fragmented terminology present in the literature. This chapter introduces lexicographic analysis as a means to systematically classify and interpret the key terms and emerging themes related to integration, with the ultimate goal of fostering greater clarity, coherence, and analytical precision in both academic and practical contexts.

Lexicographic analysis is a mapping technique based on content analyses conducted on a text corpus (Harber and Leroy, 2017; Mendes et al., 2019). Lexicographic analysis, in this context, refers to the structured examination of how language is used to construct and communicate concepts within scientific discourse. Rather than assuming fixed or universally agreed-upon definitions, lexicographic analysis involves the study of words, their meanings, contextual usages, and evolution across various contexts (Zheng and Cui, 2020).

Methodologically, the process typically involves the collection of a representative body of texts, such as speeches, peer-reviewed articles, policy briefs, or professional guidelines, followed by the identification of key terms, associated contexts, and cooccurrence with other relevant concepts. Analytical tools, including frequency analysis, collocation networks, and semantic field mapping, are often used to detect patterns, trends, and relationships among terms (Biber et al., 1998). This approach yields multiple benefits. First, it promotes terminological transparency, making explicit the assumptions and meanings attached to different terms. Second, it supports comparative analysis, allowing researchers to contrast how integration is conceptualized across disciplines, regions, or time periods. Third, it provides a foundation for the development of a common lexicon, which, while not eliminating all ambiguity, facilitates more precise communication and collaboration among stakeholders.

Moreover, unlike other techniques, lexicographic analysis offers a transparent and replicable method that can be applied across disciplines. It is particularly suited to health services research, where clarity, consistency, and practical relevance are essential. Ultimately, lexicographic analysis unifies language and practice. By mapping the discursive structure of integration, it equips researchers, policymakers, and practitioners with a clearer view of the field, its priorities, blind spots, and emerging directions. As such, it contributes not only to the academic coherence of integration studies but also to the design of more aligned, context-sensitive, and communicatively robust healthcare strategies.

The utility of this method is best illustrated through its application in various health services research contexts, where it has helped to resolve conceptual differences.

For example, a study by Carvalho et al. (2020) on the use of IRaMuTeQ in regulatory processes at the Brazilian National Agency demonstrates the methodological foundation. This article highlights how software based approach allows researchers to systematically categorize and interpret large volumes of text. It's a tool, but also a method for revealing underlying themes and conceptual structures.

Brambilla et al. (2025) also put into practice this methodology on the Triple Helix model in the Brazilian context. The Triple Helix represents a model of collaboration between universities, government, and industry. By using lexicographic analysis on a body of text (likely a corpus of academic papers, policy documents, and institutional reports), the researchers showed that one can:

- Deconstruct core concepts: The analysis can reveal which of the three helices is most prominent in the discourse. By examining the frequency of specific terms, researchers can determine whether the focus is, for example in this case, if the text focuses more on the role of the government, or on the university, or on the industry.
- Map conceptual relationships: Lexicographic analysis can show the cooccurrence of terms. For instance, if one term consistently appears alongside another, it provides a data-driven understanding of how the roles of the terms are perceived and linked together.
- Identify context-specific dynamics: The analysis might identify a high frequency of terms related to concepts that are not part of the original theoretical model, for example, a part from the triple helix, terms related to social inclusion. This suggests that the model is being adapted or expanded to fit the specific political, social, or cultural context.

By lexicographic analysis of the discourse, it uncovers the conceptual and contextual nuances that might otherwise remain hidden. This makes it a potent tool for understanding complex and multifaceted systems like healthcare, where terminology is often fluid and context-dependent.

In the context of community pharmacy and primary care, where conceptual confusion can hinder effective integration, lexicographic analysis can illustrate/guide how terms such as "integration", "collaboration", "interprofessional care", or "coordination" are being used in the literature. This, in turn, enables a more nuanced understanding of the conceptual terrain.

Consequently, and given the demonstrated capacity of this methodology to reveal conceptual structures and context-specific dynamics, we selected this analytical tool for the current study. Rather than relying on subjective qualitative reviews, our aim was to use an objective, data-driven approach to systematically uncover how integration is constructed and communicated within the specific context of community pharmacy and primary care. The details of this methodological approach are outlined below.

2 Methods

This study applied lexicographic analysis to a selected corpus of scientific texts addressing healthcare integration, with a particular focus on the context of integrating community pharmacy and primary care. This approach, deeply rooted in the study of language as it is actually used (corpus linguistics) and advanced computational techniques (natural language processing, NLP), allowed for the systematic unraveling of how concepts are constructed and communicated through textual data. Unlike more subjective qualitative reviews, lexicographic analysis offers an objective, data-driven methodology to reveal the hidden structures within language, identify ambiguities, and track conceptual evolution over time.

2.1 Theoretical underpinnings of lexicographic analysis

Fundamentally, lexicographic analysis involves the empirical examination of textual data. Instead of relying on predefined notions, the actual text from scientific publications is analyzed to reveal how terms are being used. This method provides a robust empirical foundation. It offers a way to examine the evidence of how words are truly employed, rather than merely assuming a shared meaning. This objective, reproducible approach is crucial for understanding whether conceptual consensus has been reached, identifying areas of ambiguity, and observing how the understanding of integration has evolved. It presents a direct challenge to the implicit assumption that complex terms like "integration" carry a single, clear meaning across all contexts.

2.2 Corpus construction and preprocessing

To ensure robust findings, a comprehensive textual corpus was constructed, comprising literature indexed in PubMed that specifically addresses healthcare integration (Urionagüena et al., 2024a). The corpus was compiled through a meticulously designed search strategy involving 10 distinct searches. Specifically, four of these searches utilized controlled vocabulary [Medical Subject Heading (MeSH) terms], while the remaining six employed flexible free-text terms. This hybrid approach was essential to capture both articles using established indexing and those employing newer or more diverse terminology in their titles and abstracts. Ultimately, the titles and abstracts of all retrieved publications constituted the raw material for the subsequent analysis.

The preparation of this extensive text volume constituted a fundamental step. This involved transforming the raw textual data into a format suitable for quantitative analysis, thereby reducing the "noise" inherent in natural language to highlight the most significant lexical units and their relationships. This process involved several key operations:

- **Cleaning the text:** Removing punctuation and special characters, and converting all text to lowercase for uniformity.
- **Removing "stop-words":** Eliminating common words (e.g., "the", "a", or "is") that, while necessary for language, carry little unique semantic weight and could otherwise obscure meaningful patterns.
- **Tokenization and lemmatization:** Breaking the text down into individual words or phrases (tokens) and then reducing words to their root form (lemma); for example, "running" and "ran" both become "run".
- **Identifying n-grams:** Crucially, focus was placed on identifying sequences of words that consistently appear together and function as a single conceptual unit (e.g., "primary care", "integrated care"). Treating these "n-grams" as single lexical units was vital for capturing compound concepts that would not be fully understood if only individual words were analyzed.

Dedicated NLP libraries (such as those available in R/RStudio) were utilized to perform these complex preprocessing steps, ensuring the data was consistent and ready for deep analysis.

2.3 Lexicographic analysis techniques

With the corpus prepared, the core of the lexicographic analysis was commenced, applying a suite of sophisticated techniques to identify patterns and relationships among terms. This comprehensive application of analytical techniques allowed for the robust exploration of the nuanced dimensions of the integration concept:

- **Frequency analysis:** Frequency analysis, conducted with Excel, was an initial step involved in identifying the most common terms, providing a broad understanding of the prominent concepts discussed in the literature.
- **Temporal trend analysis:** Temporal trend analysis involved examining the frequency of specific terms over time, utilizing tools such as Excel, to observe the evolution of the discussion around integration and its associated terminology.
- **Cooccurrence analysis:** Cooccurrence analysis, performed using software like Gephi and R/RStudio, examined which words frequently appeared together. Consistent cooccurrence indicates conceptual linkage, revealing semantic associations and subtle nuances within the discourse.
- **Topic modeling:** Topic modeling, implemented with tools such as IRaMuTeQ, moved beyond simple word counts to uncover hidden thematic clusters of words that tended to appear together across different documents. These clusters represent the underlying conceptual areas within the literature.
- **Descending hierarchical classification (DHC):** DHC, performed using IRaMuTeQ, is a powerful statistical method that groups words into coherent "lexical classes", organizing the vast vocabulary into a hierarchical structure. This method reveals inherent groupings of words, each representing a distinct facet of integration. The most distinctive words within each class were identified, which then guided the naming of these conceptual groupings.
- **Correspondence analysis:** Correspondence analysis, also conducted using IRaMuTeQ, was employed to visually map the relationships between these lexical classes and other contextual factors (such as specific search terms or publication year). This provided a rich, spatial understanding of how different aspects of integration connect and change.

This meticulous application of lexicographic analysis has allowed for the unveiling of emergent conceptual structures directly from the text, without imposing preconceived notions. It provides a solid and irrefutable empirical basis for discussing the terminology and conceptualization of healthcare integration, ultimately guiding towards a more consistent and precise use of language in this critical field.

3 Discussion

The empirical application of this methodology, as detailed in the preceding section and consistent with the study by Urionagüena et al. (2024b), has yielded substantial insights into the terminological landscape of healthcare integration, confirming its multifaceted nature and the prevalent inconsistencies in its conceptualization.

3.1 Key findings from the lexicographic analysis

The comprehensive lexicographic analysis, performed on a corpus of 42,479 articles published between 1943 and 2023 in 4469 different journals, revealed several critical observations regarding the use of "integration" and its associated terminology in healthcare literature. Of these articles, 7.7% were retrieved by both MeSH and Title/Abstract (TIAB) searches, 39.6% only by MeSH, and 52.7% only by TIAB searches (See table Table 4.3). The MeSH "Delivery of Health Care, Integrated" was the most productive search, retrieving 33.7% of total articles and 22.6% of articles not found in any other search.

Firstly, the analysis identified that the term "integration" (n = 15,357) and the MeSH "Delivery of Health Care, Integrated" were the most frequently used terms. While "Delivery of Health Care, Integrated" was highly used since its inception in 1996 (See Fig. 4.1 and Fig. 4.2). This finding underscores the concept's prominence in health services research and suggests these terms as preferred options for clear communication.

Secondly, cooccurrence analysis revealed "care" as having the highest centrality and high cooccurrence with words like "integrated". Among the list of highly relevant words, only "integration", "integrated", and "collaborative" appeared in the cooccurrence network, highlighting their central role in the discourse (See Fig. 4.3).

TABLE 4.3 Results of the 10 searches performed, retrieved articles and their percentage of total articles retrieved.

	Search 1	Search 2	Search 3	Search 4	Search 5	Search 6	Search 7	Search 8	Search 9	Search 10
Articles retrieved (%)	590 (1.4)	2453 (5.8)	14,298 (33.7)	2955 (7)	7524 (17.7)	5883 (13.8)	6837 (16.1)	4243 (10)	1026 (2.4)	2497 (5.9)
Exclusive articles (%)	519 (1.2)	2227 (5.2)	11,285 (26.6)	2608 (6.1)	5862 (13.8)	4577 (10.8)	4088 (9.6)	3683 (8.7)	922 (2.2)	1520 (3.6)

Search 1. MeHS: "Systems Integration" [MH] AND "Professional Practice" [MH].
Search 2. MeSH: "Intersectoral Collaboration" [MH].
Search 3. MeSH: "Delivery of Health Care, Integrated" [MH].
Search 4. MeSH: "Cooperative Behavior" [MH] AND "Professional Practice" [MH].
Search 5. (Collaboration): "interprofessional collaboration"[TIAB] OR "collaborative care"[TIAB] or "collaborative practice"[TIAB].
Search 6. (Integration): "integration proessional"[TIAB: ~ 3] OR "integrated care"[TIAB: ~ 3].
Search 7. (Integrated care): "integrated care"[TIBA].
Search 8. (Collaboration): "coordination professionals"[TIAB: ~ 3] OR "coordination practice"[TIAB: ~ 3] OR "coordinated practice"[TIAB: ~ 3] OR "coordinated care"[TIAB: ~ 3].
Search 9. (Cooperation): "cooperation profesional"[TIAB: ~ 3] OR "cooperation interprofessional"[TIAB: ~ 3] OR "cooperative care"[TIAB: ~ 3].
Search 10. (Interprofessional care): "interprofessional care"[TIAB: ~ 3].

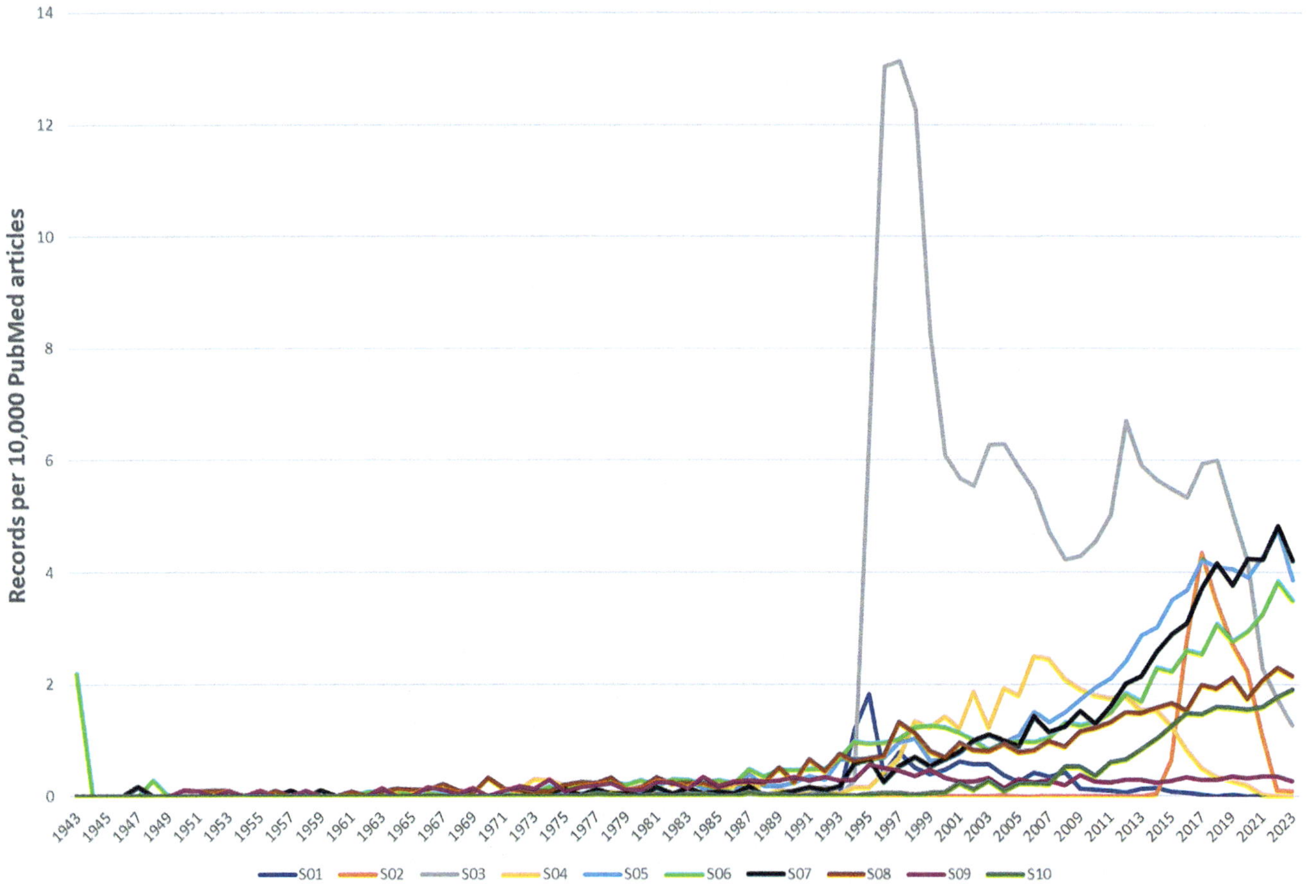

FIG. 4.1 Time trend of the productivity of different searches. The line graph compares the time-based productivity for different search methods between 1943 and 2023. The data shows a clear divergence in performance, with Search 3 having a drastic increase in 1996, Searches 5, 6, and 7 gradually rising from 1997, and Searches 1 and 9 remaining stable with low productivity.

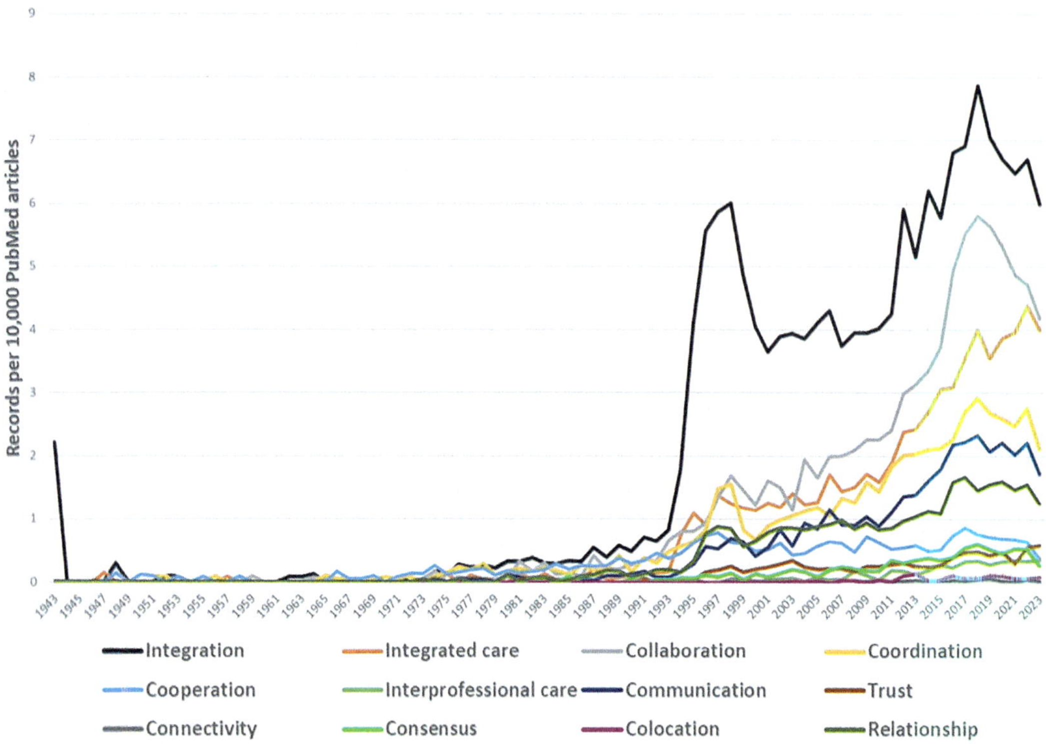

FIG. 4.2 Utilization time trends of the highly relevant words (meaningful terms around integration selected by researchers). The line graph compares the time-based productivity for different meaningful terms around integration selected by researchers. The data shows a drastic increase of "integration" in 1993, while "collaboration", "integrated care" and "coordination" increase gradually since 1997. On the other hand, terms like "consensus", "colocation", "trust", "interprofesional care" or "cooperation" remain constant with low productivity over time.

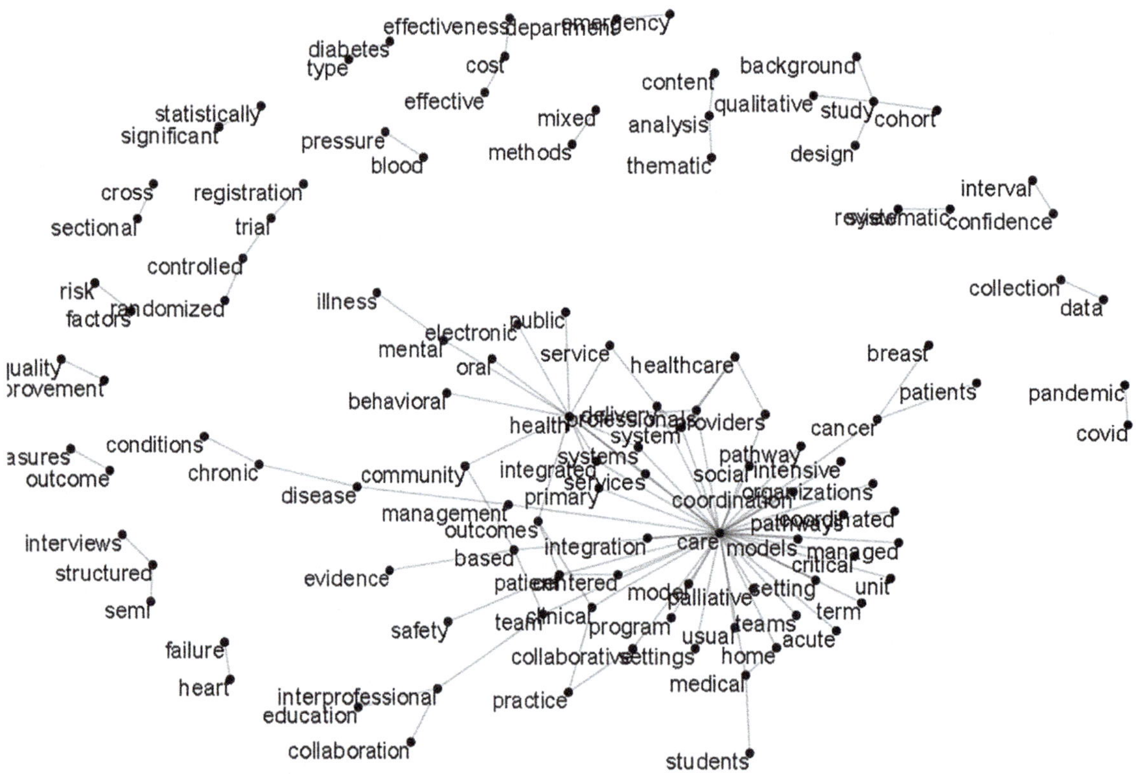

FIG. 4.3 The most frequent bigrams found in the corpus text. This visualization displays the most frequent bigrams extracted from the text corpus. The strong connections and prominent size of the terms "health" and "care" highlight their dominance and centrality in the overall subject matter of the analyzed text.

Thirdly, the DHC, performed on the lemmatized corpus, resulted in the identification of seven distinct lexical classes or conceptual clusters. These classes represent different dimensions through which integration is discussed in the literature: (1) evidence and implementation, (2) quantitative research, (3) professional education, (4) qualitative research, (5) governance and leadership, (6) clinical research and (7) financial resources (See Fig. 4.4 and Fig. 4.5).

These distinct lexical classes unequivocally underscore that "integration" is a complex concept with many interconnected themes surrounding it, yet often separately emphasized dimensions as empirically reflected in the literature.

Finally, the association between the seven classes and the articles retrieved in each of the 10 searches was largely weak or nonexistent, demonstrating a lack of a standard pattern of term use in the literature regarding healthcare integration. However, some specific associations were identified: a strong association between Class #7 (Financial resources) and search #2 (Intersectoral collaboration), and moderate associations between Class #3 (Professional education) and searches #5 (Collaboration) and #10 (Interprofessional care), as well as between Class #2 (Quantitative research) and search #7 (Integrated care). In addition, a strong association was found between Class #3 (Professional education) and the word "collaboration", and moderate associations between Class #5 (Governance and leadership) and the word "integration", and between Class #2 (Quantitative research) and "integrated care"(Brambilla et al., 2025).

3.2 Discussion of findings

The empirical findings from this lexicographic analysis echoed the challenges articulated in the chapter's introduction regarding the complex, often ambiguous, conceptualization of "integration".

The lack of term standardization observed in this study could be attributed to the widespread dispersion of publications across over 4000 journals from various disciplines and scopes, with few journals being highly productive (Rotta et al., 2017; Pinto et al., 2021; Meshcheryakov et al., 2022). The diverse backgrounds of editorial boards and reviewers in these journals may introduce limitations and bias, further confounding terminology standardization in editorial processes (Fernandez-Llimos et al., 2023; da Costa F et al., 2025).

The variation in terms and definitions for integration may also stem from differences in healthcare systems (Martin and Knowles, 2019). A lack of commonly agreed-upon definitions and terminology for healthcare integration has been identified as a significant barrier to measuring and comparing integration outcomes (Armitage et al., 2009; Shigayeva et al., 2010). This absence of standardized terminology creates an additional difficulty for evidence synthesis, complicating systematic searches (McGowan and Sampson, 2005). Without standardized terms, there is a risk of missing relevant papers in systematic reviews. This mapping exercise demonstrated that the low overlap and significant exclusivity among the 10 searches were necessary to comprehensively retrieve the existing literature on integration. While using controlled vocabularies like MeSH can increase search efficiency (DeMars and Perruso, 2022), MeSH terms are typically created after consistent use of terms in the literature (Fernandez-Llimos and Garcia-Cardenas, 2022). Despite the MeSH "Delivery of Health Care, Integrated" providing the best results, it only retrieved 34% of articles and showed a negative trend over time, indicating a need for further analysis to identify additional appropriate MeSH terms for cataloging integration literature.

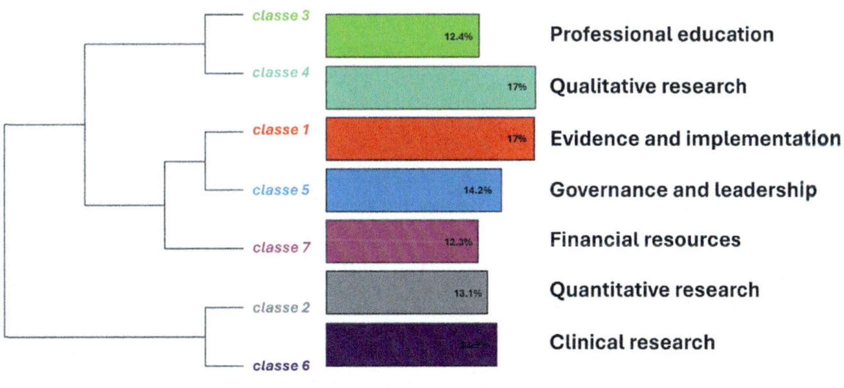

FIG. 4.4 Descendent hierarchic cluster analysis. The dendrogram depicts the hierarchical grouping of thematic areas within the integration literature. The structure shows an initial split between quantitative research (Class 2) and clinical research (Class 6). This is followed by the differentiation of professional education (Class 3) and qualitative research (Class 4), and then the separation of financial resources (Class 7). The smallest conceptual distance is observed between evidence and implementation (Class 1) and governance and leadership (Class 5), which are the last classes to differentiate.

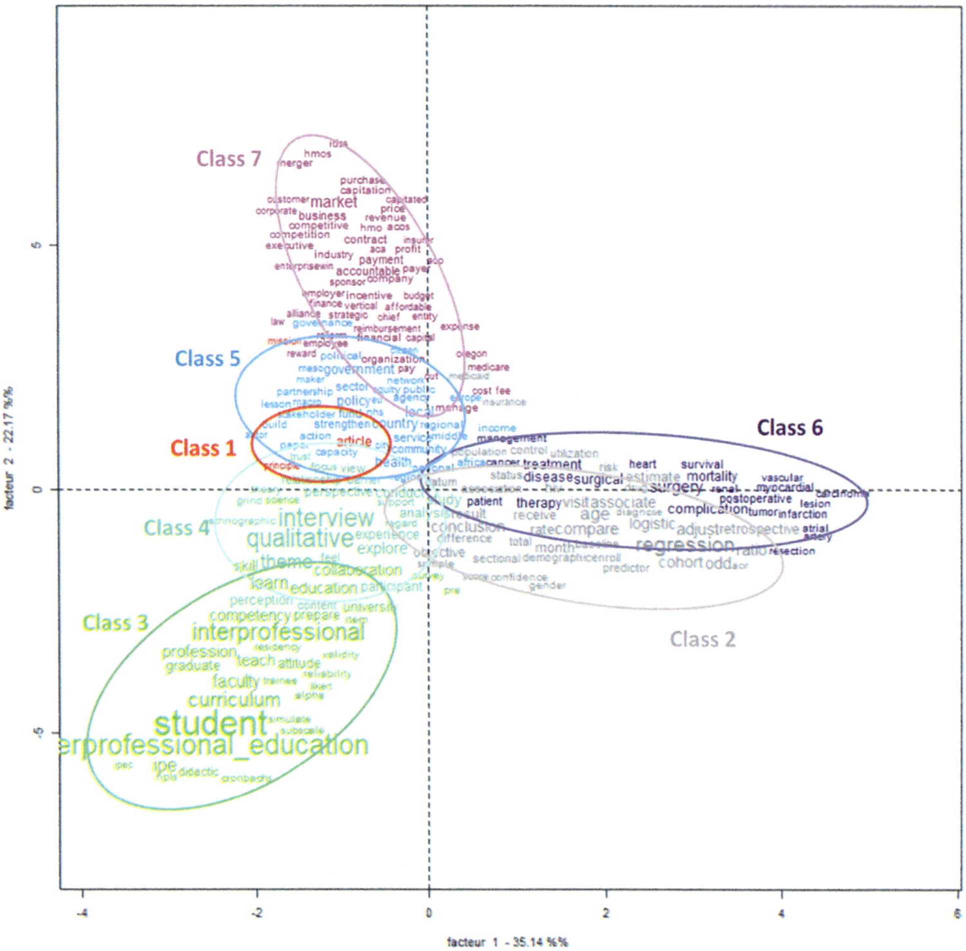

FIG. 4.5 Correspondence analysis of the text corpus resulting in 7 classes. The two-dimensional correspondence analysis plot visualizes the distribution of the seven thematic classes. The proximity between classes indicates a conceptual overlap within the corpus. Classes 1 and 5 (center-left) are highly overlapped, signifying the maximum conceptual similarity. Classes 6 and 2 (center-right) are quite close but show less proximity than the 1 and 5 pairing. Classes 3 and 4 (bottom-left) are more distinctly separated, with Class 3 positioned furthest from the plot center. Class 7 is located in the top-left area.

The complexity in terminology may partly be attributed to the slightly different concepts/ideas hidden within the specific areas of integration we looked at. Nevertheless, NLP and topic modeling techniques are effective in identifying such underlying factors from text (Brookes and McEnery, 2019).

The study's analysis of healthcare integration terminology revealed a clear structure, with its identified seven lexical classes distributed into three main regions. Three of these classes focused primarily on research (qualitative, clinical, and quantitative). Another three classes represented a policy component (governance and leadership, evidence and implementation, and financial resources). The last class identified was professional education. Interestingly, these classes generally were not strongly tied to specific search terms or individual words. This suggests there is often no logical reason to use different terms for quite similar concepts that are equally distributed among all the factors. However, there were a few exceptions: "Intersectoral collaboration" showed a strong link to "Financial resources" class, possibly because of its placement in the MeSH thesaurus "Health Services Administration" branch. The word "collaboration" was also strongly associated with Class #3 (Professional education), likely reflecting its importance in educational activities promoting integration. Finally, "integration" had an intermediate association with Class #5 (Governance and leadership), probably because policymakers frequently use it to describe the necessity of joint work in health systems (Sandhu et al., 2021; Department of Health & Social Care, 2025).

Among the 12 terms relevant to this mapping exercise, "integration" was not only the most prevalent in the 42,479 titles and abstracts but also showed the clearest increase in use over time. Interestingly, the term "integrated care" has experienced rapid growth in the past decade. This coincides with the highest prevalence of the MeSH "Delivery of Health Care, Integrated" (created in 1995, two years after the surge of "integration"). This suggests that "integration" could function as a preferred term that unifies separate but interconnected topic components (Ahgren and Axelsson, 2005). While the literature describes integration as a continuum of stages, including collaboration and coordination (Leutz, 1999; Bradley et al., 2012; Wihlman et al., 2008), and it can imply incorporating different components into a unique system, there are instances, such as public-private integration, that do not require a single entity as an outcome (Sekhri et al., 2011). Integration fundamentally represents the degree to which functions and activities are managed across operating units, irrespective of their location, ownership, or physical characteristics (Gillies et al., 1993).

The implications for fields like community pharmacy, as highlighted in the introduction, are significant. As community pharmacy's role in integrated care continues to evolve, a clear and consistent conceptualization of integration is paramount. The insights from this lexicographic analysis can inform the development of a more precise vocabulary that facilitates the structured integration of community pharmacy services into primary care and broader healthcare systems, ensuring that their contributions are accurately defined and understood. This mapping exercise has been invaluable in discerning the different subareas within the concept of integration and identifying which terms (free text words or MeSH) should be prioritized in future systematic searches aiming to gather evidence about healthcare integration. However, further research is necessary to refine search queries and achieve optimal strategies, especially considering the weak or null associations between MeSH terms/free text words and the seven classes. Future studies should also investigate the appropriate assignment of existing MeSH terms to integration-related articles and consider suggesting new MeSH terms to differentiate the subareas based on frequently used free text terms within each class.

4 Questions for further discussion

The insights gleaned from this lexicographic analysis, highlighting the multidimensional and often inconsistent conceptualization of healthcare integration, open several avenues for further inquiry and discussion.

These avenues include exploring how lexical classes found in the study can be used to develop a more standardized vocabulary, not only for consistent communication among stakeholders but also to properly index scientific contributions. Furthermore, it prompts a deeper examination of the tangible consequences of observed terminological inconsistencies and conceptual ambiguities on health policy formulation, interprofessional collaboration and integration, and the design and evaluation of integrated care initiatives.

Methodologically, there is a need to refine lexicographic applications, considering the impact of including full-text articles or gray literature. It's also important to address these conceptual gaps in professional education, especially for new roles, like community pharmacies getting involved in the integration of health systems.

Finally, further discussion should focus on how contextual and comparative analyses can show changes in terminology across different healthcare systems or for different diseases as well as how lexicographic analysis can inform the development of more precise metrics for measuring the successful implementation and effectiveness of integration models.

Key questions for further discussion:

- How should current educational programs for health professionals, particularly those training for new integrated roles (e.g., community pharmacists), be adapted to address and bridge these conceptual gaps in integration terminology?
- How can the insights from this analysis be used to develop a more standardized vocabulary that ensures consistent communication among all stakeholders?
- What are the tangible consequences of the observed terminological inconsistencies and conceptual ambiguities on health policy formulation, and the design and evaluation of integration initiatives?

5 Application exercise/scenario

Lexicographic analysis is an essential methodological tool for mapping the field and deriving practical recommendations. To illustrate the direct implications of evidence-based terminological prioritization from this analysis, a practical exercise has been designed. It compares two versions of an abstract to show how the choice of words and descriptors affects the visibility, retrievability, and potential impact of research in databases like PubMed. The objective is to move towards a shared and optimized vocabulary for the field of health integration.

TABLE 4.4 Comparison of two abstracts applying the lexicographic analysis.

Version 1: Without Terminological Prioritization	Version 2: With Prioritized Terminology (Based on Lexicographical Analysis)—Terms Changed in Bold
Title: Study on the coordination between healthcare professionals to improve quality of care in diabetes management. **Abstract:** **Background:** Interprofessional work and collaboration between pharmacists and primary care are crucial for optimizing outcomes in chronic diseases. It is necessary to evaluate the barriers to a better articulation of services. Despite the increasing adoption of these models, there is a lack of evidence regarding the specific structural and policy determinants that ensure the sustainability of care coordination. **Methods:** A qualitative approach was applied to analyze the perceptions of 30 professionals on the task coordination in five health centers. The study included focus groups and individual interviews. Data analysis followed a thematic approach, focusing on identifying common obstacles and facilitators regarding how different services interact on a day-to-day basis. **Results:** The main barriers identified were the lack of time and problems with interdisciplinary communication. Only 15% of the respondents reported clear protocols for information transfer. Furthermore, professionals frequently mentioned a lack of shared vision regarding patient pathways, often referring to a "silo" mentality rather than a structured system. **Conclusions:** It is necessary to promote collaboration and teamwork in primary care to improve outcomes. Simple measures like shared meetings and communication workshops could be beneficial, but a broader strategy is needed to define clear roles for all providers involved in care. **MeSH indexing:** community pharmacy services, health services research, Chronic disease management.	**Title:** Study on **integration** between healthcare professionals to improve quality of care in diabetes management. **Abstract:** **Background: Healthcare integration** or **integrated care** between community pharmacists and physicians are crucial for optimizing outcomes in chronic disease management. It is necessary to evaluate the barriers to a better **integration of services**. Despite the increasing adoption of these models, there is a lack of evidence regarding the specific structural and policy determinants that ensure the sustainability of **integrated care.** **Methods:** A qualitative approach was applied to analyze the perceptions of 30 professionals on the **integrated care models** in five health centers. The study included focus groups and individual interviews. Data analysis followed a thematic approach, focusing on identifying common obstacles and facilitators regarding how different services interact on a day-to-day basis. **Results:** The main barriers identified were the lack of time and problems with **governance and leadership**. Only 15% of the respondents reported clear protocols for information **continuity of care**. Furthermore, professionals frequently mentioned a lack of shared vision regarding patient pathways, often referring to a "silo" mentality rather than a structured system. **Conclusions:** It is necessary to promote **health service integration** and **integrated care models** in primary care to improve outcomes. Simple measures like shared meetings and communication workshops could be beneficial, but a broader strategy is needed to define clear roles for all providers involved in care. **MeSH indexing: Delivery of health care, integrated**, community pharmacy services, health services research, chronic disease management.

Practical activity

Version 1 uses less prevalent and generalist terminology, while Version 2 has been revised to incorporate the terms (highlighted in bold) that this lexicographical analysis identified as more prevalent or better associated with the key dimensions of integration (See Table 4.4).

References

Ahgren, B., Axelsson, R., 2005. Evaluating integrated health care: a model for measurement. Int. J. Integr. Care. 5 (3). doi:10.5334/ijic.134.

Allen, L.N., Rasanathan, K., Mash, R., Villar Uribe, M., Martinez-Bianchi, V., Kidd, M., 2025. Models of global primary care post-2030. The Lancet Primary Care 1 (3), 100027. doi:10.1016/j.lanprc.2025.100027.

Andueza, I.R. Euskadi admite que tiene "dificultades serias" para encontrar personal para los ambulatorios y no sólo en la pandemia. Published online 2022. Accessed May 24, 2025. https://www.eldiario.es/euskadi/euskadi-admite-dificultades-serias-encontrar-personal-ambulatorios-no-pandemia_1_8681454.html

Armitage, G.D., Suter, E., Oelke, N.D., et al., 2009. Health systems integration: state of the evidence. Int. J. Integr. Care. 9, e82. doi:10.5334/ijic.316.

Armitage, P., 1983. Joint working in primary health care. Nurs. Times. 79 (43), 75–78.

Biber, D., Reppen, R., Conrad, S. (Eds.), 1998. Lexicography. In: Corpus Linguistics: Investigating Language Structure and Use. Cambridge Approaches to Linguistics, Cambridge University Press, pp. 21–54. doi:10.1017/CBO9780511804489.003.

Bradley, F., Ashcroft, D.M., Noyce, P.R., 2012. Integration and differentiation: a conceptual model of general practitioner and community pharmacist collaboration. Res. Soc. Adm. Pharm. 8 (1), 36–46. doi:10.1016/j.sapharm.2010.12.005.

Brambilla, M.A., MLGGR, E., Sartori, V., 2025. Triple helix and its implications in the Brazilian context. Innov. Manag. Rev. Published online, 1–14. doi:10.1108/INMR-02-2024-0034.

Brookes, G., McEnery, T., 2019. The utility of topic modelling for discourse studies: a critical evaluation. Discourse Stud. 21 (1), 3–21. doi:10.1177/1461445618814032.

Carvalho, T.S., Mota, D.M., Saab, F., 2020. Utilização do software IRaMuTeQ na análise de contribuições da sociedade em processo regulatório conduzido pela Agência Nacional de Vigilância Sanitária. Vigilância Sanitária Em Debate 8 (1), 10–21. doi:10.22239/2317-269X.01429.

Contandriopoulos', A.P., Denis, J.L., Touati, N., et al., The integration of health care: dimensions and implementation. Published online 2003. Accessed June 17, 2025. http://catalogue.iugm.qc.ca/GED_IUG/194387991256/gris.PDF

Cutler, D.M., 2023. Health system change in the wake of COVID-19. JAMA Health Forum. 4 (10), e234355. doi:10.1001/jamahealthforum.2023.4355.

da Costa F, A., Fernandez-Llimos, F., Desselle, S., et al., 2025. The international collaboration of pharmacy journal editors (ICPJE) formally constituted to foster quality around clinical and social pharmacy practice research publications. Res. Soc. Adm. Pharm. 21 (2), 71–73. doi:10.1016/j.sapharm.2024.10.001.

de Ries, K.E., Schaap, H., van Loon, A.M.M.J.A.P., et al., 2022. A literature review of open-ended concept maps as a research instrument to study knowledge and learning. Qual. Quant. 56 (1), 73–107. doi:10.1007/s11135-021-01113-x.

De Vries, N., Lavreysen, O., Boone, A., et al., 2023. Retaining healthcare workers: a systematic review of strategies for sustaining power in the workplace. Healthcare 11 (13), 1887. doi:10.3390/healthcare11131887.

DeMars, M.M., Perruso, C., 2022. MeSH and text-word search strategies: precision, recall, and their implications for library instruction. J. Med. Libr. Assoc. 110 (1), 23–33. doi:10.5195/jmla.2022.1283.

Department of Health & Social Care. Integration and innovation: working together to improve health and social care for all. GOV.UK. 2025. Accessed July 3, 2025. https://www.gov.uk/government/publications/working-together-to-improve-health-and-social-care-for-all/integration-and-innovation-working-together-to-improve-health-and-social-care-for-all-html-version

DiPietro Mager, N, Bright, D., 2023. Advancing public health through community pharmacy practice. Pharmacy 11 (2), 56. doi:10.3390/pharmacy11020056.

Evans, J.M., Baker, R.G., Berta, W., et al., 2014. The Evolution Of Integrated Health Care Strategies. In: Annual Review of Health Care Management: Revisiting the Evolution of Health Systems Organization, Vol. 15, Emerald Group Publishing Limited, pp. 125–161. doi:10.1108/S1474-8231.

Fernandez-Llimos, F., Desselle, S., Stewart, D., et al., 2023. Improving the quality of publications in and advancing the paradigms of clinical and social pharmacy practice research: the Granada statements. Res. Soc. Adm. Pharm. 19 (5), 830–835. doi:10.1016/j.sapharm.2023.01.007.

Fernandez-Llimos, F., Garcia-Cardenas, V., 2022. The importance of using standardized terminology in titles and abstracts of pharmacy practice articles. Res. Soc. Adm. Pharm. 19 (2), 190–192. doi:10.1016/j.sapharm.2022.08.017.

Gillies, R.R., Gillies,, Shortell, S.M., et al., 1993. Conceptualizing and measuring integration: findings from the health systems integration study. J. Healthc. Manag. 38 (4), 467.

Graham, H., White, P.C.L., 2016. Social determinants and lifestyles: integrating environmental and public health perspectives. Public Health. 141, 270–278. doi:10.1016/j.puhe.2016.09.019.

Gray, C.S., Wodchis, W.P., Baker, G.R., et al., 2018. Mapping for conceptual clarity: exploring implementation of integrated community-based primary health care from a whole systems perspective. Int. J. Integr. Care. 18 (1). doi:10.5334/ijic.3082.

Gröne, O., Garcia-Barbero, M., WHO European Office for Integrated Health Care Services. Integrated care: a position paper of the WHO european office for integrated health care services. Int. J. Integr. Care. 2001;1e21.

Harber, P., Leroy, G., 2017. Feasibility and utility of lexical analysis for occupational health text. J. Occup. Environ. Med. 59 (6), 578–587. doi:10.1097/JOM.0000000000001035.

Hepler, C.D., 1985. Pharmacy as a clinical profession. Am. J. Hosp. Pharm. 42 (6), 1298–1306.

Hepler, C.D., Strand, L.M., 1990. Opportunities and responsibilities in pharmaceutical care. Am. J. Hosp. Pharm. 47 (3), 533–543.

Hudon, C., Chouinard, M.C., Pluye, P., et al., 2019. Characteristics of case management in primary care associated with positive outcomes for frequent users of health care: a systematic review. Ann. Fam. Med. 17 (5), 448–458. doi:10.1370/afm.2419.

Hughes, L.S., Cohen, D.J., RL Jr, P., 2022. Strengthening primary care to improve health outcomes in the US—creating oversight to address invisibility. JAMA Health Forum. 3 (9), e222903. doi:10.1001/jamahealthforum.2022.2903.

Johansen, O., 1993. Introduccion a La Teoria General de Sistemas (8th ed.). Editorial Limusa (Grupo Noriega Editores), Mexico City.

Kodner, D.L., Spreeuwenberg, C., 2002. Integrated care: meaning, logic, applications, and implications–a discussion paper. Int. J. Integr. Care. 2, e12. doi:10.5334/ijic.67.

Lalani, M., Wytrykowski, S., Hogan, H., 2023. Approaches to improving patient safety in integrated care: a scoping review. BMJ Open. 13 (4), e067441. doi:10.1136/bmjopen-2022-067441.

Lawrence, P.R., Lorsch, J.W. (1986). Organization and Environment: Managing Differentiation and Integration, 1st. Harvard Business School Press.

Leutz, W.N., 1999. Five laws for integrating medical and social services: lessons from the United States and the United Kingdom. Milbank Q. 77 (1), 77–110. doi:10.1111/1468-0009.00125.

Lucero-Prisno III, D.E., Shomuyiwa, D.O., Kouwenhoven, M.B.N., et al., 2025. Top 10 public health challenges for 2024: charting a new direction for global health security. Public Health Chall. 4 (1), e70022. doi:10.1002/puh2.70022.

Mahtani, K.R., Abrams, R., 2025. General practice must be the foundation of primary care reform. BMJ 390, r1851. doi:10.1136/bmj.r1851.

Martin, L., Knowles, E.E., 2019. Model for an integrated health system. J. Integr. Care. 28 (2), 161–170. doi:10.1108/JICA-08-2019-0034.

Martín, R., Aldecoa, S., Galir, G., et al., 2023. La transformación de la Atención Primaria pasa por un nuevo modelo organizativo y de gestión. Aten Primaria 55 (4), 102609. doi:10.1016/j.aprim.2023.102609.

Maslin-Prothero, S.E., Bennion, A.E., 2010. Integrated team working: a literature review. Int. J. Integr. Care. 10, e043.

Matthews, K., Hughes, L., Sprott, C., Barnett, K.G., 2025. Primary care: a crucial catalyst to build a healthier USA. The Lancet Primary Care 1 (1), 100026. doi:10.1016/j.lanprc.2025.100026.

McGowan, J., Sampson, M., 2005. Systematic reviews need systematic searchers. J. Med. Libr. Assoc. 93 (1), 74–80.

Mendes, A.M., Tonin, F.S., Buzzi, M.F., et al., 2019. Mapping pharmacy journals: a lexicographic analysis. Res. Soc. Adm. Pharm. 15 (12), 1464–1471. doi:10.1016/j.sapharm.2019.01.011.

Meshcheryakov, B.G., Ponomareva, V.V., Shvedovskaya, A.A., 2022. A bibliometric analysis of scientific publications on cultural-historical psychology from 2010 to 2020: dynamics, Geography, and Key Ideas. Psychol Russ State Art 15 (4), 188–214. doi:10.11621/pir.2022.0412.

Nolte, E., McKee, M., 2008. Integration and chronic care: a review, In: Caring for People with Chronic Conditions: A Health System Perspective, Vol. 71, 1st, Open University Press, pp. 64–91.

Pinto, G.O., da, S.J.L.C.S., Assad, D.B.N., et al., 2021. Trends in global greywater reuse: a bibliometric analysis. Water Sci. Technol. 84 (10-11), 3257–3276. doi:10.2166/wst.2021.429.

Piquer-Martinez, C., Urionagüena, A., Benrimoj, S.I., et al., 2024a. Theories, models and frameworks for health systems integration. A scoping review. Health Policy. 141, 104997. doi:10.1016/j.healthpol.2024.104997.

Piquer-Martinez, C., Urionagüena, A., Benrimoj, S.I., et al., 2024b. Strategic interventions and a novel model for the integration of community pharmacy and primary care in Spain: qualitative insights. BMJ Open. 14 (12), e086285. doi:10.1136/bmjopen-2024-086285.

Rotenstein, L., Gitomer, R., 2023. Advancing team-based primary care: the importance and challenges in 2023. Am. J. Accountable Care. 11 (3), 33–35.

Rotta, I., Souza, T.T., Salgado, T.M., et al., 2017. Characterization of published randomized controlled trials assessing clinical pharmacy services around the world. Res. Soc. Adm. Pharm. 13 (1), 201–208. doi:10.1016/j.sapharm.2016.01.003.

Sandhu, S., Sharma, A., Cholera, R., et al., 2021. Integrated health and social care in the united states: a decade of policy progress. Int. J. Integr. Care. 21 (S2). doi:10.5334/ijic.5687.

Sawicki, O.A., Mueller, A., KlaaBen-Mielke, R., Glushan, A., Gerlach, F.M., Beyer, M., et al., 2021. Strong and sustainable primary healthcare is associated with a lower risk of hospitalization in high risk patients. Sci. Rep. 11 (1), 4349. doi:10.1038/s41598-021-83962-y.

Sekhri, N., Feachem, R., Ni, A., 2011. Public-private integrated partnerships demonstrate the potential to improve health care access, quality, and efficiency. Health Aff. 30 (8), 1498–1507. doi:10.1377/hlthaff.2010.0461.

Shigayeva, A., Atun, R., McKee, M., et al., 2010. Health systems, communicable diseases and integration. Health Policy Plan. 25 (Suppl 1), i4–20. doi:10.1093/heapol/czq060.

Shortell, S.M., Gillies, R.R., Anderson, D.A., 1994. The new world of managed care: creating organized delivery systems. Health Aff. 13 (5), 46–64. doi:10.1377/hlthaff.13.5.46.

Simoens, S., Scott, A., 2005. Integrated primary care organizations: to what extent is integration occurring and why? Health Serv. Manage. Res. 18 (1), 25–40. doi:10.1258/0951484053051951.

Singer, S.J., Burgers, J., Friedberg, M., et al., 2011. Defining and measuring integrated patient care: promoting the next frontier in health care delivery. Med. Care Res. Rev. 68 (1), 112–127. doi:10.1177/1077558710371485.

Starfield, B., Shi, L., Macinko, J., 2005. Contribution of primary care to health systems and health. Milbank Q. 83 (3), 457–502. doi:10.1111/j.1468-0009.2005.00409.x.

Suter, E., Oelke, N.D., Adair, C.E., et al., 2009. Ten key principles for successful health systems integration. Healthc Q. 13 (Spec No), 16–23. doi:10.12927/hcq.2009.21092.

Tichenor, M., Sridhar, D., 2017. Universal health coverage, health systems strengthening, and the World Bank. BMJ 358 (j3347). doi:10.1136/bmj.j3347.

Urionagüena, A., Piquer-Martinez, C., Benrimoj, S.I., et al., 2024a. Community pharmacy & primary care integration: qualitative study on stakeholders' opinions and interventions. J. Pharm. Policy Pract. 17 (1), 2395551. doi:10.1080/20523211.2024.2395551.

Urionagüena, A., Piquer-Martinez, C., Benrimoj, S.I., et al., 2024b. Mapping the concept of health care integration: a lexicographic analysis of scientific literature. Res. Soc. Adm. Pharm. 20 (5), 506–511. doi:10.1016/j.sapharm.2024.01.013.

Urionagüena, A., Piquer-Martinez, C., Gastelurrutia, M.Á., et al., 2023. Community pharmacy and primary health care - Types of integration and their applicability: a narrative review. Res. Soc. Adm. Pharm. 19 (3), 414–431. doi:10.1016/j.sapharm.2022.10.007.

Valentijn, P.P., Schepman, S.M., Opheij, W., et al., 2013. Understanding integrated care: a comprehensive conceptual framework based on the integrative functions of primary care. Int. J. Integr. Care. 13, e010. doi:10.5334/ijic.886.

Wihlman, U., Lundborg, C.S., Axelsson, R., et al., 2008. Barriers of inter-organisational integration in vocational rehabilitation. Int. J. Integr. Care. 8, e52. doi:10.5334/ijic.234.

World Health Organization. Constitution of the World Health Organization. Published online 1948. Accessed May 24, 2025. https://www.who.int/about/governance/constitution

World Health Organization, 2016a. Integrated Care Models: An Overview. World Health Organization, Regional Office for Europe, https://www.euro.who.int/__data/assets/pdf_file/0005/322475/Integrated-care-models-overview.pdf.

World Health Organization. Framework on integrated, people-centred health services. Published online 2016b. Accessed May 26, 2025. https://www.integratedcare4people.org/ipchs-framework/

World Health Organization. *Integrating health services: brief.* World Health Organization, regional office for Europe; 2018. Accessed June 24, 2025. https://iris.who.int/handle/10665/326459

World Health Organization. Primary health care. 2022. Accessed June 27, 2025. https://www.who.int/news-room/questions-and-answers/item/primary-health-care

World Health Organization. Services organization and integration. Accessed June 24, 2025. https://www.who.int/teams/integrated-health-services/clinical-services-and-systems/service-organizations-and-integration

Zheng, F., Cui, L. A lexical-based formal concept analysis method to identify missing concepts in the NCI thesaurus. Proc IEEE Int Conf Bioinforma Biomed. 2020; doi:10.1109/bibm49941.2020.9313186

Zonneveld, N., Driessen, N., Stüssgen, R.A.J., et al., 2018. Values of integrated care: a systematic review. Int. J. Integr. Care. 18 (4), 9. doi:10.5334/ijic.4172.

CHAPTER

5

Methodological quality and risk of bias of meta analyses of pharmacy services: A systematic review

Aline de Fátima Bonetti[a,d], *Suelem Tavares da Silva Penteado*[b], *Ana Flávia Redolfi Oliota*[c], *and Antonio Matoso Mendes*[a,d]

[a]Pharmacy Department, Federal University of Paraná, Curitiba, Brazil
[b]Paraná State Department of Health, Curitiba, Brazil
[c]State University of Western Paraná, Cascavel, Brazil
[d]Clinical Pharmacy Unit, Clinics Hospital Complex, Federal University of Paraná, Curitiba, Brazil

CHAPTER OBJECTIVES

- To assess the reporting quality of meta analyses of pharmacy services
- To evaluate the methodological quality of meta analyses of pharmacy services
- To examine the risk of bias in meta analyses of pharmacy services
- To identify which attributes of pharmacy services studies are associated with higher quality, lower susceptibility to bias, and more reliable evidence

1 Introduction

Between 1986 and 2015, approximately 266,782 systematic reviews (SRs) and 58,611 meta analyses were indexed in PubMed, with an annual growth between 1991 and 2014 of over 2700% for SRs and 2600% for meta analyses, while the overall growth of PubMed items was only 153% (Ioannidis, 2016). These publications represent secondary studies with a high level of evidence, capable of answering questions that individual primary studies cannot clarify. However, Ioannidis et al. (2016) identified poor methodological quality in many published SRs, highlighting the absence of preregistered protocols, limited search strategies, and lack of risk of bias assessment of primary studies. These factors compromise confidence in the conclusions, making them more susceptible to bias and of reduced utility for clinical decision-making. Added to this is the duplication of efforts, with several SRs addressing the same clinical question without plausible justification, which contributes to the saturation of the literature (Ioannidis, 2016).

In parallel, studies on pharmacy services have also increased in recent decades, representing a relevant advance in pharmaceutical practice within healthcare. According to Moullin et al. (2013), a pharmacy service can be defined as actions carried out or organized by health services and provided by pharmacists, with the aim of optimizing care and improving health outcomes (Moullin et al., 2013). In 2014, the Pharmaceutical Care Network Europe defined pharmaceutical care as

Contemporary Research Methods in Pharmacy and Health Services - Volume 2
https://doi.org/10.1016/B978-0-443-44607-8.00013-3

"the pharmacist's contribution to optimizing the use of medicines and improving health outcomes"(Allemann et al., 2014). These definitions reinforce the clinical role of the pharmacist, which is aimed at the safe and effective use of medicines.

The growth of primary studies was accompanied by the increase in SRs and meta analyses on pharmacy services, which seek to synthesize evidence to support health decisions (Rotta et al., 2015; Tonin et al., 2019; Bonetti et al., 2020). However, if primary studies are poorly conducted, the results obtained in SRs and meta analyses may lead to biased conclusions, underestimating or overestimating results, with a negative impact on clinical practice and health decision-making. In this scenario, a large proportion of published SRs can be considered unnecessary, redundant, or of limited utility, while high-quality and truly informative meta analyses represent the minority within this wide set of publications (Ioannidis, 2016).

Most SRs and meta analyses on pharmacy services present favorable results for interventions. Although this may reflect real benefits, it may also stem from publication bias and significant methodological limitations. Overly positive conclusions, without considering the quality and consistency of the evidence, may lead to disproportionate clinical and policy recommendations. Furthermore, it is extremely important to understand the reasons for this predominance and critically assess the robustness of SRs so that health decisions are based on solid and balanced evidence (Rotta et al., 2015; Tonin et al., 2019; Bonetti et al., 2020).

The evaluation of methodological quality and risk of bias is, therefore, an essential step in evidence synthesis, as it determines the reliability of findings and their clinical applicability. Several tools have been developed for this purpose, each with a specific scope and objectives.

The Preferred Reporting Items for SRs and Meta analyses (PRISMA) guidelines are widely used to ensure transparency in the conduct and reporting of reviews. The updated version, PRISMA 2020, revised the 2009 guideline, incorporating methodological advances and expanding its applicability (PRISMA Statement, n.d.). It consists of 27 items that guide what should be reported in each section of the review, from the introduction and study rationale to search methods, eligibility criteria, data analysis, and presentation of results. It also includes a flowchart for visualization of the study inclusion process (Page et al., 2021). It should be emphasized that PRISMA does not define how a review should be conducted but rather how the methods and results should be described. Its use promotes greater methodological rigor and is required by journals and research institutions. Furthermore, specific extensions have been developed, such as Preferred Reporting Items for Systematic Reviews and Meta-Analyses extension for Scoping Reviews (PRISMA-ScR) (Tricco et al., 2018) for scoping reviews, Preferred Reporting Items for Systematic Review and Meta-Analysis Protocols (PRISMA-P) (Moher et al., 2015) for review protocols, and Preferred Reporting Items for Systematic Reviews and Meta-Analyses of Individual Participant Data (PRISMA-IPD) (Stewart et al., 2015) for reviews with individual participant data, maintaining the principles of the guideline but adapted to the particularities of each study type.

The A Measurement Tool to Assess SRs tool (AMSTAR) (Shea et al., 2007), published in 2007, consists of 11 items that assess the methodological quality of SRs, providing criteria to verify the robustness and transparency of the processes adopted. Subsequently, in 2017, the revised version, AMSTAR-2 (Shea et al., 2017), was launched, expanding the applicability of the instrument to cover not only SRs of randomized controlled trials but also SRs including observational studies. This version, composed of 16 items (seven considered critical), does not yield a numerical score but provides a qualitative classification of confidence in results (high, moderate, low, or critically low), offering a more detailed assessment adapted to the current requirements of evidence synthesis. In addition, the revised AMSTAR tool (Kung et al., 2010) was developed by Kung and collaborators in 2010 to improve the methodological quality assessment of SRs. Like the original AMSTAR, this instrument is composed of 11 items, but its main innovation is the attribution of a quantitative score from 1 to 4 for each item, increasing precision, reproducibility, and comparability among reviews. R-AMSTAR evaluates central aspects such as the presence of a protocol, defined inclusion criteria, study quality, and synthesis methods, constituting a useful tool to identify more consistent and well conducted SRs.

The Risk of Bias in SRs tool (ROBIS), published in 2016 and updated in 2018, was created to identify potential sources of bias in the conduct of SRs and to assess the credibility of their results and conclusions. It can be applied to reviews with or without metaanalysis and is used by assessors trained in research methodology (Whiting et al., 2018, 2016). The tool is structured into three phases: (1) optional verification of the review's relevance to the research question; (2) analysis of four methodological domains—eligibility criteria, search and selection of studies, data collection and appraisal, and synthesis of results; and (3) final judgment of risk of bias (low, high, or unclear). With this structure, ROBIS allows for a clear and systematic assessment of the confidence that can be placed in the conclusions of a review, making it useful for researchers, health professionals, and developers of clinical guidelines.

Despite their value, these tools still lack international standardization regarding the weighting of their domains and are often applied through summative scores without considering the relative importance of each criterion, which may mask critical flaws in the review process. Thus, the careful choice and application of these tools are essential to ensure the validity of SRs used in policy formulation and clinical decision-making.

Given the growing production of SRs and meta analyses in pharmacy services, it becomes essential that these evidence syntheses are conducted with methodological rigor and transparency. The absence of critical assessments of evidence quality and the limited use of guidelines such as PRISMA, AMSTAR, and ROBIS may compromise the reliability of results and lead to the adoption of ineffective or harmful interventions. Thus, this chapter seeks to contribute to the strengthening of evidence-based practice by analyzing the methodological quality and risk of bias of meta analyses on pharmacy services in order to support safer and more evidence-based clinical, managerial, and policy decisions.

2 Methods

This chapter was developed from an article previously published by Bonetti and collaborators (Bonetti et al., 2022), exploring its hypotheses and results, as well as the bibliographic references cited by the authors. For the elaboration of the chapter, fidelity to the methodological design employed in the original study was maintained, with adaptations made to suit a book chapter format, including more detailed conceptual explanations and integration with complementary literature.

The original study (Bonetti et al., 2022) critically evaluated the methodological quality, risk of bias, and reporting quality of meta analyses on pharmacy services. To ensure transparency and reproducibility, it followed the PRISMA guidelines and the methodological recommendations described in the Cochrane Handbook for SRs of Interventions (Higgins et al, 2024). The review process carried out by the article comprised four sequential stages: screening of titles and abstracts, full-text appraisal, data extraction, and quality assessment. Each stage was independently performed by two reviewers to ensure methodological rigor. Discrepancies were resolved through consensus, with the input of a third reviewer when necessary.

A comprehensive search strategy was implemented across three major bibliographic databases—PubMed (including MEDLINE and PubMed Central), Scopus, and Web of Science—to identify meta analyses comparing clinical pharmacy services with either alternative interventions or usual care. No restrictions were imposed on language or publication date, allowing for the broadest possible inclusion of relevant literature. The search was last updated on February 5, 2020, and the complete strategies are provided in Supplementary material 1, available online at http://dx.doi.org/10.1016/B978-0-443-44607-8.00013-3.

SRs without metaanalysis, outdated versions of previously published reviews (keeping only the most recent version), and those evaluating multiprofessional interventions without a clear distinction of the pharmacist's role were excluded. Additional details on the search strategies are available in the Supplementary material of the original study at http://dx.doi.org/10.1016/B978-0-443-44607-8.00013-3 (Bonetti et al., 2022).

A standardized extraction form was used to collect the following information: authorship and year of publication; presence of international collaboration; journal impact factor (2018 *Journal Citation Reports*); number of primary studies included in the review and in the metaanalysis of the primary outcome; direction and statistical significance of the pooled result; availability of raw data; and whether the conclusions explicitly discussed the quality of evidence, methodological quality assessment (e.g., Risk of Bias for randomized controlled trials, Newcastle–Ottawa for nonrandomized studies), heterogeneity, or the need for further research. Funding sources and conflict-of-interest statements were also recorded.

The PRISMA checklist was applied to all studies published after July 2009 to assess reporting quality. Each item adequately addressed by the authors was scored as 1, and those judged as incomplete or absent were scored as 0, yielding a maximum possible score of 27.

Methodological quality was evaluated using the R-AMSTAR tool, which rates 11 domains on a scale from 1 to 4: (1) specification of an "a priori" design; (2) duplication of study selection and data extraction; (3) comprehensiveness of the literature search; (4) inclusion of additional sources (e.g., gray literature); (5) appropriate inclusion/exclusion criteria; (6) description of included study characteristics; (7) assessment of the scientific quality of included studies; (8) consideration of study quality when drawing conclusions; (9) appropriateness of synthesis methods; (10) assessment of publication bias; and (11) disclosure of conflicts of interest. The total score was used as the global indicator of methodological quality.

Risk of bias was assessed using the ROBIS tool, which is designed specifically for SRs. This process involved three phases: (1) optional assessment of relevance; (2) evaluation of potential concerns across four domains—eligibility criteria, identification and selection of studies, data collection and appraisal, and synthesis of results; and (3) an overall judgment of risk of bias (low, unclear, or high) based on the findings from phase 2.

All variables (PRISMA, R-AMSTAR, and ROBIS) were subjected to descriptive analysis. Data normality was examined using the Shapiro–Wilk test and visual inspection of Q–Q plots. For not normally distributed continuous variables, results were presented as median and interquartile range (IQR), with between-group differences assessed using the Mann–Whitney *U* test. Categorical variables were reported as absolute and relative frequencies.

Associations between PRISMA and R-AMSTAR scores were explored using Spearman's correlation coefficient, while the linear-by-linear association test was applied to ROBIS results. The following covariates were examined: year of publication; journal impact factor; whether the primary outcome favored interventions led by pharmacists international collaboration status; inclusion in the conclusions of comments on methodological quality, quality of evidence, heterogeneity, the primary outcome, or the need for further studies; and disclosure of conflicts of interest or funding sources. A *P*-value < 0.05 was considered statistically significant. All statistical analyses were performed using IBM SPSS Statistics, version 24.0.

3 Summary findings

This section is based on the findings previously published by Bonetti and collaborators (Bonetti et al., 2022). To ensure coherence with the methodological framework described in the preceding section, the results are presented here in a concise and integrative manner, highlighting the most relevant quantitative and qualitative findings that support the subsequent discussion. The complete set of data, statistical outputs, and replication analyses can be consulted in the original article (Bonetti et al., 2022), which provides the full methodological and analytical details underlying the summarized results below.

A total of 109 meta analyses evaluating pharmacy services met the inclusion criteria. Most were published between 2016 and 2020 (median year: 2017; IQR: 2014–2018), reflecting a steady growth in scientific production over the last decade. Among these, 49 were conducted through international collaboration, and the median impact factor of the 61 journals in which they were published was 3.03 (IQR: 2.37–4.51).

3.1 Reporting quality (PRISMA)

Among the meta analyses evaluated for reporting quality (n = 102), the median PRISMA score was 24 (IQR 21.75–25), representing 88.8% of the maximum score. The main deficiencies were related to the summary of evidence (26.5%), protocol registration (39.2%), and reporting of complete search strategies (60.8%). No association was found between PRISMA scores and publication year (P = 0.315). A weak positive correlation was observed with the journal impact factor (rho = 0.313; P = 0.002), and higher scores were observed in reviews that reported evidence quality (P = 0.018) and acknowledged the need for further studies (P = 0.011).

3.2 Methodological quality (R-AMSTAR)

The mean R-AMSTAR score was 30 (IQR 27–32.5), equivalent to 68.2% of the maximum score, indicating moderate methodological quality among the included meta analyses. The lowest-rated domains were consideration of scientific quality in conclusions (82.6%), assessment and documentation of study quality (77.9%), criteria for search and selection (64.2%), and the list of excluded articles (63.3%). In contrast, higher scores were observed for duplicate data extraction (69.7%), comprehensive literature search (71.6%), description of included studies (65.1%), and data synthesis methods (81.7%).

The R-AMSTAR scores remained stable over time (P = 0.223) but were higher in reviews published in journals with greater impact factors (rho = 0.338; P = 0.001), in those that reported evidence quality (P = 0.002), and in studies that mentioned quality analyses in their conclusions (P = 0.046). Overall, methodological rigor was moderate, with better performance associated with higher-impact journals and greater transparency in reporting evidence quality.

3.3 Risk of bias (ROBIS)

According to the ROBIS tool evaluation, 76.1% (n = 83) of the reviews had a high risk of bias, 13.8% (n = 15) had a low risk, and 10.1% (n = 11) were unclear. The highest-risk domains were eligibility criteria (64.2%) and study identification methods (62.7%), mainly due to search restrictions by language or publication date. In the synthesis of results domain, 60.6% showed a high risk for not reporting predefined analyses, funnel plots, or sensitivity analyses. No correlation was found between ROBIS classification and publication year (P = 0.282) or journal impact factor (P = 0.329). Reviews that acknowledged the need for further studies had a significantly lower risk of bias (P = 0.041).

3.4 Overall summary

This synthesis of findings, derived from the evaluation conducted by Bonetti and collaborators (Bonetti et al., 2022), summarizes the methodological performance and reporting quality of meta analyses on pharmacy services assessed through the PRISMA, R-AMSTAR, and ROBIS tools.

In general, the studies demonstrated a notable increase in scientific production and growing international collaboration, accompanied by acceptable levels of reporting quality and moderate methodological rigor. However, important limitations were consistently observed, particularly regarding transparency, completeness of documentation, and control of potential sources of bias. The overall pattern revealed that, while reporting practices tend to follow established guidelines, methodological consistency and risk management remain challenges for the field.

4 Discussion

SRs and meta analyses occupy the top of the evidence hierarchy, but their methodological quality can vary considerably. When rigorously conducted, they allow verification of whether interventions truly produce relevant clinical, economic, or humanistic effects. However, low-quality reviews—those without a registered protocol, with limited search strategies, inadequate risk of bias assessments, or biased interpretations—may compromise decisions in clinical practice (Kung et al., 2010).

The adoption of pharmacy services based on weak evidence may overestimate benefits, consume time and resources without generating concrete improvements in health outcomes, and even put patient safety at risk. Furthermore, such methodological fragility may negatively impact the health system, leading to inefficient use of human and financial resources, hindering service sustainability, and compromising the credibility and integration of pharmacists in healthcare teams (Rotta et al., 2015; Tonin et al., 2019; Bonetti et al., 2020). Bonetti and collaborators (Bonetti et al., 2022) identified that most studies on pharmacy services fail to report essential elements necessary for the critical interpretation of evidence. The article indicates that fewer than 20% of studies discussed methodological quality, quality of evidence, or heterogeneity in their conclusions. Specifically, only 14.3% of studies explored the impact of heterogeneity. Moreover, most meta analyses on pharmacy services did not explicitly describe the methodological limitations of the included studies, as only 17.4% mentioned the methodological quality of the included studies, and 14.7% discussed the quality of evidence. The need for future studies was discussed in 62.4% of conclusions.

The study also observed that weaker meta analyses were associated with more exaggerated conclusions, and that those which did not mention the quality of evidence had lower scores in the PRISMA and R-AMSTAR instruments. Likewise, meta analyses that did not recognize the need for new studies obtained lower PRISMA scores and a higher risk of bias. These findings indicate that the absence of a critical analysis of limitations may directly impact methodological quality and the credibility of conclusions (Bonetti et al., 2022).

In many of the meta analyses evaluated, the conclusions did not consider essential points necessary to correctly interpret the results, such as heterogeneity among studies, quality of evidence, and methodological rigor. It is essential that conclusions are critical, well-founded, and consistent with the strength and consistency of the available evidence (Bonetti et al., 2022).

In addition, the study classified most SRs and meta analyses (76.1%) as having a high risk of bias according to the ROBIS tool, while only 13.8% were classified as low risk. The main domains that contributed to this classification were "eligibility criteria" and "methods of study identification." Most studies (60.6%) were considered at high risk of bias due to failures in reporting sensitivity analyses, absence of publication bias assessments (such as funnel plots), or failure to address bias in primary studies. These findings reinforce that a considerable proportion of published studies lack sufficient methodological rigor to support reliable clinical recommendations, even when their results favor pharmacy services (Bonetti et al., 2022).

Finally, regarding the risk of bias (assessed by ROBIS), the only statistically significant association was observed with the mention of the need for more studies in the conclusion ($P = 0.041$), with SRs that recognized this need showing a lower risk of bias. This may indicate that SRs more aware of their limitations are also those less likely to present bias in the conduct and synthesis of findings (Bonetti et al., 2022).

A relevant methodological aspect pointed out by the authors of the article (Bonetti et al., 2022) refers to the use of summative scores in the applied tools (PRISMA, R-AMSTAR, and ROBIS) without assigning relative weights to the evaluated domains. This approach, although practical and frequently used in secondary studies, disregards heterogeneity in the relative importance of different domains for the internal and external validity of SRs, which may mask critical flaws in the review process. This methodological limitation has already been discussed in the literature and highlights the lack of robust international standardization to assign weight to domains according to their relevance for the reliability of findings (Tonin et al., 2019; Whiting et al., 2016). Furthermore, applying a total score tends to oversimplify complex judgments and ignores potential interactions between domains, such as the influence of primary study quality on the interpretation of pooled effects.

In this sense, the need to develop more sophisticated evaluation systems is emphasized, incorporating weightings based on expert consensus, empirical validations, and adaptations to the context of pharmacy services, which are still little addressed in major international methodological frameworks.

Regarding the promotion of international collaboration, in this review, only 45% of meta analyses on pharmacy services involved international collaboration—a proportion considered low compared to other biomedical areas (Wagner et al., 2015; Li et al., 2016). Although no statistically significant association was found between the presence of international collaboration and scores of methodological quality or risk of bias ($P = 0.085$ for PRISMA, 0.545 for R-AMSTAR, and 0.135 for ROBIS), the literature indicates that international collaboration, consisting of multicenter teams, tends to produce more robust, comprehensive, and generalizable syntheses. The lack of collaboration among different countries may limit the scope and applicability of results, as reviews conducted only by local groups tend to reflect more the specific context in which they were performed. On the other hand, international partnerships favor the inclusion of more diverse data, allow consideration of different health systems, and broaden cultural and professional perspectives on the subject. For example, differences in clinical protocols, health policies, or drug availability among countries may enrich analysis and expand the validity of findings. These factors strengthen methodological quality, reduce bias, and make conclusions more useful and relevant to different realities (Bonetti et al., 2022).

In addition, editors and reviewers may value studies involving multicenter teams, suggest collaborations when appropriate, and make clear in editorial policies that diversity of authorship is a positive aspect. Such actions not only increase visibility and scientific impact but also help consolidate evidence synthesis as a decision-support tool in healthcare with greater global representativeness (Bonetti et al., 2022; Wagner et al., 2015; Li et al., 2016).

These results reinforce the importance of practices such as critical discussion of evidence quality, acknowledgment of knowledge gaps, use of appropriate tools for risk of bias assessment, and methodological transparency. Although the number of SRs and meta analyses on pharmacy services has increased, methodological quality and transparency have not kept pace, compromising the robustness of conclusions and limiting their clinical applicability. In this context, the reliability of evidence-based practice directly depends on the quality of the studies used, making the careful application of recognized methodological tools essential to ensure internal and external validity. Furthermore, it is necessary to integrate scientific findings with clinical experience and patient values, stimulating the development of critical appraisal skills among pharmacists, especially in shared decision-making contexts. Systematic use of instruments such as ROBIS or AMSTAR-2 and prioritization of reviews registered in databases such as International Prospective Register of Systematic Reviews (PROSPERO), with transparent protocols, may increase the accuracy and safety of decisions. Together, these factors strengthen the reliability, applicability, and utility of conclusions, allowing SRs to achieve high standards of quality and support clinical practice more effectively (Bonetti et al., 2022; Wagner et al., 2015; Li et al., 2016).

To ensure the quality of an SR, some essential factors must be considered:

- **Methodological quality of primary studies:** The inclusion of methodologically sound studies strengthens the reliability of results, as well conducted reviews may have their conclusions compromised if based on low-rigor research. However, excluding primary studies with low methodological quality or high risk of bias from SRs is not recommended; instead, conclusions must take into account the identified biases so that results are interpreted with caution (Higgins et al., 2024).
- **Rigor in the conduct of the review:** SRs should be conducted according to a protocol formulated before the start of the search, which is fundamental to ensuring transparency and quality of the review. The protocol should explicitly contain the research question, inclusion and exclusion criteria, and a description of the methods to be used (search strategy, selection, extraction, and data analysis). Prior registration of the protocol ensures transparency and reproducibility and can be performed on platforms such as the PROSPERO or the Open Science Framework, or through the publication of the protocol as a scientific article (Higgins et al., 2024).
- **Broad and rigorous bibliographic search:** The literature search must be broad and utilize more than one database, chosen according to the research question. There are general databases such as PubMed/Medline, Embase, and Scopus, as well as more specialized ones, including national databases or those focused on thematic areas. Furthermore, it is important to use search strategies that combine appropriate terms and keywords, ensuring the search is both sensitive and specific, thereby reducing the risk of missing relevant

studies and minimizing bias (Higgins et al., 2024).

- **Consistent and transparent critical appraisal:** The analysis of available evidence quality is essential for evidence-based practice, and in this context, the proper use of specific tools is fundamental. To assess the risk of bias in SRs, the ROBIS tool is highlighted, identifying potential sources of bias that may compromise the validity of results and conclusions. Meanwhile, the R-AMSTAR and AMSTAR-2 tools are aimed at assessing the methodological quality of reviews, verifying whether they were conducted according to rigorous standards. The use of these tools favors the appropriate interpretation of evidence quality and contributes to safer decisions in clinical practice (Bonetti et al., 2022; Higgins et al., 2024).
- **Clarity and completeness in the presentation of results:** It is essential that SRs present in detail the characteristics of included studies, as this facilitates data interpretation and enables relevant comparisons. This transparency increases the utility of the review for clinical practice (Higgins et al., 2024).
- **Recognition and management of heterogeneity:** Differences in methods, populations, interventions, or outcomes should be identified, described, and properly managed to avoid misinterpretations or misleading conclusions. Heterogeneity can be clinical, methodological, or statistical, with the latter often assessed through the I^2 test and visual inspection of *forest plots*. When present, strategies such as subgroup analyses, metaregression, or exclusion of high risk of bias studies should be considered. Failure to recognize heterogeneity may lead to overestimation or underestimation of effects, compromising the applicability of results in clinical practice (Bonetti et al., 2022; Higgins et al., 2024).
- **Periodic updating of the review:** Regardless of topic, new studies are continuously published, and incorporating this evidence into the SR is essential to maintain its relevance and ensure that conclusions reflect the current state of knowledge. Failure to update may lead to clinical decisions based on outdated or incomplete evidence (Higgins et al., 2024).

In summary, the reliability of SRs and meta analyses directly depends on methodological rigor and transparency in conduct and reporting. Improving these practices is essential for evidence synthesis to fulfill its role in guiding healthcare decisions in a safe, efficient, and relevant manner.

5 Questions for further discussion

Why do so many SRs on pharmacy services present a high risk of bias?

The high risk of bias in pharmacy services may be related to the authors' lack of familiarity with adequate methods of conducting and reporting, including the formulation of well-structured questions, the definition of inclusion/exclusion criteria, and the correct use of methodological assessment tools. Inexperience in applying guidelines such as PRISMA or instruments such as ROBIS also contributes to failures in the process.

In addition, many primary studies have fragile methodological designs, with small samples, the absence of a control group, or incomplete data, which compromises the reliability of findings and increases the risk of bias in SRs.

Another relevant factor is the low use of previously registered protocols, such as PROSPERO, which may lead to selectivity in the choice of studies or outcomes analyzed.

Finally, the pressure to publish and the lack of multidisciplinary teams experienced in research methodology and statistics often result in SRs being conducted without the necessary rigor, reducing the validity and clinical applicability of the results.

- **How can pharmacists contribute to improving the quality of SRs in their field?**

To improve the quality of SRs in pharmacy services, it is essential that pharmacists who use this evidence pay attention to all stages of the process, ensuring rigorous compliance with established recommendations. In addition, it is crucial that they have knowledge of health technology assessment and are able to perform consistent critical appraisal of evidence. Expertise in areas such as pharmacy, pharmacology, therapeutics, and medication safety is also indispensable to add value to reviews.

Specifically, pharmacists developing these syntheses may contribute at the following stages:

1. **Formulation of the research question:** Ensuring that the question is clear, relevant, and applicable to clinical practice.
2. **Selection and critical appraisal of studies:** Properly applying inclusion/exclusion criteria, conducting careful analysis of selected studies, assessing methodological quality, evaluating the applicability of results in daily practice, and determining relevance to the research question.

3. **Synthesis and interpretation of studies:** Extracting relevant data and analyzing results objectively, identifying clinical implications, and methodological limitations. Pharmacists may provide important contributions to interpreting findings related to medications, pharmacy practice, and interactions, always focusing on the safety and usefulness of conclusions.
4. **Review and standardization of reporting:** Ensuring that the review follows predefined protocols for reporting results, such as PRISMA, thereby guaranteeing transparency and reproducibility.
5. **Dissemination and practical application of results:** Translating SR findings into clinical practice is one of the most relevant functions, as this is the point where knowledge transforms into real impact, whether in direct patient care or in decision-making within health institutions.

- **What is the role of editors and reviewers in ensuring methodological quality?**
  Editors and reviewers have a fundamental role in ensuring the quality of SRs and should:

- Confirm prior registration of the protocol on platforms such as PROSPERO and verify whether it was followed as planned.

Assess the clarity, rationale, and relevance of the research question.

1. Analyze the search strategy, verifying whether it was comprehensive, sensitive, specific, relevant to the topic, and adequately described. They should also verify whether the chosen databases were appropriate and whether the strategies were adapted for each database.
2. Assess study selection and data extraction, ensuring independent review to reduce errors and bias.
3. Analyze the synthesis of results, ensuring that narrative or metaanalytical methods are appropriate and justified.
4. Ensure that conclusions answer the original research question and are aligned with the findings and limitations of the studies, providing reliable results while avoiding extrapolations or misinterpretations.
5. Check the correct use of tools for risk of bias and methodological quality assessment.
6. Ensure reporting follows recognized guidelines, such as PRISMA, and provides complete and transparent information.

Such careful assessment by editors and reviewers contributes to the reliability, scientific integrity, and applicability of published evidence.

- **How can the PRISMA, R-AMSTAR, and ROBIS tools be integrated into the routine process of producing and evaluating SRs?**
  Integration of PRISMA, R-AMSTAR, and ROBIS tools into the routine of SRs should begin at the planning stage, not just at the final evaluation stage. To make this feasible, it is essential to offer training and promote the dissemination of best practices among researchers responsible for conducting studies.

In addition to training, another important strategy is to make the use of these tools a prerequisite for the submission or acceptance of scientific articles. This requirement would encourage authors to incorporate them into their daily practice, thereby strengthening SR quality from the earliest stages. For this measure to be effective, journal author guidelines should provide clear instructions and support for the correct application of these tools.

Integrated adoption of these tools, from planning to publication, brings evident benefits: it promotes greater transparency, increases confidence in conclusions, and ensures more methodological rigor. At the same time, it strengthens shared responsibility among authors, reviewers, and editors, with the aim of continuously improving SR quality and making them increasingly useful and applicable to clinical practice.

6 Application exercise/scenario

6.1 Scenario 1: Public health

You work as a pharmacist in a Primary Health Care (PHC) team and have been assigned to evaluate the feasibility of implementing a medication review service for patients with type 2 diabetes, aiming to improve glycemic control and reduce associated complications.

The coordinator requested that the decision be based on robust scientific evidence, and for this purpose, you selected two SRs with meta analyses on the topic.

However, upon analyzing the documents, you noticed that they present important methodological differences, including differences in reporting evidence quality, search methods, and risk of bias assessment.

6.1.1 SR A

- PRISMA: 25/27
- R-AMSTAR: 33/44
- ROBIS: High risk of bias
- Conclusion: "The medication review service appears promising for reducing HbA1c, but included studies presented risk of bias and high heterogeneity."

6.1.2 SR B

- PRISMA: 21/27
- R-AMSTAR: 26/44
- ROBIS: Low risk of bias
- Conclusion: "Moderate-quality evidence suggests that the medication review service may reduce HbA1c in patients with T2DM in PHC. Further studies are needed for confirmation."

Questions and Answers:

1. *One of the selected reviews presents a high PRISMA score but was classified as high risk of bias by ROBIS. How would you interpret this situation?*

This indicates that the SR was well-reported but poorly conducted from a methodological perspective. PRISMA assesses reporting quality, i.e., whether authors clearly described methods, results, and limitations. However, good reporting does not guarantee adequate or unbiased methods. ROBIS, on the other hand, specifically evaluates the risk of bias in review conduct, considering aspects such as inclusion criteria, the study selection process, critical appraisal of primary studies, and data synthesis. Therefore, a high PRISMA score associated with a high ROBIS risk of bias reveals that, although the review was transparently presented, its conclusions may be compromised by substantial methodological flaws.

2. *Based on these data, which review would you consider more appropriate to support your recommendation for PHC coordination? Justify your choice.*

SR B is more appropriate to support the recommendation, even with slightly lower PRISMA and R-AMSTAR scores. This is justified by two main factors: (1) a low risk of bias according to ROBIS, meaning the methods were more rigorous and the study was more reliably conducted; (2) a more cautious conclusion aligned with the level of certainty of the evidence, indicating moderate quality and the need for further studies, demonstrating methodological integrity and scientific transparency.

In clinical practice, evidence reliability is more important than reporting completeness. SRs with a low risk of bias, even if they do not report all PRISMA items, tend to produce more reliable conclusions than well-reported but methodologically flawed studies. Therefore, Review B represents a stronger basis for supporting an informed, safe, and proportionate decision, especially for a new service to be implemented in PHC.

6.2 Scenario 2: Hospital

You are a hospital manager and have been designated to evaluate whether there is robust evidence to implement a medication reconciliation service at hospital discharge as part of patient safety strategies. A recent metaanalysis shows positive results; however, you decide to critically evaluate the study using the PRISMA, R-AMSTAR, and ROBIS tools. You identify that the review does not report evidence quality, omits heterogeneity data, and lacks a registered protocol.

Questions and Answers:

1. *Is the evidence sufficiently robust to support the decision?*

No, it is not sufficient. Although the metaanalysis presents positive results, the absence of essential information compromises evidence robustness and reliability. The lack of tools such as GRADE to classify evidence quality, the omission of heterogeneity in the included studies, and the absence of a registered protocol are critical flaws identified by PRISMA, R-AMSTAR, and ROBIS. These factors increase the risk of bias, hinder the reproducibility of the study, and reduce transparency in evidence synthesis. For evidence to be considered robust, it must be based on a rigorous synthesis of the best available evidence, critically assessed for risk of bias and consistency of findings, and applicable to the local clinical context.

2. *What are the main risks of relying solely on this metaanalysis?*

Relying exclusively on this metaanalysis may entail the following risks:

- Decision-making based on low-quality evidence may compromise the effectiveness of the implemented intervention (in this case, medication reconciliation).
- Inefficient allocation of human and financial resources occurs if the service does not yield the expected benefits.
- False sense of institutional safety, leading managers and teams to believe that the intervention is validated by reliable evidence.
- Negative impacts on patient safety may arise if reconciliation is not well-structured, properly trained, and effectively monitored.
- Reputational and ethical risks, especially in public institutions, arise if questioned about justifying interventions based on questionable science.

3. *What actions would you recommend taking before making a policy decision?*
   Before deciding to implement the service, it is recommended to:

- Seek higher-quality SRs, preferably with Grading of Recommendations Assessment, Development and Evaluation (GRADE) evaluation, a registered protocol, and explicit heterogeneity assessment.
- Consult reliable clinical guidelines, such as those published by World Health Organization (WHO), National Institute for Health and Care Excellence (NICE), or Agency for Healthcare Research and Quality (AHRQ).
- Consider conducting a rapid evidence synthesis or consulting a health technology assessment unit to deepen the analysis in the short term.

6.3 Scenario 3: Community pharmacy

You work as a pharmacist in a community pharmacy and have been invited to participate in a screening program for hypertension and diabetes, offering blood pressure and capillary glucose measurements, with referrals to primary care in suspected cases. To support your decision, you consult two SRs on screening in community pharmacies.

6.3.1 SR A

- PRISMA: 23/27
- R-AMSTAR: 29/44
- ROBIS: High risk of bias
- Conclusion: "Screening in community pharmacies appears to improve the detection of undiagnosed cases of hypertension and diabetes; however, the included studies presented a high risk of bias and significant variation in outcomes."

6.3.2 SR B

- PRISMA: 20/27
- R-AMSTAR: 32/44
- ROBIS: Low risk of bias
- Conclusion: "Moderate-quality evidence indicates that screening may contribute to the early detection of hypertension and diabetes, although long-term studies are needed to assess the impact on clinical outcomes."

Questions and Answers:

1. *What does it mean to find a review with a high risk of bias, even if it presents a good PRISMA score?*
   PRISMA evaluates the transparency of reporting but does not guarantee methodological quality. ROBIS identifies flaws such as poorly defined inclusion criteria, the absence of risk of bias assessments of primary studies, or inadequate analyses. Thus, an SR may be well-reported but still methodologically limited.
2. *Which review would be more appropriate to support the decision to implement the screening service?*
   Review B is more appropriate, as it presents a low risk of bias and more balanced conclusions. Despite the slightly lower PRISMA score, its methodological conduct was more rigorous, conferring greater reliability to support the decision.
3. *What additional aspects should be considered before implementing the screening program?*

- Availability of clear and standardized protocols
- Training of pharmacy staff
- Integration with PHC for referral and follow-up
- Cost-effectiveness evaluation, still little explored
- Impact on relevant clinical outcomes, such as the reduction of cardiovascular complications

The incorporation of pharmacy services in different settings—primary care, hospitals, and community pharmacies—requires decisions supported by high-quality scientific evidence. Although SRs and meta analyses are valuable sources, their utility depends on the critical evaluation of methodological rigor and risk of bias.

Tools such as PRISMA, R-AMSTAR, and ROBIS allow for the analysis of both reporting transparency and the robustness of review conduct, showing that good reporting may hide critical flaws, just as a methodologically solid review may lack transparency.

For pharmacists, adopting this critical perspective is fundamental to distinguishing reliable evidence from weak evidence, strengthening decision-making, increasing service safety, and amplifying the impact of clinical practice. Assessing evidence quality is, therefore, not optional but a core competence to align professional practice with the best available science and with the needs of patients and health systems.

AI disclosure

During the preparation of this work, the author(s) used ChatGPT for English translation, grammar, and spelling correction. After using this tool/service, the author(s) reviewed and edited the content as needed and take(s) full responsibility for the content of the publication.

Appendix Supplementary material

Supplementary material related to this chapter can be found online at http://dx.doi.org/10.1016/B978-0-443-44607-8.00013-3.

References

Allemann, S.S., Van Mil, J.W.F., Botermann, L., Berger, K., Griese, N., Hersberger, K.E., 2014. Pharmaceutical care: the PCNE definition 2013. Int. J. Clin. Pharm. 22107703. 36 (3), 544–555. Available from: http://springerlink.metapress.com/content/2210-7703/. doi:10.1007/s11096-014-9933-x.

Bonetti, A.F., Della Rocca, A.M., Lucchetta, R.C., Tonin, F.S., Fernandez-Llimos, F., Pontarolo, R., 2020. Mapping the characteristics of meta-analyses of pharmacy services: a systematic review. Int. J. Clin. Pharm. 22107711. 42 (5), 1252–1260. Available from: http://springerlink.metapress.com/content/2210-7703/. doi:10.1007/s11096-020-01058-5.

Bonetti, A.F., Tonin, F.S., Rocca, A.M.D., Lucchetta, R.C., Fernandez-Llimos, F., Pontarolo, R., 2022. Methodological quality and risk of bias of meta-analyses of pharmacy services: a systematic review. Res. Soc. Adm. Pharm. 15517411. 18 (3), 2403–2409. Available from: http://www.journals.elsevierhealth.com/periodicals/rsap. doi:10.1016/j.sapharm.2020.12.011.

Higgins, J.P.T., Thomas, J., Chandler, J., 2024. Cochrane Handbook for Systematic Reviews of Interventions, Version 6.5. Cochrane. Available from: https://www.cochrane.org/authors/handbooks-and-manuals/handbook.

Ioannidis, J.P.A., 2016. The mass production of redundant, misleading, and conflicted systematic reviews and meta-analyses. Milbank Q. 14680009. 94 (3), 485–514. Available from: http://onlinelibrary.wiley.com/journal/10.1111/(ISSN)1468-0009. doi:10.1111/1468-0009.12210.

Kung, J., Chiappelli, F., Cajulis, O.O., Avezova, R., Kossan, G., Chew, L., Maida, C.A., 2010. From systematic reviews to clinical recommendations for evidence-based health care: validation of revised assessment of multiple systematic reviews (R-AMSTAR) for grading of clinical relevance. Open Dent. J. 1874-2106. 4 (1), 84–91. doi:10.2174/1874210601004010084.

Li, L., Catalá-López, F., Alonso-Arroyo, A., Tian, J., Aleixandre-Benavent, R., Pieper, D., Long, G., Yao, L., Wang, Q., Yang, K., Hayasaka, S., 2016. The global research collaboration of network meta-analysis: a social network analysis. PLOS ONE. 1932-6203. 11 (9), e0163239. doi:10.1371/journal.pone.0163239.

Moher, D., Shamseer, L., Clarke, M., Ghersi, D., Liberati, A., Petticrew, M., Shekelle, P., Stewart, L.A., 2015. Preferred reporting items for systematic review and meta-analysis protocols (PRISMA-P) 2015 statement. Syst. Rev. 2046-4053. 4 (1). doi:10.1186/2046-4053-4-1.

Moullin, J.C., Sabater-Hernández, D., Fernandez-Llimos, F., Benrimoj, S.I., 2013. Defining professional pharmacy services in community pharmacy. Res. Soc. Adm. Pharm. 15517411. 9 (6), 989–995. doi:10.1016/j.sapharm.2013.02.005.

Page, M.J., McKenzie, J.E., Bossuyt, P.M., Boutron, I., Hoffmann, T.C., Mulrow, C.D., Shamseer, L., Tetzlaff, J.M., Akl, E.A., Brennan, S.E., Chou, R., Glanville, J., Grimshaw, J.M., Hróbjartsson, A., Lalu, M.M., Li, T., Loder, E.W., Mayo-Wilson, E., McDonald, S., McGuinness, L.A., Stewart, L.A., Thomas, J., Tricco, A.C., Welch, V.A., Whiting, P., Moher, D., 2021. The PRISMA 2020 statement: an updated guideline for reporting systematic reviews. BMJ. 17561833. 372. Available from: http://www.bmj.com/. doi:10.1136/bmj.n71.

PRISMA Statement, n.d. Available from: https://www.prisma-statement.org.

Rotta, I., Salgado, T.M., Silva, M.L., Correr, C.J., Fernandez-Llimos, F., 2015. Effectiveness of clinical pharmacy services: an overview of systematic reviews (2000–2010). Int. J. Clin. Pharm. 22107711. 37 (5), 687–697. Available from: http://springerlink.metapress.com/content/2210-7703/. doi:10.1007/s11096-015-0137-9.

Shea, B.J., Grimshaw, J.M., Wells, G.A., Boers, M., Andersson, N., Hamel, C., Porter, A.C., Tugwell, P., Moher, D., Bouter, L.M., 2007. Development of AMSTAR: a measurement tool to assess the methodological quality of systematic reviews. BMC Med. Res. Methodol. 14712288. 7. doi:10.1186/1471-2288-7-10.

Shea, B.J., Reeves, B.C., Wells, G., Thuku, M., Hamel, C., Moran, J., Moher, D., Tugwell, P., Welch, V., Kristjansson, E., Henry, D.A., 2017. AMSTAR 2: a critical appraisal tool for systematic reviews that include randomised or non-randomised studies of healthcare interventions, or both. BMJ. 0959-8138. 358, j4008. doi:10.1136/bmj.j4008.

Stewart, L.A., Clarke, M., Rovers, M., Riley, R.D., Simmonds, M., Stewart, G., Tierney, J.F., 2015. Preferred reporting items for a systematic review and meta-analysis of individual participant data: the PRISMA-IPD statement. JAMA. 15383598. 313 (16), 1657–1665. Available from: http://jama.jamanetwork.com/article.aspx?articleid=2279718. doi:10.1001/jama.2015.3656.

Tonin, F.S., Borba, H.H., Leonart, L.P., Mendes, A.M., Steimbach, L.M., Pontarolo, R., Fernandez-Llimos, F., 2019. Methodological quality assessment of network meta-analysis of drug interventions: implications from a systematic review. Int. J. Epidemiol. 14643685. 48 (2), 620–632. Available from: http://ije.oxfordjournals.org/. doi:10.1093/ije/dyy197.

Tricco, A.C., Lillie, E., Zarin, W., O'Brien, K.K., Colquhoun, H., Levac, D., Moher, D., Peters, M.D.J., Horsley, T., Weeks, L., Hempel, S., Akl, E.A., Chang, C., McGowan, J., Stewart, L., Hartling, L., Aldcroft, A., Wilson, M.G., Garritty, C., Lewin, S., Godfrey, C.M., MacDonald, M.T., Langlois, E.V., Soares-Weiser, K., Moriarty, J., Clifford, T., Tunçalp, Ö., Straus, S.E., 2018. PRISMA extension for scoping reviews (PRISMA-ScR): checklist and explanation. Ann. Intern. Med. 15393704. 169 (7), 467–473. Available from: http://annals.org/aim/fullarticle/2700389/prisma-extension-scoping-reviews-prisma-scr-checklist-explanation. doi:10.7326/M18-0850.

Wagner, C.S., Park, H.W., Leydesdorff, L., Glanzel, W., 2015. The continuing growth of global cooperation networks in research: a conundrum for national governments. PLOS ONE. 1932-6203. 10 (7), e0131816. doi:10.1371/journal.pone.0131816.

Whiting, P., Savović, J., Higgins, J., 2018. ROBIS: tool to assess risk of bias in systematic reviews—guidance on how to use ROBIS. Guidance document. University of Bristol, School of Social and Community Medicine, Bristol. https://www.bristol.ac.uk/media-library/sites/social-community-medicine/robis/robisguidancedocument.pdf. (Acessed 29 June 2026).

Whiting, P., Savović, J., Higgins, J.P.T., Caldwell, D.M., Reeves, B.C., Shea, B., Davies, P., Kleijnen, J., Churchill, R., 2016. ROBIS: a new tool to assess risk of bias in systematic reviews was developed. J. Clin. Epidemiol. 18785921. 69, 225–234. Available from: www.elsevier.com/locate/jclinepi. doi:10.1016/j.jclinepi.2015.06.005.

CHAPTER

6

Developing high-quality research questions

Jordan R. Covvey[a], Michael R. Gionfriddo[b], Melissa A. Kalarchian[c], David A. Nolfi[d], and Chyna McClendon[a]

[a]Duquesne University, School of Pharmacy, Pittsburgh, PA, United States
[b]Geisinger College of Health Sciences, Scranton, PA, United States
[c]Duquesne University, School of Nursing, Pittsburgh, PA, United States
[d]Duquesne University, Gumberg Library, Pittsburgh, PA, United States

CHAPTER OBJECTIVES

- Identify the value of detailed research questions within pharmacy research
- Develop fully articulated research questions using the PICO framework
- Evaluate research questions for iterative quality improvement using the FINER criteria

1 Introduction

Research is a fundamental and necessary process to advance the science and practice of pharmacy. This process involves many steps (Fig. 6.1), and at each step, researchers must take care to ensure their project is designed in such a way that the findings can be trusted. This chapter (along with our corresponding chapter on literature searching) is not intended to be a comprehensive guide to conducting high-quality research. It will, however, help researchers develop fundamental skills so that their research begins with a solid foundation. Given that all research starts with an idea, this chapter will specifically guide you through the process of converting that idea into a well-formulated research question. By following this method, pharmacy researchers can develop a more detailed research proposal, feeling confident in the foundation of their project.

Writing quality research questions may seem simplistic compared to other sophisticated methods used by pharmacy researchers and described throughout this book. However, research questions are not merely the first step; they are the foundation on which a rigorous study is built (Covvey et al., 2024). A well-crafted research question, grounded in the literature, directly informs the study's design and methods. Without one, researchers risk producing results that are irrelevant and contribute to waste in research. These shortcomings often come to light at the conclusion of a project during the dissemination stage, when researchers struggle to justify their key decisions: "*Why did you choose this population or method? Why did you study this instead of that? What is the value of this work within today's practice?*" Even experienced researchers may find themselves tempted to rush through this initial step in the

Contemporary Research Methods in Pharmacy and Health Services - Volume 2
https://doi.org/10.1016/B978-0-443-44607-8.00008-X

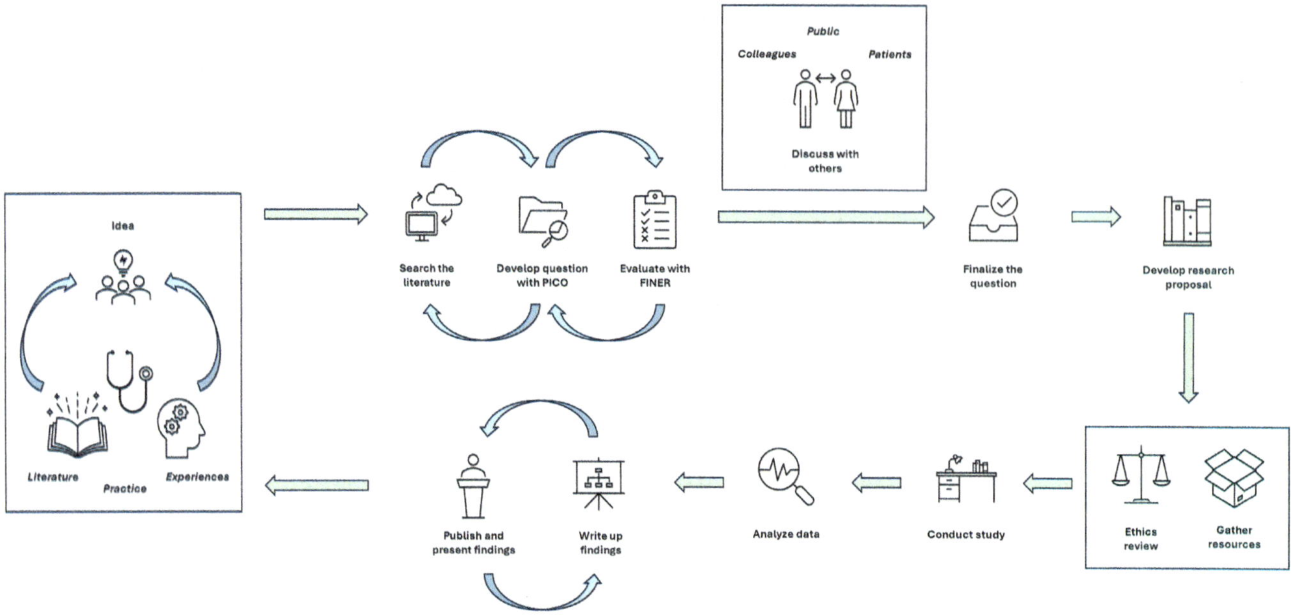

FIG. 6.1 The scientific research process. Research begins with an idea, which is operationalized into a research question using PICO/FINER and a thorough literature review. Subsequent steps in the process include the development of a research proposal, an ethics review, gathering resources, conducting the study, analyzing data, writing up the findings, and publishing or presenting the findings.

research process, which can undermine the coherence and impact of the work. Therefore, we advocate for time and effort spent carefully crafting research questions to prevent issues downstream.

2 Method

There are many types of research questions (Kamper, 2020). Some questions are focused on formal hypothesis testing, while others are aimed at more open exploration and discovery. They can vary in their goals, including descriptive, associative/predictive, and causal aims. No matter the type, the research question should serve as a framework that will guide the design, conduct, analysis, and reporting of the research. Having a clear and well-specified research question will help inform what design may be best, what methods may be most appropriate, what data is necessary to collect, and how to analyze the data. This coherence across all aspects of a study helps to contribute to the quality of the research, as well as improve the ability of the researcher to effectively and efficiently conduct the research. The process of developing a sound question is highly iterative; documentation is, therefore, essential to success (Box 6.1).

For example, many pharmacy researchers have an impulse to collect as many different variables as possible, particularly given the complicated nature of patient care. Less often, there is a clear plan for why they are collecting these variables, how they will be analyzed, and how they will contribute to the overall conclusions. If the researcher is conducting a study requiring manual review of the data, each additional data point impacts the feasibility of conducting the study. If the data is collected but there is no clear thought regarding the variables used and the relationships between them, the researcher risks integrating questionable research practices (e.g., p-hacking) or failing to adjust for confounding factors.

2.1 Where research questions come from

Research ideas arise from a variety of places. Informally, these may include experiences a researcher has had professionally (e.g., interesting past projects) or personally (e.g., individual situations), or they may be based on discussions with friends, mentors, or colleagues. Within the healthcare environment, ideas can arise from various care processes (Box 6.2); pharmacy researchers commonly draw from experiences with patients where the existing

BOX 6.1

Documentation for research questions

As you iteratively develop a research question, remember that rigorous research should be reproducible. Creating clear, detailed documentation can help you during the development of a question, but it can also help you as you conduct, analyze, or publish your findings to remember why you made certain decisions. Consider keeping a physical or electronic notebook where you can jot down ideas on items such as:

- What inspired the research idea?
- What is already documented in the literature?
- The gap your question will address
- What ideas have you eliminated, and why?
- Exemplar or pilot studies you have already identified
- Justification for how to operationalize and measure different variables
- Pros/cons of different methodological approaches
- Resources to support the chosen approach (e.g., methods papers)
- Potential funders and deadlines

BOX 6.2

Research questions within clinical environments

- Clinical evidence: synthesizing clinical findings
- Diagnosis: interpreting results
- Prognosis: predicting patient outcomes
- Therapy: choosing effective treatments
- Prevention: lessening the risk of disease
- Education: communicating essential information

From Richardson, W. Scott, Wilson, Mark C., Nishikawa, Jim & Hayward, Robert S.A. (1995). The well-built clinical question: a key to evidence-based decisions. ACP Journal Club, 123(3). https://doi.org/10.7326/acpjc-1995-123-3-a12

evidence was unclear. Increasingly, generative artificial intelligence (AI) is being utilized as a mechanism for researchers to brainstorm ideas, contributing to another source of inspiration. Concerns, however, have been raised about its role in the many tasks it is increasingly used for, such as the potential for the creation of "echo chambers" within information retrieval (Goswami, 2025). From each of these sources of inspiration, researchers should consider how their position, experiences, and background influence what questions are asked and the potential for bias within their development of questions (Greco et al., 2016), particularly given the homogeneity of the research community itself (Clair et al., 2022). Furthermore, researchers often compose questions that are familiar to them, assuming certain interventions and outcomes without fully and impartially exploring the area of interest. As researchers develop their questions, they should critically assess their assumptions and the extent to which they may negatively affect the development of a fair and objective research question (University of Alaska Fairbanks, 2025).

While research questions can be inspired by individual experiences, more often, ideas come from "the literature," or the existing collection of scientific work that has been published. Scientific papers are being published at an exponential rate. Data from the National Science Foundation estimated a global output of over 3.3 million publications in science and engineering in 2022, with health sciences representing the largest proportion (25%) of publications (National Science Foundation., 2023). In 2010, it was estimated that 75 trials and 11 systematic reviews were published daily (Bastian et al., 2010), while in 2021, this estimate had grown to 80 systematic reviews per day (Hoffmann et al., 2021). Researchers are tasked with understanding what this literature communicates (in their given area of science) and designing their own research to complement it. A careful review of the literature can help researchers identify gaps and their question's place in addressing those gaps; however, similar to drawing on personal experiences, researchers should be mindful of biases in how research is published and identified through literature searches.

2.2 Characteristics of a good research question

Good research questions specify the "who," "what," "why," and "how" of a given project. Although an idea or topic area can be broad and nebulous, a research question is specific and refined. It essentially operationalizes an idea into something actionable. To assist researchers in composing questions, a variety of formalized frameworks have been developed (Booth et al., 2019; Davies, 2011; Food and Drug Administration; Health Evidence; Hulley et al., 2013; Hosseini et al., 2024). These frameworks guide researchers on the different elements they should include in their research questions. The most common framework is **P**atient, **I**ntervention, **C**omparison, and **O**utcome (**PICO**) (or one of several variations, including PICOT ((including **t**iming) (Riva et al., 2012), PICOTS (including **t**iming and **s**etting) (Food and Drug Administration), or PECO (with E for exposure) (Morgan et al., 2018)). This framework is well-suited to assist in composing most quantitative-based questions in pharmacy-related research. Other frameworks can be utilized for qualitative, mixed-methods, or evaluation research, using similar schemes (Table 6.1). For the purposes of this chapter, we will focus on PICO-driven questions.

2.2.1 P—patient

Research questions begin with clearly defining the patient group, or more generally, "who" you intend to study. This assists the research proposal downstream because the choices made here impact methodological decisions later, including the target population and sample. Choosing a patient group requires a researcher to delineate the inclusion/exclusion criteria (Capili, 2021), which generates consideration of how selection bias may impact the study and its goals. Consider the use of hormone replacement therapy (HRT) for cardiovascular disease (CVD), where early observational studies suggested a benefit, but later randomized trials demonstrated harm (Rossouw et al., 2002). Populations in observational studies of patients who took HRT were more likely to have protective factors for CVD (e.g., exercise) that contributed to the resulting difference (Humphrey et al., 2002). Accordingly, this aspect of the research question is important in determining whether a chosen sample is likely to be systematically different in important ways from the population to which the researcher wants to apply their results.

TABLE 6.1 Frameworks for specifying research questions.

Framework	Primary usage	Components	Brief description
PICO (Richardson et al., 1995)	Quantitative research	Patient	The subjects of interest
		Intervention	The action being tested
		Comparison	What the process is being tested against
		Outcome	The result of interest
SPIDER (Cooke et al., 2012)	Qualitative and mixed-methods research	Sample	The subjects of interest
		Phenomenon of interest	The how and why are being studied
		Design	How the method is created/implemented
		Evaluation	The measurement of the outcome
		Research type	The specific approach
SPICE (Booth, 2006)	Project/service evaluation	Setting	The context of the question
		Perspective	Interested parties (potential or actual)
		Intervention/interest/exposure	The action taken
		Comparison	The alternative action
		Evaluation	Measurement of the success
ECLIPSE (Wildridge and Bell, 2002)	Policy/service evaluation	Expectation	Outcome targeted for improvement
		Client group	Who the policy/service targets
		Location	Where the policy/service is located
		Impact	What change is being investigated
		Professionals	Who is involved in delivering
		Service	Kind of service/policy

2.2.2 *I—intervention*

The intervention, or more generally "what" you are proposing to study, may include items such as medication, behavioral interventions, educational interventions, pharmacy services, or systems-level strategies to improve the uptake of evidence-based practices. It may also include exposures rather than interventions (as referenced within the similar PECO framework (Morgan et al., 2018); language related to interventions is utilized in experimental studies, whereas language related to exposures is used in observational studies. When specifying the intervention/exposure, it is important to be clear and specific about the components, defining any empirical or theoretical foundations that underpin the choice.

For interventions involving medications, specification often includes factors such as the dose, frequency, and route, but it could also include factors such as timing, strength, or dosage form. For other types of interventions, helpful guidance has been developed to assist researchers in specifying their treatment or implementation strategies (Proctor et al., 2013; Hoffmann et al., 2014). The process of specifying an intervention or exposure should help clarify important aspects of the study design, conduct, and analysis. The questions that arise when developing an intervention can help refine a researcher's thinking about what they intend to study and will also help later on when assessing the feasibility of doing so.

2.2.3 *C—comparison*

Although not all studies require or use a comparison or control group, they remain important in many research designs, as the use of a control can help isolate the effect of the intervention from other effects (Grimes and Schulz, 2005). These other effects may include the natural progression of disease, cooccurring interventions, or chance. There are many different types of comparisons that can be used, and these are often incompletely described in studies (Webster et al., 2019). In pharmacy-based research, these often include placebos, sham treatments, standard of care, or no treatment, to name a few. When specifying the comparison, a researcher should use similar guidance to that provided for interventions so that the control or comparison condition is clear and supports reproducibility. This is particularly important since the description of controls has been identified as inadequate across analyses of published research (Mills et al., 2004, 2005; Yu et al., 2018).

Careful consideration of the control or comparison is essential to defining other aspects of the study design. Consider the choice between parallel and cross-over studies; the former requires the recruitment of a larger sample, while the latter enables participants to serve as their own control. The choice of comparison may also impact the blinding or masking procedures, such as the need to incorporate a double-dummy procedure when comparing oral versus intravenous medications. The choice of comparison can also affect the interpretation of a study. Many pharmacy-based studies evaluate a new service against usual care, commonly defined as the standard or routine method by which a healthcare service is delivered. However, usual care can differ across healthcare institutions and practices, and it can evolve significantly over time (de Bruin et al., 2009). Finally, the choice of comparison can influence the applicability of your study, especially if inappropriate or inferior comparators are used (Hilal et al., 2019). For example, if a clinical trial finds that a medication is better than usual care, but the dose of the control medication is below what would be considered the standard of care, the result would only be applicable to the use of a suboptimal dose not used in routine care.

2.2.4 *O—outcome*

Outcomes in studies can target one potential effect or may span multiple outcome domains. They may include clinical outcomes ("*medical events that occur as a result of disease or treatment*"), economic outcomes (costs of the intervention, which may include direct medical, direct nonmedical, indirect, or intangible costs), humanistic outcomes ("effects of *disease or treatment on patient functional status or quality of life*"), and implementation outcomes ("*effects of deliberate and purposive actions to implement new treatments, practices, and services*") (Proctor et al., 2011; Kozma et al., 1993). For some research questions, there may be core outcome sets to consider when defining your outcomes of interest—these are collections of outcomes, typically judged by panels of experts, to be important for generating evidence for a condition (Williamson et al., 2017). Choosing outcomes depends on the target audience, what the research aims to change, and what evidence that audience needs to make decisions regarding whether that change should be made (Iwashyna and McPeake, 2018). In many instances, researchers need to choose a primary outcome upon which to base the statistical power of the study. However, decisions in practice are often informed by the totality of the evidence; as such, secondary or exploratory outcomes are also important to consider for relevant end users. For instance, trials of new medications often evaluate efficacy as the primary outcome of interest, but clinicians, patients, and regulators are also interested in the safety of the intervention.

When defining the outcomes, a researcher should consider when and how outcomes will be measured (Coster, 2013). The timing of outcome assessment should be long enough after receiving the intervention to reasonably observe an effect, but not so long that unmeasured confounding may obscure the effect. For example, consider the impact of in-hospital care on hospital readmissions. Typical quality measures use 30-day readmissions as a benchmark; however, studies have suggested that out-of-hospital effects are more likely to influence readmissions than in-hospital care after about seven days (Chin et al., 2016). In addition to the timing of the outcome assessment, researchers need to consider how to measure the outcome. This includes the data source (e.g., self-report, insurance claims, records documentation, or objective evidence), the collection approach (e.g., using trained data extractors with quality checks), and the assessment method used (e.g., choosing between various scales or measurement approaches).

2.2.5 Bringing it all together

PICO essentially provides a framework for researchers to operationalize their research idea. Although a research question is often summarized in a single sentence, it references a deeper and more detailed plan within its composition. By individually working through each domain, a researcher must confront a variety of questions about how they plan to design and execute their research (Table 6.2). Clear specification is important as researchers embark on the next step in the process, which is self-evaluation.

TABLE 6.2 An example using PICO.

Component	Example questions to consider	Linked considerations
Consider an example of a researcher interested in studying GLP-1 agonists in diabetes.		
P (Patients)	• Will you focus on type 2 diabetes mellitus (the labeled indication), or will you also include patients with type 1 or latent adult-onset diabetes (off-label indications)? • When identifying patients with diabetes, will you use self-reported diagnoses, ICD coding from medical records, or diagnostic laboratory results as recorded in the EMR? • Do you want to include patients initiating the medication with well-controlled or poorly controlled diabetes? Should the patients be treatment-experienced or newly diagnosed? • Will you place restrictions on age, gender, race/ethnicity, or other factors to define the sample? How might you manage patients with comorbid conditions (e.g., obesity) that may impact the achievement of the outcome?	• Helps to define the inclusion/exclusion criteria and determine the external validity • Impacts the design of the study (retrospective vs. prospective) and the ideal setting (primary care vs. specialist care).
I (Intervention) C (Control)	• Are you interested in a specific care process related to treatment with GLP-1 agonists (e.g., a pharmacist-led diabetes service), or only the medication itself? Will you include all GLP-1 agonists or specific medications within the class (e.g., semaglutide, liraglutide, etc.)? • Will you evaluate it against another medication, such as SGLT-2 inhibitors, for comparison? • What doses will you study, particularly given that this medication is often titrated according to patient tolerance and effects over time? What routes and regimens are you interested in, given the availability of both oral and subcutaneous formulations? • Given that diabetes is often treated with complex regimens, what other treatments are patients allowed to receive alongside the intervention or control of interest during the study? • Will you track patient adherence to the intervention? If so, will this be done using patient self-report, EMR prescribing data, pharmacy fill data, or direct observation?	• Impacts the design of the study (observational vs. experimental) and how potential confounders can be handled • Relates to external validity and whether the study's conclusions are likely to reflect what clinicians observe or perform in real-world practice
O (Outcome)	• What timeframe will you use for the primary outcome? Is this better suited for surrogate outcomes like BG/HgbA1c, or macrovascular outcomes like CVD? • Will you measure secondary outcomes in other domains, such as patient satisfaction, quality of life, or symptom burden? • What tools or sources of data will be used to assess the outcome(s)? Are they valid and reliable? Have they been used previously for similar analyses? • How will you manage patients who drop out of the study in the final analysis (particularly if it is due to adverse effects)? What strategy will be employed for handling missing data?	• Connects to the duration of the study required to measure the chosen outcomes (days, months, or years) • Influences sample size calculations and the statistical power of the study

BG = blood glucose; CVD = cardiovascular disease; EMR = electronic medical record; HgbA1c = hemoglobin A1c; ICD = International Classification of Diseases; GLP-1 = glucose-like peptide-1; SGLT-2 = sodium-glucose cotransporter 2.

2.3 Self-evaluation of research questions

Once a researcher has ensured that the question they want to investigate is clear and well-specified, it is time to evaluate whether: (1) the question can be answered with the resources available, (2) the researcher (and others) are interested in answering the question, (3) the question has been answered before, (4) the question raises any ethical concerns, and finally, (5) what impact answering this question will have upon the field at large. These considerations, captured in the mnemonic **F**easible, **I**nteresting, **N**ovel, **E**thical, and **R**elevant (**FINER**), can be used by researchers to critically appraise their drafted research questions (Table 6.3) (Elsevier Author Services; Farrugia et al., 2010; Fandino, 2019; Kwiatkowski and Silverman, 1998).

2.3.1 *F—feasible*

The first component (F) addresses the practicality of the research question. Arguably, the most important evaluation question is whether a researcher has the necessary resources to conduct the proposed research. Resources should be considered broadly, including items such as time, finances, personnel, expertise, physical space, necessary equipment, data, and participants. It is not uncommon for investigators to embark on a research project only to find later that they lacked the resources to properly complete it (Sica, 2002; Goldberg et al., 2022). If, after inventorying existing resources or the availability of additional resources, a researcher finds that their project is not feasible, they should revisit the research question and assess whether anything can be modified to increase feasibility (without compromising the project overall). For example, if the initial design was prospective but the researcher faces time constraints, it is worthwhile to consider whether a retrospective design is appropriate. Similarly, if a researcher is measuring an outcome that takes time to manifest (e.g., death in primary prevention of CVD) or is difficult to measure (e.g., directly observed medication adherence), they may consider the use of surrogate markers (e.g., cholesterol) or more feasible methods of data collection (e.g., use of claims data). There are many ways that researchers can design a given study, and feasibility often influences these choices. When making trade-offs, however, researchers need to have honest dialogs about how such changes impact what their study is able to achieve.

Finally, it is important to consider the scope of the question and whether it can be broken down into smaller, more feasible components. In modifying the question to improve feasibility, a researcher will often, but not always, face tradeoffs involving the internal and external validity of the study. When evaluating these tradeoffs, consider whether the redesigned question is likely to meaningfully contribute to the body of evidence, as well as whether the refined question meets the other components of FINER.

2.3.2 *I—interesting*

As mentioned previously, research projects are often resource-intensive endeavors. To effectively and continually mobilize those resources requires immense interest in the research question. Initially, this interest should come from the researcher. Are they interested enough to devote the resources needed to properly craft a research question? As

TABLE 6.3 Definitions and self-assessment using the FINER criteria.

Component	Definition	Self-assessment questions
Feasible	Can the research question be answered, given the available resources?	Do you have the items needed for the research? Do you have the skills to execute the research? Is the planned time frame appropriate for the work?
Interesting	Is the research question exciting to you and the scientific community?	Are you personally interested or engaged in your project? Is the project of interest to the broader scientific community? Does your project align with the funding agency's priorities?
Novel	Does the research question aim to address an existing gap in knowledge?	What is known, and what is unknown? What are the limitations in existing research in the field? Has it been done before?
Ethical	Does the research question protect and respect the subjects of interest?	Does your research minimize potential harm? Are you working with a vulnerable population or researching an area with specific ethical concerns? Have you engaged in ethical oversight processes?
Relevant	Will the research question lead to societal improvements?	What is the potential impact of your research? What are the needs of the interested parties? Are you providing value for money?

they craft that question and consider the project's feasibility, are they still interested, recognizing that many projects require months to years to complete? In addition to their own interest, researchers should identify whether collaborators, funders, and the broader community of researchers are also interested in the research question. This provides an external viewpoint that is ultimately needed for the research to generate scientific or clinical value once completed. It also impacts feasibility, given that a lack of interest from funders can mean the requisite resources for a given question are not available. Assessing interest can be determined through conversations with relevant parties, a review of current funding opportunities, or past funded projects.

Finally, consider whether the question is of interest to the end user of the research, who are often patients or the general public. In fact, patient and public involvement is now required by many funders (e.g., Patient-Centered Outcomes Research Institute (PCORI)) and journals (e.g., British Medical Journal (*BMJ*)), and it may improve the feasibility, acceptability, applicability, validity, and relevance of research projects (Lammons et al., 2025). Indeed, the phrase *"nothing about us without us"* has been adapted over the years for many purposes but, in this context, reinforces the value that community inclusion brings to research development (Chu et al., 2016; Gionfriddo et al., 2025; Oliver et al., 2009; Boote et al., 2014).

2.3.3 N—*novel*

The ideal research question, if answered, adds clarity to a phenomenon. This clarity can come from discovering something new about the phenomenon or from gaining additional resolution on a known phenomenon by reducing uncertainty through increased statistical precision or methodological rigor. The National Institutes of Health (NIH) particularly values novelty with regard to research funding, supporting innovative research that pushes biomedicine forward (Packalen and Bhattacharya, 2020). However, there is a balance to be struck between the incremental versus breakthrough nature of science, with both pursuits essential to progress (Falkenberg et al., 2022).

Judging the novelty of a research question requires engagement with the existing literature to understand which phenomena or aspects of a phenomenon could benefit from additional clarity (Ioannidis et al., 2014). For example, while searching the literature may confirm a lack of research in an area, often the search may uncover many studies. At this point, a researcher needs to consider whether (1) the existing studies address their specific proposed question (by comparing PICOs), (2) the existing evidence base could be improved through additional studies with enhanced statistical precision (i.e., through meta-analysis or conducting a primary study that can then be meta-analyzed), or (3) the proposed study approach will address methodological issues in the existing evidence. For example, in this last case, researchers may identify concerns in the existing evidence about the replicability of a result and propose to repeat a study. Replications have value but should be undertaken deliberately and thoughtfully so as not to waste resources (Engineering National Academies of Sciences, 1991).

Consider the classic case of streptokinase for myocardial infarction. Between 1959 and 1988, there were 32 trials published examining this question; yet, if a metaanalysis had been conducted, clear evidence of effect would have been identified in 1973 after only eight trials were published (Lau et al., 1992). This phenomenon of not reviewing or synthesizing the existing research when embarking on a research project is common, with the percentage of reports using systematic reviews to justify new studies ranging from 16% to 87% (Andreasen et al., 2022). Alternatively, consider that replication can also raise questions about the reliability of the original findings. Sometimes this can lead to moderation of the initially observed effect, while other times it can lead to contradictory results, which may arise due to chance, study limitations, or misconduct (Prasad et al., 2013; Alahdab et al., 2018; Ioannidis, 2005).

2.3.4 E—*ethical*

Researchers need to consider not only how their research question is composed but also whether it should be conducted. A research question may be appropriate in design but still generate concerns relevant to its methodology. There are cases where a placebo control is not appropriate from an ethical perspective, whereas in other cases, a higher level of informed consent procedures is needed to prevent coercion of a vulnerable population (Gordon, 2020). There are a number of specialized areas across research that warrant special consideration, such as work with embryonic stem cells, cloning, AI, and private health data.

To ensure the ethical conduct of research, there are well-defined regulatory mechanisms (National Commission for the Protection of Human Subjects of Biomedical and Behavioral Research., 1979), such as institutional review boards (IRBs). These mechanisms have arisen from numerous historical abuses of human rights within science (e.g., the Tuskegee study of syphilis, the Willowbrook study of hepatitis, the Stateville Penitentiary study of malaria, and Nazi experimentation) and aim to prevent such atrocities from happening again (Beecher, 1966; Jones et al., 2016). Although the time and effort associated with navigating ethical safeguards may sometimes feel frustrating for researchers, it is essential to the research process. Ethics in science should not be viewed as just an administrative hurdle. Researchers have a responsibility beyond formal approval from bodies like IRBs to ensure that they are investing time and resources into endeavors that are worthwhile. For instance, researchers with funding from the NIH and other federal agencies are entrusted with public funds supported by taxation; ethical use of these funds not only requires adherence to regulations, policies, and procedures but also ensuring that the money being spent is used judiciously through rigorous research that will benefit the public good.

2.3.5 *R—relevant*

Finally, research questions should be crafted such that, by answering them, the researcher can generate a significant impact. This impact will look different depending on the type of research being conducted. For example, for a pharmacologist, it may involve establishing the mechanism of action or target of a novel compound (e.g., which may lead to the identification of a compound with therapeutic potential). For a clinical researcher, it may involve establishing the efficacy of that compound (e.g., which, if efficacious may lead to new treatments for disease). For a pharmacovigilance researcher, it may involve identifying rare but serious side effects (e.g., to ultimately inform regulatory or clinical decision-making). Finally, for health services researchers, this may involve understanding the barriers to the use of evidence-based treatment (e.g., to ultimately inform interventions to facilitate the use of these treatments).

Although the research question may not always have a direct impact on health, practice, or policy, careful consideration of the relevance of a research question, how it advances knowledge, and the practical implications of that knowledge is important to support the translation of those findings toward the ultimate goal of advancing human flourishing. When considering whether a question is relevant, it is important to consider who the end users of the evidence are. That is, the evidence generated by answering the question should be relevant to and inform their decision-making. Failure to consider the relevance of a research project contributes to research waste, may delay translation, and may generate evidence that does not meet the needs of the end-users. For example, one analysis found that education and self-help were judged as a higher priority than medications for research for patients with osteoarthritis, yet the majority of trials are on medications (Chalmers et al., 2014; Tallon et al., 2000). Accordingly, community-engaged research is increasingly encouraged within healthcare (Michener et al., 2012).

As discussed previously, the generation of research questions can be influenced by researchers' personal biases, which may contribute to questions relevant to certain groups not being asked (impacting both relevance and ethics). Researchers should recognize that many groups have been systematically excluded from research and scientific advancement (e.g., women, racial/ethnic minorities, 2SLGBTQIA +, etc.) or that investigation in these populations was not deemed as important as other pursuits. Consequently, we encourage researchers, as they develop their questions, to carefully reflect on the extent to which their research efforts will inform meaningful improvements for those most in need.

3 Discussion

The information laid out in this chapter can provide a framework for researchers developing research questions. Researchers seeking to apply this framework should be mindful of several considerations. First, research is often a collaborative endeavor, and the development of a research question benefits from discussions with colleagues involved in the work, as well as colleagues external to the work who can provide helpful insights. Engagement in professional groups and local, regional, and national networking can also be invaluable to this process. Sometimes they will validate your ideas, and other times they may offer a new perspective. Gathering multiple perspectives, including those of stakeholders, will help pharmacy researchers gauge the interest and relevance of their question and may strengthen the feasibility by connecting the researcher with potential collaborators or funders. Interested parties in the scientific research process include, but are not limited to, the public, patients, family members, providers, payers, and policy makers.

Second, the framework described here must be applied critically. Research (and researchers) are susceptible to bias (Pannucci and Wilkins, 2010). Throughout the process of developing a question, researchers should ask critical questions (many of which we have provided in this chapter) about each component of their question and consider the extent to which taking the proposed approach may introduce bias. Furthermore, pharmacy researchers should self-reflect on the choices they are making, consider what is influencing those choices, and evaluate the impact of those choices. For example, are they asking a question in such a way that it will generate the answer they want (e.g., by using selective inclusion/exclusion criteria, unfair comparisons, or inappropriate outcome measures) (Baldwin et al., 2022)? Are they being honest about how potential conflicts of interest may impact their research goals and ultimate work (Ostengaard et al., 2020)? Reflexivity, or reflecting on potential partiality, as well as transparency in documenting key decisions, is essential to maintaining rigor in pharmacy research and minimizing bias (Finlay, 2002). The goal is not to eliminate bias but to document limitations and potential sources of bias throughout the research process.

Third, it is rare for a researcher to generate a research idea fully formed; as emphasized here, the idea will often undergo several rounds of revision. Thus, researchers should expect the process of developing a research question using this framework to include feedback loops as a result of critical reflection, collaboration with others, or emergent evidence. Application of the FINER criteria can be invaluable. For example, a clinician may witness a situation within their practice [*a patient taking a glucose-like peptide (GLP)-1 agonist who loses interest in social alcohol consumption*] and be inspired to develop a research idea based on it. They then search the literature and find that, while their original idea has already been evaluated, the relevant literature calls for additional research around a specific aspect of the clinical problem (*the influence of GLP-1 agonists on heavy drinking days among patients with alcohol use disorder*). The researcher then begins to sketch out a research question based on that gap and, after evaluating the feasibility at their institution, realizes they do not have the resources (*access to patients within the psychiatric clinic*) to conduct a robust study to answer the question as originally posed. However, after discussing the matter with a mentor, they realize that through collaboration (*with a psychiatric pharmacist colleague*) and by leveraging some funding (*targeting quality improvement projects at their institution*), they can increase the feasibility of executing a study to answer that new question.

This example illustrates the iterative nature of generating a research question. Although iteration is important during question development, once a study has been initiated, researchers should avoid changing their questions in response to data. For example, changing the primary outcome or statistical analysis plan, as well as selectively reporting the findings, would be inappropriate (Nagy et al., 2025; Goldacre et al., 2019a, 2019b). Solid research questions in pharmacy form the foundation to support rigorous scientific research that can move the field forward and have a public health impact.

4 Questions for further discussion

- What have been the most common sources of research questions throughout your career?
- How do collaboration and team-based science improve the generation of research questions?
- How do you balance the creation of desired and optimal research questions with real-world feasibility?
- In what ways can you purposefully engage interested parties in your research earlier in the process during research question generation? What value can that provide to planning?

5 Application exercise/scenario

An ambulatory care pharmacist in a primary care clinic conducts a review of records from the past year and discovers that a considerable proportion of the clinic's adult patients with hypertension have been prescribed antihypertensive medications yet continue to have high blood pressure. They engage a team through their health system to investigate antihypertensive prescribing and patient adherence.

1. Map out a potential research question using the PICO framework for this scenario.
2. What information (beyond the scenario) would you need to further specify your question and study?
3. What skills and resources would your team need to execute your proposed study?
4. How might the FINER criteria assist in refining your research question?
5. In what ways is your proposed research question interesting to the profession of pharmacy?

AI disclosure

During the preparation of this work, the author(s) used Microsoft Copilot to assist in abstract generation for this chapter. After using this tool/service, the author(s) reviewed and edited the content as needed and take full responsibility for the content of the publication.

References

Alahdab, F., Farah, W., Almasri, J., Barrionuevo, P., Zaiem, F., Benkhadra, R., Asi, N., Alsawas, M., Pang, Y., Ahmed, A.T., Rajjo, T., Kanwar, A., Benkhadra, K., Razouki, Z., Murad, M.H., Wang, Z., 2018. Treatment effect in earlier trials of patients with chronic medical conditions: a meta-epidemiologic study Mayo Clin Proc. 93 (3), 278–283. Available from: https://pubmed.ncbi.nlm.nih.gov/29477781/. doi:10.1016/j.mayocp.2017.10.020.

Andreasen, J., Norgaard, B., Draborg, E., Juhl, C.B., Yost, J., Brunnhuber, K., Robinson, K.A., Lund, H., 2022. Justification of research using systematic reviews continues to be inconsistent in clinical health science-A systematic review and meta-analysis of meta-research studies. PLoS One. 1932-6203. 17 (10), e0276955. Available from: https://www.ncbi.nlm.nih.gov/pubmed/36315526. doi:10.1371/journal.pone.0276955.

Baldwin, J.R., Pingault, J.B., Schoeler, T., Sallis, H.M., Munafo, M.R., 2022. Protecting against researcher bias in secondary data analysis: challenges and potential solutions. Eur. J. Epidemiol. 1573-7284. 37 (1), 1–10. Available from: https://www.ncbi.nlm.nih.gov/pubmed/35025022. doi:10.1007/s10654-021-00839-0.

Bastian, H., Glasziou, P., Chalmers, I., 2010. Seventy-five trials and eleven systematic reviews a day: how will we ever keep up? PLoS Med. 1549-1676. 7 (9), e1000326. Available from: https://www.ncbi.nlm.nih.gov/pubmed/20877712. doi:10.1371/journal.pmed.1000326.

Beecher, H.K., 1966. Ethics and clinical research. N. Engl. J. Med. 0028-4793. 274 (24), 1354–1360. Available from: https://www.ncbi.nlm.nih.gov/pubmed/5327352. doi:10.1056/NEJM196606162742405.

Boote, J.D., Dalgleish, M., Freeman, J., Jones, Z., Miles, M., Rodgers, H., 2014. 'But is it a question worth asking?' A reflective case study describing how public involvement can lead to researchers' ideas being abandoned. Health Expect. 1369-7625. 17 (3), 440–451. Available from: https://www.ncbi.nlm.nih.gov/pubmed/22646745. doi:10.1111/j.1369-7625.2012.00771.x.

Booth, A., 2006. Clear and present questions: formulating questions for evidence based practice. Library Hi Tech 24 (3), 355–368.

Booth, A., Noyes, J., Flemming, K., Moore, G., Tuncalp, O., Shakibazadeh, E., 2019. Formulating questions to explore complex interventions within qualitative evidence synthesis. BMJ Glob. Health. 2059-7908. 4 (Suppl 1), e001107. Available from: https://www.ncbi.nlm.nih.gov/pubmed/30775019. doi:10.1136/bmjgh-2018-001107.

Capili, B., 2021. Selection of the study participants. Am. J. Nurs. 1538-7488. 121 (1), 64–67. Available from: https://www.ncbi.nlm.nih.gov/pubmed/33350703. doi:10.1097/01.NAJ.0000731688.58731.05.

Chalmers, I., Bracken, M.B., Djulbegovic, B., Garattini, S., Grant, J., Gulmezoglu, A.M., Howells, D.W., Ioannidis, J.P., Oliver, S., 2014. How to increase value and reduce waste when research priorities are set. Lancet. 1474-547X. 383 (9912), 156–165. Available from: https://www.ncbi.nlm.nih.gov/pubmed/24411644. doi:10.1016/S0140-6736(13)62229-1.

Chin, D.L., Bang, H., Manickam, R.N., Romano, P.S., 2016. Rethinking thirty-day hospital readmissions: shorter intervals might be better indicators of quality of care. Health Aff. (Millwood. 2694-233X. 35 (10), 1867–1875. Available from: https://www.ncbi.nlm.nih.gov/pubmed/27702961. doi:10.1377/hlthaff.2016.0205.

Chu, L.F., Utengen, A., Kadry, B., Kucharski, S.E., Campos, H., Crockett, J., Dawson, N., Clauson, K.A., 2016. "Nothing about us without us"-patient partnership in medical conferences. BMJ. 1756-1833. 351, i3883. Available from: https://www.ncbi.nlm.nih.gov/pubmed/27628427. doi:10.1136/bmj.i3883.

Clair, C.A., Melvin, T.J., Taylor, J.L., Saylor, M.A., 2022. "Researcher" bias: how our assumptions on technology affect research of older adults. Front. Public Health. 1034497. 2296-2565(10), Available from https://www.ncbi.nlm.nih.gov/pubmed/36407974 10.3389/fpubh.2022.1034497.

Cooke, A., Smith, D., Booth, A., PICO, B., 2012. The SPIDER tool for qualitative evidence synthesis. Qualitative Health Research. 15527557. 22 (10), 1435–1443. doi:10.1177/1049732312452938.

Coster, W.J., 2013. Making the best match: selecting outcome measures for clinical trials and outcome studies. Am. J. Occup. Ther. 1943-7676. 67 (2), 162–170. Available from: https://www.ncbi.nlm.nih.gov/pubmed/23433270. doi:10.5014/ajot.2013.006015.

Covvey, J.R., McClendon, C., Gionfriddo, M.R., 2024. Back to the basics: guidance for formulating good research questions. Res. Social Adm. Pharm. 1934-8150. 20 (1), 66–69. Available from: https://www.ncbi.nlm.nih.gov/pubmed/37838572. doi:10.1016/j.sapharm.2023.09.009.

Davies, K.S., 2011. Formulating the evidence based practice question: a review of the frameworks. Evid. Based Libr. Inf. Pract. 6 (2), 75–80. doi:10.18438/B8WS5N.

de Bruin, M., Viechtbauer, W., Hospers, H.J., Schaalma, H.P., Kok, G., 2009. Standard care quality determines treatment outcomes in control groups of HAART-adherence intervention studies: implications for the interpretation and comparison of intervention effects. Health Psychol. 1930-7810. 28 (6), 668–674. Available from: https://www.ncbi.nlm.nih.gov/pubmed/19916634. doi:10.1037/a0015989.

Elsevier Author Services. Navigating the research landscape: A deep dive into the FINER method. https://scientific-publishing.webshop.elsevier.com/research-process/finer-research-framework/

Engineering National Academies of Sciences, 1991. Duplication, replication, and complementarity: Challenges in organization research and service programs in the PHS, 109–118. https://www.ncbi.nlm.nih.gov/books/NBK234549/.

Falkenberg, R., Fochler, M., Sigl, L., Burstmayr, H., Eichorst, S., Michel, S., Oburger, E., Staudinger, C., Steiner, B., Woebken, D., 2022. The breakthrough paradox: how focusing on one form of innovation jeopardizes the advancement of science: how focusing on one form of innovation jeopardizes the advancement of science. EMBO Rep. 1469-3178. 23 (7), e54772. Available from: https://www.ncbi.nlm.nih.gov/pubmed/35620860. doi:10.15252/embr.202254772.

Fandino, W., 2019. Formulating a good research question: pearls and pitfalls. Indian J Anaesth. 0019-5049. 63 (8), 611–616. Available from: https://www.ncbi.nlm.nih.gov/pubmed/31462805. doi:10.4103/ija.IJA_198_19.

Farrugia, P., Petrisor, B.A., Farrokhyar, F., Bhandari, M., 2010. Practical tips for surgical research: research questions, hypotheses and objectives. Can. J. Surg. 1488-2310. 53 (4), 278–281. Available from https://www.ncbi.nlm.nih.gov/pubmed/20646403.

Finlay, L., 2002. "Outing" the researcher: the provenance, process, and practice of reflexivity. Qual. Health Res. 1049-7323. 12 (4), 531–545. Available from: https://www.ncbi.nlm.nih.gov/pubmed/11939252. doi:10.1177/104973202129120052.

Food and Drug Administration Using the PICOTS framework to strengthen evidence gathered in clinical trials - guidance from the AHRQ's Evidence-based Practice Centers https://www.fda.gov/media/109448/download

Gionfriddo, M.R., McClendon, C., Nolfi, D.A., Kalarchian, M.A., Covvey, J.R., 2025. The importance of rigor in pharmacy research: challenges and solutions. Res. Social Adm. Pharm. 1934-8150. 21 (5), 424–430. Available from: https://www.ncbi.nlm.nih.gov/pubmed/39948010. doi:10.1016/j.sapharm.2025.02.005.

Goldacre, B., Drysdale, H., Dale, A., Milosevic, I., Slade, E., Hartley, P., Marston, C., Powell-Smith, A., Heneghan, C., Mahtani, K.R., 2019a. COMPare: a prospective cohort study correcting and monitoring 58 misreported trials in real time. Trials. 1745-6215. 20 (1), 118. Available from: https://www.ncbi.nlm.nih.gov/pubmed/30760329. doi:10.1186/s13063-019-3173-2.

Goldacre, B., Drysdale, H., Marston, C., Mahtani, K.R., Dale, A., Milosevic, I., Slade, E., Hartley, P., Heneghan, C., 2019b. COMPare: qualitative analysis of researchers' responses to critical correspondence on a cohort of 58 misreported trials. Trials. 1745-6215. 20 (1), 124. Available from: https://www.ncbi.nlm.nih.gov/pubmed/30760328. doi:10.1186/s13063-019-3172-3.

Goldberg, A., Bakhireva, L.N., Page, K., Henrie, A.M., 2022. A qualitative scoping review of early-terminated clinical trials sponsored by the Department of Veterans Affairs Cooperative Studies Program from 2010 to 2020. Epidemiol. Rev. 1478-6729. 44 (1), 110–120. Available from: https://www.ncbi.nlm.nih.gov/pubmed/36193844. doi:10.1093/epirev/mxac009.

Gordon, B.G., 2020. Vulnerability in research: basic ethical concepts and general approach to review. Ochsner J. 1524-5012. 20 (1), 34–38. Available from: https://www.ncbi.nlm.nih.gov/pubmed/32284680. doi:10.31486/toj.19.0079.

Goswami, G., 2025. AI echo chambers: how algorithms shape reality, influence democracy, and fuel misinformation. TechRxiv. doi:10.36227/techrxiv.174059950.03385147/v1.

Greco, A.N., Wharton, R.M., Brand, A., 2016. Demographics of scholarly publishing and communication professionals. Learn. Publ. 29 (2), 97–101. doi:10.1002/leap.1017.

Grimes, D.A., Schulz, K.F., 2005. Compared to what? Finding controls for case-control studies. Lancet. 1474-547X. 365 (9468), 1429–1433. Available from: https://www.ncbi.nlm.nih.gov/pubmed/15836892. doi:10.1016/S0140-6736(05)66379-9.

Health Evidence, Developing an efficient search strategy using PICO https://healthevidence.org/practice-tools.aspx#PT2

Hilal, T., Sonbol, M.B., Prasad, V., 2019. Analysis of control arm quality in randomized clinical trials leading to anticancer drug approval by the US Food and Drug Administration. JAMA Oncol. 2374-2445. 5 (6), 887–892. Available from: https://www.ncbi.nlm.nih.gov/pubmed/31046071. doi:10.1001/jamaoncol.2019.0167.

Hoffmann, F., Allers, K., Rombey, T., Helbach, J., Hoffmann, A., Mathes, T., Pieper, D., 2021. Nearly 80 systematic reviews were published each day: observational study on trends in epidemiology and reporting over the years 2000-2019. J. Clin. Epidemiol. 1878-5921. 138, 1–11. Available from: https://www.ncbi.nlm.nih.gov/pubmed/34091022. doi:10.1016/j.jclinepi.2021.05.022.

Hoffmann, T.C., Glasziou, P.P., Boutron, I., Milne, R., Perera, R., Moher, D., Altman, D.G., Barbour, V., Macdonald, H., Johnston, M., Lamb, S.E., Dixon-Woods, M., McCulloch, P., Wyatt, J.C., Chan, A.W., Michie, S., 2014. Better reporting of interventions: template for intervention description and replication (TIDieR) checklist and guide. BMJ. 1756-1833. 348, g1687. Available from: https://www.ncbi.nlm.nih.gov/pubmed/24609605. doi:10.1136/bmj.g1687.

Hosseini, M.S., Jahanshahlou, F., Akbarzadeh, M.A., Zarei, M., Vaez-Gharamaleki, Y., 2024. Formulating research questions for evidence-based studies. J. Med. Surg. Pub. Health 2 (100046). doi:10.1016/j.glmedi.2023.100046.

Hulley, S.B., Cummings, S.R., Browner, W.S., Grady, D.G., Newman, T.B., Cummings, S.R., Browner, W.S., Hulley, S.B., 2013, Conceiving the Research Question and Developing the Study Plan Designing Clinical Research, 4ed. Lippincott Williams & Wilkins, Philadelphia.

Humphrey, L.L., Chan, B.K., Sox, H.C., 2002. Postmenopausal hormone replacement therapy and the primary prevention of cardiovascular disease. Ann. Intern. Med. 1539-3704. 137 (4), 273–284. Available from: https://www.ncbi.nlm.nih.gov/pubmed/12186518. doi:10.7326/0003-4819-137-4-200208200-00012.

Ioannidis, J.P., 2005. Contradicted and initially stronger effects in highly cited clinical research. JAMA. 1538-3598. 294 (2), 218–228. Available from: https://www.ncbi.nlm.nih.gov/pubmed/16014596. doi:10.1001/jama.294.2.218.

Ioannidis, J.P., Greenland, S., Hlatky, M.A., Khoury, M.J., Macleod, M.R., Moher, D., Schulz, K.F., Tibshirani, R., 2014. Increasing value and reducing waste in research design, conduct, and analysis. Lancet. 1474-547X. 383 (9912), 166–175. Available from: https://www.ncbi.nlm.nih.gov/pubmed/24411645. doi:10.1016/S0140-6736(13)62227-8.

Iwashyna, T.J., McPeake, J., 2018. Choosing outcomes for clinical trials: a pragmatic perspective. Curr. Opin. Crit. Care. 1531-7072. 24 (5), 428–433. Available from: https://www.ncbi.nlm.nih.gov/pubmed/30074502. doi:10.1097/MCC.0000000000000532.

Jones, D.S., Grady, C., Lederer, S.E., 2016. "Ethics and clinical research"–the 50th anniversary of Beecher's bombshell. N. Engl. J. Med. 1533-4406. 374 (24), 2393–2398. Available from: https://www.ncbi.nlm.nih.gov/pubmed/27305197. doi:10.1056/NEJMms1603756.

Kamper, S.J., 2020. Types of research questions: descriptive, predictive, or causal. J. Orthop. Sports Phys. Ther. 1938-1344. 50 (8), 468–469. Available from: https://www.ncbi.nlm.nih.gov/pubmed/32736498. doi:10.2519/jospt.2020.0703.

Kozma, C.M., Reeder, C.E., Schulz, R.M., 1993. Economic, clinical, and humanistic outcomes: a planning model for pharmacoeconomic research. Clin. Ther. 0149-2918. 15 (6), 1121–1132. discussion 1120, Available from https://www.ncbi.nlm.nih.gov/pubmed/8111809.

Kwiatkowski, T., Silverman, R., 1998. Research fundamentals: II. Choosing and defining a research question. Acad. Emerg. Med. 1069-6563. 5 (11), 1114–1117. Available from: https://www.ncbi.nlm.nih.gov/pubmed/9835477. doi:10.1111/j.1553-2712.1998.tb02673.x.

Lammons, W., Buffardi, A.L., Marks, D., 2025. Measuring impacts of patient and public involvement and engagement (PPIE): a narrative review synthesis of review evidence. Res. Involv. Engagem. 2056-7529. 11 (1), 76. Available from: https://www.ncbi.nlm.nih.gov/pubmed/40616180. doi:10.1186/s40900-025-00748-6.

Lau, J., Antman, E.M., Jimenez-Silva, J., Kupelnick, B., Mosteller, F., Chalmers, T.C., 1992. Cumulative meta-analysis of therapeutic trials for myocardial infarction. N. Engl. J. Med. 0028-4793. 327 (4), 248–254. Available from: https://www.ncbi.nlm.nih.gov/pubmed/1614465. doi:10.1056/NEJM199207233270406.

Michener, L., Cook, J., Ahmed, S.M., Yonas, M.A., Coyne-Beasley, T., Aguilar-Gaxiola, S., 2012. Aligning the goals of community-engaged research: why and how academic health centers can successfully engage with communities to improve health. Acad. Med. 1938-808X. 87 (3), 285–291. Available from: https://www.ncbi.nlm.nih.gov/pubmed/22373619. doi:10.1097/ACM.0b013e3182441680.

Mills, E., Loke, Y.K., Wu, P., Montori, V.M., Perri, D., Moher, D., Guyatt, G., 2004. Determining the reporting quality of RCTs in clinical pharmacology. Br. J. Clin. Pharmacol. 0306-5251. 58 (1), 61–65. Available from: https://www.ncbi.nlm.nih.gov/pubmed/15206994. doi:10.1111/j.1365-2125.2004.2092.x.

Mills, E., Wu, P., Gagnier, J., Heels-Ansdell, D., Montori, V.M., 2005. An analysis of general medical and specialist journals that endorse CONSORT found that reporting was not enforced consistently. J. Clin. Epidemiol. 0895-4356. 58 (7), 662–667. Available from: https://www.ncbi.nlm.nih.gov/pubmed/15939216. doi:10.1016/j.jclinepi.2005.01.004.

Morgan, R.L., Whaley, P., Thayer, K.A., Schunemann, H.J., 2018. Identifying the PECO: a framework for formulating good questions to explore the association of environmental and other exposures with health outcomes. Environ. Int. 1873-6750. 121 (Pt 1), 1027–1031. Available from: https://www.ncbi.nlm.nih.gov/pubmed/30166065. doi:10.1016/j.envint.2018.07.015.

Nagy, T., Hergert, J., Elsherif, M.M., Wallrich, L., Schmidt, K., Waltzer, T., Payne, J.W., Gjoneska, B., Seetahul, Y., Wang, Y.A., Scharfenberg, D., Tyson, G., Yang, Y.F., Skvortsova, A., Alarie, S., Graves, K., Sotola, L.K., Moreau, D., Rubinova, E., 2025. Bestiary of questionable research practices in psychology. Adv. Method Pract. Psychol. Sci. 8 (3). doi:10.1177/25152459251348431.

National Commission for the Protection of Human Subjects of Biomedical and Behavioral Research. The Belmont Report: ethical principles and guidelines for the protection of human subjects of research. 1979 https://www.hhs.gov/ohrp/regulations-and-policy/belmont-report/read-the-belmont-report/index.html

National Science Foundation. 2023. Publications output: US trends and international comparisons. Publication output by country, region, or economy and scientific field. Published October, https://ncses.nsf.gov/pubs/nsb202333/publication-output-by-region-country-or-economy-and-by-scientific-field.

Oliver, S., Armes, D.G., Gyte, G., 2009. Public involvement in setting a national research agenda: a mixed methods evaluation. Patient. 1178-1653. 2 (3), 179–190. Available from: https://www.ncbi.nlm.nih.gov/pubmed/22273169. doi:10.2165/11314860-000000000-00000.

Ostengaard, L., Lundh, A., Tjornhoj-Thomsen, T., Abdi, S., Gelle, M.H.A., Stewart, L.A., Boutron, I., Hrobjartsson, A., 2020. Influence and management of conflicts of interest in randomised clinical trials: qualitative interview study. BMJ. 1756-1833. 371, m3764. Available from: https://www.ncbi.nlm.nih.gov/pubmed/33109515. doi:10.1136/bmj.m3764.

Packalen, M., Bhattacharya, J., 2020. NIH funding and the pursuit of edge science. Proc. Natl. Acad. Sci. U. S. A. 1091-6490. 117 (22), 12011–12016. Available from: https://www.ncbi.nlm.nih.gov/pubmed/32430336. doi:10.1073/pnas.1910160117.

Pannucci, C.J., Wilkins, E.G., 2010. Identifying and avoiding bias in research. Plast. Reconstr. Surg. 1529-4242. 126 (2), 619–625. Available from: https://www.ncbi.nlm.nih.gov/pubmed/20679844. doi:10.1097/PRS.0b013e3181de24bc.

Prasad, V., Vandross, A., Toomey, C., Cheung, M., Rho, J., Quinn, S., Chacko, S.J., Borkar, D., Gall, V., Selvaraj, S., Ho, N., Cifu, A., 2013. A decade of reversal: an analysis of 146 contradicted medical practices. Mayo Clin. Proc. 1942-5546. 88 (8), 790–798. Available from: https://www.ncbi.nlm.nih.gov/pubmed/23871230. doi:10.1016/j.mayocp.2013.05.012.

Proctor, E.K., Powell, B.J., McMillen, J.C., 2013. Implementation strategies: recommendations for specifying and reporting. Implement. Sci. 1748-5908. 8, 139. Available from: https://www.ncbi.nlm.nih.gov/pubmed/24289295. doi:10.1186/1748-5908-8-139.

Proctor, E., Silmere, H., Raghavan, R., Hovmand, P., Aarons, G., Bunger, A., Griffey, R., Hensley, M., 2011. Outcomes for implementation research: conceptual distinctions, measurement challenges, and research agenda. Adm. Policy Ment. Health. 1573-3289. 38 (2), 65–76. Available from: https://www.ncbi.nlm.nih.gov/pubmed/20957426. doi:10.1007/s10488-010-0319-7.

Richardson, W.S., Wilson, M.C., Nishikawa, J., Hayward, R.S., 1995. The well-built clinical question: a key to evidence-based decisions. ACP J. Club. 1056-8751. 123 (3). Available from https://www.ncbi.nlm.nih.gov/pubmed/7582737.

Riva, J.J., Malik, K.M., Burnie, S.J., Endicott, A.R., Busse, J.W., 2012. What is your research question? An introduction to the PICOT format for clinicians. J. Can. Chiropr. Assoc. 1715-6181. 56 (3), 167–171. Available from https://www.ncbi.nlm.nih.gov/pubmed/22997465.

Rossouw, J.E., Anderson, G.L., Prentice, R.L., LaCroix, A.Z., Kooperberg, C., Stefanick, M.L., Jackson, R.D., Beresford, S.A., Howard, B.V., Johnson, K.C., Kotchen, J.M., Ockene, J., 2002. Investigators Writing Group for the Women's Health Initiative, Risks and benefits of estrogen plus progestin in healthy postmenopausal women: principal results From the Women's Health Initiative randomized controlled trial. JAMA. 0098-7484. 288 (3), 321–333. Available from: https://www.ncbi.nlm.nih.gov/pubmed/12117397. doi:10.1001/jama.288.3.321.

Sica, D.A., 2002. Premature termination of clinical trials–lessons learned. J. Clin. Hypertens. (Greenwich). 1524-6175. 4 (3), 219–225. Available from: https://www.ncbi.nlm.nih.gov/pubmed/12045375. doi:10.1111/j.1524-6175.2002.01094.x.

Tallon, D., Chard, J., Dieppe, P., 2000. Relation between agendas of the research community and the research consumer. Lancet. 0140-6736. 355 (9220), 2037–2040. Available from: https://www.ncbi.nlm.nih.gov/pubmed/10885355. doi:10.1016/S0140-6736(00)02351-5.

University of Alaska Fairbanks, Understanding biased and unbiased research questions. Published March 13, 2025 https://ctl.uaf.edu/2025/03/13/understanding-biased-and-unbiased-research-questions/

Webster, R.K., Howick, J., Hoffmann, T., Macdonald, H., Collins, G.S., Rees, J.L., Napadow, V., Madigan, C., Price, A., Lamb, S.E., Bishop, F.L., Bokelmann, K., Papanikitas, A., Roberts, N., Evers, A.W.M., 2019. Inadequate description of placebo and sham controls in a systematic review of recent trials. Eur. J. Clin. Invest. 1365-2362. 49 (11), e13169. Available from: https://www.ncbi.nlm.nih.gov/pubmed/31519047. doi:10.1111/eci.13169.

Wildridge, V., Bell, L., 2002. How CLIP became ECLIPSE: a mnemonic to assist in searching for health policy/ management information. Health Info. Libr. J. 1471-1834. 19 (2), 113–115. Available from: https://www.ncbi.nlm.nih.gov/pubmed/12389609. doi:10.1046/j.1471-1842.2002.00378.x.

Williamson, P.R., Altman, D.G., Bagley, H., Barnes, K.L., Blazeby, J.M., Brookes, S.T., Clarke, M., Gargon, E., Gorst, S., Harman, N., Kirkham, J.J., McNair, A., Prinsen, C.A.C., Schmitt, J., Terwee, C.B., Young, B., 2017. The COMET Handbook: version 1.0. Trials. 1745-6215. 18 (Suppl 3), 280. Available from: https://www.ncbi.nlm.nih.gov/pubmed/28681707. doi:10.1186/s13063-017-1978-4.

Yu, A.M., Balasubramanaiam, B., Offringa, M., Kelly, L.E., 2018. Reporting of interventions and "standard of care" control arms in pediatric clinical trials: a quantitative analysis. Pediatr. Res. 1530-0447. 84 (3), 393–398. Available from: https://www.ncbi.nlm.nih.gov/pubmed/29899384. doi:10.1038/s41390-018-0019-7.

CHAPTER

7

Executing high-quality literature searches

Jordan R. Covvey[a], *Michael R. Gionfriddo*[b], *Melissa A. Kalarchian*[c], *David A. Nolfi*[d], *and Chyna McClendon*[a]

[a]Duquesne University, School of Pharmacy, Pittsburgh, PA, United States
[b]Geisinger College of Health Sciences, Scranton, PA, United States
[c]Duquesne University, School of Nursing, Pittsburgh, PA, United States
[d]Duquesne University, Gumberg Library, Pittsburgh, PA, United States

CHAPTER OBJECTIVES

- Identify the value of literature searches within pharmacy research
- Recognize available sources and methods for literature searches
- Develop a structured approach to literature searches in preparation for conducting research

1 Introduction

Scientific knowledge and publications are growing at an unprecedented rate. It is impossible for any researcher to stay current on the work in their field without regular examination of the literature, given the pace at which new knowledge is generated. Research can be designed with a variety of goals in mind—to purposely replicate existing work, to adapt previous work in new environments and/or settings, or to generate something completely novel. Regardless of the nature of the research, a literature search helps situate new research within the existing body of knowledge. Although literature searches are commonplace among most researchers, our experience has shown that even experienced researchers may benefit from a focused review on this topic, as it is often conducted with less consideration than other aspects of project design. Accordingly, this chapter will provide guidance on how to search the literature efficiently and effectively.

A clear grasp of the literature helps researchers in multiple aspects of the research process. Specifically, it can provide insight into the nature and scope of the clinical problem the research aims to address, as well as the strengths and limitations of the existing evidence, including important unanswered questions. Failure to search the literature may have several consequences depending on the stage of the research. If not conducted at the start of a research project, it may lead to research waste and potential harm through unnecessarily redundant studies. Many research studies fail to cite relevant existing literature, including randomized trials (Robinson and Goodman, 2011)

Contemporary Research Methods in Pharmacy and Health Services - Volume 2
https://doi.org/10.1016/B978-0-443-44607-8.00011-X

and systematic reviews (Clarke and Hopewell, 2013; Andreasen et al., 2022), often because researchers were unaware that such literature existed (Cooper et al., 2005). It may also result in the research being noncompetitive for funding if it fails to represent a novel or significant advancement. Overlooking key studies may negatively impact study design by applying outdated estimates of effect, unreliable outcome measures, or interventions known to be ineffective. It is also advisable to search the literature after the conclusion of the research, as placing your contributions in the context of what is known is an important component of a manuscript, using a problem/gap/hook heuristic (Lingard, 2015). Even if the literature was searched at project initiation, most research takes significant time to complete, during which new studies may be published, and failure to address these in the discussion section of a manuscript may cause issues during peer review.

Despite these recommendations, researchers have undoubtedly found themselves in peer review situations where they have read manuscripts or grants and had more questions than answers: "*What about the study by Smith* et al., *published last year on this very topic? Why is this important to investigate, given what we already know? What is the knowledge gap revealed by existing studies in this area?*" Often, such questions are a sign that more attention to a literature search is needed. Similar to composing research questions, what may seem like a straightforward step in the research process often lacks full investment by even experienced researchers. Accordingly, we advocate that renewing one's focus on literature searching is a worthwhile endeavor for any pharmacy researcher.

2 Method

Researchers spend considerable time identifying and reading literature for different reasons. In some cases, they stumble upon literature on the internet that catches their attention. In other cases, they search for assistance in solving a targeted problem in the classroom, clinical environment, or scholarly setting. More often, they purposely seek literature to learn something new or to add to their existing knowledge on a given topic. On an almost daily basis, these situations help them build informal skills in locating the information they need and identifying sources they can trust.

For pharmacy-based researchers, searching scientific literature is an essential step in the conceptualization and design of new research (Jha et al., 2022). The platforms we use to find information and the strategies we employ to search ultimately impact the results we gather and the decisions we make based on them. Using a more structured approach, with thoughtful consideration of what to search for, where to search, and how to search, will lead to more efficient and effective searches. Furthermore, careful documentation of how the search is conducted and how the results will be synthesized improves the rigor and reproducibility of the search (Box 7.1).

2.1 What to search for

We search the literature in a broad effort to seek knowledge. For novice researchers or those embarking on a new research direction, a literature search may be conducted to provide an overview of a specific topic (e.g., medication adherence measures, risk factors for diabetes mellitus). Established researchers or those preparing an introduction or discussion section of a manuscript may search the literature to stay up to date on the most recent developments in their field (e.g., new phase 3 study results, novel research methodologies). Researchers may also search the litera-

BOX 7.1

Documentation for literature searches

As you iteratively develop a literature search in tandem with refining your question, keep the goal of your search in mind. Although a literature search is commonly conducted at the start of a project, it should be repeated along the way, given the pace at which new studies are published. In order to replicate that search, documentation is essential. Consider items such as:

- Important keywords and/or index terms of interest
- Potential A&I databases
- Scientific/clinical journals of targeted interest
- Exemplary articles on what you are searching for
- Systematic/scoping reviews in your topic area
- Trial-and-error search syntax and result sets
- Use of recurring searches stored on online platforms

ture for a specific fact (e.g., how many prescriptions for atorvastatin were dispensed in the last year, in what year tirzepatide was approved by the Food and Drug Administration [FDA]). In addition, researchers may be interested in conducting a focused search of the literature to either answer a specific research question or support the development of a novel research question.

Knowledge can broadly be conceptualized as either background or foreground information (Steele, 2015). Background information generally refers to the broad, contextual knowledge on a given topic. This exists in a variety of formats, including books, websites, clinical resources, narrative reviews, and more. Foreground information, on the other hand, is the more specific, in-depth knowledge relating to a given inquiry. This is more likely to be found within primary peer-reviewed literature, such as a clinical trial published in a major biomedical journal. Both of these information types are essential to the work of pharmacy researchers. For example, in the preparation of a scientific manuscript, a researcher often uses background information to introduce the reader to the clinical issue at hand, summarizing relevant definitions, epidemiology, and context. Then, in an effort to delineate the need for their own research, researchers utilize foreground information to describe the evolution of knowledge in the specific area and where recent and evolving research is driving progress. Although the recommendations within this chapter can be utilized to seek both types of information, we will primarily focus on the latter. As a researcher looking to develop a question, identifying appropriate foreground knowledge is an essential and foundational step of the process, as reflected by the "Novel" component within the **F**easible, **I**nteresting, **N**ovel, **E**thical, and **R**elevant criteria (as discussed in our chapter on research questions) (Kwiatkowski and Silverman, 1998; Farrugia et al., 2010; Fandino, 2019). This formalized literature search to support the development of research should be composed with a specific goal in mind and use an approach that limits bias and favors knowledge-seeking.

It is worth distinguishing between literature searches (the focus of this chapter) and literature reviews, despite the fact that these terms are often used interchangeably within science. Literature searching refers to the broad process of locating relevant materials for a given topic or objective. This is only a single step within a literature review, which further includes steps related to analyzing, synthesizing, and organizing the results of the search in a manner that aims to communicate that knowledge (Patrick and Munro, 2004; Baker, 2016; Goodfellow, 2023). There are many different types of literature reviews (Grant and Booth, 2009), with common types shown below (Table 7.1). Most pharmacy researchers are most familiar with the systematic review, a transparent and documented approach to identifying, selecting, and critically appraising literature related to a specific research question. There are calls for wider adoption of systematic reviews in the planning of new research (Chalmers et al., 2014) and ample guidance on how to compose them (Higgins et al., 2024; Khan et al., 2003). However, these are not always possible or necessary; as such, researchers are advised to consider which type of literature review best fits the needs related to their research, given that pharmacy research covers a diverse array of needs.

TABLE 7.1 Common types of literature reviews in pharmacy research.

Review type	Characteristics	Pros and cons
Narrative (Sukhera, 2022)	Summarizes relevant background information	• Allows for a broader scope and flexibility in execution • Less resource-intensive to conduct and write • Prone to bias due to the subjective selection of data
Scoping (Mak and Thomas, 2022)	Maps and defines the available literature on a topic	• Exploratory in nature and good for assessing feasibility • Often includes a limited synthesis of the data
Rapid (Moons et al., 2021)	Prioritize relevant evidence on a topic	• Faster and more efficient turnaround time to produce • May omit relevant literature due to time constraints
Integrative (Dhollande et al., 2021)	Provides a holistic understanding of complex topics	• Incorporates diverse methodologies and theories • Less standardized methodology to conduct • Often complex and requiring specialized skillsets
Systematic (Yuan and Hunt, 2009)	Comprehensively synthesizes evidence on a specific question	• Rigorous, transparent, and reproducible methodology • Can include qualitative or quantitative (meta-analysis) synthesis • Time and resource-intensive to conduct
Umbrella (Belbasis et al., 2022)	Summarizes and evaluates findings from existing systematic reviews and metaanalyses	• Comprehensive yet rapid review of a body of literature • Highlights the consistency or lack thereof in a body of literature • Limited by the questions asked in the included studies and their quality

2.2 Where to search

There are many places to search, including search engines, abstracting and indexing (A&I) databases, and other sources such as grey literature. When considering where to search, researchers should consider the relevance of the source within the context of the search goal(s), the availability of the source, and the reliability of the source.

2.2.1 *Search engines*

Search engines (e.g., Google, Bing, DuckDuckGo) are widely available and commonly used tools among pharmacy researchers. They provide a familiar and comfortable way to locate relevant sources on a topic. Often, they connect to the more specific A&I databases described next. These engines, however, may produce results that are difficult to reproduce. This is due to sponsored and tailored listings based on the user's search history, which means that result sets using the same search syntax differ across users. As such, search engines are not recommended for use in systematic reviews due to a lack of reproducibility (Giustini and Boulos, 2013; Halevi et al., 2017). However, they can be useful for researchers looking for background information on a topic as well as for identifying relevant sources of grey literature (also discussed shortly).

Many of these search engines have now incorporated various artificial intelligence (AI) technologies to assist users (Jin et al., 2024). Researchers should be cautious about relying solely on these tools, given limitations such as the inclusion of biased or out-of-date training data, a tendency to "hallucinate" sources, sensitivity to prompt language, and lack of reproducibility. Furthermore, many websites now block web crawlers, which feed into these technologies, additionally limiting their usefulness for researchers performing more technical tasks.

2.2.2 *Abstracting and indexing databases*

A&I databases are specialized platforms that provide summaries (abstracts) and catalog (indexing) of scholarly literature; they essentially make scholarly literature discoverable within specific disciplines. A variety of different A&I databases exist within the realm of biomedicine, each unique in its composition, coverage, and accessibility (Table 7.2) (Gionfriddo et al., 2024; Bramer et al., 2017). Databases index different journals (usually with some level of overlap), meaning that the literature located in one database may differ from that in another. Depending on the researcher's purpose for searching the literature, searching a more specialized database (e.g., International Pharmaceutical Abstracts (IPA)) may result in fewer but more relevant results than a more general scientific database (e.g., Scopus). In addition, the researcher should consider searching several databases to improve the chances of finding relevant literature.

Beyond the relevance to the purpose of their search, researchers should also consider the availability of the database. Although there are several freely available options (e.g., PubMed), many require subscriptions, necessitating that a researcher incorporate consideration of their institutional resources into their decision. Finally, while the listings in A&I databases should be accurate and up to date, there are some limitations. For example, depending on the database, there may be an indicator that a given article has been retracted or comes from a source with poor publication practices. In addition, the presence of a record in an A&I database is not an indicator of the rigor of the research; accordingly, researchers should carefully evaluate the validity and applicability of the study findings to their research question, just as they would with any other source.

2.2.3 *Grey literature*

Most A&I databases focus on studies published in peer-reviewed literature. Although this source is critical for pharmacy researchers, data that have not been published or data that have been published outside of traditional academic channels may also be relevant (Paez, 2017). This is known as grey literature, and it is especially important for background information (Pappas and Williams, 2011). A mapping study within hospital pharmacy literature found that, on average, 13% of the literature in five selected hospital pharmacy journals came from sources other than journal articles (Barrett et al., 2016).

The use of grey literature is important in areas that rely on work done outside traditional academic sectors, including governmental bodies, nongovernmental organizations, and private/public companies, among others. Searching grey literature may also be particularly valuable in areas where publication bias is documented, such as in the case of clinical studies for medications, where peer-reviewed literature is known to highlight studies with positive results, but unpublished data submitted to the FDA reveals a different story (Hart et al., 2012). Finally, some areas of science rely on sources commonly published outside journal articles; for instance, many studies and theories in sociology, psychology, and anthropology are published as books (Savage and Olejniczak, 2022).

Although much of the grey literature is found using search engines, some A&I databases do include sources of grey literature. For example, when two of the authors conducted a study examining media coverage of semaglutide related to weight loss (Gionfriddo et al., 2025), they leveraged a combination of searches in ProQuest US Newsstream

TABLE 7.2 Common A&I databases used by pharmacy researchers.

A&I database	Access and availability	Types of literature indexed	Useful tips
PubMed	Free US NLM	• Biomedical journal articles (38 million +) • Books from PubMed Bookshelf (13,000 +)	• For best results, use clinical or scientific terms when searching • Initially, avoid using truncation or phrase searching because they disable PubMed's automatic term mapping (search translation) • Check Advanced Search to see how PubMed translates your searches, and manually modify them as needed
Embase	Paid Elsevier, Ovid	• Biomedical journal articles (46 million +) • Preprints and conference abstracts • Clinical trials (new in 2025)	• Provides extensive subheadings for drug terms, enabling more detailed searches for pharmacy researchers • Elsevier version includes a "PV Wizard" that facilitates pharmacovigilance searching • Elsevier version's PICO search option simplifies the use of Emtree index terms and the identification of alternate keywords
Scopus	Paid Elsevier, Ovid	• Science, health science, social science, and arts/humanities journal articles (100 million + dating back to 1995) • Preprints and conference abstracts • Books & book chapters	• Includes most articles from PubMed, Embase, and other databases • Incorporates subject indexing terms from other databases but does not have tools to help you use them more effectively • Enables you to easily find publications citing the articles you have found • Comparable to Web of Science, but it indexes a larger (more inclusive) number of journals
APA PsycInfo	Paid APA, EBSCO, Ovid, ProQuest	• Psychology and mental health journal articles (5 million +) • Book chapters and dissertations (psychology)	• The "APA Thesaurus of Terms" helps build extremely specific searches for psychological concepts • Provides a "Tests and Measures" filter that facilitates finding articles describing or using scales/research instruments
CINAHL	Paid EBSCO	• Nursing, allied health professions, and selected medical journal articles (number varies with version) • Books and dissertations (primarily nursing)	• Provides a smaller number of pharmacy-specific journals compared to PubMed and Embase • CINAHL is offered in five different versions with varying coverage and full text. Note the version used when reporting literature searches in published reviews
Web of Science	Paid Clarivate, Ovid (Core Collection only)	• Science, health science, social science, and arts/humanities journal articles (235 + million, dating back to 1864) • Preprints and conference abstracts • Books and book chapters	• Enables you to easily find publications that cite the articles you have found. • Comparable to Scopus, but it indexes a smaller (and more exclusive) number of journals
SciFinder^{n}	Paid ACS	• Chemistry, science, engineering, and health sciences journal articles (57 million + dating back to 1907) • Chemical reactions and substances • Patents, books, dissertations	• Includes most articles in PubMed, enabling simultaneous searching of health sciences, broader sciences, and engineering literature • Provides extensive tools for chemical structure searches • Authoritative source for chemical names and structures, including CAS Registry Numbers used to identify chemical substances
International Pharmaceutical Abstracts	Paid APA, Clarivate, EBSCO, Ovid, ProQuest	• Pharmaceuticals and the pharmaceutical industry journals (500,000 + articles dating back to 1970) • Conference abstracts	• Database is smaller than the others listed • If you are considering subscribing, ask for a trial to see if it meets your needs

ACS: American Chemical Society; *APA*: American Psychological Association; *ASHP*: American Society of Health-System Pharmacists; *CAS*: Chemical Abstracts Service; *CINAHL*: Cumulated Index in Nursing and Allied Health Literature; *EBSCO*: Elton B. Stephens Company; *MeSH*: medical subject headings; *NLM*: National Library of Medicine.

(an A&I database) and websites of highly accessed news sources (via search engines) to isolate data for the study. There are also repositories like OpenGrey (a search portal for European grey literature), the National Technical Information Service (containing U.S. government-funded data), the World Health Organization Library (containing governing and technical documents), and preprint servers (e.g., medRxiv.org), which may be useful. Within pharmacy practice, formulary guidelines, internal hospital or clinic reports, or drug safety bulletins can provide real-world data that may not appear in the peer-reviewed literature.

Regardless of how grey literature is identified, researchers should be mindful that the sources found in grey literature are rarely peer-reviewed. Accordingly, they may vary significantly in their rigor. Although quality assessment of literature from any source is essential in any literature search (whether formal or informal), data derived from grey literature may warrant particular scrutiny.

2.3 How to search

Although the specifics of how to search will differ by source, there are general approaches that can be used to improve the efficiency and effectiveness of a literature search. Here, we illustrate these techniques within PubMed (Table 7.3), given that it is often a chosen source among pharmacy researchers due to the relevance of its content, the depth of its coverage, and the ease of its controlled vocabulary.

2.3.1 Generating keywords and index terms

The core of any search is keywords, or the text typed in the search bar of the database. Although many keywords are single words (e.g., *diabetes*), others are actually phrases (e.g., *"medication therapy management"*). Searching for phrases as opposed to the individual keywords making up a phrase can be helpful to avoid irrelevant results. In PubMed, this is accomplished using quotation marks around the phrase. Researchers should be mindful, however, that using phrase searching in certain A&I databases may affect the search in other potentially unintended ways. For example, in PubMed, when keywords are searched, PubMed automatically checks if those keywords map to

TABLE 7.3 Working with different elements within PubMed searches.

Element	Description	Examples in PubMed	Example search strings in PubMed
Keywords	Words, topics, or phrases that assist in locating relevant information in an A&I database	Author-generated based on the topic of interest, with "x x" used around phrases	Type 2 diabetes Ozempic
Index terms[a]	Controlled vocabulary is used by individual A&I databases to describe and catalog content	Using MeSH, a hierarchical vocabulary produced by the NLM	"diabetes mellitus, type 2"[MeSH] semaglutide[supplementary concept]
Boolean operators	Mechanisms to combine and connect search terms in A&I databases	AND: narrow a search, requiring results to contain all of the terms combined through the operator OR: Broaden a search by requiring the results to contain at least one of the terms NOT: recommended to be used sparingly, as it can eliminate relevant articles in ways that are not always predictable	("type 2 diabetes" OR "diabetes mellitus"[MeSH]) AND (Ozempic OR semaglutide[supplementary concept])
Field tags	Identifiers are used in A&I databases to partition different fields within a publication record	[AU] for author, [TI] for title, [TIAB] for title/abstract (and author keywords), [DP] for publication date	("type 2 diabetes"[TIAB] OR "diabetes mellitus"[MeSH]) AND (Ozempic[TIAB] OR semaglutide[supplementary concept])
Filters/limits	Mechanisms to narrow result sets in an A&I database	Article type: specific types of study designs, such as case reports, systematic reviews, and clinical trials Publication date: specific publication date range Age: patient groups (child, adult, aged)	Limit to systematic reviews conducted from December 2017 onward (when semaglutide received FDA approval)

A&I: abstracting and indexing; *FDA*: Food and Drug Administration; *MeSH*: medical subject headings; *NLM*: National Library of Medicine.

[a]*Drug-related index terms within PubMed are operationalized in different formats, including MeSH (when the drug is well-established in the literature), supplementary concepts (newer terms that need to be added quickly and have not yet achieved MeSH status), and pharmacological action (substances that have known pharmacologic effects) (National Library of Medicine).*

existing index terms. Searching for a phrase in PubMed turns off automatic term mapping, and thus, while the results may be more sensitive to your phrase of interest, you may also exclude potentially relevant records that use related but different keywords.

Index terms, sometimes called controlled vocabulary, can be used to supplement the use of keywords in a search. These terms are the formal terms used to organize records within A&I databases. Index terms are often database-specific and assigned by A&I database staff who scan articles upon publication and indexing, consulting with author-supplied keywords. For instance, within PubMed, index terms are known as medical subject headings (MeSH). As the process and method used to index articles are also variable across databases (e.g., MeSH versus Emtree), researchers may need to utilize different search strategies across databases (although there are tools to assist with search translation (Kung, 2022). Using a combination of keywords and index terms is recommended, as index terms are not always comprehensive or accurate.

For searches related to research, a starting place for generating keywords should be the research question. Consider breaking the research question down into concepts or component parts (guided by frameworks such as **P**atient, **I**ntervention, **C**omparison, and **O**utcome (Richardson et al., 1995). For each concept, consider synonyms or related terms used in the literature to describe the concept (e.g., hypertension and high blood pressure). Brainstorm terms that are less commonly used or may exist in different formats internationally [e.g., paracetamol (globally) vs. acetaminophen (in the United States)]. Consider how wildcards may help to capture multiple relevant and related terms; within PubMed, this is achieved through the use of an asterisk (e.g., pharm* to search pharmacist, pharmacy, pharmaceutical, etc.). During this stage of a search, it may be helpful to review existing literature on hand or discuss potential keywords with colleagues or librarians. When reviewing the available literature, be mindful that keywords can appear in different places, including embedded in the article itself (near the abstract), on the journal website for the article (including author keywords), or in the A&I database record linking to the article.

In addition to facilitating the capture of relevant results, the generation of keywords will help researchers identify the appropriate index terms from the A&I database, as sometimes the initial keyword may not directly translate into an index term. To identify the appropriate index term for a concept in the chosen A&I database, most databases have a dedicated search function for index terms. In that search, researchers can enter their keyword(s), and the A&I database will generate potentially relevant index terms. For example, in PubMed, there is a dedicated and searchable MeSH database connected to a function to start auto-building your search in PubMed (MeSHNational Library of Medicine (MeSH)). Once a potentially relevant index term is identified, researchers should review the description to confirm the relevance of the index term. In addition, the record for the index term will often contain the keywords that are mapped to that index term, which can be used to identify additional keywords.

2.3.2 *Incorporating boolean operators*

After the generation of search concepts using a combination of keywords and index terms, researchers can use Boolean operators to combine those concepts in meaningful ways (Fig. 7.1). The most common Boolean operators are AND, OR, and NOT. These operators work in most major search engines and A&I databases (many databases require you to type the Boolean operators in all capital letters), and, depending on how they are incorporated, they can be used to either expand or limit a search. AND is used to connect search concepts and returns results that contain the connected concepts. OR returns results that contain any one of the connected concepts and is commonly used within concepts to connect related keywords or index terms.

Finally, NOT is used to exclude certain concepts from a search. Caution is recommended when using the NOT operator, as it may exclude potentially relevant results. For example, a pharmacist might be interested in non-opioid pain management due to concerns about dependence or addiction. However, if the query includes "pain management NOT opioids," all articles that include the term "opioids" will be excluded. Because many articles could discuss *both* opioid and non-opioid approaches to pain management, this search could inadvertently exclude many relevant publications, such as studies that might compare opioids to other approaches, such as Nonsteroidal antiinflammatory drugs (NSAIDs). Both AND and NOT will result in narrower search results, while OR will expand the number of results returned. Importantly, most sources read search strings left to right, so when using multiple Boolean operators, parentheses should be used to establish the order of operations for the search.

2.3.3 *Leveraging field tags and search filters*

In addition to using the Boolean operators AND/NOT to narrow search results, pharmacy researchers can also use field tags and search filters. Databases, including those behind search engines and A&I databases, consist of a collection of records, with each record being a collection of fields. Many sources allow searching based on these fields. For example, a researcher might use "New England" as a keyword in their search. This is likely to capture a

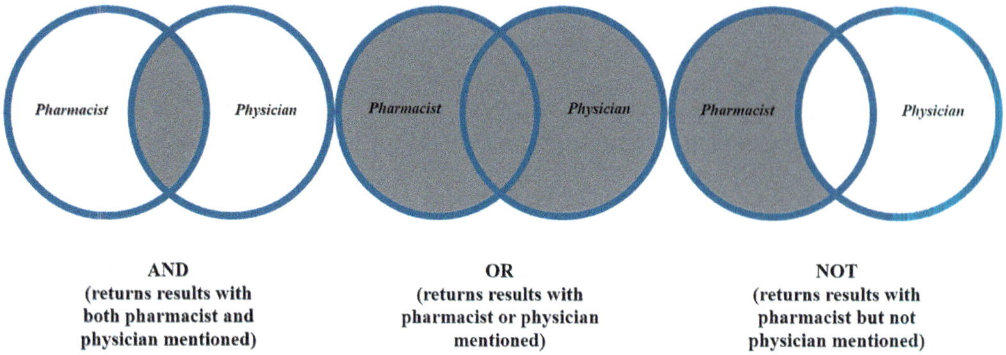

FIG. 7.1 **Visual representation of Boolean operators.** Three Venn diagrams demonstrate the differences in AND, OR, and NOT in how they return result sets within A&I databases.

broad result set, including studies set in New England geographically, as well as articles published within the *New England Journal of Medicine*. If searching this keyword with a field tag specific to a journal, it will only return results published in the journal of interest. Field tags can also be useful when researchers search for specific articles, such as when they remember a specific author and search within that specific field.

Experimenting with field tags can be an efficient way to optimize a literature search. In PubMed, for example, search syntax without field tags will return the highest number of articles (since the database is searching all available fields and automatically translating terms without quotes or asterisks). Using a field tag to search only titles or abstracts returns a smaller result set, and finally, searching only in the title field returns the smallest result set. However, while narrower search result sets may seem desirable, researchers should consider the implications. Searching only the title field will improve specificity but dampen the sensitivity of the search. Although this approach may be useful for researchers trying to identify the most up-to-date review on a topic, it may miss potentially relevant articles for researchers interested in a more comprehensive view of a field.

Search filters can also be used to limit a result set. Instead of limiting a search to a given field, filters limit a result set to those with a certain value in a given field. While field tags are applied as part of the search, filters can be applied either as part of the search or after the results are returned. Although most sources have similar filter functions, field tags may be implemented differently across databases. Similar to the use of index terms, these tools should be used with caution, as they are dependent upon accurate record entry into the database.

3 Discussion

The strategies within this chapter can assist researchers in developing and executing effective and efficient searches. While additional methodological guidance on literature is available elsewhere for developing and evaluating searches (McGowan et al., 2016; Bramer et al., 2018), in applying these techniques, researchers should be mindful of additional considerations. Namely, this includes the importance of iteration and critical reflection in search development, the dangers of confirmation bias, the importance of having a low threshold for curiosity, how the current publishing landscape affects accessible science, and the value of collaboration with experts and the use of technology.

3.1 The importance of iteration

Similar to the process of creating a research question, the execution of a literature search should be iterative in nature, incorporating self-evaluation. Often, this begins with a simple scanning of the results returned from a search. Is the result set too large or returning records that are not relevant to the search goals? Or is the result set too small, missing important literature that the researcher knows exists? Although there is not a "correct" number of results that a search should return, researchers should critically evaluate the scope of their results and the impact of making adjustments. For instance, a draft search that is too broad may benefit from incorporating filters or limits, or reconsidering whether the chosen keywords or index terms are specific enough for the intended purpose. A draft search that is too narrow may need additional terms added to the search to see how the result set is impacted and whether the additional records are of interest and value.

3.2 Confirmation bias

Without a standardized approach, literature searching can be particularly vulnerable to confirmation bias (Kaanders et al., 2022; Suzuki and Yamamoto, 2021). Often, researchers search for what they already know or believe the answer to be. Search engines (and AI tools) reinforce this bias through result sets tailored to the researcher's behavior. To support rigorous science, researchers should use predefined protocols and appropriate methods for conducting formal literature reviews (Page et al., 2021, PLoS Medicine Editors, 2011). When conducting a more informal search (e.g., looking for background information), researchers should make efforts to either find well-done reviews on the subject (e.g., high-quality systematic reviews) or make explicit efforts to verify the accuracy and quality of, as well as the heterogeneity surrounding, a given question.

For example, clinicians and researchers often may only read the abstract of an article (Saint et al., 2000; Shiely et al., 2024), which can present an incomplete or misleading picture of the evidence (Chiu et al., 2017; Khan et al., 2019). If this picture is uncritically accepted, pharmacy researchers risk drawing unfounded conclusions. Before using a source to inform a manuscript or their research, researchers should critically evaluate the quality of the evidence using one of several available guides (Ma et al., 2020). Another strategy to mitigate confirmation bias is to specifically search for disconfirming evidence. For example, if a researcher believes that a treatment works, they can try to identify any evidence suggesting the treatment may not be effective. Researchers can then discuss this heterogeneity in their manuscript, which may actually serve as justification for future studies.

3.3 Predatory journals and open-access publishing

Globally, much of science remains behind paywalls, requiring a subscription or one-time payment (Stromberg et al., 2023). For individuals in resource-constrained environments, this limits their ability to access and properly utilize a large portion of the literature. To address this challenge, there is a large and growing movement for open science—a movement to make research freely available. Yet, the practical implementation of this ideal has been hindered by high open-access (OA) fees along with the rise of predatory publishers. Predatory publishers, or *"entities that prioritize self-interest at the expense of scholarship and are characterized by false or misleading information, deviation from best editorial and publication practices, a lack of transparency, and/or the use of aggressive and indiscriminate solicitation practices"* (Grudniewicz et al., 2019) pollute the literature with poor-quality studies (Elmore and Weston, 2020; Laine et al., 2025). Further complicating this issue is the fact that reputable OA publishers exist that uphold standards related to quality. It is therefore critical for pharmacy researchers to develop skills to identify trustworthy publishers. One initiative that may assist in this endeavor is Think.Check.Submit, which provides a tool for researchers to assess the suitability of a source (Think. Check. Submit.). Furthermore, the Open Access Scholarly Publishing Association utilizes a code of conduct that may help researchers distinguish between predatory journals and reputable OA journals based on membership (Open Access Scholarly Publishing Association).

Given that subscription journals have fees that are often out of reach for many individuals and institutions, there are many initiatives aimed at making research more accessible. PubMed Central is a free archive of full-text biomedical science, serving as a repository for publications resulting from publicly funded research within the United States (containing about five million records compared to 30 + million within PubMed (National Library of Medicine). ResearchGate is a scholarly social networking website that facilitates direct sharing of publications between researchers (ResearchGate), albeit with the responsibility for researchers to consider publisher copyright limitations associated with sharing. An additional challenge arises when researchers endeavor to publish their findings, as even legitimate OA journals may have publication fees that are not feasible for many pharmacy researchers. This shifting of the financial burden of publishing from the consumers to the producers of research may contribute to publication bias; however, preprint repositories such as medRxiv (medRxiv) and similar repositories in other academic fields (Directory of Open Access Preprint Repositories) and government initiatives such as Open Research Europe may facilitate publication in the peer-reviewed literature (European Union).

3.4 The value of medical librarians

Developing the skill of literature searching is critical for pharmacy researchers. However, navigating the ever-evolving landscape of databases and technologies can be challenging. To help address these challenges, most academic institutions and larger health systems employ a health sciences librarian. These individuals are specially trained in literature searching and can be an invaluable resource for research and literature reviews specifically (Geda, 2021). In fact, studies have found that formalized searches (such as systematic reviews) that include a health sciences librarian are, on average, of higher quality than those conducted without the involvement of a medical librarian (Rethlefsen et al., 2015). Accordingly, their involvement is highly recommended for researchers who have access to them within their institutions.

3.5 Leveraging technology

A variety of tools exist to support researchers' efforts to efficiently search the literature (Jin et al., 2024; Patterson, 2025; Siemens et al., 2025). These include tools to facilitate finding relevant literature, accessing identified literature, organizing findings from a literature search, and keeping up with the literature. The growth of artificial intelligence

TABLE 7.4 Selected technology tools for literature searches.

Resource	Cost	Functionality	Sources
Consensus https://consensus.app/	Free minimal access Paid premium access for individuals, teams, and large organizations	• AI-enhanced • Simple Google-like searching or natural language searching • Finds relevant studies, synthesizes study results, links to studies, and evaluates the level of consensus across studies • Additional features include assistance with drafting outlines and creating tables	Semantic Scholar; OpenAlex; additional unspecified scholarly websites
Elicithttps://elicit.com/	Free minimal access Paid options for individuals, small teams, and large teams	• AI-enhanced • Natural language searching • Summarizes up to 50 (free) or 500 (paid) papers • Prepares extraction tables and develops its own extraction criteria (population, conditions, study design, study size, etc.) • Develop a report that you can "chat" with	Semantic Scholar; OpenAlex; Preprint repositories (arXiv, bioRxiv, etc.)
Epistomenokoshttps://www.epistemonikos.org/	Free	• Simple Google-like searching or natural language searching • Nine languages available • Categorizes results as broad syntheses, systematic reviews, structured summaries, and primary studies • Search option for titles, abstracts, and authors	Cochrane Database of Systematic Reviews; PubMed; Embase; CINAHL; APA PsycInfo; LILACS; other databases that are no longer updated
OpenAlex-https://openalex.org/	Free with database updated monthly Paid options with hourly updates and priority for users Institutional paid includes training	• Simple Google-like searching or natural language searching • Searches 250 million + papers • Provides filters for publication type, institution, topic, and more • Improved coverage of "diamond open access" journals compared to A&I databases • Attempts to improve the coverage of research produced in the Global South	Microsoft Academic Graph; CrossRef; ORCID; ROR; DOAJ; Unpaywall; PubMed; PMC; ISSN International Center; preprint repositories (e.g., arXiv, Zenodo, etc.)
PubMed.aihttps://www.pubmed.ai/	Free	• AI-enhanced • Natural language searching (with the option to switch to traditional PubMed using filters) maps searches to MeSH (but does not show the mapping) • Provides a brief search results summary and an "AI Research Co-Pilot" that synthesizes the results of 20 papers • Links to papers in PubMed	PubMed
Semantic Scholarhttps://www.semanticscholar.org/	Free	• Simple/Google-like search interface • Searches 228 million + papers • Links to free full text and can connect with library subscriptions • Includes API options for individuals with coding skills	PubMed; preprint servers (medRxiv, bioRxiv, etc.); publishers (SpringerNature, Wolters Kluwer, etc.); see website for full list

AI: artificial intelligence; *APA*: American Psychological Association; *API*: application programming interface; *CINAHL*: Cumulated Index in Nursing and Allied Health Literature; *DOAJ*: Directory of Open Access Journals; *ISSN*: international standard serial number; *LILACS*: Latin American and Caribbean Health Sciences Literature; *MeSH*: medical subject headings; *ORCID*: Open Researcher and Contributor ID; *PMC*: PubMed Central; *ROR*: Research Organization Registry.

BOX 7.2

Saving and automating searches in PubMed

Researchers can register an account with the National Center for Biotechnology Information (NCBI), enabling them to save searches within PubMed and other NCBI databases. They can also set up automatic email alerts related to specific search results, which can assist in the longitudinal repetition of literature searches across a research project.

and related technologies has created numerous tools that can help researchers quickly find relevant articles (Table 7.4); this space is currently experiencing rapid expansion, with changes in tool availability and associated access. When using these tools, researchers should be mindful of the limitations of the current generation of AI-enabled tools: namely, bias, accuracy, and reproducibility. Thus, any output from an AI-enabled resource should be checked for accuracy (i.e., ensuring that the citation actually exists) and that the source is relevant and high-quality (i.e., critically appraised to understand strengths and limitations).

There are also technologies to facilitate access to relevant articles. Many institutions support browser plug-ins or other technologies that link their institutional accounts to users, ensuring that any article available to the institution is accessible to the user. In addition, there are technologies that facilitate finding and accessing the literature, as well as numerous tools that assist in organizing the results of a literature search. These tools include reference managers (e.g., EndNote, Zotero, Mendeley) and more specialized tools designed to facilitate systematic reviews of the literature (e.g., Covidence, DistillerSR). Most A&I databases support the exporting of search results into reference managers, where researchers can sort, tag, filter, or otherwise organize their results. Reference managers are also useful when writing up results, as they help properly format cited references based on journal styles. Finally, many A&I databases (and journals) support automated searches that can be delivered at specified intervals (Box 7.2). Using this type of tool can help researchers stay up to date in their area of interest.

4 Questions for further discussion

- What have been your "go-to" sources for finding research throughout your career?
- In what ways do you stay abreast of the latest research developments in your field?
- What role does critical thinking play when you are planning a literature review strategy?
- How can a robust literature search help to focus a research question?
- How can interdisciplinary collaboration during the literature search process lead to more innovative approaches to research?
- How have you integrated technology into your literature searches in recent years?

5 Application exercise/scenario

A pharmacy clinical specialist has been working with a patient struggling with adherence to their insulin regimen. They start an informal Google search and quickly become overwhelmed by the sheer volume of information on this broad topic. They discover that medication adherence is related to cultural beliefs, health literacy, regimen complexity, medication costs, healthcare professional support, adverse effects, and a host of other factors. They decide they need a more targeted search, particularly after a colleague recently mentioned the opportunity to collaborate on a research study the clinic is initiating in this area.

1. What would be some ways in which you could narrow your search?
2. What data sources would you search, and what keywords or index terms could be utilized?
3. How would your search differ if it were to support evidence-based practice versus to design research?
4. How can you engage interested parties in the process to make your literature search more relevant?
5. How might you work to ensure your conclusions are based on high-quality studies?

References

Andreasen, J., Norgaard, B., Draborg, E., Juhl, C.B., Yost, J., Brunnhuber, K., Robinson, K.A., Lund, H., 2022. Justification of research using systematic reviews continues to be inconsistent in clinical health science-A systematic review and meta-analysis of meta-research studies. PLoS One. 1932-6203. 17 (10), e0276955. Available from: https://www.ncbi.nlm.nih.gov/pubmed/36315526. doi:10.1371/journal.pone.0276955.

Baker, J.D., 2016. The purpose, process, and methods of writing a literature review. AORN J. 1878-0369. 103 (3), 265–269. Available from: https://www.ncbi.nlm.nih.gov/pubmed/26924364. doi:10.1016/j.aorn.2016.01.016.

Barrett, A., Helwig, M., Neves, K., 2016. Mapping the literature of hospital pharmacy. J. Med. Libr. Assoc. 1558-9439. 104 (2), 118–124. Available from: https://www.ncbi.nlm.nih.gov/pubmed/27076798. doi:10.3163/1536-5050.104.2.005.

Belbasis, L., Bellou, V., Ioannidis, J.P.A., 2022. Conducting umbrella reviews. BMJ Med. 2754-0413. 1 (1), e000071. Available from: https://www.ncbi.nlm.nih.gov/pubmed/36936579. doi:10.1136/bmjmed-2021-000071.

Bramer, W.M., de Jonge, G.B., Rethlefsen, M.L., Mast, F., Kleijnen, J., 2018. A systematic approach to searching: an efficient and complete method to develop literature searches. J. Med. Libr. Assoc. 1558-9439. 106 (4), 531–541. Available from: https://www.ncbi.nlm.nih.gov/pubmed/30271302. doi:10.5195/jmla.2018.283.

Bramer, W.M., Rethlefsen, M.L., Kleijnen, J., Franco, O.H., 2017. Optimal database combinations for literature searches in systematic reviews: a prospective exploratory study. Syst. Rev. 2046-4053. 6 (1), 245. Available from: https://www.ncbi.nlm.nih.gov/pubmed/29208034. doi:10.1186/s13643-017-0644-y.

Chalmers, I., Bracken, M.B., Djulbegovic, B., Garattini, S., Grant, J., Gulmezoglu, A.M., Howells, D.W., Ioannidis, J.P., Oliver, S., 2014. How to increase value and reduce waste when research priorities are set. Lancet. 1474-547X. 383 (9912), 156–165. Available from: https://www.ncbi.nlm.nih.gov/pubmed/24411644. doi:10.1016/S0140-6736(13)62229-1.

Chiu, K., Grundy, Q., Bero, L., 2017. 'Spin' in published biomedical literature: a methodological systematic review. PLoS Biol. 1545-7885. 15 (9), e2002173. Available from: https://www.ncbi.nlm.nih.gov/pubmed/28892482. doi:10.1371/journal.pbio.2002173.

Clarke, M., Hopewell, S., 2013. Many reports of randomised trials still don't begin or end with a systematic review of the relevant evidence. J. Bahrain Med. Soc. 24 (3), 145–148.

Cooper, N.J., Jones, D.R., Sutton, A.J., 2005. The use of systematic reviews when designing studies. Clin. Trials. 1740-7745. 2 (3), 260–264. Available from: https://www.ncbi.nlm.nih.gov/pubmed/16279149. doi:10.1191/1740774505cn090oa.

Dhollande, S., Taylor, A., Meyer, S., Scott, M., 2021. Conducting integrative reviews: a guide for novice nursing researchers. J. Res. Nurs. 1744-988X. 26 (5), 427–438. Available from: https://www.ncbi.nlm.nih.gov/pubmed/35251272. doi:10.1177/1744987121997907.

Directory of Open Access Preprint Repositories. Respositories. https://doapr.coar-repositories.org/repositories/.

Elmore, S.A., Weston, E.H., 2020. Predatory journals: what they are and how to avoid them. Toxicol. Pathol. 1533-1601. 48 (4), 607–610. Available from: https://www.ncbi.nlm.nih.gov/pubmed/32319351. doi:10.1177/0192623320920209.

European Commission. Open Research Europe. https://open-research-europe.ec.europa.eu/

Fandino, W., 2019. Formulating a good research question: pearls and pitfalls. Indian J. Anaesth. 0019-5049. 63 (8), 611–616. Available from: https://www.ncbi.nlm.nih.gov/pubmed/31462805. doi:10.4103/ija.IJA_198_19.

Farrugia, P., Petrisor, B.A., Farrokhyar, F., Bhandari, M., 2010. Practical tips for surgical research: research questions, hypotheses and objectives. Can. J. Surg. 1488-2310. 53 (4), 278–281. Available from https://www.ncbi.nlm.nih.gov/pubmed/20646403.

Geda, F.A., 2021. The roles of medical library in information seeking behavior of health care professionals: a review of the literature. J. Hosp. Librarian 21 (4), 405–416. doi:10.1080/15323269.2021.1982263.

Gionfriddo, M.R., McClendon, C., Nolfi, D.A., Kalarchian, M.A., Covvey, J.R., 2024. Back to the basics: guidance for designing good literature searches. Res. Social Adm. Pharm. 1934-8150. 20 (4), 463–468. Available from: https://www.ncbi.nlm.nih.gov/pubmed/38272775. doi:10.1016/j.sapharm.2024.01.009.

Gionfriddo, M.R., Owens, K.M., Banks, H., Sherigar, A., Covvey, J.R., 2025. An analysis of national news coverage of semaglutide for weight loss. J. Am. Pharm. Assoc. 1544-3450. 65 (1), 102297. Available from https://www.ncbi.nlm.nih.gov/pubmed/39580054. doi:10.1016/j.japh.2024.102297.

Giustini, D., Boulos, M.N., 2013. Google Scholar is not enough to be used alone for systematic reviews. Online J. Public Health Inform. 1947-2579. 5 (2), 214. Available from: https://www.ncbi.nlm.nih.gov/pubmed/23923099. doi:10.5210/ojphi.v5i2.4623.

Goodfellow, L.T., 2023. An overview of how to search and write a medical literature review. Respir. Care. 1943-3654. 68 (11), 1576–1584. Available from: https://www.ncbi.nlm.nih.gov/pubmed/37339890. doi:10.4187/respcare.11198.

Grant, M.J., Booth, A., 2009. A typology of reviews: an analysis of 14 review types and associated methodologies. Health Info Libr. J. 1471-1834. 26 (2), 91–108. Available from: https://www.ncbi.nlm.nih.gov/pubmed/19490148. doi:10.1111/j.1471-1842.2009.00848.x.

Grudniewicz, A., Moher, D., Cobey, K.D., Bryson, G.L., Cukier, S., Allen, K., Ardern, C., Balcom, L., Barros, T., Berger, M., Ciro, J.B., Cugusi, L., Donaldson, M.R., Egger, M., Graham, I.D., Hodgkinson, M., Khan, K.M., Mabizela, M., Manca, A., Milzow, K., Mouton, J., Muchenje, M., Olijhoek, T., Ommaya, A., Patwardhan, B., Poff, D., Proulx, L., Rodger, M., Severin, A., Strinzel, M., Sylos-Labini, M., Tamblyn, R., van Niekerk, M., Wicherts, J.M., Lalu, M.M., 2019. Predatory journals: no definition, no defence. Nature. 1476-4687. 576 (7786), 210–212. Available from: https://www.ncbi.nlm.nih.gov/pubmed/31827288. doi:10.1038/d41586-019-03759-y.

Halevi, G., Moed, H., Bar-Ilan, J., 2017. Suitability of Google Scholar as a source of scientific information and as a source of data for scientific evaluation—Review of the Literature. J. Informetics 11 (3), 823–834. doi:10.1016/j.joi.2017.06.005.

Hart, B., Lundh, A., Bero, L., 2012. Effect of reporting bias on meta-analyses of drug trials: reanalysis of meta-analyses. BMJ. 1756-1833. 344, d7202. Available from: https://www.ncbi.nlm.nih.gov/pubmed/22214754. doi:10.1136/bmj.d7202.

Higgins, J.P.T., Thomas, J., Chandler, J., Cumpston, M., Li, T., Page, M.J., Welch, V.A., Cochrane handbook for systematic reviews of interventions version 6.5. Updated August 2024, Cochrane (2024), Available from: http://www.cochrane.org/handbook.

Jha, R., Sondhi, V., Vasudevan, B., 2022. Literature search: simple rules for confronting the unknown. Med. J. Armed Forces India. 0377-1237. 78 (Suppl 1), S14–S23. Available from: https://www.ncbi.nlm.nih.gov/pubmed/36147432. doi:10.1016/j.mjafi.2022.07.009.

Jin, Q., Leaman, R., Lu, Z., 2024. PubMed and beyond: biomedical literature search in the age of artificial intelligence. EBioMedicine. 104988. 2352-3964(100), Available from https://www.ncbi.nlm.nih.gov/pubmed/38306900 10.1016/j.ebiom.2024.104988.

Kaanders, P., Sepulveda, P., Folke, T., Ortoleva, P., De Martino, B., 2022. Humans actively sample evidence to support prior beliefs. Elife. 2050-084X. 11. Available from: https://www.ncbi.nlm.nih.gov/pubmed/35404234. doi:10.7554/eLife.71768.

Khan, K.S., Kunz, R., Kleijnen, J., Antes, G., 2003. Five steps to conducting a systematic review. J. R. Soc. Med. 0141-0768. 96 (3), 118–121. Available from: https://www.ncbi.nlm.nih.gov/pubmed/12612111. doi:10.1177/014107680309600304.

Khan, M.S., Lateef, N., Siddiqi, T.J., Rehman, K.A., Alnaimat, S., Khan, S.U., Riaz, H., Murad, M.H., Mandrola, J., Doukky, R., Krasuski, R.A., 2019. Level and prevalence of spin in published cardiovascular randomized clinical trial reports with statistically nonsignificant primary outcomes: a systematic review. JAMA Netw. Open. 2574-3805. 2 (5), e192622. Available from: https://www.ncbi.nlm.nih.gov/pubmed/31050775. doi:10.1001/jamanetworkopen.2019.2622.

Kung, J.Y., 2022. Polyglot search translator. J. Can. Health Libr. Assoc. 43 (1), 35–39. doi:10.29173/jchla29600.

Kwiatkowski, T., Silverman, R., 1998. Research fundamentals: II. Choosing and defining a research question. Acad. Emerg. Med. 1069-6563. 5 (11), 1114–1117. Available from: https://www.ncbi.nlm.nih.gov/pubmed/9835477. doi:10.1111/j.1553-2712.1998.tb02673.x.

Laine, C., Babski, D., Bachelet, V.C., Barnighausen, T.W., Baethge, C., Bibbins-Domingo, K., Frizelle, F., Gollogy, L., Kleinert, S., Loder, E., Monteiro, J., Rubin, E.J., Sahni, P., Wee, C.C., Yoo, J.H., Zakhama, L., 2025. Predatory journals: what can we do to protect their prey? Lancet. 1474-547X. 405 (10476), 362–364. Available from: https://www.ncbi.nlm.nih.gov/pubmed/39788137. doi:10.1016/S0140-6736(24)02863-0.

Lingard, L., 2015. Joining a conversation: the problem/gap/hook heuristic. Perspect. Med. Educ. 2212-2761. 4 (5), 252–253. Available from: https://www.ncbi.nlm.nih.gov/pubmed/26346497. doi:10.1007/s40037-015-0211-y.

Ma, L.L., Wang, Y.Y., Yang, Z.H., Huang, D., Weng, H., Zeng, X.T., 2020. Methodological quality (risk of bias) assessment tools for primary and secondary medical studies: what are they and which is better? Mil Med Res. 2054-9369. 7 (1), 7. Available from: https://www.ncbi.nlm.nih.gov/pubmed/32111253. doi:10.1186/s40779-020-00238-8.

Mak, S., Thomas, A., 2022. An introduction to scoping reviews. J. Grad. Med. Educ. 1949-8357. 14 (5), 561–564. Available from: https://www.ncbi.nlm.nih.gov/pubmed/36274758. doi:10.4300/JGME-D-22-00620.1.

McGowan, J., Sampson, M., Salzwedel, D.M., Cogo, E., Foerster, V., Lefebvre, C., 2016. PRESS peer review of electronic search strategies: 2015 guideline statement. J. Clin. Epidemiol. 1878-5921. 75, 40–46. Available from: https://www.ncbi.nlm.nih.gov/pubmed/27005575. doi:10.1016/j.jclinepi.2016.01.021.

MedRxiv. The preprint server for health sciences. https://www.medrxiv.org/.

Moons, P., Goossens, E., Thompson, D.R., 2021. Rapid reviews: the pros and cons of an accelerated review process. Eur. J. Cardiovasc. Nurs. 1873-1953. 20 (5), 515–519. Available from: https://www.ncbi.nlm.nih.gov/pubmed/34007994. doi:10.1093/eurjcn/zvab041.

National Library of Medicine. MeSH (MeSH). https://www.ncbi.nlm.nih.gov/mesh/.

National Library of Medicine. PMC FAQs. https://pmc.ncbi.nlm.nih.gov/about/faq/#q1.

National Library of Medicine. Topic searching in PubMed®: using the medical subject headings (MeSH®) https://www.nlm.nih.gov/oet/ed/pubmed/mesh/index.html

Open Access Scholarly Publishing Association. Code of conduct. https://www.oaspa.org/membership/code-of-conduct/.

Paez, A., 2017. Gray literature: an important resource in systematic reviews. J. Evid. Based Med. 1756-5391. 10 (3), 233–240. Available from: https://www.ncbi.nlm.nih.gov/pubmed/28857505. doi:10.1111/jebm.12266.

Page, M.J., McKenzie, J.E., Bossuyt, P.M., Boutron, I., Hoffmann, T.C., Mulrow, C.D., Shamseer, L., Tetzlaff, J.M., Akl, E.A., Brennan, S.E., Chou, R., Glanville, J., Grimshaw, J.M., Hrobjartsson, A., Lalu, M.M., Li, T., Loder, E.W., Mayo-Wilson, E., McDonald, S., McGuinness, L.A., Stewart, L.A., Thomas, J., Tricco, A.C., Welch, V.A., Whiting, P., Moher, D., 2021. The PRISMA 2020 statement: an updated guideline for reporting systematic reviews. BMJ. 1756-1833. 372, n71. Available from: https://www.ncbi.nlm.nih.gov/pubmed/33782057. doi:10.1136/bmj.n71.

Pappas, C., Williams, I., 2011. Grey literature: its emerging importance. J. Hosp. Librarian 11 (3), 228–234. doi:10.1080/15323269.2011.587100.

Patrick, L.J., Munro, S., 2004. The literature review: demystifying the literature search. Diabetes Educ. 0145-7217. 30 (1). Available from: https://www.ncbi.nlm.nih.gov/pubmed/14999892. doi:10.1177/014572170403000106.

Patterson, B., 2025. Can AI help with that? The limitations of AI tools for information discovery, search and reviews. J. Electron. Resource Med. Libr. 1542-4065. 22 (1-2), 56–59. doi:10.1080/15424065.2025.2496622.

PLoS Medicine Editors, Best practice in systematic reviews: the importance of protocols and registration, 2011. PLoS Med. 1549-1676. 8 (2), e1001009. Available from https://www.ncbi.nlm.nih.gov/pubmed/21364968. doi:10.1371/journal.pmed.1001009.

ResearchGate. https://www.researchgate.net/

Rethlefsen, M.L., Farrell, A.M., Trzasko, L.C.O., Brigham, T.J., 2015. Librarian co-authors correlated with higher quality reported search strategies in general internal medicine systematic reviews. J. Clin. Epidemiol. 1878-5921. 68 (6), 617–626. Available from: https://www.ncbi.nlm.nih.gov/pubmed/25766056. doi:10.1016/j.jclinepi.2014.11.025.

Richardson, W.S., Wilson, M.C., Nishikawa, J., Hayward, R.S., 1995. The well-built clinical question: a key to evidence-based decisions. ACP J. Club. 1056-8751. 123 (3). Available from https://www.ncbi.nlm.nih.gov/pubmed/7582737.

Robinson, K.A., Goodman, S.N., 2011. A systematic examination of the citation of prior research in reports of randomized, controlled trials. Ann. Intern. Med. 1539-3704. 154 (1), 50–55. Available from: https://www.ncbi.nlm.nih.gov/pubmed/21200038. doi:10.7326/0003-4819-154-1-201101040-00007.

Saint, S., Christakis, D.A., Saha, S., Elmore, J.G., Welsh, D.E., Baker, P., Koepsell, T.D., 2000. Journal reading habits of internists. J. Gen. Intern. Med. 0884-8734. 15 (12), 881–884. Available from: https://www.ncbi.nlm.nih.gov/pubmed/11119185. doi:10.1046/j.1525-1497.2000.00202.x.

Savage, W.E., Olejniczak, A.J., 2022. More journal articles and fewer books: publication practices in the social sciences in the 2010's. PLoS One. 1932-6203. 17 (2), e0263410. Available from: https://www.ncbi.nlm.nih.gov/pubmed/35113974. doi:10.1371/journal.pone.0263410.

Shiely, F., Gallagher, K., Millar, S.R., 2024. How, and why, science and health researchers read scientific (IMRAD) papers. PLoS One. 1932-6203. 19 (1), e0297034. Available from: https://www.ncbi.nlm.nih.gov/pubmed/38252646. doi:10.1371/journal.pone.0297034.

Siemens, W., von Elm, E., Binder, H., Böhringer, D., Eisele-Metzger, A., Gartlehner, G., Hanegraaf, P., Metzendorf, M.-I., Mosselman, J.-J., Nowak, A., Qureshi, R., Thomas, J., Waffenschmidt, S., Labonté, V., Meerpohl, J.J., 2025. Opportunities, challenges and risks of using artificial intelligence for evidence synthesis. BMJ Evid.-Based Med. 2515-446X bmjebm-2024-113320. 10.1136/bmjebm-2024-113320.

Steele, R., 2015. 'Background' and 'foreground' knowledge: targeting learning materials to trainees' needs. BJPsych Bull. 2056-4694. 39 (4), 206–207. Available from: https://www.ncbi.nlm.nih.gov/pubmed/26755959. doi:10.1192/pb.39.4.206a.

Stromberg, A., Norekval, T.M., Moons, P., Lauck, S., 2023. Open Access publishing: benefits and challenges. Eur. J. Cardiovasc. Nurs. 1873-1953. 22 (8), e115–e117. Available from: https://www.ncbi.nlm.nih.gov/pubmed/37874910. doi:10.1093/eurjcn/zvad099.

Sukhera, J., 2022. Narrative reviews: flexible, rigorous, and practical. J. Grad. Med. Educ. 1949-8357. 14 (4), 414–417. Available from: https://www.ncbi.nlm.nih.gov/pubmed/35991099. doi:10.4300/JGME-D-22-00480.1.

Suzuki, M., Yamamoto, Y., 2021. Characterizing the influence of confirmation bias on web search behavior. Front. Psychol. 1664-1078. 12, 771948. Available from https://www.ncbi.nlm.nih.gov/pubmed/34938242. doi:10.3389/fpsyg.2021.771948.

Think. Check. Submit. Identify trusted publishers for your research. https://www.thinkchecksubmit.org

Yuan, Y., Hunt, R.H., 2009. Systematic reviews: the good, the bad, and the ugly. Am. J. Gastroenterol. 1572-0241. 104 (5), 1086–1092. Available from: https://www.ncbi.nlm.nih.gov/pubmed/19417748. doi:10.1038/ajg.2009.118.

CHAPTER

8

Synthesizing the scatter: Conducting purposeful scoping reviews in pharmacy education

Cherie Lucas

Faculty of Medicine and Health, University of NSW (UNSW) Sydney, Sydney, NSW, Australia

CHAPTER OBJECTIVES

The learning objectives for this chapter are:

- **Explain** when to apply a scoping review strategy over other strategies, such as systematic review methodologies; and **identify** its applications in pharmacy/health education
- **Describe** the key steps in conducting a high-quality scoping review using the JBI and Prisma-ScR guidelines
- **Critically evaluate** the strengths, limitations, and transparency issues associated with scoping reviews
- **Apply** practical tools and strategies (e.g., grey literature searches, protocol registration, platform choices) to enhance the methodological rigor of scoping reviews
- **Reflect** on methodological "lessons learned" from conducting scoping reviews to inform future practice
- **Design** a preliminary scoping review plan suitable for research or curriculum evaluation in pharmacy or health education

1 Introduction

Scoping reviews have become increasingly popular in pharmacy and other health professions education due to their utility to map emerging evidence, particularly in novel fields. The first scoping review framework was introduced in 2005 (Arksey and O'Malley, 2005) and has since been modified with iterations, which have informed the most current Joanna Briggs Institute (JBI) guidelines (2020) and forming a JBI scoping review methodology working

Contemporary Research Methods in Pharmacy and Health Services - Volume 2
https://doi.org/10.1016/B978-0-443-44607-8.00009-1

group for conducting scoping reviews (Khalil et al., 2021; Peters et al., 2024). In pharmacy and health education, fields typified by rapidly evolving pedagogical and technological innovations, scoping reviews provide a valuable lens for identifying trends, gaps, and future research priorities and directions. These types of reviews are typically conducted without emphasizing critical appraisal and are aimed to inform future practice, health education, training programs, and policy (Colquhoun et al., 2014; Lucas and Desselle, 2024).

The scoping review strategy is not the only option for researchers. The decision for a researcher on the selection of a review strategy usually requires careful consideration (Lucas and Desselle, 2024). Review strategies may include frameworks for systematic reviews, rapid reviews, narrative reviews, as well as scoping reviews, notwithstanding emerging review strategies in the pipeline.

It is important to note that the most established of all the review strategies are the systematic reviews, first described in the 1970s under the term "metaanalysis" (History of systematic reviews, n.d.). These types of reviews have long been deemed instrumental; however, this type of review strategy is usually undertaken by researchers when there has been a great deal of research conducted in the topic area. This leaves a gap for a review strategy for those emerging and novel topic areas, such as topics related to generative artificial intelligence (GenAI) and new scopes of practice, as in the example by Mortlock and Lucas (2024). This is where scoping reviews have become a key contender as a research strategy.

This chapter offers guidance for the novice researcher and outlines each phase of the scoping review process, from protocol development to data analysis and dissemination. It discusses practical considerations, including platform selection and grey literature search processes. Reflections on the "dos" and don'ts" drawn from lived research experience by the author (an experienced pharmacy education researcher with a PhD in pharmacy education focusing on reflective practice strategies) are also provided to support advanced learners in designing and conducting their own scoping review research. As such, throughout this chapter, reflective prompts are presented in sidebar boxes. These are designed to support scholarly reflexivity, encouraging readers, particularly PhD candidates and early career researchers, to critically engage with their own review processes. They align with the principles of reflective practice, enhancing thoughtful inquiry into methodological choices, assumptions, and research positioning.

2 Methods

2.1 Considerations for the methods section?

The methodological discussion in this Methods section of the chapter is anchored in the Arksey and O'Malley's framework, expanded by Levac et al.'s refinements (Levac et al., 2010) and the JBI (Arksey and O'Malley, 2005) guidelines (Tricco et al., 2018). This section covers the importance of: developing a protocol using the Population, Concept, Context (PCC) approach (Chan et al., 2024) (Fig. 8.1); considerations around documenting protocols

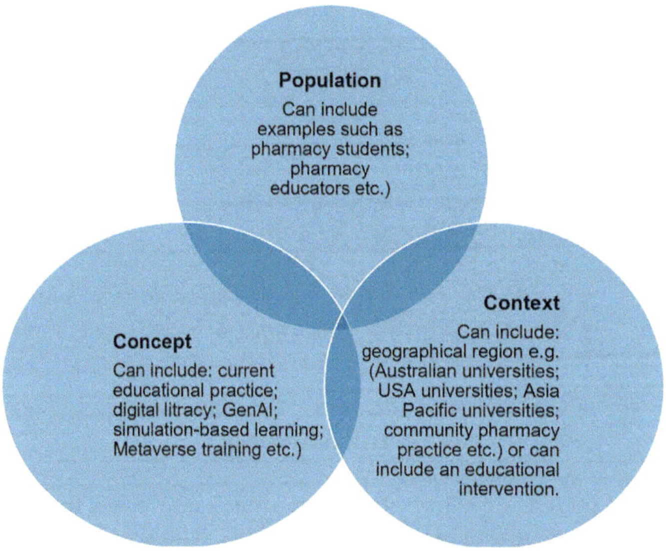

FIG. 8.1 Anchoring your scoping review in the PCC (population, concept, context) framework. Considerations of the PCC framework: Population, concept and context.

including platforms to submit a developed protocol; ensuring that the inclusion and exclusion criteria are clear and transparent, identifying the appropriate scientific database(s) and grey literature sources; screening processes; and the use of tools such as Covidence (2025c); data extraction methods, thematic categorization, and synthesis strategies.

This chapter also includes a table representation of the stages that a researcher would work through to conduct a robust scoping review (see Table 8.1).

2.1.1 *Choosing the type of review strategy*

Before you start the processes, you and your research team need to decide if a scoping review is the most appropriate review strategy. Scoping reviews are different from the more traditional review strategies, such as systematic reviews. While both review options use different approaches to extracting evidence, that evidence serves different purposes. For example, scoping reviews categorize, map, or group evidence often from emerging, novel, and evolving fields, and the evidence is not typically critically appraised (Lucas and Desselle, 2024). Hence, scoping reviews often extract both scientific literature and grey literature. Grey literature (also known as "records" or "documents") is not traditionally indexed in scientific databases (Godin et al., 2017); however, they may be useful to access and utilize (and timely) to inform policy changes and future practice for educational institutions or professional bodies. Typically, as scoping reviews involve topic areas that are novel, emerging, or evolving, both scientific database searches and grey literature search strategies are often adopted (Lucas and Desselle, 2024).

TABLE 8.1 Key methodological stages, elements and tools utilized when conducting a scoping review.

Stage	Description	Examples/tools
Protocol development	Define topic, research questions and objectives, consider the PCC Framework; Discuss with your research team and apply inclusion and exclusion criteria	PCC framework; review JBI Guidelines, undertake consultation with your research team
Protocol registration and/ or publication	Decide on a platform to register your protocol or publish your protocol in a journal with a manuscript type indicating "research protocol"	Public platforms include: OSF; researchgate, figshare Journals with manuscript type "research protocol"
Data selection	Identify and select appropriate scientific databases and grey literature sources	Scientific databases may include: pubmed, ERIC, scopus, etc. Grey literature sources may include institutional documents, policy (Figshare, 2025a; Rayyan, 2025b; Covidence, 2025c; Researchgate, 2025d; Khalil et al., 2021; Peters et al., 2024; Colquhoun et al., 2014; Lucas and Desselle, 2024; History of systematic reviews, n.d.; Mortlock and Lucas, 2024; Tsingos et al., 2014; Tsingos, 2013; Tsingos-Lucas et al., 2016; Mantzourani et al., 2019; Le et al., 2019; Deslandes et al., 2018; Lucas et al., 2019; Tsingos et al., 2015; Arksey and O'Malley, 2005; Levac et al., 2010; Tricco et al., 2018; Chan et al., 2024; Godin et al., 2017; Gopalakrishnan and Ganeshkumar, 2013; Tricco et al., 2016; McGowan et al., 2020; Munn et al., 2018; Aly et al., 2020; Sharma et al., 2022; Open Science Framework (OSF), n.d.; Kastner et al., 2012; Kolb, 2015; Schön, 2016; Holmes and Desselle, 2004; Jackson et al., 2017) documents, websites, opinion articles from blogs that may not be located in the scientific literature
Screening and data extraction	Title and abstract review; full text selection; data charting	Covidence software; rayyan software; excel
Data synthesis	Collate, collaborate with the research team and summarize descriptive and/or thematic categorization; visual mapping; narrative summaries	Conceptual themes; visual tables
Reporting and transparency	Document search strategies (scientific and grey literature search strategies); use reporting standards	Visual representation flow charts e.g., PRISMA-ScR
Disseminate findings	Reflect on future directions	School, faculty, institution, professional bodies, national and international conference presentations, publications

Systematic reviews do not utilize grey literature sources; however, they utilize reproducible methods to mitigate bias and systematically synthesize evidence, where critical appraisal of that evidence is pivotal to the process (Gopalakrishnan and Ganeshkumar, 2013). That is not to say that scoping reviews do not use a systematic approach in selecting and extracting evidence; however, it is more flexible in that approach. For example, the scientific literature may be accessed first, followed by the grey literature or vice-versa, or follow a more structured approach with their search strategy, which may be tailored towards the needs of the decision and/or policy makers (Tricco et al., 2016; McGowan et al., 2020). Hence, some authors describe their scoping review, which utilizes a more structured approach, as a "systematic scoping review" rather than simply describing it as a "scoping review" (Munn et al., 2018). Aly et al. (2020) is an example of a systematic scoping review in pharmacy education, where the approach to data selection and extraction follows a more structured process. There are guidelines for scoping reviews that follow a structured approach to the search strategy, and recommendations indicate that these should be formed in collaboration with other independent reviewers of the research team (Sharma et al., 2022). For examples of the type of topic areas and review choices, Lucas and Desselle (2024) provide some exemplar published studies aligned to either a scoping review or systematic review strategy in pharmacy education (Lucas and Desselle, 2024).

2.1.2 *Developing a protocol or not?*

The decision to develop a research protocol or not depends on a range of factors. For example, time constraints in developing a protocol and conducting a full scoping review in order to inform timely decisions may be a consideration. Are there any time constraints for decisions to be made to change guidelines or policies? If not, then protocol development is an essential component of the scoping review process. Protocols for scoping reviews typically outline the background for conducting the review, follow the PCC framework (Fig. 8.1), outline the search strategy for data extraction, including the reasons for inclusion and exclusion criteria and the type and breadth of sources that will be sought, how the data will be analyzed; and the impact and purpose for conducting the scoping review. There is also an additional purpose for registering and/ or publishing a protocol, as this shows transparency by the researcher(s) and research team, enhancing the rigor in the research as to what data is being collected and over what timeframe. With this transparency, there is the potential that data could be shared with the permission of the lead researcher/ chief investigator. Furthermore, this type of transparency is important because other researchers can see what research is being undertaken and, therefore, may consider not spending their time conducting similar research. In addition, other information can also be transparent, such as grant funding acknowledgements, any conflicts of interest by any of the research team members, or any other acknowledgements with the development of the protocol (Lucas and Desselle, 2024). It is difficult to know where to publish a protocol; however, some journals offer a manuscript type tailored towards a research protocol. Not all journals offer this manuscript type. When this is the case, there are a few other considerations, such as publicly available platforms that are useful for registering a research protocol and have been utilized for data sharing and collaboration. These include platforms such as Open Science Framework (OSF) (n.d.), ResearchGate (2025d), and Figshare (2025a). As a researcher, if you cannot locate a suitable journal that would accept a research protocol as a publication or have opted for not using one of the other platforms to register the protocol, it is still an important part of the scoping review process to develop a research protocol prior to commencing the research and this should be noted in your methods section for any future publication. Kastner and colleagues provide an example of a research protocol that was developed to explore the most appropriate knowledge synthesis methods to conduct a review (Kastner et al., 2012). One could argue the impact of registering a protocol or publishing a protocol could be considered a limitation and have an impact on a blinded review process, however, in the spirit of sharing information before starting the data collection, this process could save valuable researchers' time and efforts especially if other researchers are currently in the process or have collected data related to the same area of research. At which point, the researchers who have identified that same or similar research is being conducted could then be redirected in their data collection to other underexplored intersections of the literature, or alternatively could reach out and contact the researchers who have registered their protocol, in view of potential future collaboration (Fig. 8.1).

2.1.3 *Commence with a generalized six-step framework*

In 2005, Arksey and O'Malley described a six-step process for conducting a purposeful scoping review (Arksey and O'Malley, 2005), which has since had iterations that are now captured in the first reporting guidelines tailored for scoping reviews, namely, the Extension for Scoping Reviews (Preferred Reporting Items for Systematic Reviews and Meta-Analyses (PRISMA)-ScR] (Tricco et al., 2018). The original six-step framework included identification and clarification of the research question(s); identification of the relevant evidence and studies; selection of the appropriate studies/evidence; charting the evidence (data); collating and reporting; and consulting with relevant stakeholders (Arksey and O'Malley, 2005).

2.1.4 Carefully select the search terms aligned to your research question(s)

This stage of the process is probably the most critical of all stages. Education and, in particular, pharmacy education, is considered a low-consensus discipline when it comes to search terms and defined definitions. This means that many terms are used interchangeably causing confusion with terminology. This is further coupled with some researchers deciding on the generation of new terms that are not all that different from the ones that are previously established (Martin et al., 2020). Understanding and having clear search terms is particularly important because if the search terms are not clearly identified, some of the important data may be missed in the extraction process.

2.1.5 Data selection and extraction

The processes for data selection and data extraction work well when using software that prompts the researcher(s) to consider inclusion and exclusion criteria plus enables the research team to have shared data, navigate the screening process, and facilitate consensus. Software such as Covidence (2025c) and Rayyan (2025b) could be used for this purpose and, if your institution does not hold licenses to use such software, then Microsoft Excel could also be considered for this purpose.

2.1.6 Writing up stage and data reporting

Presenting methodology in research protocols, publications, and conference presentations involves clearly outlining the steps for the search strategies. This includes the steps taken to select and extract records from the scientific databases as well as how grey literature sources were searched and utilized (Lucas and Desselle, 2024). Furthermore, it is important to write about how consensus for the selection of data was achieved.

Presenting results from your research can have its challenges. The skill here is to know what is required to be displayed. At a minimum, a PRISMA flow chart is required, which differs slightly depending on the review strategy. In the case for displaying results for a scoping review, the PRISMA-ScR, as outlined in the PRISMA flow diagram for scoping reviews, should be utilized (Tricco et al., 2018; McGowan et al., 2020). This flow chart is a visual representation of the databases searched, the inclusion and exclusion criteria applied, number of data extracted, and the records/data excluded that did not meet the eligibility criteria.

A table of results, also known as a "data extraction table", can be a useful display for further detail. For example, a table may include the following: date of source, authorship, study country of origin, type of study methodology (quantitative/ qualitative/ mixed methods/ other), thematic findings, and key outcomes or impact.

In addition, if your search involved a grey literature search strategy then another table should be included within the methods section outlining the search strategy for the grey literature sources; and the outcome of the types of data extracted (type of record) should be included in the results section, for example institutional or professional bodies policy documents; date of record, author (if known); country of origin; and key impact or outcomes.

2.1.7 Data dissemination

The purpose of many scoping reviews in pharmacy education is to inform future practice, change of policies, and/or inform educational innovations. As such, dissemination may simply involve faculty/ institutional level/ professional body presentations to the relevant stakeholders. However, given the rigor you have applied to the research, and so that knowledge is shared, considerations for publications in high impact, Q1 top-tier reputable educational journals (Q1 journals refers to a journal that ranks in the top 25% of journals within its subject category, based on citation-based metrics such as *Impact Factor* (Clarivate's journal Citation Reports), *Cite Score* (Scopus; Web of Science), or similar ranking systems), will no doubt contribute to the body of research as well as presentations at educational conferences.

2.1.8 Publication considerations

If you do decide on a publication route, it is recommended for researchers to seek high-impact and reputable peer-reviewed journals in the field. Once a journal has been decided upon, researchers need to ensure that they are explicit and that the title of a manuscript for reviews includes the type of review strategy within the title. For example, in the manuscript titled: "Educational needs of community pharmacy staff in minor ailments service delivery: a systematic scoping review," it clearly states in the title that a systematic scoping review strategy was employed (Aly et al., 2020). The manuscript titled "Generative artificial intelligence (GenAI) in pharmacy education: Utilization and Implications for Academic Integrity: A Scoping Review", clearly acknowledges the review strategy as scoping (Mortlock and Lucas, 2024).

3 Reflective prompts

3.1 Reflective prompt: Framing the research question

What assumptions am I making in the way I have defined my research question? How might these shape the boundaries of my review?

Consider how your positionality or educational context may influence what you consider a relevant research focus.

3.2 Reflective prompt: Choosing databases and platforms

Do the platforms and databases I have chosen reflect the diverse perspectives and contexts required for the research, or might they privilege certain types of knowledge?

Reflect on the consequences of favoring peer-reviewed versus *grey literature and the potential exclusion criteria involved.*

3.3 Reflective prompt: Collaboration and selecting the research team

What considerations am I making when selecting the research team? Have I considered the diverse skill set of the potential research team members?

Consider how different limitations of research team members' expertise can be optimally harnessed, and if additional researchers (who may have other expertise in analysis or synthesis) are required to be invited to the research team.

3.4 Reflective prompt: What to do if consensus is not met by the research team members?

Who has been allocated the role to extract the data, and how many independent reviewers are reviewing the data?

What are the reasons for a lack of consensus? Have there been any differences in interpreting the data?

What methods am I applying to ensure clear communication among the research team, and in instances where there is disagreement, how is nonconsensus dealt with to achieve final consensus?

Reflect on your processes as a researcher and any limitations for the study. Consider a process when nonconsensus for inclusion and exclusion criteria, and ensure that this process is documented in a protocol and future publication.

3.5 Reflective prompt: Missing voices

Whose perspectives are missing in the literature I have mapped? How might their absence influence the understanding of the topic?

Reflect on missing voices and consider how inclusion might be improved in future reviews.

3.6 Reflective prompt: Transparency

In what ways could I make my review process more transparent and replicable for others in the field? Have I considered a platform to register my research protocol?

Reflect on the ethical and scholarly value of sharing protocols, data extraction, or frameworks publicly.

3.7 Reflective prompt: Communicating the findings

Who is my audience? How might they use these findings? Am I presenting these findings in a way that supports decision-making or future inquiry?

Revisit your review's purpose and assess whether the presentation of results serves that intended purpose effectively.

4 Case vignettes, teaching points, and further reflective prompts

The following five case vignettes offer some likely scenarios that you may be presented with, with teaching points and reflective considerations, many of which focus on clarity with terminology. When reading through these examples, it is important to note that each context is different and considerations should be made based on the purpose of the review.

4.1 Case vignette 1: The overloaded question: Mapping professional identity in a sea of terms

A first-year PhD candidate, Ms. Judith Bently, wanted to explore how professional identity is conceptualized and taught in pharmacy education globally. She drafted a scoping review protocol but found her search returned thousands of articles, many of which did not align with her research question. Upon review, she realized that she had used search terms such as "professionalism", "professional", "identity" and "value system" interchangeably.

Teaching point: The importance of refining clear search terms and anchoring the concept clearly in the PCC framework to manage scope and relevance.

Reflective prompt: *How might you navigate overlapping terminology?*

4.2 Case vignette 2: Navigating the generative frontier- another case for a sea of terms

Dr. Trish Skoutas is an early-career pharmacy educator and research academic, and she noticed a sudden shift in student assessment submissions. Essays appeared more polished, reflective prompts more generic, and citations, strangely, more consistent. It became clear that some students used GenAI agents without acknowledgement, and there were concerns among the faculty regarding risk to academic integrity. Dr. Skoutas proposed conducting a scoping review to explore how GenAI is being integrated, regulated, and evaluated in pharmacy education globally. However, during the initial search strategy design, she encountered a major hurdle: the terminology was inconsistent; some studies referred to "large language models", others referred to "AI tools" or "AI agents", and some used broader terms such as "digital transformation" or "e-learning innovations". Her research team debated whether blog posts, conference presentations, or institutional documents (grey literature) should be included, since peer-reviewed research in this area in pharmacy education was limited and fast-evolving.

Teaching points:

1. Scoping reviews are especially useful in emerging and rapidly evolving fields such as GenAI, but terminology inconsistency poses challenges to the search strategy design. Some studies could be missed because search terms are not chosen well or are not broad enough to capture the relevant studies and/or grey literature sources.
2. Inclusion of grey literature can offer current and emerging insights.

Reflective prompts:

1. *How might the evolving nature of GenAI impact the scope and timeline of a review in pharmacy education?*
2. *How can researchers maintain methodological rigor when definitions are inconsistent or contested within the literature?*
3. *What ethical considerations should be addressed with including grey literature or nonpeer-reviewed sources in a review on such a fluid topic?*
4. *How can pharmacy educators design assessments that remain authentic and resilient in the age of GenAI?*

4.3 Case vignette 3: Curriculum reform on a deadline: Scoping for strategy in a compressed timeframe

Associate professor Jason Chu, a curriculum and program director, was tasked with reviewing the current literature on integrating GenAI into pharmacy curriculum. A scoping review was deemed ideal given the novelty of this emerging field. However, institutional pressures demanded a turnaround in four months. He debated whether to skip the protocol development and reduce the number of databases searched.

Teaching point: Navigating methodological rigor under real-world time constraints can be a real issue.

Reflective prompt: *How might a researcher balance feasibility with integrity when they receive pressure from stakeholders? How could these limitations of the review be communicated, and what are the consequences?*

4.4 Case vignette 4: The mirage of meaningful reflection—When mapping turns meta

Dr. Aran Javed, a lecturer in experiential learning and manager for clinical placements, was passionate about embedding reflective practice into experiential pharmacy education. Inspired by shifts in competency-based frameworks, he proposed a scoping review to explore how reflection is conceptualized, taught, and assessed in pharmacy curricula globally. However, he soon found himself entangled in a plethora of literature spanning nursing, medicine, and allied health, with some pharmacy-specific studies. Moreover, "reflection" was often used ambiguously—sometimes referring to structured assessment tools, other literature addressing other areas where reflection may be engaged, such as through "peer debriefs".

His inclusion criteria became difficult to apply consistently: should he include interprofessional studies? What about articles where pharmacy was mentioned only peripherally? His initial data extraction table did not account for such nuances. Furthermore, the review team debated whether to map educational theory use—such as Kolb's experiential reflective model (Kolb, 2015) or Schön's reflective practitioner model (Schön, 2016)—or focus solely on descriptive curricula papers.

Teaching points:

1. Scoping reviews exploring pedagogical concepts (like reflection or professionalism) in discipline-specific contexts can be challenging when relevant studies span disciplines and differ in depth.
2. Defining inclusion/exclusion criteria requires careful thought, especially when the concept is broad, terminology may differ between disciplines, and the literature is either sparse or cross-disciplinary.
3. Mapping underpinning theoretical frameworks can add value, but requires consistency and a clear rationale.

Reflective prompts:

1. When your concept exists across disciplines but with different emphases, how do you draw boundaries without compromising the rich data?
2. What strategies can you use to ensure consistency and transparency in applying inclusion/exclusion criteria when terms or contexts vary across studies?
3. How might theoretical frameworks help clarify or complicate your synthesis, particularly in pedagogical reviews?

4.5 Case vignette 5: Lost in translation—differing global experiential placements and the language of cultural safety

Ms. Kaper Raj, a second-year PhD student with a background in community pharmacy practice, wanted to examine how cultural safety is taught, developed, and evaluated in pharmacy student placements. She was especially interested in how programs prepare students for cross-cultural communication.

Her initial scoping review protocol seemed solid—framed by the PCC model and informed by previous global health studies and literature. She had decided that the countries she would focus on were Australia, Canada, and New Zealand. Yet, when piloting her search strategy, she encountered a cascade of confusingly broad and inconsistent terminology. Some studies used "cultural competence", others "cultural sensitivity", "cultural awareness", and/ or "cultural safety". Many articles referred to "cultural differences and communication preparedness" without clear definitions. Furthermore, terminology related to First Peoples differed in different countries, with some published manuscripts referring to Indigenous Peoples, First Nations Peoples, Aboriginal and/ or Torres Strait Islander Peoples, all of which needed consideration to capture all relevant data.

Further, pharmacy was often grouped with broader health sciences in global placement literature, with pharmacy-specific insights hard to disaggregate. She also indicated that there were challenges with how to treat experiential program evaluation reports or unpublished training materials shared by other universities.

Teaching points:

1. Terminology related to cultural safety is often used interchangeably but can carry very different meanings; clarity in concept definition is essential.
2. Pharmacy education research on global placements may be embedded within broader interprofessional or medical education studies, requiring nuanced screening decisions.
3. Grey literature, including program evaluations, can hold valuable insights—especially in underresearched areas

Reflective prompts:

1. *How might differences in cultural safety terminology affect the clarity and reproducibility of your review?*
2. *What are the ethical considerations when including or excluding pharmacy-adjacent data in global or interprofessional studies?*

3. *How can a researcher justify the inclusion of grey literature in culturally complex or underresearched areas of pharmacy education?*

5 Discussion

Scoping reviews occupy a unique space within the broader spectrum of evidence synthesis, offering a methodological flexibility that is particularly beneficial in underexplored or evolving domains, such as in pharmacy education. Selecting this approach over a systematic review research strategy often hinges on the nature of the research question. Scoping reviews are often employed when addressing broad, exploratory inquiries where a comprehensive understanding of the landscape (literature) is more valuable than a critical appraisal.

One key consideration in pharmacy education is its status as a "low-consensus" discipline,as education is generally regarded as low-consensus (Jackson et al., 2017), unlike other fields such as chemistry or physics, where terminologies are considered "high consensus". That is, they have widely accepted definitions, standardized methods, and consensus as to what constitutes valid knowledge or evidence. This, therefore, amplifies the complexity of the pharmacy researcher in navigating diverse terminologies and conceptual frameworks as well as reinforces the need for well-defined objectives and inclusion/ exclusion criteria, grounded in the PCC framework. This is because a key to the successful conduct (and meaningful results) of a scoping review is that there are well-defined, clear terms used to define the review (Lucas and Desselle, 2024). The iterative process of refining search terms also becomes crucial, as overly narrow or ambiguous terminology can limit the scope and breadth of evidence.

Another notable challenge is balancing comprehensiveness with feasibility. Grey literature, such as policy documents, institutional reports, and professional body statements, can provide essential insights, yet are more difficult to locate and evaluate. With some grey literature not being made publicly available or having iterations that require updating, some of these insights may be missed in a scoping review. However, establishing search strategies that incorporate both scientific literature and grey literature is not just beneficial but often necessary to ascertain the "bigger picture" for the education trends and gaps, often required for future policy and educational program changes.

As a pharmacy education researcher and reflecting on the conduct of my own review processes, I have found that early collaboration and specific task allocations across the research team enhanced both efficiency and consistency with all the review processes. Using shared platforms such as Covidence (2025c), enables us to streamline the screening and data extraction processes with several coinvestigators and also provides a platform to meet consensus. One practical insight was the value of documentation at every step, including rationale for excluding specific sources, as this becomes especially important when revisiting earlier decisions or responding to peer reviewers.

Finally, the utility of scoping reviews in informing future research agendas cannot be overstated. In pharmacy education, where rapid curriculum design aligned with evolving scopes of practice, coupled with technological change, is inevitable, these reviews provide a valuable snapshot of current knowledge, gaps, and emerging priorities. They also support educators and policymakers in making informed decisions grounded in evidence. Although scoping reviews do not traditionally appraise the study quality, their methodological rigor lies in their reproducibility (protocol development), transparency (protocol publication or registration), and the clarity of the conceptual focus.

6 Questions for further discussion

1. In what context is a scoping review preferable to a systematic or other type of review in educational research?
2. How can transparency be enhanced when publishing scoping review protocols and findings?
3. What challenges arise from conducting reviews, and how may these be mitigated?
4. How might scoping reviews be used to drive and inform curriculum innovations and reform in health professions education?
5. What role do stakeholder perspectives (e.g., educators, students, policy makers) play in shaping the scope and utility of a scoping review? Should there be considerations for codesign processes and practical relevance?
6. What considerations have you made regarding differences in the terminology of search terms?

References

Aly, M., Schneider, C.R., Sukkar, M.B., Lucas, C., 2020. Educational needs of community pharmacy staff in minor ailment service delivery: a systematic scoping review. Curr. Pharm. Teach. Learn. 18771300. 12 (10), 1269–1287. Available from: http://www.elsevier.com/wps/find/journaldescription.cws_home/718643/description#description. doi:10.1016/j.cptl.2020.05.013.

Arksey, H., O'Malley, L., 2005. Scoping studies: towards a methodological framework. Int. J. Soc. Res. Methodol. 1364-5579. 8 (1), 19–32. doi:10.1080/1364557032000119616.

Chan, S.L., Ho, C.Z.H., Khaing, N.E.E., Ho, E., Pong, C., Guan, J.S., Chua, C., Li, Z., Lim, T., Lam, S.S.W., Low, L.L., How, C.H., 2024. Frameworks for measuring population health: a scoping review. PLoS ONE. 19326203. 19 (2). Available from: https://journals.plos.org//plosone/article?id=10.1371/journal.pone.0278434. doi:10.1371/journal.pone.0278434.

Colquhoun, H.L., Levac, D., O'Brien, K.K., Straus, S., Tricco, A.C., Perrier, L., Kastner, M., Moher, D., 2014. Scoping reviews: time for clarity in definition, methods, and reporting. J. Clin. Epidemiol. 18785921. 67 (12), 1291–1294. Available from: www.elsevier.com/locate/jclinepi. doi:10.1016/j.jclinepi.2014.03.013.

Covidence, 2025c. Available from: https://www.covidence.org/.

Deslandes, R., Lucas, C., Hughes, M.L., Mantzourani, E., 2018. Development of a template to facilitate reflection among student pharmacists. Res. Social Adm. Pharm. 15517411. 14 (11), 1058–1063. doi:10.1016/j.sapharm.2017.11.010.

Figshare, 2025a. Available from: https://figshare.com/.

Godin, K.M., Kirkpatrick, S.I., Hanning, R.M., Stapleton, J., Leatherdale, S.T., 2017. Examining guidelines for school-based breakfast programs in Canada: a systematic review of the grey literature. Can. J. Diet. Pract. Res. 1486-3847. 78 (2), 92–100. doi:10.3148/cjdpr-2016-037.

Gopalakrishnan, S., Ganeshkumar, P., 2013. Systematic reviews and meta-analysis: understanding the best evidence in primary healthcare. J. Fam. Med. Prim. Care. 2249-4863. 2 (1), 9. doi:10.4103/2249-4863.109934.

History of systematic reviews, n.d. Available from: https://eppi.ioe.ac.uk/cms/Resources/EvidenceInformedPolicyandPractice/HistoryofSystematicReviews/tabid/68/Default.aspx#:~:text=Critical%20appraisal%20and%20synthesis%20of%20research%20findings%20in,1980%29%20and%20class%20size%20%28Glass%20and%20Smith%201979%29.

Holmes, E.R., Desselle, S.P., 2004. Is scientific paradigm important for pharmacy education? Am. J. Pharm. Educ. 00029459. 68 (5), 1–10. Available from: http://www.ajpe.org/page/about. doi:10.5688/aj6805118.

Jackson, J.K., Latimer, M., Stoiko, R., 2017. The dynamic between knowledge production and faculty evaluation: perceptions of the promotion and tenure process across disciplines. Innov. High. Educ. 15731758. 42 (3), 193–205. Available from: http://www.springerlink.com/content/0742-5627. doi:10.1007/s10755-016-9378-3.

Kastner, M., Tricco, A.C., Soobiah, C., Lillie, E., Perrier, L., Horsley, T., Welch, V., Cogo, E., Antony, J., Straus, S.E., 2012. What is the most appropriate knowledge synthesis method to conduct a review? Protocol for a scoping review. BMC Med. Res. Methodol. 14712288. 12. doi:10.1186/1471-2288-12-114.

Khalil, H., Peters, M.D., Tricco, A.C., Pollock, D., Alexander, L., McInerney, P., Godfrey, C.M., Munn, Z., 2021. Conducting high quality scoping reviews-challenges and solutions. J. Clin. Epidemiol. 18785921. 130, 156–160. Available from: www.elsevier.com/locate/jclinepi. doi:10.1016/j.jclinepi.2020.10.009.

Kolb, D., 2015. Experiential learning: experience as the source of learning and development (2nd ed.). Pearson Education, Inc.

Le, J., Mantzourani, E., Desselle, S., Lonie, J.M., Lucas, C., 2019. Enhancing future pharmacy practice through integration of reflective practice strategies to embed self-development in a medication safety culture. Res. Social Adm. Pharm. 15517411. 15 (5), e18. doi:10.1016/j.sapharm.2019.03.119.

Levac, D., Colquhoun, H., O'Brien, K.K., 2010. Scoping studies: advancing the methodology. Implement. Sci. 17485908. 5 (1). Available from: http://www.implementationscience.com/content/5/1/69. doi:10.1186/1748-5908-5-69.

Lucas, C., Desselle, S.P., 2024. Considerations for conducting a scoping review in pharmacy education. Explor. Res. Clin. Soc. Pharm. 26672766. 14, 100448. doi:10.1016/j.rcsop.2024.100448.

Lucas, C., Smith, L., Lonie, J.M., Hough, M., Rogers, K., Mantzourani, E., 2019. Can a reflective rubric be applied consistently with raters globally? A study across three countries. Curr. Pharm. Teach. Learn. 18771300. 11 (10), 987–994. Available from: http://www.elsevier.com/wps/find/journaldescription.cws_home/718643/description#description. doi:10.1016/j.cptl.2019.06.004.

Mantzourani, E., Desselle, S., Le, J., Lonie, J.M., Lucas, C., 2019. The role of reflective practice in healthcare professions: next steps for pharmacy education and practice. Res. Social Adm. Pharm. 15517411. 15 (12), 1476–1479. doi:10.1016/j.sapharm.2019.03.011.

Martin, G.P., Jenkins, D.A., Bull, L., Sisk, R., Lin, L., Hulme, W., Wilson, A., Wang, W., Barrowman, M., Sammut-Powell, C., Pate, A., Sperrin, M., Peek, N., 2020. Towards a framework for the design, implementation and reporting of methodology scoping reviews. arXiv 23318422. Available from: https://arxiv.org. doi:10.48550/arxiv.2001.08988.

McGowan, J., Straus, S., Moher, D., Langlois, E.V., O'Brien, K.K., Horsley, T., Aldcroft, A., Zarin, W., Garitty, C.M., Hempel, S., Lillie, E., Tunçalp, ö., Tricco, A.C., 2020. Reporting scoping reviews—PRISMA ScR extension. J. Clin. Epidemiol. 08954356. 123, 177–179. doi:10.1016/j.jclinepi.2020.03.016.

Mortlock, R., Lucas, C., 2024. Generative artificial intelligence (Gen-AI) in pharmacy education: utilization and implications for academic integrity: a scoping review. Explor. Res. Clin. Soc. Pharm. 26672766. 15, 100481. doi:10.1016/j.rcsop.2024.100481.

Munn, Z., Peters, M.D.J., Stern, C., Tufanaru, C., McArthur, A., Aromataris, E., 2018. Systematic review or scoping review? Guidance for authors when choosing between a systematic or scoping review approach. BMC Med. Res. Methodol. 14712288. 18 (1). Available from: http://www.biomedcentral.com/bmcmedresmethodol/. doi:10.1186/s12874-018-0611-x.

Open Science Framework (OSF), n.d. Available from: https://osf.io/.

Peters, M.D.J., Godfrey, C., McInerney, P., Munn, Z., Tricco, A.C., Khalil, H., n.d. 2024. Scoping reviews (2020 version). In: Aromataris, E., Lockwood, C., Porritt, K., Pilla, B. and Jordan, Z. (Eds.), JBI Manual for Evidence Synthesis 2024. Adelaide: JBI, Chapter 10. Available from: https://synthesismanual.jbi.global. doi:10.46658/JBIMES-24-09.

Rayyan, 2025b. Available from: https://www.rayyan.ai/.

Researchgate, 2025d Available from: https://www.researchgate.net/.

Schön, D.A., 2016. The reflective practitioner: how professionals think in action.

Sharma, N., Arahna, V.P., Saxena, S., Ateef, M., Samuel, A.J., 2022. Scoping out the scope of scoping reviews in neonatal and pediatric pain management: a scoping review methodological framework. J. Pediatr. Surg. 15315037. 57 (8), 1599–1608. Available from: http://www.elsevier.com/inca/publications/store/6/2/3/1/4/8/index.htt. doi:10.1016/j.jpedsurg.2021.11.012.

Tricco, A.C., Lillie, E., Zarin, W., O'Brien, K., Colquhoun, H., Kastner, M., Levac, D., Ng, C., Sharpe, J.P., Wilson, K., Kenny, M., Warren, R., Wilson, C., Stelfox, H.T., Straus, S.E., 2016. A scoping review on the conduct and reporting of scoping reviews. BMC Med. Res. Methodol. 14712288. 16 (1). Available from: http://www.biomedcentral.com/bmcmedresmethodol/. doi:10.1186/s12874-016-0116-4.

Tricco, A.C., Lillie, E., Zarin, W., O'Brien, K.K., Colquhoun, H., Levac, D., Moher, D., Peters, M.D.J., Horsley, T., Weeks, L., Hempel, S., Akl, E.A., Chang, C., McGowan, J., Stewart, L., Hartling, L., Aldcroft, A., Wilson, M.G., Garritty, C., Lewin, S., Godfrey, C.M., MacDonald, M.T., Langlois, E.V., Soares-Weiser, K., Moriarty, J., Clifford, T., Tunçalp, Ö., Straus, S.E., 2018. PRISMA extension for scoping reviews (PRISMA-ScR): checklist and explanation. Ann. Intern. Med. 15393704. 169 (7), 467–473. Available from: http://annals.org/aim/fullarticle/2700389/prisma-extension-scoping-reviews-prisma-scr-checklist-explanation. doi:10.7326/M18-0850.

Tsingos-Lucas, C., Bosnic-Anticevich, S., Schneider, C.R., Smith, L., 2016. The effect of reflective activities on reflective thinking ability in an undergraduate pharmacy curriculum. Am. J. Pharm. Educ. 00029459. 80 (4), 65. doi:10.5688/ajpe80465.

Tsingos, C., 2013. Reflective practice: learning from experience. J. Pharm. Pract. Res. 1445937X. 43 (3), 249–250.

Tsingos, C., Bosnic-Anticevich, S., Lonie, J.M., Smith, L., 2015. A model for assessing reflective practices in pharmacy education. Am. J. Pharm. Educ. 00029459. 79 (8), 124. doi:10.5688/ajpe798124.

Tsingos, C., Bosnic-Anticevich, S., Smith, L., 2014. Reflective practice and its implications for pharmacy education. Am. J. Pharm. Educ. 00029459. 78 (1), 18. doi:10.5688/ajpe78118.

SECTION II

Designing and evaluating interventions in pharmacy research

CHAPTER

9

Investigating the impact of agile methods on psychological safety perception in pharmaceutical practice: A multidimensional approach

Dragana Jocic[a] *and Valentina Marinkovic*[b]

[a]Faculty of Pharmacy, Novi Sad, Serbia

[b]Faculty of Pharmacy, Belgrade, Serbia

CHAPTER OBJECTIVES

This chapter aims to:

- Explore the concept of psychological safety in healthcare, with a specific focus on community pharmacy settings and the distinct challenges faced by pharmacists
- Emphasize the role of psychological safety in enhancing team collaboration, professional efficiency, and patient safety within pharmacy practice
- Analyze how psychological safety relates to pharmacists' individual outcomes, specifically job satisfaction, stress management, and protection against burnout
- Investigate the impact of different professional development approaches—namely, agile coaching and traditional education—on pharmacists' perceptions of psychological safety
- Present the design and implementation of an experimental study conducted in community pharmacies, employing validated psychometric instruments to assess changes in perceived psychological safety over time
- Discuss key methodological considerations in evaluating psychological constructs in real-world healthcare contexts, including participant sampling, intervention delivery, and data interpretation
- Offer insights into the methodological integration of agile approaches within healthcare intervention research, providing a practical model for future studies

1 Introduction

Psychological safety, as conceptualized by Edmondson (1999, 2018), refers to a shared belief within a workgroup that the environment is safe for interpersonal risk-taking. This means that employees feel comfortable expressing their thoughts, asking questions, admitting mistakes, and challenging existing norms without fear of humiliation or reprisal. This construct has increasingly been recognized as a critical determinant of team effectiveness, learning, innovation, and overall organizational health—particularly in complex and high-stakes environments such as healthcare (Carmeli et al., 2009; Carmeli and Gittell, 2009; Cochrane et al., 2017). Importantly, in pharmacy practice,

https://doi.org/10.1016/B978-0-443-44607-8.00010-8

psychological safety extends beyond team dynamics and organizational performance, as it directly influences patient safety. When pharmacists are able to speak up about potential errors, uncertainties, or system flaws without fear of negative consequences, the likelihood of medication errors decreases and the overall quality of patient care improves.

Within healthcare, psychological safety is essential for fostering environments where frontline professionals collaborate openly, share critical information, and engage in continuous learning to improve patient outcomes. The absence of psychological safety has been linked to communication breakdowns, errors, and adverse events, thus directly impacting patient safety and care quality (Edmondson, 2018; Carmeli and Gittell, 2009). In this respect, psychological safety is not merely a "soft" organizational climate factor but a vital component of healthcare reliability and resilience (Cochrane et al., 2017).

Pharmacy practice, particularly in community settings, presents a unique context where psychological safety plays a pivotal role. Community pharmacists serve as the most accessible healthcare professionals to the public, delivering medication therapy management, patient education, and counseling services while navigating complex regulatory, organizational, and social demands (Cochrane et al., 2017; Newman et al., 2017). Their responsibilities often require rapid decision-making, error prevention, and multidisciplinary coordination, frequently within time-pressured and resource-constrained environments. Such conditions elevate the risk of stress, job dissatisfaction, and burnout—phenomena increasingly documented among pharmacists globally (O'Donovan et al., 2020; Jocić et al., 2018; Jocić and Krajnović, 2014).

Psychological safety within pharmacy teams is, therefore, not only about creating a positive workplace culture but also about safeguarding the mental health and professional wellbeing of pharmacists, which, in turn, is linked to higher-quality patient care. Pharmacists who experience psychological safety report greater job satisfaction, reduced stress levels, and lower burnout rates (Jocić and Krajnović, 2014; Lackie et al., 2023; Jocić and Marinković, 2024). The relationship between psychological safety and these outcomes can be further understood through its protective function in demanding work environments, such as community pharmacies. A psychologically safe climate enables pharmacists to cope more effectively with workload intensity and role complexity, thereby reducing perceived stress and supporting sustainable job satisfaction. In contrast, the absence of psychological safety increases the likelihood of emotional exhaustion and disengagement, ultimately contributing to burnout. As highlighted in the literature, psychological safety thus represents a critical organizational resource that not only safeguards professional wellbeing but also reinforces resilience and the capacity to maintain high-quality patient care (Jocić et al., 2018; Jocić and Krajnović, 2014; Jocić and Marinković, 2024). These outcomes promote workforce sustainability and contribute to improved patient safety by facilitating open communication, error reporting, and collaborative problem-solving (Edmondson, 1999, 2018; Jocić and Marinković, 2024). The relationship between psychological safety and these outcomes can be further understood through its protective function in demanding work environments, such as community pharmacies. A psychologically safe climate enables pharmacists to cope more effectively with workload intensity and role complexity, thereby reducing perceived stress and supporting sustainable job satisfaction. In contrast, the absence of psychological safety increases the likelihood of emotional exhaustion and disengagement, ultimately contributing to burnout (Jocić et al., 2018; Jocić and Krajnović, 2014; Jocić and Marinković, 2024).

Moreover, the interplay between psychological safety and professional development is an emerging area of interest. Traditional education models in pharmacy emphasize knowledge acquisition, adherence to established protocols, and structured learning environments but may not fully address the socio-emotional competencies and adaptive capacities necessary for dynamic team environments (Jocić and Marinković, 2024). In contrast, agile coaching prioritizes continuous feedback, reflection, iterative learning cycles, and adaptability to real-world clinical challenges. Agile approaches foster empowerment, resilience, and collaborative problem-solving among pharmacy professionals—qualities closely tied to fostering psychological safety (Jocić and Marinković, 2024). The choice between these approaches depends on the learning objectives, the complexity of professional tasks, and the balance desired between procedural competence and adaptive socio-emotional skills. Despite the recognized benefits of agile coaching, its application in community pharmacy remains largely unexplored. Existing training approaches often focus primarily on procedural knowledge and adherence to protocols, which may not sufficiently develop socio-emotional competencies, adaptability, or collaborative problem-solving—key factors in fostering psychological safety (Jocić and Marinković, 2024; Jocic, 2024).

The learner-centered and iterative structure of agile coaching contrasts with conventional didactic methods by enabling contextualized learning aligned with pharmacists' immediate professional challenges. This responsiveness enhances engagement and facilitates the internalization of psychological safety principles as lived experiences rather than abstract concepts. By nurturing a growth mindset and a collaborative orientation toward problem-solving, agile coaching can directly contribute to creating psychologically safe work environments in community pharmacies.

Studying these relationships calls for rigorous and context-sensitive methodological approaches. Experimental study designs are well-suited for this purpose because they allow researchers to manipulate independent variables—in this case, different professional development interventions—and observe their causal effects on psychological safety perceptions and related outcomes (Edmondson, 1999; Verma et al., 2024). This level of control is particularly important in healthcare settings, where multifactorial influences on team behavior and safety perceptions can obscure causal inferences in purely observational studies.

Given the complex and multifaceted nature of psychological safety as a phenomenon, a multidimensional methodological approach is most appropriate. This approach allows for capturing the various interacting factors and contextual influences that shape psychological safety perceptions in community pharmacy settings, providing a more comprehensive and nuanced understanding than single-method designs (Verma et al., 2024; Buvik and Tkalich, 2021).

Measurement of psychological safety in healthcare settings poses significant challenges. Given its subjective and multifaceted nature, accurate assessment demands validated psychometric instruments that are sensitive to contextual nuances (O'Donovan et al., 2020). Surveys based on Edmondson's psychological safety scale have been widely used and adapted for healthcare professionals, including pharmacists, with demonstrated reliability and validity (Edmondson, 1999; O'Donovan et al., 2020). However, relying solely on quantitative survey data risks overlooking rich contextual factors such as team dynamics, leadership behavior, and organizational culture.

To address this, mixed-method approaches incorporating observational data or qualitative interviews have been advocated (O'Donovan et al., 2020; Lackie et al., 2023). Observational methods, for example, can capture real-time behaviors indicative of psychological safety, such as the willingness to speak up or support colleagues during stressful events. Integrating multiple data sources strengthens construct validity and provides a more comprehensive picture of psychological safety in practice.

Furthermore, methodologically sound sampling and data collection procedures are crucial for generalizability and replicability. The study described in this chapter targets community pharmacies with diverse demographic and organizational characteristics to reflect the heterogeneity of practice settings. Intervention fidelity is ensured through standardized training protocols and ongoing supervision of coaches and educators, while repeated measurements at multiple time points allow for the assessment of change trajectories and intervention sustainability.

A distinctive feature of this research is the integration of agile principles not only within the content of the intervention but also in the study design itself. Agile methodologies emphasize iterative cycles of planning, action, evaluation, and adaptation. Applying these principles methodologically enhances flexibility in responding to emergent challenges during intervention delivery, such as participant feedback or contextual shifts (Jocić and Marinković, 2024; Verma et al., 2024). This adaptive research design facilitates continuous improvement of the intervention and optimizes engagement and relevance for participants.

The present study thus contributes methodologically by demonstrating how agile frameworks can be employed in healthcare research to study complex psychosocial constructs, such as psychological safety. This approach may serve as a model for future research aiming to implement and evaluate behavioral interventions in dynamic, real-world healthcare environments.

In summary, psychological safety represents a critical foundation for effective, sustainable, and high-quality pharmacy practice. Its systematic promotion through targeted professional development interventions—especially those utilizing agile coaching—is a promising strategy to enhance pharmacist wellbeing, team collaboration, and ultimately patient care quality (DuBose, 2023; Carrillo et al., 2024; Todaro-Franceschi, 2024; Motta, 2024). Employing a rigorous experimental design with validated measurement tools and agile methodological principles provides a robust framework for advancing both scientific understanding and practical application of psychological safety in community pharmacy settings (Jocić and Marinković, 2024).

The following sections will elaborate on the study's experimental design, psychometric measures, intervention protocols, and analytical strategies to provide replicable, evidence-based insights into fostering psychological safety in pharmacy teams.

2 Methods

2.1 Study design

This section outlines the methodology best suited to investigate the perception of psychological safety among pharmacists in community pharmacy settings, especially when comparing two different educational approaches, such as agile coaching and traditional training. Given the complex and multifaceted nature of psychological safety, the specific characteristics of the pharmaceutical sector and community pharmacy work, as well as the need to rigorously evaluate and compare intervention effects, a multidimensional methodological approach is most appropriate. This approach enables a comprehensive assessment that captures both the nuanced psychological phenomena and the practical realities of pharmacy practice, while providing a robust framework to directly compare the impacts of agile coaching versus traditional education methods. The methodologies discussed in this chapter provide valuable insights into how psychological safety can be measured and how different interventions may influence its perception in real-world pharmacy environments.

2.2 Participants and sampling

The study included pharmacists working in community pharmacy settings, with participants allocated to either agile coaching or traditional education groups according to the study design.

Determining the appropriate sample size is a critical step in designing both experimental and longitudinal observational studies to ensure sufficient statistical power to detect meaningful effects (Althubaiti, 2023; Politi et al., 2023).

For the experimental design, sample size calculations typically focus on detecting differences between groups (e.g., agile coaching versus traditional education) on key outcome measures such as psychological safety. The calculation requires specifying the expected effect size, desired statistical power (commonly 0.80), and significance level (usually $\alpha = 0.05$) (Politi et al., 2023; Julious, 2023).

For the longitudinal observational design, the sample size calculation additionally considers the repeated measurements over time and the potential correlations among these repeated observations within subjects. The design requires accounting for within-subject variance and potential attrition during follow-up.

Details of the sample size calculations for both the experimental and longitudinal studies are provided in Box 9.1.

By carefully calculating sample sizes based on these considerations, the study design aims to optimize resource use while maximizing the validity and reliability of the findings.

2.3 Interventions (agile versus traditional)

2.3.1 *Comparing agile coaching and traditional education methods*

To examine the effectiveness of agile coaching versus traditional education methods in enhancing psychological safety, a comparative analysis can be performed using both experimental and observational research designs. Agile coaching and traditional education differ not only in instructional format but also in their underlying assumptions about learning, motivation, and interpersonal dynamics (Fernandez and Fernandez, 2008). While traditional education is typically content-driven, hierarchical, and structured around standardized knowledge transfer, agile coaching adopts a more flexible, iterative, and learner-centered approach that emphasizes team collaboration, psychological empowerment, and adaptive learning (Fernandez and Fernandez, 2008; Klünder et al., 2022; López-Alcarria et al., 2019).

In the context of pharmacy practice, where rapid changes, high accountability, and complex interpersonal communication are common, these differences may have significant implications for psychological safety (Jocić and Marinković, 2024). Agile coaching encourages open dialog, continuous feedback, and collective problem-solving, which can foster trust and a climate of interpersonal risk-taking. On the other hand, traditional education may be

BOX 9.1

Sample size calculation for experimental and longitudinal studies

Experimental study: An a priori power analysis was performed using parameters such as an expected medium effect size (Cohen's $d = 0.5$), $\alpha = 0.05$, and power = 0.80. This analysis determined the minimum number of participants required in each group to reliably detect group differences in psychological safety scores (Althubaiti, 2023; Politi et al., 2023; Julious, 2023). Resulting sample size: n = XX per group.

Longitudinal observational study: Sample size calculation incorporated the number of measurement points, expected correlation between repeated measures, and effect sizes based on previous literature or pilot data. This ensured adequate power to detect changes over time and between intervention conditions (Althubaiti, 2023; Politi et al., 2023; Julious, 2023). Resulting sample size: n = XX participants.

less effective in promoting psychological safety if it lacks mechanisms for addressing relational dynamics, reflective practice, or emotional support (Bäcklander, 2019; Hunt et al., 2021).

Research comparing these two approaches typically involves multidimensional assessment strategies that capture both objective outcomes (e.g., behavioral indicators, error reporting rates) and subjective experiences (e.g., perceived team support, openness to feedback). Mixed-methods designs are particularly valuable as they allow for triangulation of data and a deeper understanding of contextual influences (Rajasekar and Verma, 2013).

Ultimately, the choice between agile coaching and traditional methods should be informed by the desired learning outcomes, the specific context of professional practice, and the psychosocial conditions that support safety, engagement, and growth among healthcare professionals (Jocić and Marinković, 2024; Stray et al., 2020). For instance, agile coaching may be particularly beneficial in dynamic team environments where ongoing problem-solving, adaptation to change, and open communication are critical. In contrast, traditional methods might be preferred for ensuring compliance with regulatory requirements, acquiring technical knowledge, or standardizing procedural skills. In many settings, a combination of both approaches can optimize learning outcomes by addressing both technical proficiency and team-based competencies (Edmondson, 1999, 2018; Jocić and Marinković, 2024).

Table 9.1 summarizes the key differences between agile coaching and traditional education methods in terms of their impact on psychological safety.

Agile coaching was delivered over six weeks, with weekly 90 min sessions led by trained coaches. The program included structured activities such as iterative feedback, collaborative problem-solving, reflective team exercises, and techniques to enhance psychological empowerment and interpersonal risk-taking. Traditional education sessions, in contrast, were instructor-led, lecture-based, and focused on regulatory knowledge, technical skills, and standardized procedures (Jocic, 2024). These findings suggest that agile coaching offers a more effective approach to enhancing psychological safety in healthcare settings, where collaboration and adaptability are paramount (Jocic, 2024). However, it is important to note that traditional education methods still have their place in providing foundational knowledge and technical skills that are necessary for pharmacists to perform their roles effectively. Thus, a hybrid model that integrates elements of both approaches could potentially yield the best outcomes in terms of improving psychological safety and overall team performance.

2.4 Measures (quantitative and qualitative)

Psychological safety can be effectively measured using a variety of quantitative and qualitative research methods, each offering distinct advantages in capturing both individual perceptions and team dynamics. The measurement of psychological safety is crucial for understanding the underlying factors that influence learning behaviors, team cohesion, and organizational performance in healthcare environments.

2.4.1 Quantitative measures

Psychological safety can be assessed using a variety of general quantitative approaches, such as self-report surveys capturing perceptions of team support, openness, and risk-taking behaviors. While these measures provide useful insights into the overall team climate, they are often less specific to individual experiences of psychological safety (Jocić and Marinković, 2024; Plouffe et al., 2023; Liu et al., 2024). For this reason, the Psychological Safety Scale (PSS), developed by Edmondson (2018) and Edmondson et al. (2004), has been widely used in studies, as it focuses directly on individuals' comfort with interpersonal risk-taking, making it particularly suitable for the pharmacy context. The scale includes items designed to assess the extent to which team members feel comfortable taking

TABLE 9.1 Comparison of agile coaching and traditional education methods.

Aspect	Agile coaching	Traditional education
Methodology	Iterative, collaborative, feedback-driven	Top-down, structured, instructor-led
Focus	Team collaboration, continuous improvement	Knowledge transfer, skill acquisition
Psychological safety impact	High (encourages openness and risk-taking)	Lower (limited opportunity for feedback and expression)
Engagement	High (active involvement in problem-solving)	Moderate (passive learning environment)
Flexibility	High (adaptable to team needs and feedback)	Low (predefined curriculum)
Evaluation approach	Ongoing, reflective, includes self- and peer-assessment	Periodic, summative, focused on testing, and external grading

such risks in their work environment (Edmondson, 2018; Edmondson et al., 2004). These risks may include voicing concerns, sharing ideas, and admitting mistakes. Participants rate statements related to their comfort in engaging in these behaviors without fear of negative consequences. The scale has been widely validated across industries and is frequently used in healthcare research (Plouffe et al., 2023; Liu et al., 2024; Edmondson, 2018; Edmondson et al., 2004).

Table 9.2 provides an overview of the items included in a version of the PSS, developed during the scale creation process in the context of the study (Jocic, 2024), along with the corresponding dimensions measured.

The items in Table 9.2 illustrate the core elements of the PSS, reflecting team members' perceptions of risk-taking, support, respect, openness, inclusion, humility, and transparency. In the context of pharmacy, psychological safety remains a crucial construct for promoting effective teamwork, open communication, and high-quality patient care (Jocić and Marinković, 2024; Jocic, 2024). It represents the shared belief among professionals that they can voice concerns, ask questions, or acknowledge mistakes without fear of embarrassment, rejection, or punishment (Edmondson, 2018).

In community pharmacy settings, psychological safety relates to the confidence of pharmacists to voice concerns, ask questions, and acknowledge mistakes without fear of negative consequences. The scale items were interpreted in light of the specific dynamics, responsibilities, and interactions characteristic of pharmacy teams.

To ensure that psychological safety is assessed appropriately among pharmacists, the measurement approach should capture the specific psychological and organizational characteristics of the pharmacy work environment. Table 9.3 presents the key domains and areas that a context-sensitive scale should address, which are further elaborated below.

As outlined in Table 9.3, the first crucial domain to be assessed is the extent to which pharmacists feel comfortable speaking up. This includes their ability to express concerns about patient safety or workflow inefficiencies and report near-misses without fear of negative consequences. Scales should include items that explore whether indi-

TABLE 9.2 Overview of psychological safety scale (PSS) items.

Item	Dimension	Example statement
I feel safe to take risks in my team.	Risk-Taking	"I feel safe taking risks in my team."
If I make a mistake, it is not held against me.	Supportiveness	"If I make a mistake, I am not criticized or reprimanded."
Members of my team value my input.	Respect	"My team values my contributions."
I am able to express my opinions without fear.	Openness	"I can express my ideas without fearing judgment."
Team members are supportive when someone voices a different opinion.	Inclusion	"Different viewpoints are welcomed and respected by the team."
I can admit when I don't know something without feeling inadequate.	Humility safety	"I feel comfortable acknowledging a lack of knowledge in front of my team."
Difficult issues can be discussed openly in my team.	Transparency	"We can talk openly about problems without blame or defensiveness."

TABLE 9.3 Key domains for assessing psychological safety among pharmacists.

Domain	Focus area	Contextual relevance in pharmacy practice
1. Comfort in speaking up	Freedom to ask questions, express opinions, and report errors	Encourages openness in daily work and supports patient safety through early error identification
2. Team respect and inclusion	Equal voice regardless of hierarchy	Promotes trust among pharmacists, technicians, and supervisors, essential for cohesive team functioning
3. Response to mistakes	Treatment of errors as learning opportunities	Reduces blame culture and enhances reflective practice and continuing education
4. Support in patient interactions	Feeling backed by colleagues and organization during complex patient communication	Increases confidence in addressing adherence issues, misinformation, and sensitive topics
5. Communication with other professionals	Comfort in raising concerns to physicians and other healthcare providers	Enhances interprofessional collaboration and safeguards therapeutic decisions
6. Autonomy and decision-making	Freedom to apply professional judgment in nonstandard situations	Supports individualized patient care and professional development

viduals perceive that their voice is genuinely heard and considered by others in the team (Jocić and Marinković, 2024; Critical Appraisal Skills Programme, 2021; Babbie et al., 2022). Equally important is the perception of respect and inclusion within the team. Regardless of hierarchy or role, all team members, including junior pharmacists and pharmacy technicians, should feel their contributions are valued (Jocić and Marinković, 2024). When such psychological inclusiveness is present, it fosters stronger interpersonal bonds and enhances collaborative decision-making (Edmondson et al., 2004).

How mistakes are handled within the team is another key element. Scales must assess whether the environment supports viewing errors as a natural part of the learning process. In psychologically safe teams, discussing and analyzing mistakes leads to better protocols and improved service quality rather than punishment or stigma (Edmondson, 2018; Edmondson et al., 2004).

In pharmacy practice, communication with patients can be highly demanding. Whether it involves educating patients about complex therapies or managing dissatisfaction, pharmacists must feel supported by colleagues and supervisors (Jocić and Marinković, 2024). A sense of psychological safety in these interactions reduces stress and burnout and encourages pharmacists to engage more deeply with patients' concerns (Jocić et al., 2018; Jocić and Krajnović, 2014).

Furthermore, interprofessional communication represents a vital dimension. Pharmacists often need to clarify prescriptions, suggest alternatives, or question drug interactions (Jocić and Marinković, 2024). The ability to do so safely—especially when interacting with physicians or specialists—is a strong indicator of psychological safety and professionalism in a collaborative care model (Jocić and Marinković, 2024).

Finally, the scale should address autonomy and the capacity for independent decision-making. Pharmacists often rely on their clinical judgment in situations where guidelines may not provide clear answers. Feeling trusted and supported in applying that judgment, even when it challenges existing norms, is central to both professional fulfillment and patient-centered care (Jocić and Marinković, 2024).

Together, these domains provide a comprehensive framework for constructing and validating psychological safety scales in pharmacy practice. By aligning measurement tools with the unique demands and social dynamics of pharmacy work, organizations can obtain meaningful insights that guide interventions to foster safer, more inclusive, and more effective practice environments.

2.4.2 *Qualitative measures*

Qualitative methods, such as semistructured interviews and focus groups, can provide deeper insights (Rajasekar and Verma, 2013; Bhattacharyya, 2006; Brunswik, 2023; Kazdin, 2021; Kumar and Praveenakumar, 2025) into individual experiences and team dynamics that influence psychological safety. These methods allow participants to share personal narratives about how they perceive their work environment, the extent to which they feel supported by their colleagues and supervisors, and the impact of team communication on their overall sense of safety. Thematic analysis of the data gathered from these interviews can reveal key factors contributing to or detracting from psychological safety in the workplace.

Table 9.4 presents an example of the qualitative interview guide that could be used to gather insights on psychological safety. The semistructured interview guide was developed by the authors and informed by the study objectives.

TABLE 9.4 Example of semistructured qualitative interview guide.

Topic	Sample question
Team dynamics	"How would you describe the way team members interact and communicate during daily work activities?"
Support from colleagues	"Can you share an example when you felt supported by your colleagues in a challenging situation?"
Openness to feedback	"To what extent do you feel comfortable expressing disagreement or offering suggestions for change?"
Risk-taking in the team environment	"How does your team respond when someone makes a mistake or takes an initiative that doesn't succeed?"
Leadership approach	"How would you describe your supervisor's role in fostering trust and open dialogue within the team?"
Conflict resolution	"When disagreements occur, how are they typically addressed in your team?"
Inclusion and participation	"Do you feel that everyone's voice is equally valued in team decisions? Can you elaborate?"
Psychological safety moments	"Can you recall a recent moment when you felt either especially safe or unsafe to speak up?"

A mixed-methods approach is often used to combine the strengths of both quantitative and qualitative data collection (Rajasekar and Verma, 2013; Bhattacharyya, 2006; Brunswik, 2023). By integrating surveys with interviews, researchers can gain a well-rounded understanding of how psychological safety operates in community pharmacies while also capturing nuanced perspectives that might not emerge from quantitative data alone.

2.5 Procedure

2.5.1 Experimental design

An experimental design is a structured approach used to examine causal relationships by systematically manipulating one or more independent variables while controlling for potential confounding factors. Participants are typically randomly assigned to different intervention groups, allowing researchers to attribute changes in outcome variables directly to the intervention (Babbie et al., 2022; Bhattacharyya, 2006).

In psychological and organizational research within healthcare, such as community pharmacy settings, this design can be applied to evaluate the effectiveness of educational interventions. For example, an experimental study may randomly assign pharmacy teams to receive either agile coaching or traditional educational training (Jocić and Marinković, 2024). Measurements of psychological safety, job satisfaction, and burnout are collected before and after the intervention to assess its impact.

Although often associated with biomedical research, randomized controlled trials (RCTs) are increasingly used in behavioral and educational sciences to investigate the effects of psychosocial interventions. As demonstrated in recent pharmacy research (Jocic, 2024), RCTs can effectively evaluate agile interventions aimed at enhancing psychological safety, even when no pharmacological component is involved. Therefore, the terminology and methodology of controlled trials are not limited to clinical drug testing but are equally applicable to complex interventions in workplace and organizational settings (Babbie et al., 2022).

By employing repeated measurements and addressing multiple psychological constructs, this design enables a robust evaluation of the outcomes and mechanisms of change associated with each intervention type. The longitudinal structure allows for both short-term and sustained effects to be captured, ensuring that the evidence generated is relevant for long-term strategic planning in healthcare education (Babbie et al., 2022).

Random assignment enhances the internal validity of the findings by reducing selection bias, while standardized procedures and consistent measurement tools support the reliability of cross-group comparisons. Including both individual-level and team-level data enriches the understanding of how educational approaches influence workplace dynamics and professional well-being.

Ultimately, the experimental design outlined here provides a strong foundation for evidence-based decision-making by enabling systematic comparisons of agile coaching and traditional training. Its applicability across different healthcare contexts makes it a valuable methodological choice for evaluating interventions aimed at improving psychological safety, organizational culture, and workforce sustainability.

2.5.2 Observational design

The longitudinal observational design involves the repeated collection of data from the same participants over a specified period, allowing for the examination of changes and trends in psychological safety and related outcomes within real-world pharmacy settings without manipulating the intervention (Critical Appraisal Skills Programme, 2021; Faul et al., 2007; Goundar, 2012; Schulz et al., 2010). Alternatively, a longitudinal observational design could be used to track psychological safety perceptions over time among pharmacy teams that are already utilizing either agile coaching or traditional educational methods. This design could involve observing natural variations in psychological safety before and after the introduction of either intervention, with regular assessments at various points throughout the year.

A longitudinal observational design can serve as a valuable approach for exploring changes in psychological safety over time in naturalistic healthcare settings. In this proposed design, data would be collected across several key phases to monitor the effects of educational interventions without experimental manipulation.

The baseline phase, occurring at Month 0, involves the initial assessment of psychological safety before any intervention begins. By Month 1, the educational approaches—such as agile coaching or traditional education—are introduced organically, based on existing institutional practices. A mid-intervention follow-up around Month 3 helps track early changes and emerging trends. Finally, a postintervention measurement at Month 6 captures more stable, longer-term outcomes (Jocic, 2024; Bhattacharyya, 2006; Faul et al., 2007). Longer follow-up periods (e.g., 12 months or more) may be considered to assess the sustainability of intervention effects over time.

This design enables researchers to observe naturally occurring developments over time, facilitating the analysis of intervention effects in real-world conditions without the need for randomization or strict experimental control. Furthermore, it allows for the systematic tracking of changes in psychological safety perceptions, which is particularly valuable for understanding the long-term impact of different educational approaches (Bhattacharyya, 2006).

The "Baseline" phase represents the initial measurement of psychological safety before any intervention is implemented. This baseline data serves as a critical reference point for subsequent comparisons and the assessment of intervention effects. The "Intervention Start" phase marks the point when participants begin receiving either agile coaching or traditional educational workshops. This is a crucial moment, defining the onset of the educational approach's influence on the work environment and the psychological state of employees. The "Mid-Intervention" phase represents a midpoint during the intervention period, allowing for the collection of preliminary data on potential changes or trends in psychological safety perception. This phase is important for identifying timely insights that may suggest the need for adjustments or additional support during the program. The "postintervention" phase corresponds to the final data collection after the intervention is completed. This phase is essential for evaluating the overall effects of the intervention, including the sustainability of changes in psychological safety and other relevant variables.

The longitudinal design as a whole enables the analysis of changes over time, providing a deeper understanding of how educational methods, such as agile coaching and traditional training, affect psychological safety among community pharmacists. It also facilitates the evaluation of the durability of these effects, which is crucial for developing sustainable improvement programs and informing practice recommendations. The duration of a longitudinal study can vary depending on research objectives, resources, and context. Longer follow-up periods allow for a more comprehensive assessment of sustained effects and the evolution of psychological safety over time, whereas shorter studies may focus on immediate and short-term impacts. This flexibility distinguishes longitudinal designs from purely experimental approaches, providing unique insights into temporal dynamics and intervention sustainability. It is important to acknowledge that external factors and confounders, independent of the educational interventions, may also influence psychological safety outcomes, which represents a limitation of the observational design.

2.6 Data analysis

Data collected through various methods can be analyzed using a combination of quantitative statistical techniques and qualitative thematic analysis, offering a multifaceted understanding of how different educational interventions may influence psychological safety and related outcomes (Bock et al., 1998; Nussbaum, 2024; Bihani and Patil, 2014).

Quantitative data may be examined using inferential statistical techniques, such as paired t-tests or repeated measures Analysis of Variance (ANOVA), to compare preintervention and postintervention scores and assess potential changes over time (Bock et al., 1998; Bihani and Patil, 2014). Given that pharmacists are nested within teams, multilevel modeling may also be employed to account for hierarchical data structures and intra-team correlations. These methods help determine whether interventions—such as agile coaching or traditional training—are associated with statistically significant differences in outcomes like psychological safety, job satisfaction, or burnout. Regression analyses can further explore predictive relationships, while correlation analyses assess the strength and direction of associations between key constructs, such as burnout and psychological safety.

Qualitative data, collected through interviews or focus groups, are analyzed using thematic analysis (Bock et al., 1998; Bihani and Patil, 2014). Qualitative coding will be conducted independently by two researchers, with interrater reliability assessed using software such as NVivo or Atlas.ti to ensure consistency and rigor in theme identification. This involves systematically coding and interpreting participants' responses to identify recurring themes related to workplace climate, communication patterns, perceived organizational support, and barriers to psychological safety. Such qualitative insights provide context and depth to the quantitative results, revealing nuanced factors that may affect the success or limitations of the interventions.

By integrating these analytical approaches, the study design supports a comprehensive evaluation of the interventions' effects, capturing both measurable outcomes and the lived experiences of participants. This mixed-methods approach allows researchers to triangulate findings and develop a more holistic understanding of how educational strategies impact psychological safety and related workplace factors in community pharmacy teams.

Table 9.5 provides a detailed summary of the proposed statistical analysis plan, outlining the types of data collected, the analytical methods applied, and the intended purpose of each analysis. This structured plan ensures clarity and rigor in interpreting both quantitative and qualitative results.

This combined analytical strategy facilitates a robust and nuanced understanding of intervention impacts, supporting the development of evidence-based recommendations for future educational practices aimed at enhancing psychological safety and well-being among healthcare professionals.

TABLE 9.5 Statistical analysis plan.

Data type	Analysis method	Research purpose
Quantitative (Psychological safety scores)	Paired *t*-test/Repeated measures ANOVA	To assess changes in psychological safety levels before and after the intervention
Quantitative (Job satisfaction)	Regression analysis	To explore the predictive relationship between job satisfaction and psychological safety
Quantitative (Burnout measures)	Correlation analysis	To examine associations between burnout symptoms and psychological safety perceptions
Qualitative (interview and focus group data)	Thematic analysis	To identify key themes related to workplace dynamics, barriers, and safety enablers
Quantitative (Organizational commitment)	Structural equation modeling (SEM)	To investigate the mediating role of psychological safety in commitment-related outcomes

2.7 Ethical considerations and procedures in psychological safety research

Given the sensitive nature of psychological safety research involving human participants, strict adherence to ethical standards is crucial to protect participants' rights and wellbeing. Ethical considerations extend beyond general principles to include specific procedural steps and the handling of potential dilemmas throughout the research process (Gregory, 2003).

Researchers must ensure that all participants receive clear, comprehensive information about the study's purpose, methods, potential risks, and benefits prior to participation. This is typically provided through an informed consent form, which should be written in accessible language and include (Gregory, 2003; Tauginienė et al., 2021):

- Explanation of the voluntary nature of participation and the right to withdraw at any time without penalty
- Assurance of confidentiality and data protection, including how data will be anonymized or de-identified, is essential
- Description of any potential harms (e.g., emotional discomfort during interviews) and available support resources
- Contact information for the research team and the ethics committee overseeing the study
- How the collected data will be reported, used, and shared, including publication plans and potential secondary analyses

In some contexts, consent may be obtained verbally (e.g., in telephone interviews), but documentation must be maintained according to institutional guidelines. For vulnerable populations or when using digital platforms, additional safeguards may be necessary (Gregory, 2003).

Psychological safety research can raise ethical dilemmas, such as (Lefkowitz, 2021; Taquette and Borges da Matta Souza, 2022; Knapp and Fingerhut, 2024):

- Managing participant distress: Participants may disclose sensitive or distressing experiences. Researchers must be trained to recognize signs of distress and provide immediate support or referrals to counseling services if needed.
- Confidentiality breaches: Especially in team-based settings like community pharmacies, maintaining anonymity is challenging. Researchers should use coding systems, limit access to raw data, and explicitly communicate confidentiality limits during consent.
- Power dynamics: Given the hierarchical structures in healthcare workplaces, participation may be influenced by perceived pressure. Ensuring voluntary and anonymous feedback mechanisms can mitigate coercion.

When dilemmas arise, researchers should consult the institutional review board or ethics committee for guidance and have predefined protocols to address unforeseen issues. Prior to commencing data collection, all research protocols must be reviewed and approved by an institutional review board or equivalent ethics committee. This process ensures that the study meets ethical standards consistent with national and international guidelines, such as the Declaration of Helsinki or the Belmont Report (Gregory, 2003; Nagai et al., 2022; Tariq, 2025).

Regular reporting and adherence to approved protocols are mandatory. Any amendments, adverse events, or breaches must be promptly reported to the committee.

Researchers are responsible for securely storing data in accordance with data protection laws (e.g., General Data Protection Regulation). Access should be restricted, and data anonymized wherever possible to prevent the identification of participants (Rochel, 2021; Milossi et al., 2021).

Upholding ethical standards in psychological safety research safeguards participants, enhances the quality and credibility of findings, and fosters trust between researchers and healthcare communities. Clear procedures for informed consent, sensitive management of dilemmas, and strict adherence to oversight mechanisms are foundational to ethically sound research.

3 Discussion

The methodologies outlined in this chapter provide a robust and comprehensive framework for examining the effects of agile coaching versus traditional educational methods on psychological safety within community pharmacy teams. By integrating quantitative longitudinal and experimental designs with qualitative analyses, researchers are equipped to capture a multidimensional picture (Östlund et al., 2011) of how different intervention strategies influence pharmacists' well-being, team dynamics, and organizational outcomes in real-world practice. However, this methodological framework is not without limitations. Self-reported measures of psychological safety may be subject to response biases, randomization can be challenging in small community pharmacy settings, and the generalizability of findings across different healthcare systems and cultural contexts may be limited.

Psychological safety is widely recognized as a foundational element of effective healthcare teams (Jocić and Marinković, 2024; Jocic, 2024). The concept of psychological safety—defined as a shared belief that the team is safe for interpersonal risk-taking—has been empirically linked to improved communication, collaboration, and innovation (Edmondson, 1999, 2018; Marder et al., 2021; Kumar, 2024; Murray et al., 2022; Ridley et al., 2021). Our framework aims to extend this understanding by systematically comparing agile coaching, with its emphasis on iterative feedback and collective problem-solving, to more traditional top-down educational interventions.

Findings from the research suggest that agile coaching creates an environment where pharmacy team members feel empowered to express concerns, share knowledge, and learn from mistakes without fear of retribution (Jocic, 2024). This inclusive and flexible approach appears to cultivate resilience and a supportive culture, enhancing individual psychological safety, team performance, and patient safety outcomes (Jocić and Marinković, 2024; Jocic, 2024). In contrast, traditional education methods, while valuable in imparting necessary knowledge and skills, may fall short in fostering the same depth of trust and openness due to their more hierarchical and didactic nature, potentially limiting candid communication and collaborative problem-solving (Jocić and Marinković, 2024). Agile coaching may further mitigate second victim experiences by providing structured debriefing sessions, fostering peer support, and promoting open communication. These mechanisms reinforce psychological safety, enabling pharmacists to discuss errors or near misses without fear of blame, thereby supporting recovery, resilience, and continuous learning. Traditional educational approaches continue to play a critical role in ensuring regulatory compliance, technical proficiency, and structured knowledge acquisition, complementing agile coaching practices (Jocić and Marinković, 2024).

The dual methodological approach, with randomized allocation in the experimental design and naturalistic follow-up in the observational design, enables both causal inference and contextual understanding (Östlund et al., 2011). The longitudinal aspect is particularly important, as psychological safety is dynamic and may evolve as teams adapt to ongoing challenges and interventions over time. By tracking these changes across multiple measurement points, the study captures not only immediate effects but also the sustainability of intervention impacts. This temporal dimension is crucial because transient improvements in psychological safety may not translate into lasting cultural change without continued support and reinforcement (Rotman Devaraj et al., 2021; Gunasekare, 2016). To enhance sustainability, concrete strategies such as peer learning groups, regular retrospectives, and communities of practice can be implemented to support ongoing development and reinforcement of psychological safety (Jocić and Marinković, 2024).

Quantitative analyses allow for the objective assessment of changes in psychological safety perceptions, job satisfaction, burnout, and stress levels, while qualitative thematic analysis deepens insight into the lived experiences of pharmacy staff, highlighting barriers and facilitators within their work environments (Jocić and Marinković, 2024). Themes such as leadership support, team communication quality, and organizational policies emerged as critical determinants of psychological safety, suggesting areas for targeted intervention. The mixed-methods integration strengthens the validity and applicability of findings, providing actionable knowledge for practitioners and policymakers aiming to improve workplace conditions and patient care (Jocić and Marinković, 2024; Östlund et al., 2011).

Ethical rigor remains paramount throughout this type of research, with strict adherence to informed consent, confidentiality, and respect for participants' autonomy (Gregory, 2003; Rochel, 2021). Given the sensitive nature of psychological safety and workplace dynamics, establishing trust with participants is essential for accurate data collection and effective intervention implementation. Researchers must navigate potential ethical dilemmas, such as managing disclosures of workplace harassment or systemic issues, by ensuring appropriate support mechanisms and referral pathways are in place.

The implications of these findings for healthcare organizations are profound. Fostering psychologically safe environments in community pharmacies not only supports staff well-being and reduces burnout but is also crucial for the prevention of the second victim syndrome—a phenomenon where healthcare professionals experience psychological distress after involvement in adverse patient events. Psychological safety enables healthcare workers, including community pharmacists, to openly discuss errors or near misses without fear of blame or retribution, which is essential for mitigating the negative impact of second victim experiences and for promoting recovery and resilience (Zimonjić et al., 2025a, Zimonjić et al., 2025b). These practices also support patient-centered care.

Implementing agile coaching practices could be a strategic priority, offering a scalable and adaptable framework for continuous learning and improvement in pharmacy settings. Organizations may consider investing in training for agile facilitators, developing internal coaching competencies, and integrating agile principles into routine workflows to sustain gains over time. Furthermore, recognizing the legislative and organizational frameworks around the second victim phenomenon can guide the establishment of structured support systems within pharmacy practice, enhancing both staff well-being and clinical safety (Zimonjić et al., 2022).

Building psychological safety competencies through targeted training programs is essential for sustaining a supportive culture among healthcare professionals. Evidence from a recent pan-European mixed-methods study highlights the positive impact of psychological safety competency training during clinical internships, as perceived by healthcare trainee mentors across diverse healthcare settings (Carrillo et al., 2024). Such training equips future professionals with the skills needed to foster inclusive and supportive work environments, which are fundamental for both individual resilience and collective patient safety. Integrating these competency-based approaches into pharmacy education and ongoing professional development can enhance the preparedness of community pharmacists to navigate complex clinical challenges while maintaining psychological well-being and professional efficacy.

Future research directions include a deeper exploration of the mechanisms by which agile coaching fosters psychological safety, such as specific communication patterns, feedback cycles, and leadership behaviors. For instance, examining how the iterative nature of agile coaching contributes to a culture of openness and accountability can provide insights into optimizing coaching protocols. In addition, exploring the interaction between leadership styles—such as transformational, servant, or inclusive leadership—and psychological safety within agile frameworks could inform leadership development programs tailored to healthcare settings.

Further investigations into the downstream effects of psychological safety on clinical outcomes, patient satisfaction, medication safety, and workforce stability would provide a broader evidence base to guide policy and practice. Understanding these relationships may help justify organizational investment in psychological safety initiatives by linking them to tangible improvements in healthcare quality and operational efficiency.

In conclusion, this integrated methodological approach underscores the critical role of psychological safety in community pharmacies and highlights agile coaching as a promising avenue for enhancing this construct. By prioritizing psychological safety through evidence-based interventions, healthcare organizations can create more resilient, engaged, and effective pharmacy teams, ultimately improving care quality and patient outcomes. Ongoing commitment to research, ethical conduct, and practical implementation will be essential to realizing the full benefits of these strategies within the complex, evolving landscape of healthcare. Furthermore, this chapter has examined the links between psychological safety, job satisfaction, stress reduction, and burnout; evaluated traditional education and agile coaching approaches; and presented an experimental study with methodological considerations that collectively address all stated chapter objectives.

4 Questions for further discussion

1. How can the principles of psychological safety be systematically integrated into daily pharmacy practice to strengthen team cohesion, enhance communication, and improve the quality of patient care?
2. How can agile coaching techniques be adapted to healthcare settings, and how can different leadership styles—such as transformational or servant leadership—support the development of psychological safety and be integrated into manager and facilitator training?
3. What practical strategies can pharmacy managers implement to maintain and reinforce psychological safety during periods of stress, crisis, or high workload?
4. How can an ethically sustainable framework be established for interventions that influence team dynamics and perceptions of safety, especially when dealing with sensitive disclosures during interviews or group discussions?

5. How does psychological safety impact key organizational outcomes such as patient satisfaction, service quality, staff retention, and burnout prevention?
6. What are the methodological advantages and challenges of combining quantitative and qualitative approaches in the assessment of psychological safety, and which tools offer the most valid and reliable insights?
7. After a formal intervention concludes, what mechanisms can be introduced to ensure the sustainability of psychological safety—such as ongoing peer support, supervision, or self-sustaining team practices?
8. What is the cost-benefit case for investing in agile coaching to promote psychological safety in pharmacy organizations?
9. How can psychological safety be reliably measured across different cultural and organizational contexts in pharmacy practice?

5 Application exercise/scenario

Scenario: A community pharmacy recently introduced a structured counseling service for patients with chronic diseases. As part of this service, pharmacists provide individualized medication counseling, aiming to improve adherence and therapeutic outcomes. During one busy afternoon, a pharmacist notices that a colleague accidentally provided incorrect dosage instructions to a patient. Although the error was quickly corrected before any harm occurred, the observing pharmacist hesitates to address the issue with the colleague or the manager, concerned about damaging team relationships or being perceived as disloyal. The pharmacy manager, aiming to build a culture of learning and trust, decides to implement agile coaching practices to improve psychological safety and promote open communication regarding professional errors.

Exercise:

- What steps can the pharmacy manager take to ensure that pharmacists feel safe reporting and discussing errors without fear of blame or stigma?
- How can agile coaching techniques facilitate constructive dialog and continuous learning in the context of professional accountability?
- In what ways can a psychologically safe culture contribute to both error prevention and improved patient care?

Reflection and team evaluation tool: Psychological safety in pharmacy practice

After reviewing the scenario and discussing the application questions, pharmacy team members (or learners) are invited to reflect individually or as a group using the following prompts:

Individual reflection questions

1. Have I ever hesitated to report a professional concern or error? What influenced that decision?
2. How do I currently perceive psychological safety in my workplace?
3. What would make it easier for me to speak up when I notice something concerning in patient care?
4. How do I typically react when a colleague points out a mistake or offers feedback?

Team discussion questions

1. What norms currently exist in our team regarding error reporting and open discussion?
2. How can we, as a team, support each other when professional mistakes occur?
3. What would a more psychologically safe work environment look like in our pharmacy?
4. How can we integrate regular feedback and reflection into our workflow without disrupting patient care?

Team evaluation checklist Rate each statement on a scale from 1 (strongly disagree) to 5 (strongly agree):

- Team members can speak up without fear of blame or embarrassment
- Errors and near-misses are treated as learning opportunities
- Constructive feedback is welcomed and not perceived as a personal attack
- Everyone's opinion is valued, regardless of position or experience
- We regularly reflect on our practice and patient outcomes as a team

Teams can use average scores to identify strengths and areas for improvement in creating a psychologically safe and high-performing pharmacy environment.

Reflective prompts

- **Reflective prompt: Speaking up in practice**
  Have you ever experienced a situation in your professional or academic environment where you felt it was unsafe to speak up? What would have made it easier for you to express your concerns?
  Reflective prompt: Agile mindset in healthcare
  Which principles of Agile coaching do you find most applicable to your current or future role in pharmacy? How might these principles support collaboration and error prevention in high-pressure settings?
- **Reflective prompt: Responding to professional mistakes**
  Imagine a colleague makes a dispensing error. What factors would influence your response? Would psychological safety in your team affect whether you address it openly or remain silent?
- **Reflective prompt: Ethical tensions in research**
  When conducting research involving colleagues or peers, how do you balance your dual role as a researcher and insider? What safeguards would you implement to uphold ethical rigor and maintain participant trust?
- **Reflective prompt: Leadership and safety culture**
  Think of a leader or supervisor you admire. How did they contribute to a psychologically safe environment? What behaviors or communication practices stood out to you?
- **Reflective prompt: Learning from adverse events**
  After a service failure or patient-related incident, what reflective practices can support team learning rather than assigning blame? How would you lead or participate in such a debriefing session?

AI disclosure

During the preparation of this work, the author(s) used ChatGPT (OpenAI) solely for language polishing and improving readability. All scientific content and conclusions were developed independently by the author. After using this tool/service, the author(s) reviewed and edited the content as needed and take(s) full responsibility for the content of the publication.

References

Althubaiti, A., 2023. Sample size determination: a practical guide for health researchers. J. Gen. Fam. Med. 24 (2), 72–78.

Babbie, E., Wagner-Huang, W.E., Zaino, J., 2022. Adventures in Social Research: Data Analysis using IBM SPSS Statistics, Sage Publications.

Bäcklander, G., 2019. Doing complexity leadership theory: how agile coaches at Spotify practise enabling leadership. Creat. Innov. Manag. 28 (1), 42–60.

Bhattacharyya, D.K., 2006. Research Methodology, Excel Books India.

Bihani, P., Patil, S.T., 2014. A comparative study of data analysis techniques. Int. J. Emerg. Trends Technol. Comput. Sci. 3 (2), 95–101.

Bock, R.K., Krischer, W., Bock, R.K., Krischer, W., 1998. The Data Analysis Briefbook. Springer, Berlin Heidelberg, pp. 1–181.

Brunswik, E., 2023. Perception and the Representative Design of Psychological Experiments, University of California Press.

Buvik, M.P., Tkalich, A., 2021. Psychological safety in agile software development teams: work design antecedents and performance consequences. arXiv arXiv:2109.15034.

Carmeli, A., Brueller, D., Dutton, J.E., 2009. Learning behaviours in the workplace: the role of high-quality interpersonal relationships and psychological safety. Syst. Res. Behav. Sci. 26 (1), 81–98.

Carmeli, A., Gittell, J.H., 2009. High-quality relationships, psychological safety, and learning from failures in work organizations. J. Organ. Behav. 30 (6), 709–729.

Carrillo, I., Skoumalová, I., Bruus, I., Klemm, V., Guerra-Paiva, S., Knežević, B., Mira, J., 2024. Psychological safety competency training during the clinical internship from the perspective of health care trainee mentors in 11 pan-European countries: mixed methods observational study. JMIR Med. Educ. 10, (1), e64125.

Cochrane, B.S., Hagins Jr, M., Picciano, G., et al., 2017. High reliability in healthcare: creating the culture and mindset for patient safety. Healthc. Manage. Forum 30 (2), 61–68.

Critical Appraisal Skills Programme, 2021. Randomised controlled trial checklist. CASP. https://casp-uk.net/casp-tools-checklists/. (Accessed 2 May 2025).

DuBose, J.R., 2023. Interactions of Strategy, Culture, Management, and Psychological Safety in Driving Transformational Innovation, Drexel University.

Edmondson, A., 1999. Psychological safety and learning behavior in work teams. Adm. Sci. Q. 44 (2), 350–383.

Edmondson, A.C., 2018. The Fearless Organization: Creating Psychological Safety in the Workplace for Learning, Innovation, and Growth. John Wiley & Sons. ISBN: 978-1-119-47726-6.

Edmondson, A.C., Kramer, R.M., Cook, K.S., 2004. Psychological safety, trust, and learning in organizations: a group-level lens. Trust and distrust in organizations. Dilemmas Approaches 12 (2004), 239–272.

Faul, F., Erdfelder, E., Lang, A.G., Buchner, A., 2007. G*Power 3: a flexible statistical power analysis program for the social, behavioral, and biomedical sciences. Behav. Res. Methods 39 (2), 175–191.

Fernandez, D.J., Fernandez, J.D., 2008. Agile Project Management - Agilism versus traditional approaches. J. Comput. Inf. Syst. 49 (2), 10–17.
Goundar, S., 2012. Research methodology and research method. Victoria Univ. Wellington 1 (1), 1–47.
Gregory, I., 2003. Ethics in Research, A&C Black.
Gunasekare, D.U., 2016. Mixed research method as the third research paradigm: a literature review. SSRN 4 (8), 361–367.
Hunt, D.F., Bailey, J., Lennox, B.R., et al., 2021. Enhancing psychological safety in mental health services. Int. J. Ment. Health Syst. 15, 1–18.
Jocic, D., 2024. Psychological safety perception in community pharmacies: 1. A randomized controlled trial of agile interventions. Explor. Res. Clin. Soc. Pharm. 14, 100452.
Jocić, D., Đonović, N., Krajnović, D., Stefanović, S., Stojkov, S., Kocić, S., 2018. Cultural adaptation and examination of metric characteristics of the shirom-melamed burnout questionnaire (SMBQ) on a sample of pharmacists in Serbia. Indian J. Pharm. Educ. Res. 52 (1), S46–S60.
Jocić, D., Krajnović, D., 2014. State anxiety, stress and burnout syndrome among community pharmacists: relation with pharmacists' attitudes and beliefs. Indian J. Pharm. Educ. Res. 48 (2), 9–15.
Jocić, D., Marinković, V., 2024. Agile Human Resource Management as a Basis for Business Sustainability in Pharmacy. Faculty of Pharmacy, Novi Sad. ISBN: 9788680788302.
Julious, S.A., 2023. Sample Sizes for Clinical Trials, Chapman and Hall/CRC.
Kazdin, A.E., 2021. Research Design in Clinical Psychology, Cambridge University Press.
Klünder, J., Trommer, F., Prenner, N., 2022. How agile coaches create an agile mindset in development teams: Insights from an interview study. J. Softw. Evol. Process 34 (12), e2491.
Knapp, S.J., Fingerhut, R., 2024. Practical Ethics for Psychologists: A Positive Approach, American Psychological Association.
Kumar, A., Praveenakumar, S.G., 2025. Research Methodology, Authors Click Publishing.
Kumar, S., 2024. Psychological safety: what it is, why teams need it, and how to make it flourish. Chest. 165 (4), 942–949.
Lackie, K., Hayward, K., Ayn, C., et al., 2023. Creating psychological safety in interprofessional simulation for health professional learners: a scoping review of the barriers and enablers. J. Interprof. Care. 37 (2), 187–202.
Lefkowitz, J., 2021. Forms of ethical dilemmas in industrial-organizational psychology. Ind. Organ. Psychol. 14 (3), 297–319.
Liu, J.J., Ein, N., Plouffe, R.A., Gervasio, J., St. Cyr, K., Nazarov, A., Richardson, J.D., 2024. Meta-analysis and systematic review of the measures of psychological safety. MedRxiv. 2024-02.
López-Alcarria, A., Olivares-Vicente, A., Poza-Vilches, F., 2019. A systematic review of the use of agile methodologies in education to foster sustainability competencies. Sustainability. 11 (10), 2015.
Marder, B., Ferguson, P., Marchant, C., et al., 2021. 'Going agile': exploring the use of project management tools in fostering psychological safety in group work within management discipline courses. Int. J. Manag. Educ. 19 (3), 100519.
Milossi, M., Alexandropoulou-Egyptiadou, E., Psannis, K.E., 2021. AI ethics: algorithmic determinism or self-determination? The GPDR approach. IEEE Access. 9, 58455–58466.
Motta, R.W., 2024. Burnout Syndrome: Characteristics and Interventions, IntechOpen.
Murray, J.S., Kelly, S., Hanover, C., 2022. Promoting psychological safety in healthcare organizations. Mil. Med. 187 (7–8), 808–810.
Nagai, H., Nakazawa, E., Akabayashi, A., 2022. The creation of the belmont report and its effect on ethical principles: a historical study. Monash Bioeth. Rev. 40 (2), 157–170.
Newman, A., Donohue, R., Eva, N., 2017. Psychological safety: a systematic review of the literature. Hum. Resour. Manag. Rev. 27 (3), 521–535.
Nussbaum, E.M., 2024. Categorical and Nonparametric Data Analysis: Choosing the Best Statistical Technique, Routledge.
O'Donovan, R., Van Dun, D., McAuliffe, E., 2020. Measuring psychological safety in healthcare teams: developing an observational measure to complement survey methods. BMC Med. Res. Methodol. 20, 1–17.
Östlund, U., Kidd, L., Wengström, Y., Rowa-Dewar, N., 2011. Combining qualitative and quantitative research within mixed method research designs: a methodological review. Int. J. Nurs. Stud. 48 (3), 369–383.
Plouffe, R.A., Ein, N., Liu, J.J., St. Cyr, K., Baker, C., Nazarov, A., Don Richardson, J., 2023. Feeling safe at work: development and validation of the psychological safety inventory. Int. J. Sel. Assess. 31 (3), 443–455.
Politi, C., Roumeliotis, S., Tripepi, G., Spoto, B., 2023. Sample size calculation in genetic association studies: a practical approach. Life. 13 (1), 235.
Rajasekar, D., Verma, R., 2013. Research Methodology, Archers & Elevators Publishing House.
Ridley, C.H., Al-Hammadi, N., Maniar, H.S., et al., 2021. Building a collaborative culture: focus on psychological safety and error reporting. Ann. Thorac. Surg. 111 (2), 683–689.
Rochel, J., 2021. Ethics in the GDPR: a blueprint for applied legal theory. Int. Data Priv. Law. 11 (2), 209–223.
Rotman Devaraj, L., Cooper, C., Simpkin Begin, A., 2021. Creating psychological safety on medical teams in times of crisis. J. Hosp. Med. 16 (1), 47–49.
Schulz, K.F., Altman, D.G., Moher, D., 2010. Consort 2010 statement: updated guidelines for reporting parallel group randomised trials. BMJ. 340, c332.
Stray, V., Tkalich, A., Moe, N.B., 2020. The agile coach role: coaching for agile performance impact. arXiv 2010.15738.
Taquette, S.R., Borges da Matta Souza, L.M., 2022. Ethical dilemmas in qualitative research: a critical literature review. Int. J. Qual. Methods. 21, 16094069221078731.
Tariq, M.U., 2025. The belmont report: guiding ethical principles in human research. In: Robin, T. (Ed.), IRB, Human Research Protections, and Data Ethics for Researchers. IGI Global Scientific Publishing. pp. 245–268.
Tauginienė, L., Hummer, P., Albert, A., Cigarini, A., Vohland, K., 2021. Ethical challenges and dynamic informed consent. Sci. Citizen Sci. pp. 397–416.
Todaro-Franceschi, V., 2024. Compassion Fatigue and Burnout in Nursing: Enhancing Professional Quality of Life, Springer Publishing Company.
Verma, R., Verma, S., Abhishek, K., 2024. Research Methodology, Booksclinic Publishing.
Zimonjić, I., Marinković, V., Mira, J.J., Djokic, B.B., Odalović, M., 2025a. Addressing the second victim phenomenon among community pharmacists and its impact on clinical pharmacy practice: a consensus study. Int. J. Clin. Pharm. 47 (1), 68–79.

Zimonjić, I., Marinković, V., Mira, J.J., Knežević, B., Djokic, B.B., Bogavac-Stanojević, N., Odalović, M., 2025b. The second victim experience and support tool: a cross-cultural adaptation, validation and psychometric evaluation of the Serbian version for pharmacy professionals (SR-SVEST-R). Int. J. Clin. Pharm. 47, 803–814.

Zimonjić, I., Marinković, V., Odalović, M., 2022. Overview of the legislation of the Republic of Serbia regarding the second victims phenomenon at community pharmacists. Arch. Pharm. 72 (Suppl. 4), S331–S332.

CHAPTER

10

Using case study methodology to examine the role of pharmacists in residential aged care

Renly Lim[a,b], *Jun Ni Ho*[a], *and Elizabeth E. Roughead*[a]

[a]Quality Use of Medicines and Pharmacy Research Centre, School of Pharmacy and Biomedical Science, College of Health, Adelaide University, Adelaide, SA, Australia

[b]Development and Innovation, Centre for Translational Research, Institute for Research, Development and Innovation, IMU University, Kuala Lumpur, Malaysia

CHAPTER OBJECTIVES

- Demonstrate how case study methodology can be used to explore pharmacists' roles beyond routine clinical care and their effects on residents' health and quality of life.
- Equip readers with guidance on developing case studies that capture both the processes and outcomes of pharmacist-led interventions in practice.

1 Introduction

Evidence from systematic reviews and individual studies suggests that pharmacist-led services in aged care, also known as nursing homes or long-term care homes (Haider et al., 2021), can effectively address medicine-related problems (Lee et al., 2019; Ali et al., 2021; Almutairi et al., 2020; Sadowski et al., 2020; Roughead et al., 2022; Haider et al., 2023; Lim et al., 2023b). For example, a 2019 systematic review of pharmacist services in residential aged care reported overall reductions in the mean number of falls (Lee et al., 2019). The review included 52 studies using experimental or quasiexperimental methods, including randomized controlled trials (n = 13), prepost studies (n = 28), retrospective analyses (n = 6), and case-control studies (n = 5). While these studies provide evidence of effectiveness through measurable outcomes, including reductions in falls, use of inappropriate medicines, or number of hospitalizations, they offer limited insight into the detailed processes, decision-making, and resident-specific impact of pharmacist interventions. As a result, important contextual factors influencing how and why these interventions work remain insufficiently explored. Alternative methodological approaches can be useful to enable closer examination of intervention processes and decision-making in real-world settings. One such approach is the case study methodology.

A case study is one of several established methods used in social sciences research and is widely applied across disciplines such as education, public health, and implementation science (Greenhalgh, 2025; Yin, 2018).

Contemporary Research Methods in Pharmacy and Health Services - Volume 2
https://doi.org/10.1016/B978-0-443-44607-8.00005-4

As a recognized research design, a case study enables an in-depth, multifaceted exploration of complex phenomena within their real-life contexts, providing a high level of richness and contextual depth (Yin, 2018; Crowe et al., 2011). In contrast to traditional clinical formats such as case reports, case series, or grand rounds, which typically provide focused descriptions of clinical scenarios, the case study approach explores, describes, or explains an event, issue, or phenomenon in detail within its natural setting in the research context (Grimes and Schulz, 2002; Crowe et al., 2011). Table 10.1 summarizes the characteristics and comparative features of the case study, case report, and case series formats.

Although definitions vary among methodologists, case studies are generally characterized by the systematic collection and analysis of multiple data sources to generate rich descriptions and inform theory development (Mills et al., 2010). Case studies may employ qualitative, quantitative, or mixed-methods approaches and are particularly well-suited to complex situations in which the number of variables of interest exceeds the available data points (Greenhalgh, 2025; Crowe et al., 2011; Guetterman and Fetters, 2018). Case studies may be conducted for descriptive, explanatory, exploratory, or evaluative purposes and are usually presented in a narrative format (Mills et al., 2010; Yin, 2018).

This methodological strength makes case studies particularly valuable when the research aim is to develop a deeper understanding of important real-world events, complex social or policy-based interventions, or program-

TABLE 10.1 Characteristics and comparative features of case study, case report, and case series.

	Case study (Greenhalgh, 2025; Crowe et al., 2011; Yin, 2018)	**Case report (Bignall and Horton, 1995; Vandenbroucke, 1999; Kidd and Saltman, 2012; Nissen and Wynn, 2012; Albrecht et al., 2005)**	**Case series (Grimes and Schulz, 2002; Kooistra et al., 2009; Fleischmann et al., 2024; Albrecht et al., 2005)**
Aim or purpose	To describe, explain, explore, or evaluate complex processes, interventions, relationships, or phenomena within real-life contexts	To describe in detail the clinical presentation, diagnosis, treatment, and clinical outcomes of a single patient	To describe the characteristics, treatments, and clinical outcomes of multiple patients with a similar condition or exposure
Primary focus	A bounded case or system (individual, group or team, organization, program, event, process, or service)	An individual patient	A group of patients sharing a defining characteristic (e.g., disease, treatment, or exposure)
Subject of investigation	One or a small number of cases are examined in depth	A single patient, often with novel or rare characteristics	Multiple patients without a comparison group
Study design	Qualitative, quantitative, or mixed methods; descriptive, explanatory, exploratory, or evaluative	Descriptive, observational	Descriptive, observational
Contextual emphasis	Explicitly examined and reported (organizational, social, policy, and practice context)	Clinical context focused	Clinical context focused
Data sources and methods	Multiple sources (e.g., interviews, documents, observations, records, artifacts); triangulation of data sources is common	Clinical history, examination findings, investigations, diagnostic tests, treatment course, and follow-up	Aggregated clinical data from patient records, registries, or clinical observations
Comparison or control group	Generally absent; embedded comparisons may be included	None	None
Level of evidence	Low to moderate (context-rich and theory-informing)	Low (anecdotal evidence)	Low to moderate (hypothesis-generating)
Ability to infer causality	Very limited; focuses on mechanisms and processes	None	Very limited
Key strengths	Contains rich, contextual details; illuminates mechanisms, contexts, and implementation processes; supports theory development	Identifies new diseases, rare adverse events or conditions, or unexpected outcomes	Identifies patterns, generates hypotheses, and/or estimates frequencies
Key limitations	Limited generalisability; potential bias	No generalisability; potential bias	No control group; cannot establish effectiveness or causation; potential bias
Useful for addressing	Observational questions	Observational questions, therapy questions, and prognosis questions	Observational questions, therapy questions, and prognosis questions
Typical output	Scholarly research report	Published case report	Published case series

Modified from multiple sources.

based service developments or reforms (Yin, 2018; Crowe et al., 2011). Specifically, case studies may be valuable when used to:

- Explain causal relationships in complex real-world interventions that cannot be adequately addressed by surveys or experimental methods. By drawing on multiple sources of evidence and tracking processes over time, case studies may enable the identification and explanation of causal mechanisms and pathways underpinning program-based service developments or reforms, particularly where outcomes are shaped by contextual, organizational, and social factors.
- Describe interventions and the real-life contexts in which they occur, enabling detailed documentation of how interventions are delivered, experienced, or adapted in practice (e.g., documenting a patient's episode of care).
- Examine interventions where outcomes are not clearly defined or predetermined, allowing researchers to explore how the interventions can be embedded within practice settings (e.g., exploring how cultural safety training is interpreted and applied in clinical settings).
- Explore specific themes or topics within broader evaluations, providing in-depth insight into stakeholder experiences, processes, or implementation challenges associated with policy or program initiatives (e.g., examining professional experiences of a new policy initiative) (Yin, 2018; Crowe et al., 2011).

In terms of design, case studies can involve a single-case or multiple-case design. These may be holistic, focusing on a single unit of analysis, or embedded, involving multiple units of analysis (Yin, 2018). Case studies may also form part of broader mixed-methods studies (Yin, 2018). The main stages involved in planning and conducting a case study typically include defining the case, selecting the case(s) and structuring the study, collecting data, analyzing and interpreting data, and sharing and reporting findings (Yin, 2018; Crowe et al., 2011). Stepwise guidance for conducting a case study is provided in Box 10.1.

BOX 10.1

Stepwise approach to case study methodology

While often described as linear, case study methodology is inherently iterative, involving ongoing processes of planning, design, preparation, data collection, analysis, and dissemination of findings.

1. Defining the case The first step is to establish the study rationale and determine whether a case study is the most appropriate approach for addressing the research questions. This involves:

- Conducting a scoping review, critical appraisal, and evidence synthesis to identify key themes and gaps
- Formulating good research questions

2. Selecting the case(s) and structuring the study Once a case study approach is justified, attention shifts to case selection and study design:

- Developing the initial study concept
- Ensuring the appropriateness of a case study design, characterized by an in-depth examination of phenomena and the use of mixed methods and multiple data sources where appropriate
- Determining the type of case study design, including:
- Single versus multiple cases
- Single versus multiple units of analysis
- Defining the boundaries of the case(s), positioning them within their broader context, and justifying case selection

3. Collecting, analyzing, and interpreting data Researchers should familiarize themselves with data collection and analysis processes and develop a case study protocol that specifies the methods to be used:

- Selecting qualitative, quantitative, or mixed methods aligns with the research question(s) and study design
- Applying appropriate analytical techniques, such as logic models or pattern matching, is essential

4. Ensuring rigor and sharing and reporting findings The final stage involves writing the case study report, providing a comprehensive description of the case, presenting data transparently and concisely, and tailoring outputs to the intended audiences. Rigor in case study research should be demonstrated through clear documentation of data sources, analytical decisions, and the links between evidence and interpretation. Common strategies to enhance rigor include triangulation of multiple data sources, the use of theory to inform analysis, maintenance of a clear chain of evidence, and reflexive consideration of the researcher(s)'s role in data collection and interpretation.

Modified from Fàbregues and Fetters, 2019; Baker, 2011; Croweetal., 2011; Thomas, 2021; Yin, 2018

Case studies can take many forms and vary in purpose and format across social sciences, public health, and implementation science (Greenhalgh, 2025). In clinical and health services research, case study methodology broadly draws on approaches from public health and implementation science, offering a complementary perspective to experimental methods by providing rich contextual data for exploring intervention effects. For example, clinical case studies primarily focus on patients and their clinical care management, whereas health services case studies examine organizations, programs, interventions, or policies within the healthcare system (for instance, a hospital, a specific ward, or an integrated care program). The key distinction lies in the unit of analysis; however, both approaches share the use of in-depth investigation of real-world phenomena to inform practice and improve health and patient outcomes.

While frequently used for clinical learning and practical guidance, the case study approach remains relatively underutilized in health services research (Crowe et al., 2011) and is even more rarely applied in pharmacy research. Only a few reports have demonstrated the use of case study methodology in pharmacy-related research, for example, to examine pharmacists' current and potential prescribing roles in a country without formal prescribing rights(Kempen et al., 2024) (Table 10.2). The application of case study methodology in pharmacy research is becoming increasingly essential, as pharmacists' scope of practice expands across multiple settings, including long-term and aged care. The rich, narrative format of case studies enables pharmacist researchers to integrate and interpret multiple data sources into a cohesive, holistic account, capturing the complexity of real-world practice. By examining individual cases in depth, case studies can reveal how pharmacists advocate for residents, tailor interventions to personal needs, and collaborate with multidisciplinary teams in ways that are not reflected in aggregate trial data.

To provide examples of how the case study can reveal new findings and knowledge, this chapter presents eight case studies from the Australian Reducing Medicine-Induced Deterioration and Adverse Reactions (ReMInDAR) trial (Roughead et al., 2022; Lim et al., 2020). These cases were purposively selected to reflect a diversity of clinical issues encountered in the trial. The case studies showcase how regular, relationship-based pharmacist involvement can improve clinical outcomes and quality of life for residents in aged care. The examples demonstrate how ongoing, personalized interactions enabled the pharmacists to identify and resolve medicine-related problems, while also advocating for safe, more effective care for the residents. We include a case study that highlights systemic barriers, involving hierarchical dynamics and limited prescribing authority, that can constrain the pharmacist's ability to fully realize patient-centered care. Following the case studies, the chapter presents an overview of practice models for pharmacists in aged or long-term care settings across different countries. The chapter concludes with a set of discussion questions, followed by an application scenario that demonstrates how the case study approach can support pharmacists in systematically documenting and analyzing complex interventions, highlighting both clinical and person-centered outcomes. Reflection prompts are also provided to support practice.

2 Pharmacist practice model piloted in the ReMInDAR trial

2.1 Study design and setting

These case studies were selected from the ReMInDAR trial (Roughead et al., 2022; Lim et al., 2020), a multicentre, open-label, randomized controlled trial involving 39 aged care facilities in Australia, conducted between August 2018 and June 2020. The trial enrolled 248 participants, including 120 in the pharmacist-led intervention group (Roughead et al., 2022). Eight cases from the intervention group were selected to illustrate a range of clinical and nonclinical scenarios addressed by the ReMInDAR trial pharmacists.

2.2 Ethical considerations and licensing

The clinical vignette represents each case; however, names and environments have been changed to ensure individuals' anonymity. Information included in the case studies was documented by the trial pharmacists and research assistants and verified by the ReMInDAR trial research staff. Case studies have been produced with consent from trial participants. The project was approved by the University of South Australia Human Research Ethics Committee (ID: 0000036440) and the University of Tasmania Health and Medical Human Research Ethics Committee (ID: H0017022).

TABLE 10.2 Recent examples of studies using case study methodology in health services and pharmacy practice research.

Author, year, country	Study aim	Study design	Data analysis	Study setting	Study population	Pharmacists' roles or pharmaceutical care services	Key findings
McIntosh et al. (2018), nine European countries (McIntosh et al., 2018)	What initiatives exist regarding polypharmacy management in the EU; why they were or were not developed; and how the initiatives were developed, implemented, and sustained?	Holistic multiple-case study design involving nine European countries.	Research teams within each country produced a summary report, a time series analysis of key events, and a summary of lessons learned. Individual case study reports were written using a standardized template. Framework analysis was conducted to generate summary findings.	Multiple	Stakeholders and practitioners involved in polypharmacy management.	• Multiple tasks (e.g., developing patient-centered care plans, conducting medicine reviews, supporting adherence, and collaborating with healthcare teams to improve medicine safety and outcomes under regional or national guidance).	• Polypharmacy initiatives were identified in five regions and included all care settings. • Variation in professional roles and approaches was identified, with several regions lacking formal programs and others emphasizing either pharmacist-led or physician-integrated models depending on the local context. • Identified common themes in how initiatives were developed, which together demonstrate that polypharmacy management is a complex intervention shaped by diverse facilitators and barriers across various settings.
Silva and Fegadolli (2020), Brazil (Silva and Fegadolli, 2020)	Evaluate the implementation of ambulatory care pharmacy services for older adult patients.	Case study using multiple sources of data, including document analysis, participatory observation, individual interviews, and focus groups.	Thematic analysis of individual interviews, focus groups, field diaries, and document analysis was performed. Identified themes were analyzed using categories provided within the theoretical and analytical framework of the realist assessment (context, mechanism, outcome—CMO).	Ambulatory care	Health professionals, pharmaceutical care service users (older adults).	• Logistical management of medicines, including selection, planning, storage control, and care actions such as dispensing, patient education, and supporting the multiprofessional team in solving medicine-related problems. • Assisting patients referred by other professionals. • Discussing cases with the health team. • Preparing assistants to identify patients with medication issues for referral for individual pharmaceutical care	• The study identified three context–mechanism–outcome (CMO) configurations that explained how pharmaceutical care was successfully implemented. • Continuous education and training for both pharmacists and other health staff have helped overcome implementation obstacles. • Using data and indicators to document activities has increased the service's recognition both internally and externally, helping to integrate it into routine care.

Continued

TABLE 10.2 Recent examples of studies using case study methodology in health services and pharmacy practice research—cont'd

Author, year, country	Study aim	Study design	Data analysis	Study setting	Study population	Pharmacists' roles or pharmaceutical care services	Key findings
Kempen et al. (2024), the Netherlands (Kempen et al., 2024)	Explore pharmacists' current roles in prescribing and their potential for prescribing in advanced pharmacy practice.	Multiple case study approach, including participatory observation and semistructured interviews.	Interview and observation data were analyzed thematically, and a concept map was created to visualize pharmacists' current tasks, processes, and professional contacts with stakeholders and systems.	Primary care (general practices and community pharmacies)	Pharmacists, patients, physicians or nurses	• Pharmacists' role in prescribing	• Pharmacists play an active role in prescribing processes despite not having formal prescribing rights, often preparing or initiating prescriptions that are later authorized by general practitioners. • Practice-based pharmacists have a more direct clinical role (e.g., initiating therapy during consultations), while community pharmacists influence prescribing indirectly through medicine reviews, recommendations, and close collaboration with GPs and nurses. • The observed practices resemble collaborative prescribing models in other countries.

Case studies 1 to 6 are reproduced from Lim et al., "Pharmacists as patient advocates: A series of case studies illustrating the impacts of a regular pharmacist service in residential aged care (nursing homes)" (Lim et al., 2023a), licensed under CC BY 4.0 (https://creativecommons.org/licenses/by/4.0/). They have been adapted and expanded to provide additional context relevant to this book chapter.

The cases arose from a trial testing a novel pharmacist service, where residents received pharmacist visits every 8 weeks over 12 months. Each pharmacist session included four key components:

1. Review of the resident care record and medication chart to identify any new illnesses or conditions present, as well as medication changes since the last assessment, including any adverse events or any signs or symptoms noted in the care record that could be indicative of adverse events.
2. Discussion with residents and care staff to identify concerns about the residents' health or medications and to assess changes in activity and cognition.
3. Resident assessment using validated tools to detect medication-induced deterioration and adverse reactions.
4. Communication with the resident's general practitioner (GP) to discuss the resident's condition and provide recommendations for actions to take if medicine-related problems are indicated.

The detailed ReMInDAR study protocol and the trial results for primary and secondary outcomes have been published previously (Roughead et al., 2022; Lim et al., 2020).

3 Case presentations

The first four case studies, which focus primarily on clinical interventions, are presented with a single, combined commentary summarizing key lessons learned and challenges encountered. The latter four case studies discuss broader roles of pharmacists, such as advocacy, GP engagement, and education for residents or staff, each accompanied by its own commentary. By documenting these individualized interventions in detail, the case study method captures not only the clinical outcomes but also the broader impact on resident satisfaction and overall well-being. Each case is presented as a clinical vignette, beginning with the resident's background and presenting issues, followed by the pharmacist's assessment and interactions with the resident, clinical decision-making, and communication with other healthcare professionals. The cases describe the pharmacist's interventions, subsequent follow-up, and outcomes over time and, where relevant, illustrate broader roles such as resident advocacy, engagement with GPs, and education of residents or aged-care staff.

3.1 Case study 1: Mary*—"Too scared to say I'm bleeding"

88 year-old Mary has been living in residential aged-care for almost a year. Mary is a widow of many years, has several children, and dotes on her grandchildren.

Mary is quite active, with a keen interest in crafts. She is on medication to manage her atrial fibrillation and hypertension. She has never smoked. She has cataracts, which are affecting her ability to do craftwork.

Mary feared the worst, so she kept her problems to herself, The ReMInDAR pharmacist spent time with Mary, and during the first session, discovered that Mary expressed concern about sometimes having bright red blood in her stool. Mary had kept this to herself because she feared needing to undergo a colonoscopy and "suspected the worst". However, based on a review of Mary's medicines, the pharmacist suspected the bleeding might be due to the apixaban dose (5 mg twice daily). The pharmacist notified the nurse regarding the blood in the stool and contacted the GP to discuss the resident and the pharmacist's concerns.

During subsequent visits, the pharmacist noted that Mary was still experiencing blood in her stool once or twice a week. Mary was not constipated or straining while using the toilet. It appeared that a GP review to address Mary's concern had not been undertaken. Mary's vital signs, including weight, age, and laboratory results indicating kidney function (serum creatinine = 0.66 mg/dL), were checked by the pharmacist. Considering Mary's age (<60 kg) and age (>80 years old), the pharmacist contacted the GP again and recommended a reduction in the apixaban dose to 2.5 mg twice daily. The GP did not think that the bleeding could be due to apixaban, and therefore no changes to the apixaban dose were made.

Persistence in GP communications pays off. The pharmacist continued to emphasize Mary's concerns about the bleeding to the GP, and by the fourth pharmacist session, the GP finally agreed to trial reducing apixaban from 5 mg twice daily to 2.5 mg twice daily. During follow-up at the fifth pharmacist session, Mary told the pharmacist that the blood in her stool had stopped recently and that she no longer had bruising. By the sixth session, Mary confirmed that her bleeding problems had resolved completely.

3.2 Case study 2: Anita*—"The leg swelling is now gone"

Anita is an 80 year-old retired school teacher who has been residing in aged care for almost 18 months. She has two sons. Anita is a very social woman who previously enjoyed having visitors at her home and going out with her friends.

Anita has a history of anxiety and depression, gastro-esophageal reflux disease, and arthritis. During the initial pharmacist review, ankle edema and ongoing constipation were identified as additional issues for Anita. The pharmacist considered that the ongoing constipation might be attributed to amlodipine or buprenorphine.

At the second session, eight weeks later, Anita's lower leg edema was still an issue and quite concerning for her. The pharmacist identified amlodipine as a likely culprit medicine; however, complicating any recommendation surrounding the cessation of amlodipine was Anita's blood pressure, which had been elevated in recent measurements (145/73 mmHg). The pharmacist contacted Anita's GP and suggested a trial cessation of amlodipine, with a possible replacement using a beta-blocker or moxonidine if the blood pressure was not managed sufficiently. The pharmacist also suggested adding regular docusate and senna to manage the on-going constipation.

The GP agreed to cease the amlodipine In the medical review one month later, the GP noted that Anita's ankle edema had significantly improved. The GP was unsure if it was due to the cessation of amlodipine, but there did not appear to be any other changes that contributed to it. The constipation remained an issue, and the pharmacist noted that buprenorphine could be the contributing factor.

Anita continued to have significantly less ankle edema at the subsequent visits with the ReMInDAR pharmacist.

During the fifth visit, the pharmacist noted several potential medicine-related problems. There was now duplication of proton-pump inhibitor therapy (PPI); Anita was already on rabeprazole, but pantoprazole had been added to the medicine chart. The pharmacist contacted the GP to suggest removing the duplicate pantoprazole (PPI) from the medicine chart and increasing the dose of rabeprazole if necessary. The dose of buprenorphine had recently increased from 10mcg/h to 15mcg/h. Anita appeared visibly tired, which the pharmacist considered might be due to the combination of buprenorphine and diazepam, the latter of which Anita was taking to manage her anxiety. Anita indicated that she would like to try not taking diazepam to see if her tiredness reduced.

The pharmacist discussed with the GP the opportunity to reduce the dose of diazepam from 5 mg to 2 mg and to eventually cease the medicine. Pantoprazole was removed from Anita's medicine chart due to duplication of PPI. All recommendations were implemented by the GP, and Anita reported to the pharmacist that she felt much better; however, constipation remained an ongoing issue for Anita.

3.3 Case study 3: John*—"Spirits lifted and an adverse medicine reaction no more"

John is a 91 year-old man who entered residential aged care due to his medical conditions, including glaucoma, macular degeneration, constipation, short-term memory loss, hypertension, hyperlipidemia, ankle edema, back pain, arthritis, gout, and an enlarged prostate.

John complained to the ReMInDAR pharmacist about his ankle edema and said he felt depressed due to his worsening condition. When the ReMInDAR pharmacist visited John, they noted that John's health had declined over the past few weeks, and his ankle edema was significantly worse, with fluid seeping from his calves. His cognitive function (assessed using the Montreal Cognitive Assessment (MoCA) test) and grip strength had both decreased significantly compared to his baseline values recorded during his enrollment in the trial. John had also developed shortness of breath with a cough, potentially secondary to the retention of fluids in his lungs, which was not present during the pharmacist's previous visit.

John told the pharmacist repeatedly, "If my edema did not further improve, I will cease all my medicines and just wait to die". The pharmacist suspected that the worsening of edema could be due to felodipine or pregabalin and was extremely concerned about John's worsening mental state. The pharmacist attempted to contact John's GP to suggest a trial cessation of those medicines. However, the GP was overseas, so the pharmacist communicated with the facility nurse instead. In addition, the pharmacist spoke to a locum GP, who stated that he could see John "early next week". Despite the pharmacist stressing the urgency of reviewing John, he was not reviewed immediately. The pharmacist continued to make several attempts to contact the locum GP and John's GP, eventually managing to get in touch with John's GP two weeks later. The pharmacist suggested that a trial cessation of felodipine or pregabalin should be undertaken. The GP was welcoming and supportive of the trial. Although the GP was not convinced that edema was medicine-related, the GP agreed to trial a decrease in pregabalin (25 mg) from three times a day to twice daily once John's infection cleared to see if this would improve his condition.

Persistence pays off!. A follow-up was scheduled by the pharmacist to further monitor John's edema and general health. During the third session, the pharmacist noted that John's health had significantly improved since the last session and that his edema had improved since the pregabalin dosage was reduced. John had started exercising regularly, which allowed him to lose weight slowly and improve his edema. The pharmacist continued to monitor his condition and reinforced the importance of exercise to help with the edema.

3.4 Case study 4:—Betty—"No more falls: Reducing the sedative dose does it"

Betty is an 80 year-old woman who has been a resident in her aged care facility for the past two years. She never married and had lived with her sister until her sister's death.

Betty had recently been hospitalized for congestive cardiac failure. In addition to this, Betty suffers from diabetes, obesity, hyperlipidemia, chronic back pain, sciatica, cognitive impairment, double vision, poor balance, necrobiosis lipoidica, peripheral artery disease, peripheral neuropathy, recurrent chronic leg ulcers, anxiety, dementia, depression, and incontinence.

In the first session, the ReMInDAR pharmacist noted that Betty's dose of pregabalin had been increased from 225 mg twice a day to 300 mg twice a day due to pain in her right foot. She had also been prescribed temazepam (10 mg at night) to aid with sleep.

Betty felt dizzy and complained of weight gain. Betty was satisfied with her pain management; however, she indicated to the pharmacist that she felt dizzy and disliked the weight gain since the increased dosing of pregabalin. Her weight had increased by 5.5 kg within a month. Pregabalin may cause drowsiness, impaired balance, confusion, and weight gain. The pharmacist discussed with Betty the potential for pregabalin to cause these side effects and the possibility of reducing the pregabalin dose; however, Betty was reluctant to reduce the dose due to her pain.

Betty began experiencing falls. Four weeks later, Betty had a fall, and she stated that she had been feeling tired for a week before her fall. Betty acknowledged the harms associated with losing her balance; however, she was still reluctant to reduce the dose of pregabalin. The pharmacist reiterated the benefits of reducing the medication. In addition, the ReMInDAR pharmacist discussed her concerns with the aged care staff to ensure they provided the necessary care for Betty. Within six days, Betty had another fall in the bathroom and was admitted to the hospital.

At the subsequent pharmacist review visit, Betty had experienced two further falls and stated that she was "losing strength" in her legs. She was still on the same medication regimen; however, she had also started taking perindopril 4 mg daily. The ReMInDAR pharmacist noted that this medication could cause hypotension, which might contribute to her falls.

The pharmacist discussed these issues with the registered nurse, as Betty's doctor was on holiday. A follow-up communication with the nurse occurred within a month, and the doctor decreased Betty's pregabalin dose from 300 mg twice a day to 250 mg twice a day.

By the fifth pharmacist review session, Betty had not experienced any falls, and at this time, Betty's pregabalin dose was further reduced to 75 mg twice a day. Betty indicated that she would like to further decrease the pregabalin dose if possible, as long as her pain remains under control. The pharmacist noted the need to review and monitor Betty closely.

3.5 Commentary

The first four case studies collectively illustrate the role of pharmacists in recognizing, managing, and mitigating medicine-related problems in aged care residents. The cases highlight the complexity of medicine management in this population, where residents are often prescribed multiple medicines to treat coexisting chronic conditions. A common concern in older people is cumulative drug burden, including cumulative sedative load and anticholinergic burden, which has been associated with poorer physical and cognitive function, increased risk of falls, frailty, and death (Lim et al., 2023b; Ruxton et al., 2015; Taipale et al., 2012). In each case, the pharmacist was able to identify medicines contributing to adverse effects: apixaban-related bleeding in Mary, amlodipine-related edema in Anita, pregabalin and felodipine effects in John, and pregabalin and temazepam-related falls in Betty. Data from the

ReMInDAR trial also showed that most residents experience a new medicine-related problem by the fourth month after their initial assessment (Dorj et al., 2022), indicating that these adverse events are not isolated but recurring, and that ongoing monitoring is needed.

While not all adverse effects are life-threatening, their impact on residents' quality of life can be profound. Edema, for example, may appear less urgent clinically, but in John's case, it led to significant distress, with him expressing a wish to "just wait to die" if the swelling did not improve. Mary's reluctance to disclose bleeding due to her fear of colonoscopy and Betty's hesitation to reduce pregabalin because of pain show that residents' concerns and fears are deeply personal and may not always be openly discussed with GPs. The regular presence of pharmacists and the trust built through ongoing contact likely created the opportunity for these issues to be voiced and addressed.

Another recurring theme across these cases was the difficulty in contacting GPs for timely intervention. Often, multiple attempts were required before any action was taken, and in some cases, recommendations were initially dismissed. The reluctance or delay in modifying medicines reflects broader systemic challenges in aged care, where competing priorities, time pressures, and uncertainty about causality may influence prescribers' decisions (Gittus et al., 2025). In Mary's and John's cases, repeated follow-ups eventually led to dose adjustments, while in Anita's and John's cases, pharmacists persisted with their recommendations even when prescribers remained unconvinced that symptoms were linked to medicines.

Unlike aggregate findings from the ReMInDAR trial (Roughead et al., 2022), which summarize overall trends such as changes in the total number of adverse events, these case studies provide a deeper examination of the processes underlying those outcomes. By tracking each case longitudinally, the case study methodology enables detailed documentation of the context, decision-making processes, and the interactions between the residents, pharmacists, GPs, and care staff. This approach makes visible how medicine-related problems are identified, negotiated, and resolved over time, particularly in situations involving diagnostic uncertainty, competing clinical priorities, or initial resistance to change. In doing so, the case studies provide explanatory insight into the "how" and "why" of adverse event resolution, situating clinical outcomes within real-world practice processes and highlighting the value of pharmacist persistence, advocacy, and person-centered engagement in aged care.

3.6 Case study 5: Harry*—"Finally in my own bed!"

Harry is a 62 year-old client of residential aged care. In his working life, he was a town planner for the local council and an active chess player. He is married and enjoys visits from his wife and their dog. Harry moved into aged care because of his illnesses, which include incontinence, osteoarthritis, amnesia, obesity, obstructive sleep apnea, transient cerebral ischemic attacks, atrial fibrillation, cancer, dementia, depression, anxiety, and hypertension; he has also been experiencing recurrent falls.

Harry has been sleeping in his chair for the past six months. Harry had been sleeping in his armchair for the last six months, as he found his bed too narrow and was fearful he would fall out. Harry had swollen ankles and back pain, which were most probably caused by sleeping in his chair. He also thought his speech and mobility were declining. Harry was on 18 regular and eight "when required" medicines, which he was unhappy about, particularly the "big orange tablets that catch his throat and irritate him for a few hours" (Allopurinol 300 mg).

Harry did not like living in the aged care facility. He was bored, his mental health was poor, and he spent almost 24 hours a day in the same armchair. Harry appeared to willingly self-isolate, refusing to leave his room and not engaging in any wellness or social activities because they were "not interesting". He also did not interact with the facility care staff, but he did look forward to visits from his wife and his dog.

The ReMInDAR pharmacist spent time with Harry and reviewed his medicines during the first visit. The pharmacist discussed Harry's issues with his doctor during the second session. Subsequently, some of Harry's medicines were removed or substituted with smaller-sized tablets, and the dose was reduced for a few medicines. At the same time, based on concerns expressed to the staff by the pharmacist, the lifestyle coordinator made additional weekly one-on-one visits to Harry to try to find activities to improve his social engagement.

At the ReMInDAR pharmacist's third visit, Harry expressed pleasure with these outcomes, especially not having to take any more "orange pills"; however, he was still not leaving his room. Despite this, the small "win" by the pharmacist helped establish a new relationship based on trust. Harry continued to open up to the pharmacist about his problems and revealed that he had previously fallen out of his bed (unreported to staff), hence his anxiety about sleeping in the current bed.

The pharmacist told Harry she was "concerned for him and would talk with the staff about the issue of the bed" and encouraged him to get out of his room. The pharmacist continued to advocate to the facility staff on Harry's behalf about the importance of getting him a new bed.

At the fourth pharmacy visit, the pharmacist learned that Harry had purchased a recliner chair that enabled him to lie further back and elevate his feet; this reduced the swelling in his legs.

More promisingly, a new, wider bed was on order for him. By the fifth session (conducted by phone during COVID – 19 access restrictions), the pharmacist noted that Harry had remarkably improved. "In the past, he was negative about the nursing care he received, but now he seemed quite complimentary about the staff. Even when talking about a fall, he didn't want to dwell on it or look back. It seemed very different from his attitude during previous visits".

Harry is now doing exercises by himself and even going for a walk down the corridor. Although the swelling in his legs has not improved significantly, he is able to sleep for longer blocks in the chair overnight. He is very much looking forward to being able to use his new bed.

3.7 Commentary

Harry's case illustrates the broader role of pharmacists in aged care, including advocacy, trust-building, and quality-of-life interventions. Unlike the earlier case studies, which primarily focused on adverse medicine events, this case study involved intersecting physical, psychological, social, and environmental factors, including polypharmacy, fear of falls, social isolation, and disengagement from care.

Using a qualitative case study approach allowed these interacting factors to be examined holistically and over time. Rather than capturing a single clinical outcome, the case documents a sequence of pharmacist-resident interactions, observations, and follow-up actions across multiple visits. By taking time to listen and build rapport over time, the pharmacist uncovered unreported issues, such as Harry's previous falls from his bed, and gained insight into his reluctance to leave his room. His initial disengagement and self-isolation highlighted the need for patience, persistence, and creative strategies when supporting residents who are anxious or withdrawn.

From a clinical standpoint, the pharmacist's role demonstrated how medication-related discomfort can compound broader physical and psychological challenges. Harry's relief from the "orange pills" and subsequent willingness to exercise and walk showed how even small, targeted medication changes can meaningfully improve autonomy, mood, and daily functioning.

From a methodological perspective, this case exemplifies the explanatory value of case study methodology. It demonstrates not only *what* changed for Harry but also *how* those changes occurred through pharmacist advocacy, interprofessional collaboration, and sustained engagement with both the resident and facility staff. Outcomes such as improved outlook, increased physical activity, and renewed engagement with care, while meaningful to residents, are not captured in aggregate trial outcomes reported in the main ReMInDAR trial paper (Roughead et al., 2022). The case study approach, therefore, provides complementary insight by situating clinical outcomes within the lived experience of the resident and the processes of care that supported change.

3.8 Case study 6: Barbara*—"My medicines are making me 'gag'!"

Barbara was born in regional Australia, where she has lived most of her life. Now, Barbara resides in a local residential aged-care facility and uses 11 regular medicines to manage her multiple comorbidities, including hyperlipidemia, hypertension, diabetes, congestive heart failure, renal failure, and depression. She also has eight medicines prescribed for use when necessary. She has been a very active member of the facility, an avid reader, and is passionate about completing cross words.

Barbara recently had a stroke and returned from the hospital with a large number of new medications. Despite being back in the facility, Barbara was still feeling very unwell after her stroke and could no longer complete the cognitive assessments for the ReMInDAR trial, which she had been able to complete prior to her stroke. Her mood was very low.

The pharmacist asked Barbara, "What bothers you the most?" to which Barbara expressed real concern about her medicines and said that all her medicines were making her feel really nauseous.

Barbara said she was "most terrified of the sound of the nurses pushing the medicine trolley to her room each day". As Barbara could not swallow her medicines after her stroke, the nursing staff had been crushing the medicines, and the mixture was very unpalatable, making her "gag".

The ReMInDAR pharmacist reviewed and reconciled Barbara's medications and identified medicines that had been discontinued in the hospital but were still listed on the medication chart in the aged care facility. The pharmacist discussed Barbara's concerns, including the issue of gagging, with her GP, and as a result, Barbara was taken off many of her tablets, the doses of some medications were reduced, and some of her medicines were changed to liquid forms.

Barbara's spirits improved; her cognition improved. During subsequent pharmacist sessions, Barbara's spirits greatly improved, and she was once again able to complete the cognitive assessments. Barbara was visibly much happier and was very grateful to the pharmacist for intervening on her behalf. The pharmacist's advocacy significantly improved Barbara's outlook and quality of life.

3.9 Commentary

Barbara's case exemplifies the unique strengths of the case study methodology in capturing the complexities of caring for residents in aged care by making visible the interactions between clinical decisions, residents' personal experiences, and system-level processes that are often obscured in aggregate data. Rather than solely focusing on diagnoses or medicine counts, the case study enabled the resident's subjective experience to be placed at the center of the narrative. In this instance, a single, open-ended question, *"What bothers you the most?"*, uncovered Barbara's greatest concern.

From a methodological perspective, this case demonstrates how pharmacists' interventions can be documented in detail—from identifying discrepancies in her medication chart to advocating for liquid alternatives and dose reductions—and how these actions translate into immediate, tangible improvements in Barbara's quality of life. Her spirits lifted, her cognition improved, and she was once again able to enjoy the simple pleasures of reading and completing crosswords. Such insights go far beyond what aggregate trial data can show; it is only through the case study lens that we can truly appreciate the fundamental human elements that matter: autonomy, comfort, and joy in daily life.

3.10 Case study 7:—Grace—"Don't question the prescribing"

Grace is an active, widowed 91 year-old who resides in a metropolitan aged care facility. She looked after her daughter as a stay-at-home mum and still continues to "worry about her," even though she is grown up now.

Grace has had a previous heart attack and underwent coronary artery bypass graft surgery in the past. She currently suffers from a number of medical conditions, including cancer, diabetes, hypertension, hyperlipidemia, varicose veins, incontinence, temporomandibular joint dysfunction, gallbladder stones, hiatus hernia, and peptic ulcer. Her conditions are managed with 13 regular medications and three medications for use as needed.

Grace expressed concern about the number of tablets she was taking and informed the pharmacist that she wanted to discontinue esomeprazole and magnesium, which she had been using long term. The pharmacist supported Grace's decision and reassured her that he would contact the GP to discuss this.

The GP was unreceptive to the pharmacist's recommendation and told Grace that "she did not need to have a pharmacist review her medicines," instructing her to take all her medicines. Consequently, Grace continued to take all her medicines and withdrew from the ReMInDAR trial.

The challenge of effective communication between healthcare professionals impeded the opportunity for Grace's medication preferences to be considered for medication optimization and for the potential improvement of Grace's health outcomes. Grace continued to use magnesium and esomeprazole long-term without any indication for their use.

3.11 Commentary

Grace's case illustrates one of the barriers that can undermine patient-centered care. The pharmacist acted appropriately in supporting her wish to cease esomeprazole and magnesium. From a clinical perspective, discontinuation of esomeprazole was justified, as long-term use is associated with increased risks of pneumonia, enteric infections, and hip fractures (Roughead et al., 2016; Ramsay et al., 2013; Islam et al., 2018).

The pharmacist attempted to communicate this recommendation to the GP; however, the GP's lack of receptivity highlighted the limitations of the pharmacist's ability to influence medication decisions. A stronger foundation of collaboration, perhaps established through prior relationship-building and regular communication between the pharmacist and GP, might have created a space where Grace's concerns were taken more seriously.

More broadly, this case reflects a broader challenge within aged care, where residents' voices are sometimes marginalized within a hierarchical system in which prescribers hold the greatest authority. In Grace's case, the hierarchy extended not only between the prescriber and patient but also between the prescriber and pharmacist. When professional communication breaks down, residents are the ones who bear the consequences. Without genuine shared decision-making among all parties, the potential for meaningful medicine optimization, and for residents like Grace to have their preferences respected, remains limited.

Looking forward, this case highlights the need to rethink models of care so that pharmacists are recognized as equal partners in the decision-making process. In the United Kingdom, for example, pharmacist independent prescribing has been successfully implemented, enabling pharmacists to directly initiate, renew, or adapt medicines for both diagnosed and undiagnosed conditions within their scope of practice (Mesbahi et al., 2025; NHS England., 2026). This model not only enhances access to care but also ensures that patients' preferences are acted upon in a timely way, while supporting overall well-being and improving health outcomes (Holland et al., 2023; Birt et al., 2021, 2023). In Australia, while pharmacists are not yet independent prescribers, several pilot programs are underway that move in this direction. These include pharmacist prescribing pilots for urinary tract infections (Medicines and Poisons Act 2019, n.d.), continuation of oral contraceptives (Medicines and Poisons Act 2019, n.d.), and medicine management in chronic conditions (Medicines and Poisons Act 2019, n.d.). For the aged care setting, embedding pharmacists in collaborative prescribing models, supported by shared responsibility and accountability as in existing practices in Australian hospitals (Tong and Yip, 2024; Tong et al., 2020), could help prevent scenarios like Grace's, where residents' wishes were overlooked.

3.12 Case study 8—Jack—"Now I know I have medicines for when I need them

Jack is an 84 year-old man who grew up in Tasmania. He moved into his residential nursing home two years ago so that he could be around more people and be taken care of. Jack's wife visits him regularly, and he enjoys participating in the wellness and social activities at the facility.

I just put up with it. Jack has been experiencing episodes of vertigo following a stroke, which has been an issue from time to time and is something he just "puts up with".

During the ReMInDAR service, the pharmacist noted that Jack had a prescription for betahistine charted on a "when required" basis, in accordance with existing facility medication administration protocols. These protocols allowed the nursing staff to administer "when required" medicines either in response to resident requests or when symptoms were observed. However, when asked about betahistine, Jack said that he had not heard of the medicine, nor had he taken any. There were several other medicines charted for use on a "when required" basis, but Jack was not aware of any of them. Jack said, "The nurses did not offer me anything when I complained of being dizzy".

As part of the trial service, the pharmacist explained to Jack what each of his medicines was and what he could request to use for each symptom. The pharmacist also typed up a list of Jack's "when required" medicines and gave it to him as a reference (docusate sodium + sennosides, metoclopramide, macrogol, acetaminophen, betahistine, triamcinolone, ibuprofen, and diclofenac gel), including the names of the medicines, their doses, and an explanation of what the medicines are used for. Jack had an active mind and was very interested in the medicines, feeling empowered by knowing what was available to him. The pharmacist reminded Jack to ask the nursing staff for assistance if he required any of the "when required" medicines and also reminded the staff that such orders were in place for his conditions.

3.13 Commentary

Jack's case demonstrates pharmacists' role in bridging information gaps and empowering residents through education. While the medicines themselves were charted and technically "available," the absence of clear communication meant that Jack had no awareness of their purpose or potential benefit, leaving him to "just put up with" symptoms like vertigo. This disconnect between what is prescribed and what the patient knows is a common challenge in aged care, where medicines intended for symptom relief often go unused because residents are uninformed or hesitant to request them.

From a methodological perspective, this case study highlights that even when residents are prescribed many "when required" medicines, some may never use them. In the ReMInDAR trial, residents often had long lists of "when required" medicines: some used these medicines frequently, while others were unaware they even had access to them. The administration of "when required" medicines is frequently not captured in aggregated trial data. The pharmacist's simple act of explaining Jack's "when required" medicines, together with a personalized written list, changed his understanding and provided him with a greater sense of control over his care.

4 Discussion

These eight case studies demonstrate how case study methodology captures the nuanced impact of pharmacist-led services in aged care by enabling detailed, longitudinal examination of individual resident experiences within their real-world care contexts. This approach reveals the clinical, social, and emotional dimensions of care, such as residents' fears, preferences, communication barriers, and system-level constraints, which are often invisible in aggregated trial data. Case studies allow for a detailed understanding of how interventions unfold over time.

The ReMInDAR trial case studies illustrate the breadth of scenarios encountered in aged care, ranging from high-risk adverse events to subtler issues that affect daily quality of life, such as sleep, comfort, and autonomy. While diverse, the cases can be broadly grouped into two categories: those with high potential for serious adverse events and those that, although less likely to result in immediate harm, still have a significant impact on residents' well-being. Serious adverse events, such as hospital admissions or falls, are easy to capture in aggregated trial data. However, for residents with declining health or reduced capacity for self-determination, these "minor" issues, such as being pain-free, feeling safe, or enjoying a good night's sleep, are often overlooked in trials and rarely appear in aggregate data. From a methodological standpoint, the case study approach allows these experiences to be documented, capturing the dynamic interactions between the resident, pharmacist, and the broader care team, and providing rich insights that quantitative data alone cannot reveal.

The case studies presented in this chapter are all clinical case studies focused on a medicine-related problem. Where multiple case studies examine the same type of medicine-related problem or the same outcome, it would be possible to create a case series, similar to those frequently undertaken for pharmacovigilance (Croteau et al., 2024; Wang et al., 2024). Coroners' reports of deaths due to medicine misadventure also provide an example of this approach. Beyond individual clinical cases, the case study methodology is also appropriate for analyses of systems and for designing and evaluating interventions. For example, case study methodology has been used to explore pharmacists' roles in bridging gaps in care and adapting services to meet patient needs in specific contexts, such as contraceptive access or medicines information codesign (Leszczynski et al., 2025; Hynes-Ryan et al., 2025). Similarly, case study methods have been applied to document patterns of medicine use and changes in practice over time in population health contexts, demonstrating their value in understanding the interplay between practice, policy, and outcomes at system or program levels (Roughead et al., 1999).

A further strength of the case study approach is its ability to explore not only outcomes but also the processes through which complex interventions are implemented (Paparini et al., 2020). Through detailed narratives, we can see how small, targeted actions over time can produce meaningful improvements in residents' physical health, mental well-being, and engagement in social and recreational activities. For instance, in "Harry's" case, the pharmacist addressed not only medicine-related issues but also his physical discomfort, anxiety about falls, disrupted sleep, and social isolation. The intervention involved identifying unreported problems, liaising with the GP to adjust medicines, reorganizing his care environment, and working with staff to support "Harry" to sleep safely in his own bed. This multifaceted approach required ongoing trust-building with "Harry", repeated follow-ups, and collaboration with both care staff and the GP, demonstrating how case studies can capture the intricate interplay of actions that go far beyond simple medicine changes.

Beyond individual experiences, case studies also highlight how pharmacists can serve as resident advocates, bridging communication gaps and building trust. The ongoing advocacy of pharmacists is evident across multiple cases: "Mary", who was initially too frightened to report bleeding; "Harry", who regained the ability to sleep in his own bed; and "John", whose desire to withdraw treatment was only reconsidered because of continuous pharmacist involvement. Case studies also uncover systemic barriers, such as hierarchical dynamics between prescribers and pharmacists, which can affect the success of interventions. Without the lens of a case study, these advocacy efforts, challenges, and their cumulative effects on resident outcomes would remain largely invisible.

The findings from the case studies support calls for integrating pharmacists more fully into multidisciplinary teams and exploring models such as pharmacist independent prescribing (Holland et al., 2023; Norman et al., 2023; Hughes and Lapane, 2011), which can strengthen residents' voices in medicine management. From a research perspective, the case study methodology emphasizes the importance of capturing the human and contextual factors that shape outcomes, highlighting the limitations of relying solely on aggregated trial data to understand the real-world impact of pharmacist services. The case studies demonstrate person-centered care, aligning with the World Health Organization's 'Medication Without Harm' initiative (World Health Organization., 2026.) and the vision of the Seven-Star Pharmacist (WHO Consultative Group on the Role of the Pharmacist in the Health Care System., 1997), particularly in the roles of caregiver, communicator, and decision-maker in promoting safe, person-centered care for residents. To illustrate these distinctions, Fig. 10.1 presents a conceptual model of pharmacist roles uncovered through case study methodology.

4.1 Pharmacist-led interventions and medicine-related problems in aged or long-term care settings

By linking case study insights to measurable outcomes from effectiveness trials, it becomes clear why pharmacist-led interventions are essential in addressing medicine-related problems in aged care. Residents in these settings often have multiple chronic conditions, functional decline, and frailty (Dorj et al., 2022; Gutiérrez-Valencia et al.,

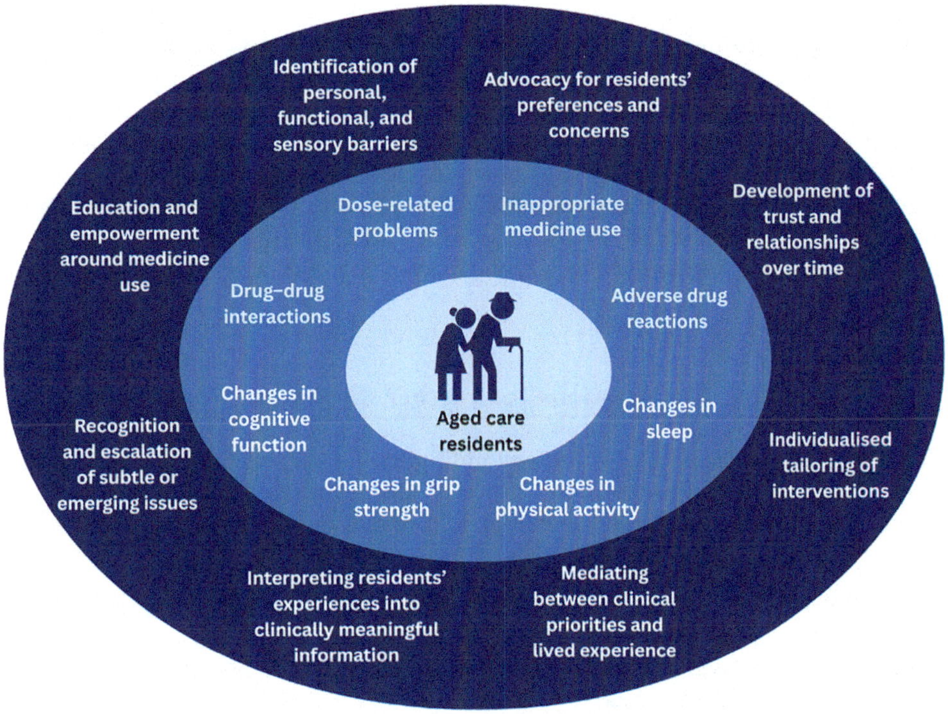

FIG. 10.1 **Conceptual model illustrating pharmacist roles uncovered through case study methodology.** The inner circle represents aged care residents at the center of pharmacist services. The middle circle depicts outcomes and issues typically captured in aggregated data, with the upper segment representing what is usually measured in routine medicine reviews or clinical trials, and the lower segment reflecting outcomes specifically assessed in the ReMInDAR trial. The outer circle highlights pharmacist roles and insights revealed through case study methodology, capturing activities that are rarely visible in routine datasets. Together, this model demonstrates how case study methodology extends understanding beyond aggregate data, providing a richer picture of pharmacist-led interventions in practice.

2018; Chen et al., 2021; Li et al., 2022), all of which increase their risk of polypharmacy, inappropriate prescribing, medication errors, adverse medication events, and adverse outcomes such as hospitalizations and reduced survival (Al-Jumaili and Doucette, 2018; Lim et al., 2022; Handler et al., 2006). The prevalence of polypharmacy in this population is high (Delara et al., 2022; Nicholson et al., 2024; Hajjar et al., 2007; Jokanovic et al., 2015), and managing complex medication regimens becomes increasingly challenging as disease burden rises. Given these patient-related challenges, pharmacists play a unique and vital role in addressing medication harms through comprehensive medication reviews, collaboration with multidisciplinary teams, and resident education. Pharmacist-led interventions or services in aged care are increasingly recognized as essential in modern pharmacy practice (Ali et al., 2021; Sadowski et al., 2020; Kim et al., 2024; McGrory and Elnaem, 2025), highlighting the importance and need for integrating pharmacists into aged care models to improve resident health outcomes and quality of life.

The role of pharmacists in geriatric care has expanded to include chronic disease management, medication reconciliation, adherence support, deprescribing (Haider et al., 2021; Lee et al., 2019; Gonçalves et al., 2025), and, in some jurisdictions, independent or collaborative prescribing (Holland et al., 2023; Norman et al., 2023; Hughes and Lapane, 2011). To support these roles, various practice models have been implemented internationally to optimize medication management in aged care (Haider et al., 2021; Lee et al., 2019). Pharmacist-led interventions that have been tested include structured medication reviews (Lee et al., 2019; Lenander et al., 2018; Bitter et al., 2019), multidisciplinary case conferencing (Baqir et al., 2014), the use of clinical decision support technologies (Almutairi et al., 2020; Loganathan et al., 2011), and the development of medication review tools through consensus-based methods (Disalvo et al., 2020).

5 Conclusion

The cases presented in this chapter demonstrate the value of the case study methodology as an approach for examining pharmacist-led services. By focusing on individual medicine-related problems within their real-world contexts, the case studies illustrate how pharmacist interventions unfold over time and how clinical decisions, interactions, and contextual factors shape outcomes. This methodological approach enables the examination of aspects of practice, including communication processes, decision-making, and care coordination, that are not readily captured through aggregated trial outcomes.

The case study approach uniquely captures both outcomes and the processes underlying them, providing insights into how pharmacists identify medicine-related problems, advocate for residents, and collaborate with care staff and prescribers to implement change. By documenting these processes in detail, case studies offer a richer understanding of how pharmacist-led services operate in practice and complement effectiveness data from clinical trials. They also highlight how pharmacists build meaningful relationships with residents and their care teams, providing a powerful lens for understanding and showcasing the real-world impact of pharmacist-led interventions.

6 Questions for further discussion

Case study methodology provides a lens for understanding the real-world complexities of pharmacist-led interventions in aged care. The following questions are designed to encourage learners and practitioners to reflect on how case studies can inform practice, highlight barriers, and reveal opportunities for patient advocacy and interdisciplinary collaboration:

1. How can case study research help identify structural changes, including funding and training, that are needed to enable pharmacists to practice to their full scope in aged care?
2. In what ways can case studies reveal how the resident voice is, or is not, effectively integrated into the decision-making process regarding their care?
3. How can digital tools or documentation strategies be leveraged in case studies to enhance pharmacist advocacy, particularly in remote or underserved settings?
4. Which outcome measures—clinical, process-related, or patient-centered—are best captured through case study research to evaluate the effectiveness of pharmacist-led interventions in improving resident outcomes and quality of life?

7 Application exercise: Developing a case study from your practice

Scenario: You are a newly appointed pharmacist at a 50-bed aged care facility in a regional area. One resident, "Mr. Smith", aged 82, is a retired farmer who lived on a large farm in rural Australia with his wife, eldest son, and his family before moving into aged care after becoming nonverbal following a stroke. His wife has moved into the town near the aged-care facility, and she visits daily, along with his son, who visits weekly. Mr. Smith's stroke has resulted in increased frailty, and he has developed stage 4 kidney disease.

He is currently prescribed the following medications:

- Aspirin 100 mg once daily
- Atorvastatin 80 mg once daily
- Perindopril 4 mg once daily
- Amlodipine 5 mg once daily
- Metformin 500 mg twice daily
- Paracetamol 500 mg every 6 hours as needed (maximum 4 g/day).
- Oxybutynin 5 mg twice daily
- Lansoprazole 30 mg once daily
- Gabapentin 100 mg, three times daily
- Loratadine 10 mg once daily
- Lorazepam 0.5 mg, as needed, up to twice daily
- Senna 7.5 mg once daily
- Calcium carbonate 600 mg with vitamin D 1000 IU, once daily

This scenario includes common challenges encountered in the aged care setting: complex medication regimens, communication barriers, the need for clinical review, and the need to include family members.

Your task: Using this scenario as an example, identify a real case from your own practice that shares similar challenges. Develop a case study based on that resident, focusing on:

- Gathering insights from the resident, family, and multidisciplinary team provides context
- Documenting clinical interventions and your role as a pharmacist and advocate
- Strategies you would use if other clinicians were hesitant to implement changes

The goal of this exercise is to demonstrate how real-life clinical scenarios can be transformed into robust case studies that capture both the outcomes and the processes underpinning the interventions. By documenting not only what changed but also how and why decisions were made, the cases illustrate how person-centered care, interprofessional collaboration, and pharmacist advocacy can improve residents' health, well-being, and quality of life.

Reflection questions for practice:

- What approaches support gathering insights from the family and the multidisciplinary team to provide richer context?
- How can clinical interventions be documented in a way that captures both your role as a pharmacist and your role as an advocate, providing evidence for case study analysis?
- If the GP is hesitant to implement changes, what strategies can you employ to advocate effectively for the resident while documenting the decision-making process?

AI disclosure

During the preparation of this work, the author(s) used ChatGPT to make some sentences clearer and better structured. After using this tool/service, the author(s) reviewed and edited the content as needed and take full responsibility for the content of the publication.

References

Al-Jumaili, A.A., Doucette, W.R., 2018. A systems approach to identify factors influencing adverse drug events in nursing homes. J. Am. Geriatr. Soc. 1532-5415. 66 (7), 1420–1427. Available from: http://onlinelibrary.wiley.com/journal/10.1111/(ISSN)1532-5415. doi:10.1111/jgs.15389.

Albrecht, J., Meves, A., Bigby, M., 2005. Case reports and case series from Lancet had significant impact on medical literature. J. Clin. Epidemiol. 0895-4356. 58 (12), 1227–1232. Available from: https://www.sciencedirect.com/science/article/pii/S0895435605001885. doi:10.1016/j.jclinepi.2005.04.003.

Ali, S., Salahudeen, M.S., Bereznicki, L.R.E., Curtain, C.M., 2021. Pharmacist-led interventions to reduce adverse drug events in older people living in residential aged care facilities: a systematic review. Br. J. Clin. Pharmacol. 1365-2125. 87 (10), 3672–3689. Available from: http://onlinelibrary.wiley.com/journal/10.1111/(ISSN)1365-2125. doi:10.1111/bcp.14824.

Almutairi, H., Stafford, A., Etherton-Beer, C., Flicker, L., 2020. Optimisation of medications used in residential aged care facilities: a systematic review and meta-analysis of randomised controlled trials. BMC Geriatr. 1471-2318. 20 (1). doi:10.1186/s12877-020-01634-4.

Baker, G.R., 2011. The contribution of case study research to knowledge of how to improve quality of care. BMJ Qual. Saf. 2044-5415. 20 (Suppl 1), i30. doi:10.1136/bmjqs.2010.046490.

Baqir, W., Barrett, S., Desai, N., Copeland, R., Hughes, J., 2014. A clinico-ethical framework for multidisciplinary review of medication in nursing homes. BMJ Qual. Improv. Rep. 2050-1315. 3 (1), u203261.w2538. doi:10.1136/bmjquality.u203261.w2538.

Bignall, J., Horton, R., 1995. Learning from stories—the lancet's case reports. Lancet. 346 (8985). doi:10.1016/s0140-6736(95)91859-0.

Birt, L., Dalgarno, L., Poland, F., Wright, D., Bond, C., 2023. What happens when pharmacist independent prescribers lead on medicine management in older people's care homes: a qualitative study. BMJ Open. 2044-6055. 13 (10), e068678. doi:10.1136/bmjopen-2022-068678.

Birt, L., Dalgarno, L., Wright, D.J., Alharthi, M., Inch, J., Spargo, M., Blacklock, J., Poland, F., Holland, R.C., Alldred, D.P., Hughes, C.M., Bond, C.M., Blyth, A., Watts, L., Daffu-O'Reilly, A., 2021. Process evaluation for the care homes independent pharmacist prescriber study (CHIPPS). BMC Health Serv. Res. 1472-6963. 21 (1). Available from: http://www.biomedcentral.com/bmchealthservres/. doi:10.1186s12913-021-07062-3.

Bitter, K., Pehe, C., Krüger, M., Heuer, G., Quinke, R., Jaehde, U., 2019. Pharmacist-led medication reviews for geriatric residents in German long-term care facilities. BMC Geriatr. 1471-2318. 19 (1). doi:10.1186/s12877-019-1052-z.

Chen, Y.-Z., Huang, S.-T., Wen, Y.-W., Chen, L.-K., Hsiao, F.-Y., 2021. Combined effects of frailty and polypharmacy on health outcomes in older adults: frailty outweighs polypharmacy. J. Am. Med. Dir. Assoc. 1525-8610. 22 (3), 606.e7. doi:10.1016/j.jamda.2020.07.019.

Croteau, D., Kim, T., Chan, V., Stevens, J., Pimentel Maldonado, D.A., Baldassari, L.E., Lee, P.R., Hughes, A., Brinker, A., 2024. Progressive multifocal leukoencephalopathy associated with sphingosine-1-phosphate receptor modulators: a large case series. Mult. Scler. Relat. Disord. 2211-0348. 92, 106163. doi:10.1016/j.msard.2024.106163.

Crowe, S., Cresswell, K., Robertson, A., Huby, G., Avery, A., Sheikh, A., 2011. The case study approach. BMC Med. Res. Methodol. 1471-2288. 11 (1). doi:10.1186/1471-2288-11-100.

Delara, M., Murray, L., Jafari, B., Bahji, A., Goodarzi, Z., Kirkham, J., Chowdhury, M., Seitz, D.P., 2022. Prevalence and factors associated with polypharmacy: a systematic review and meta-analysis. BMC Geriatr. 1471-2318. 22 (1). doi:10.1186/s12877-022-03279-x.

Disalvo, D., Luckett, T., Bennett, A., Davidson, P.M., Agar, M., 2020. Multidisciplinary perspectives on medication-related decision-making for people with advanced dementia living in long-term care: a critical incident analysis. Eur. J. Clin. Pharmacol. 0031-6970. 76 (4), 567–578. doi:10.1007/s00228-019-02820-z.

Dorj, G., Lim, R., Ellett, L.K., Kelly, T.-L., Andrade, A., Widagdo, I., Pratt, N., Bilton, R., Roughead, E., 2022. Medicine-related problems: a recurrent issue among residents living in nursing homes. Front. Pharmacol. 1663-9812. 13. doi:10.3389/fphar.2022.978871.

Fàbregues, S., Fetters, M.D., 2019. Fundamentals of case study research in family medicine and community health. Fam. Med. Community Health. 7 (2). doi:10.1136/fmch-2018-000074.

Fleischmann, M., McLaughlin, P., Vaughan, B., Hayes, A., 2024. A clinician's guide to performing a case series study. J. Bodyw. Mov. Ther. 40, 211–216.

Gittus, M., O'Cathain, A., Miller, K., Oklopcic, A., Ong, A.C., Fotheringham, J., 2025. A conceptual model of factors potentially influencing prescribing decisions for chronic conditions: an overview of systematic reviews. BMC Med. 1741-7015. 23 (1). Available from: https://bmcmedicine.biomedcentral.com/. doi:10.1186/s12916-025-04194-9.

Gonçalves, J.R., Magalhães, N., Machado, S., Ramalhinho, I., Cavaco, A.M., 2025. Pharmacist-mediated deprescribing in long-term care facilities: a systematic review. Pharmacy. 2226-4787. 13 (1), 3. doi:10.3390/pharmacy13010003.

Greenhalgh, T., 2025. Case studies: a guide for researchers, educators, and implementers. BMJ Med. 4 (1). doi:10.1136/bmjmed-2025-001623.

Grimes, D.A., Schulz, K.F., 2002. Descriptive studies: what they can and cannot do. Lancet (London, England). 359 (9301), 145–149.

Guetterman, T.C., Fetters, M.D., 2018. Two methodological approaches to the integration of mixed methods and case study designs: a systematic review. Am. Behav. Sci. 0002-7642. 62 (7), 900–918. doi:10.1177/0002764218772641.

Gutiérrez-Valencia, M., Izquierdo, M., Cesari, M., Casas-Herrero, Á., Inzitari, M., Martínez-Velilla, N., 2018. The relationship between frailty and polypharmacy in older people: a systematic review. Br. J. Clin. Pharmacol. 0306-5251. 84 (7), 1432–1444. doi:10.1111/bcp.13590.

Haider, I., Kosari, S., Naunton, M., Koerner, J., Dale, M., Nizamani, S., Davey, R., 2023. The role of on-site pharmacist in residential aged care facilities: findings from the PiRACF study. J. Pharm. Policy Pract. 2052-3211. 16 (1). doi:10.1186/s40545-023-00587-4.

Haider, I., Naunton, M., Davey, R., Peterson, G.M., Baqir, W., Kosari, S., 2021. How do pharmacists practice in aged care? A narrative review of models from Australia, England, and the United States of America. Int. J. Environ. Res. Public Health 1660-4601. 18 (23). Available from: https://www.mdpi.com/1660-4601/18/23/12773/pdf. doi:10.3390/ijerph182312773.

Hajjar, E.R., Cafiero, A.C., Hanlon, J.T., 2007. Polypharmacy in elderly patients. Am. J. Geriatr. Pharmacother. 1543-5946. 5 (4), 345–351. doi:10.1016/j.amjopharm.2007.12.002.

Handler, S.M., Wright, R.M., Ruby, C.M., Hanlon, J.T., 2006. Epidemiology of medication-related adverse events in nursing homes. Am. J. Geriatr. Pharmacother. 1543-5946. 4 (3), 264–272. doi:10.1016/j.amjopharm.2006.09.011.

Holland, R., Bond, C., Alldred, D.P., Arthur, A., Barton, G., Birt, L., Blacklock, J., Blyth, A., Cheilari, S., Daffu-O'Reilly, A., Dalgarno, L., Desborough, J., Ford, J., Grant, K., Harry, B., Hill, H., Hughes, C., Inch, J., Maskrey, V., Myint, P., Norris, N., Poland, F., Shepstone, L., Spargo, M., Turner, D., Watts, L., Zermansky, A., Wright, D., 2023. Evaluation of effectiveness and safety of pharmacist independent prescribers in care homes: cluster randomised controlled trial. BMJ. 1756-1833. 380, e071883. doi:10.1136/bmj-2022-071883.

Hughes, C.M., Lapane, K.L., 2011. Pharmacy interventions on prescribing in nursing homes: from evidence to practice. Ther. Adv. Drug Saf. 2042-0994. 2 (3), 103–112. doi:10.1177/2042098611406167.

Hynes-Ryan, C., Kelleher, I., Kathryn, S., Beaudelot, C., Carolan, A., Columb, D., Donnelly, S., Gamage, N., Hill, N., Migone, M., McWilliams, S., Morning, J., O'Donoghue, B., Solan, I., Strawbridge, J., Hayden, J.C., Keating, D., 2025. Youth Med.Info: a case study in co-design of mental health medicines-information resources for children, young people and their parents/guardians. BMJ Open. 2044-6055. 15 (9), e103146. doi:10.1136/bmjopen-2025-103146.

Islam, M.M., Poly, T.N., Walther, B.A., Dubey, N.K., Ningrum, D.N.A., Shabbir, S.A., Li, Y.C., 2018. Adverse outcomes of long-term use of proton pump inhibitors: a systematic review and meta-analysis. Taiwan Eur. J. Gastroenterol. Hepatol. 1473-5687. 30 (12), 1395–1405. Available from: http://journals.lww.com/eurojgh/pages/default.aspx. doi:10.1097/MEG.0000000000001198.

Jokanovic, N., Tan, E.C.K., Dooley, M.J., Kirkpatrick, C.M., Bell, J.S., 2015. Prevalence and factors associated with polypharmacy in long-term care facilities: a systematic review. J. Am. Med. Dir. Assoc. 1525-8610. 16 (6), 535.e1. doi:10.1016/j.jamda.2015.03.003.

Kempen, T.G.H., Benaissa, Y., Molema, H., Valk, L.E., Hazen, A.C.M., Heringa, M., Kwint, H.F., Zwart, D.L.M., Kälvemark Sporrong, S., Stewart, D., van Dijk, L., 2024. Pharmacists' current and potential prescribing roles in primary care in the Netherlands: a case study. J. Interprof. Care 1469-9567. 38 (5), 787–798. Available from: http://www.tandfonline.com/loi/ijic20. doi:10.1080/13561820.2024.2374017.

Kidd, M.R., Saltman, D.C., 2012. Case reports at the vanguard of 21st century medicine. J. Med. Case Rep. 6. doi:10.1186/1752-1947-6-156

Kim, I.J., Ryu, G., Rhie, S.J., Kim, H.J., 2024. Pharmacist interventions in Asian healthcare environments for older people: a systematic review and meta-analysis on hospitalization, mortality, and quality of life. BMC Geriatr. 1471-2318. 24 (1). Available from: https://bmcgeriatr.biomedcentral.com/. doi:10.1186/s12877-024-05089-9.

Kooistra, B., Dijkman, B., Einhorn, T.A., Bhandari, M., 2009. How to design a good case series. J. Bone Joint Surg. 91 (Suppl 3), 21–26. doi:10.2106/JBJS.H.01573.

Lee, S.W.H., Mak, V.S.L., Tang, Y.W., 2019. Pharmacist services in nursing homes: a systematic review and meta-analysis. Br. J. Clin. Pharmacol. 1365-2125. 85 (12), 2668–2688. Available from: http://onlinelibrary.wiley.com/journal/10.1111/(ISSN)1365-2125. doi:10.1111/bcp.14101.

Lenander, C., Bondesson, Å., Viberg, N., Beckman, A., Midlöv, P., 2018. Effects of medication reviews on use of potentially inappropriate medications in elderly patients; a cross-sectional study in Swedish primary care. BMC Health Serv. Res. 1472-6963. 18 (1). doi:10.1186/s12913-018-3425-y.

Leszczynski, A., Bowen, B., Schultz, C.P., Herman, A., Aragon, K., Bachyrycz, A., 2025. Utilizing pharmacists to bridge gaps in contraceptive care: new Mexico as case study. J. Am. Pharm. Assoc. 1544-3191, 102926. doi:10.1016/j.japh.2025.102926.

Li, Y., Zhang, X., Yang, L., Yang, Y., Qiao, G., Lu, C., Liu, K., 2022. Association between polypharmacy and mortality in the older adults: a systematic review and meta-analysis. Arch. Gerontol. Geriatr. 0167-4943. 100, 104630. doi:10.1016/j.archger.2022.104630.

Lim, R., Bereznicki, L., Corlis, M., Ellett, L.M.K., Kang, A.C., Merlin, T., Parfitt, G., Pratt, N.L., Rowett, D., Torode, S., Whitehouse, J., Andrade, A.Q., Bilton, R., Cousins, J., Kelly, L., Schubert, C., Williams, M., Roughead, E.E., 2020. Reducing medicine-induced deterioration and adverse reactions (ReMInDAR) trial: study protocol for a randomised controlled trial in residential aged-care facilities assessing frailty as the primary outcome. BMJ Open. 2044-6055. 10 (4), e032851. doi:10.1136/bmjopen-2019-032851.

Lim, R., Bilton, R., Dorj, G., Bereznicki, L., Rowett, D., Ho, J.N., Freeman, A., Roughead, E.E., 2023a. Pharmacists as patient advocates: a series of case studies illustrating the impacts of a regular pharmacist service in residential aged care (nursing homes). Explor. Res. Clin. Soc. Pharm. 2667-2766. 10, 100268. doi:10.1016/j.rcsop.2023.100268.

Lim, R., Dumuid, D., Parfitt, G., Stanford, T., Post, D., Bilton, R., Kalisch Ellett, L.M., Pratt, N., Roughead, E.E., 2023b. Using wrist-worn accelerometers to identify the impact of medicines with anticholinergic or sedative properties on sedentary time: a 12 month prospective analysis. Maturitas. 172, 9–14. doi:10.1016/j.maturitas.2023.03.006.

Lim, R., Ellett, L.M.K., Semple, S., Roughead, E.E., 2022. The extent of medication-related hospital admissions in Australia: a review from 1988 to 2021. Drug Saf. 1179-1942. 45 (3), 249–257. Available from: http://rd.springer.com/journal/40264. doi:10.1007/s40264-021-01144-1.

Loganathan, M., Singh, S., Franklin, B.D., Bottle, A., Majeed, A., 2011. Interventions to optimise prescribing in care homes: systematic review. Age Ageing. 1468-2834. 40 (2), 150–162. doi:10.1093/ageing/afq161.

McGrory, F., Elnaem, M.H., 2025. Pharmacist-led interventions for polypharmacy management in older adults: a systematic review of strategies and outcomes in the United Kingdom and the Republic of Ireland. Pharmacy. 2226-4787. 13 (4), 109. doi:10.3390/pharmacy13040109.

McIntosh, J., Alonso, A., MacLure, K., Stewart, D., Kempen, T., Mair, A., Castel-Branco, M., Codina, C., Fernandez-Llimos, F., Fleming, G., Gennimata, D., Gillespie, U., Harrison, C., Illario, M., Junius-Walker, U., Kampolis, C.F., Kardas, P., Lewek, P., Malva, J., Menditto, E., Scullin, C., Wiese, B., Hersberger, K., 2018. A case study of polypharmacy management in nine European countries: implications for change management and implementation. PLOS ONE. 1932-6203. 13 (4), e0195232. doi:10.1371/journal.pone.0195232.

Medicines and Poisons Act 2019, n.d. Extended practice authority 'Pharmacists—community pharmacy chronic conditions management pilot'—version 1. Available from: https://www.psa.org.au/wp-content/uploads/2025/07/epa-pharmacists-community-pharmacy-chronic-conditions-mgt.pdf.

Medicines and Poisons Act 2019, n.d. Extended practice authority 'Pharmacists'—version 8. Available from: https://www.psa.org.au/wp-content/uploads/2025/07/epa-pharmacists.pdf.

Mesbahi, Z., Piquer-Martinez, C., Benrimoj, S.I., Martinez-Martinez, F., Amador-Fernandez, N., Zarzuelo, M.J., Dineen-Griffin, S., Garcia-Cardenas, V., 2025. Pharmacists as independent prescribers in community pharmacy: a scoping review. Res. Soc. Adm. Pharm. 1551-7411. 21 (3), 142–153. doi:10.1016/j.sapharm.2024.12.008.

Mills, A., Durepos, G., Wiebe, E., 2010. Encyclopedia of Case Study Research. SAGE Publications, Inc., Thousand Oaks, California. Available from: https://methods.sagepub.com/ency/edvol/encyc-of-case-study-research/chpt/quick-start-case-study-research. doi:10.4135/9781412957397.n283.

NHS England. 2026. Independent prescribing. https://www.hee.nhs.uk/our-work/pharmacy/independent-prescribing.

Nicholson, K., Liu, W., Fitzpatrick, D., Hardacre, K.A., Roberts, S., Salerno, J., Stranges, S., Fortin, M., Mangin, D., 2024. Prevalence of multimorbidity and polypharmacy among adults and older adults: a systematic review. Lancet Healthy Longev. 2666-7568. 5 (4), e287. doi:10.1016/s2666-7568(24)00007-2.

Nissen, T., Wynn, R., 2012. The recent history of the clinical case report: a narrative review. JRSM Short Rep. 3 (12). Available from: https://pubmed.ncbi.nlm.nih.gov/23476729/. doi:10.1258/shorts.2012.012046.

Norman, K., Cassim, S., Papa, V., Te-Karu, L., Clark, P., Mullins, H., Chepulis, L., 2023. "Prescribing for the whole person": a qualitative study exploring prescribing pharmacist views on type 2 diabetes management in New Zealand. BMC Health Serv. Res. 1472-6963. 23 (1). doi:10.1186/s12913-023-09877-8.

Paparini, S., Green, J., Papoutsi, C., Murdoch, J., Petticrew, M., Greenhalgh, T., Hanckel, B., Shaw, S., 2020. Case study research for better evaluations of complex interventions: rationale and challenges. BMC Med. 1741-7015. 18 (1). doi:10.1186/s12916-020-01777-6.

Ramsay, E.N., Pratt, N.L., Ryan, P., Roughead, E.E., 2013. Proton pump inhibitors and the risk of pneumonia: a comparison of cohort and self-controlled case series designs. BMC Med. Res. Methodol. 1471-2288. 13 (1). doi:10.1186/1471-2288-13-82.

Roughead, E.E., Chan, E.W., Choi, N.K., Griffiths, J., Jin, X.M., Lee, J., Kimura, M., Kimura, T., Kubota, K., Lai, E.C.C., Man, K.K.C., Nguyen, T.A., Ooba, N., Park, B.J., Sato, T., Shin, J.Y., Wang, T.T., Wong, I.C.K., Yang, Y.H.K., Pratt, N.L., 2016. Proton pump inhibitors and risk of Clostridium difficile infection: a multi-country study using sequence symmetry analysis. Expert Opin. Drug Saf. 1744-764X. 15 (12), 1589–1595. doi:10.1080/14740338.2016.1238071.

Roughead, E.E., Gilbert, A.L., Primrose, J.G., 1999. Improving drug use: a case study of events which led to changes in use of flucloxacillin in Australia. Soc. Sci. Med. 0277-9536. 48 (6), 845–853. doi:10.1016/S0277-9536(98)00405-5.

Roughead, E.E., Pratt, N.L., Parfitt, G., Rowett, D., Kalisch-Ellett, L.M., Bereznicki, L., Merlin, T., Corlis, M., Kang, A.C., Whitehouse, J., Bilton, R., Schubert, C., Torode, S., Kelly, T.L., Andrade, A.Q., Post, D., Dorj, G., Cousins, J., Williams, M., Lim, R., 2022. Effect of an ongoing pharmacist service to reduce medicine-induced deterioration and adverse reactions in aged-care facilities (nursing homes): a multicentre, randomised controlled trial (the ReMInDAR trial). Age Ageing. 1468-2834. 51 (4). Available from: http://ageing.oxfordjournals.org/. doi:10.1093/ageing/afac092.

Ruxton, K., Woodman, R.J., Mangoni, A.A., 2015. Drugs with anticholinergic effects and cognitive impairment, falls and all-cause mortality in older adults: a systematic review and meta-analysis. Br. J. Clin. Pharmacol. 80 (2), 209–220. doi:10.1111/bcp.12617.

Sadowski, C.A., Charrois, T.L., Sehn, E., Chatterley, T., Kim, S., 2020. The role and impact of the pharmacist in long-term care settings: a systematic review. J. Am. Pharm. Assoc. 1544-3450. 60 (3), 516. Available from: http://www.japha.org/issues.aspx?journalid=63. doi:10.1016/j.japh.2019.11.014.

Silva, B.B., Fegadolli, C., 2020. Implementation of pharmaceutical care for older adults in the brazilian public health system: a case study and realistic evaluation. BMC Health Serv. Res. 1472-6963. 20 (1). Available from: http://www.biomedcentral.com/bmchealthservres/. doi:10.1186/s12913-020-4898-z.

Taipale, H.T., Bell, J.S., Gnjidic, D., Sulkava, R., Hartikainen, S., 2012. Sedative load among community-dwelling people aged 75 years or older: association with balance and mobility. J. Clin. Psychopharmacol. 32 (2), 218–224. doi:10.1097/JCP.0b013e3182485802.

Thomas, G., 2021. How to Do Your Case Study, third ed. SAGE Publications. Available from: https://sk.sagepub.com/book/mono/how-to-do-your-case-study-3e/toc. doi:10.4135/9781036232238.

Tong, E.Y., Mitra, B., Yip, G., Galbraith, K., Dooley, M.J., Roman, C., Smit, D.V., Gibbs, H., Newnham, H., Kirsa, S., Weeks, G., Jones, N., Toner, P., Turner, C., Terril, D., Hua, P., 2020. Multi-site evaluation of partnered pharmacist medication charting and in-hospital length of stay. Br. J. Clin. Pharmacol. 1365-2125. 86 (2), 285–290. Available from: http://onlinelibrary.wiley.com/journal/10.1111/(ISSN)1365-2125. doi:10.1111/bcp.14128.

Tong, E.Y., Yip, G., 2024. Partnered pharmacist medication charting and prescribing in Australian hospitals. Aust. Prescr. 1839-3942. 47 (2), 48–51. Available from: https://australianprescriber.tg.org.au/assets/AP/pdf/p48-Tong-Yip.pdf. doi:10.18773/austprescr.2024.011.
Vandenbroucke, J.P., 1999. Case reports in an evidence-based world. J. R. Soc. Med. 92 (4), 159–163.
Wang, S., Zhang, R., Wang, S., Guo, Q., Yin, D., Song, Y., She, X., Wang, X., Duan, J., 2024. Osteonecrosis of the jaw in patients with clear cell renal cell carcinoma treated with targeted agents: a case series and large-scale pharmacovigilance analysis. Front. Pharmacol. 1663-9812. 15. doi:10.3389/fphar.2024.1309148.
WHO Consultative Group on the Role of the Pharmacist in the Health Care System. 1997. The role of the pharmacist in the health care system: preparing the future pharmacist: curricular development: report of a third WHO Consultative Group on the Role of the Pharmacist, Vancouver, Canada, 27-29 August 1997. World Health Organization. World Health Organization. https://iris.who.int/handle/10665/63817.
World Health Organization. 2026. Medication without harm. https://www.who.int/initiatives/medication-without-harm.
Yin, R.K., 2018. Case study research and applications : design and methods. Sixth edition (Los Angeles: SAGE).

CHAPTER

11

Using habit science in the design and delivery of a pharmacist-delivered medication adherence intervention

Matthew Witry[a] *and L. Alison Phillips*[b]

[a]Department of Pharmacy Practice and Science, University of Iowa, Iowa City, IA, United States
[b]Department of Psychology, Iowa State University, Ames, IA, United States

CHAPTER OBJECTIVES

- Examine the application of habit science in designing and implementing a pharmacist-delivered habit intervention for medication adherence
- Differentiate habits from reflective mechanisms and other automatic processes for behavior maintenance, both theoretically and practically
- Choose and justify approaches to measuring habits, including self-reported measures of automaticity and behavior tracking
- Report results of an initial pilot test of a pharmacist-led, simple, and scalable intervention for promoting medication adherence through medication-taking habit formation, compared to a standard education approach
- Evaluate the relative utility of patients' beliefs about medicines versus habit strength in predicting self-reported adherence at follow-up among patients new to a medication
- Code habit cues and backup plans were chosen and selected by patients in the pilot test

1 Introduction

The field of health psychology has a well-developed scientific basis for habit science. Scholars in this field have developed several definitions for habit, including the definition offered by Gardner and Lally (2023): Habits are automatic impulses to engage in an action when in the presence of a conditioned (learned) context or situational

Contemporary Research Methods in Pharmacy and Health Services - Volume 2
https://doi.org/10.1016/B978-0-443-44607-8.00024-8

cue for that action. Such automatic cue-response associations are formed through rewarded behavioral repetition in a stable context (Gardner and Lally, 2023). Habits can range from incidental actions, such as following a particular driving route to work from home, to complex health behaviors, such as the impulse to exercise being triggered by one's normal preexercise routine of transitioning from work to home at the end of the workday (Phillips and Mullan, 2023a).

Habits are increasingly being recognized for their role in understanding and improving the maintenance of health behaviors (Verplanken and Orbell, 2022; Wood, 2019). This is particularly important given persistent challenges with long-term health behavior maintenance across a wide range of evidence-based actions related to diet (Shams-White et al., 2023), exercise (Du et al., 2019), medication adherence (Osterberg and Blaschke, 2005) and others. The high level of nonadherence to guideline lifestyle-related health behaviors also has a significant economic burden, as lifestyle factors are estimated to be associated with 90% of the United States' $4.1 trillion in annual healthcare spending (Ramachandran, 2022). Habit science offers an important avenue to support patients and providers as they seek strategies to more reliably engage in behaviors known to improve health and decrease chronic illness.

Nonadherence to medication therapy is an area of particular interest to researchers in pharmacy. Many pharmacy researchers have focused on exploring how attitudes, motivation, and other reflective factors influence medication adherence and use theoretical models based on the influence of medication beliefs and self-efficacy (Unni and Bae, 2022) to explain adherence, design, and test interventions, while focusing less on habits and automatic processes.

This chapter introduces habit science concepts and their application to medication adherence in a pharmacy context. It describes basic concepts of habit science, including current definitions of habit, the habit formation process, habit measurement, and how habit relates to other important concepts like medication beliefs, using an example of a pharmacist-provided habit-based intervention for medication adherence.

1.1 Habit formation process

Habit formation can be conceptualized as a process involving multiple stages. Initially, behavior is goal-directed and requires conscious effort and motivation (Lally and Gardner, 2013). As the behavior is repeated (and repeatedly rewarded) in a consistent context, it becomes more automatic and less dependent on conscious control (Gardner, 2015). Studies suggest habits can become established within 2–5 months, although there is considerable variability among individuals and behaviors (Lally et al., 2010; Singh et al., 2024). Over time, some people may lose interest in maintaining their habit or face new barriers that can interfere with the habit, which presents new challenges that require motivation and revisiting cues and contexts (Kaushal et al., 2025; Wood and Neil, 2016).

Health coaches, physicians, pharmacists, and other providers can help patients identify appropriate cues and craft target behaviors into specific steps. Studies suggest that both relatively simple behaviors (e.g., taking medication) and relatively complex behaviors (e.g., regular exercise) can be maintained through habitual processes (Phillips and Mullan, 2023a). Regardless of complexity, a habit forms through repeating an action in a specific and stable context and experiencing a reward from that action. The stable context or triggering cue may be a consistent part of an existing routine (e.g., forming a habit of flossing after brushing one's teeth or exercising whenever transitioning between specific components of one's daily routine) (Labrecque et al., 2024). For medication adherence, common cues often focus on hygiene factors (e.g., brushing teeth, getting dressed) and meal-focused factors, as these are done regularly (Bolman et al., 2011). Location cues are another option and rely on visual prompts, such as having your medicines visible in a location you regularly visit. Time-based cues generally do not work as well for forming habits because time itself is not an observable cue, unless one relies on a consistent alarm for the habitual action (in which case the alarm is the cue, not the specific time of day).

Only actions that are rewarded will be conditioned or associated with a stable context and form into habits (Wiedemann et al., 2014; Gardner and Lally, 2013; Phillips and Mullan, 2023b, 2023a). This concept dates back to the original behavioral sciences in psychology, where rats were trained to develop habits of running through a particular maze and were rewarded with cheese; if the cheese was never presented or was removed, the habit either never formed or was dishabituated, respectively (Skinner, 1953). More recent research has found that intrinsically rewarded (enjoyable) behaviors will form into stronger habits with repetition in a stable context than behaviors that participants do not enjoy (Phillips et al., 2016a). Reward does not need to be enjoyment, which would be difficult to achieve with swallowing pills. Reward can be a sense of satisfaction for accomplishing a goal, behaving in line with one's identity, or adhering to one's values, among other health and goal-related pursuits (Ryan and Deci, 2000). With repetition in a stable and consistent context, a rewarded behavior can become driven by habit—or an automatic impulse to engage in the behavior upon encountering the conditioned context (Gardner and Lally, 2023).

Studies based on habit science have demonstrated that using behavior change techniques, including context-dependent repetition (habit formation), can lead to improvements in behavioral outcomes through improved and sustained behavioral maintenance. For example, establishing healthy eating habits, regular physical activity, and adherence to medical regimens can be enhanced through habit-based interventions, where a coach engages in action planning with the patient to identify personalized cues for the desired health behavior (Wood and Neil, 2016; Gardner, 2015; Conn and Ruppar, 2017; Fritz et al., 2020).

1.2 Applying habit science to medication adherence in a pharmacy setting

Observational studies have found that patients' reports of habit strength and the consistency of their medication-taking behavior (a measure of habit strength) better predict medication adherence than patients' beliefs about and attitudes toward the medicines, among other reflective factors (Phillips et al., 2013, 2016b). However, these studies have evaluated individuals already taking the medication in question. Evaluating the relative role of habit and beliefs about medicines is important in a sample new to a medication. Furthermore, experimental design, where possible, will help evaluate the efficacy of habit formation strategies. Pharmacists are well-positioned to help patients form habits for taking new medicines, given their established role as medication educators.

2 Methods

To illustrate the design decisions, development, analysis, and interpretation of a habit-based intervention, we will consider a 2025 pilot study by the chapter authors (Witry et al., 2026). The study was designed as a quasiexperimental, two-group controlled trial conducted at a single United States primary care clinic. The intervention was informed by the Extended Common-Sense Model (CSM) and aimed to promote medication adherence through habit formation compared to standard education.

2.1 Theoretical model

The extended CSM (Fig. 11.1) posits assessing both reflective and automatic factors for testing the mechanistic factors influencing the intervention outcomes. This model, from Phillips et al. (2016a), expands Leventhal's original self-regulation framework (Leventhal et al., 1998) by proposing that health behaviors are guided by two pathways: a reflective pathway (conscious attitudes, intentions, and planning) and an automatic pathway (habit formation and cue-driven behavior).

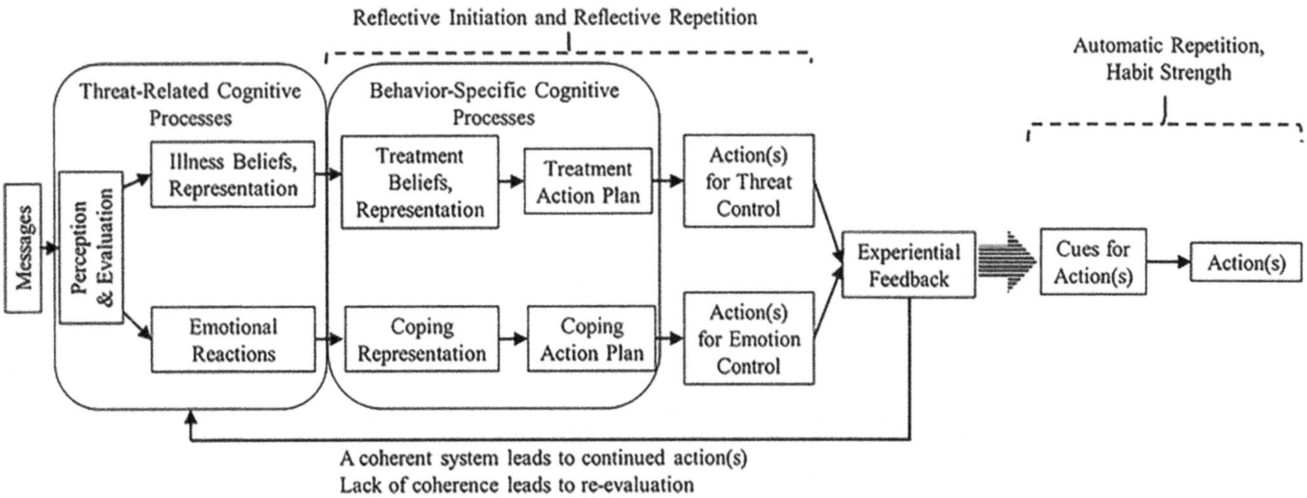

FIG. 11.1 Extended common-sense model of self-regulation. *Data from Phillips, L.A., Cohen, J., Burns, E., Abrams, J., Renninger, S., 2016. Self-management of chronic illness: the role of "habit" versus reflective factors in exercise and medication adherence. Journal of Behavioral Medicine, 39 (6), 1076–1091. https://doi.org/10.1007/s10865-016-9732-z.*

2.2 Study measures

The example study assessed the reflective portion of the Extended CSM by evaluating the patient's beliefs about medicines using the Beliefs about Medicines Questionnaire (Horne et al., 1999), which assessed the perceived necessity of the new medication and concerns about medicines in general. Example items included *"My health, at present, depends on my medicines"* and *"Having to take medicines worries me."* Responses were provided on a 5-point scale ranging from strongly disagree to strongly agree.

For the automatic portion of the model, we measured habit strength using the 4-item self-reported behavioral automaticity index (SRBAI) (Gardner et al., 2012). This is a 4-item subscale of the self-reported habit index (SRHI) (Verplanken and Orbell, 2003). The SRBAI uses a 5-point scale ranging from "Strongly disagree" to "Strongly agree" and asks how automatic or routine the behavior has become (e.g., *"Taking my medicine is something I do automatically"*). Participants were also asked, *"Do you currently have a daily routine for taking your medicines?* and used a 5-point scale—from definitely no, somewhat no, uncertain, somewhat yes, and definitely yes—to respond to this question (Vrijens et al., 2014).

These measures were chosen because the extended CSM posits that adherence is governed by both deliberate beliefs and automatic, habit-driven processes. Including both domains addresses the sequential process posited by the model for understanding behavior adoption and maintenance. Demographics were also collected at baseline to describe the sample.

The 100-day survey included the 5-item Medication Adherence Report Scale (MARS-5), which asks about five different ways a patient could be nonadherent to their therapy, such as altering a dose or forgetting to take their medicines (Fialko et al., 2008). The five response options ranged from "never" to "always." Participants were also asked to self-report how many of the last seven days they missed a dose of their medication (Fig. 11.2).

2.3 Study hypotheses

Several hypotheses guided by the extended CSM were tested in the study. Hypothesis 1 posited that patients receiving the habit-based intervention would develop stronger medication-taking habits and better medication adherence over the study period compared to patients not receiving the habit intervention. This hypothesis was based on the expectation that the habit intervention would encourage the development of an automatic medication-taking habit by facilitating action plans for cue-behavior associations. It was tested by comparing the intervention and control groups' habit strength scores, adherence (MARS-5 outcomes), and reported missed doses after approximately 100 days. Second, the team hypothesized that both reflective factors and habit (automatic) factors would play a role in adherence outcomes, but that habit strength would be a stronger predictor of adherence outcomes, as posited by the extended CSM. A stronger influence of habit (if observed) would support the model's assertion that, over time, habitual automatic processes overtake medication beliefs in maintaining health behaviors.

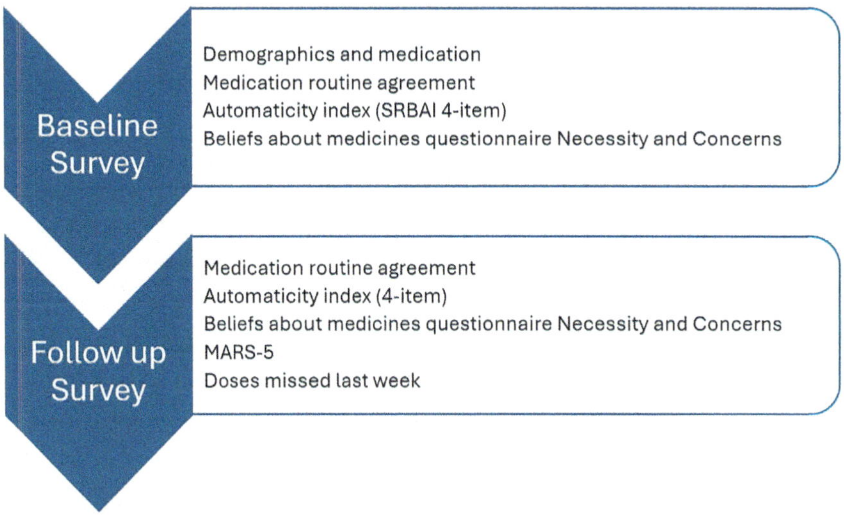

FIG. 11.2 Summary of pre and post survey measures.

2.4 Study design

Sequential, nonrandomized assignment was used, beginning with the control group, which received standard medication counseling, followed by the intervention group, which received counseling in addition to a habit worksheet. The rationale for sequential versus random assignment was to prevent the habit intervention from contaminating the pharmacists' interactions with the control patients. Participants were patients prescribed a new chronic medication, with the goal of having sixteen participants recruited for each group.

2.5 Study intervention: Habit worksheet

The study intervention focused on the patient and pharmacist collaborating to complete a habit worksheet (Fig. 11.3). The worksheet was designed to incorporate several behavior change techniques, including pairing medication-taking behavior with an existing cue (action planning, associative learning), making a commitment (goal-setting), and specifying a back-up plan (coping planning). Each of these behavior change techniques is supported by evidence (Michie et al., 2013).

The habit worksheet includes spaces for the medication name, instructions, cue identification, commitment, and a backup plan (Fig. 11.3).

2.6 Study procedures

Patients new to medication were recruited in two phases. During Phase 1, the pharmacist provided standard education (control). In Phase 2, the pharmacist added a habit-formation component by completing a habit worksheet with the patients. Surveys measuring medication beliefs, habit strength, and adherence were completed at baseline and 100 days later.

Medication-Taking Habit Worksheet

Remembering to take your medication can be tricky. Everyone gets busy and sometimes people forget to take their medication.

Picking a specific time, location, or regular activity ("cue") to pair with taking your medication can help make it a routine. After a while, you may start to notice you are taking your medicine without having to think about it.

My Medication ______________________

My Instructions ______________________

My cue for taking my new medication ______________________

Example Cues

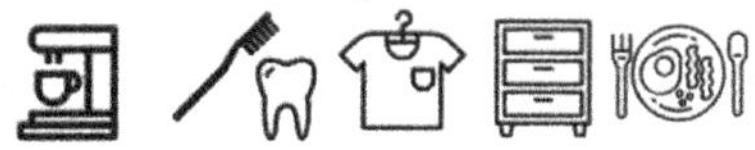

My Commitment ______________________

____

Write out your plan in words to help it stick

My Back-Up Plan ______________________

If you at first have trouble remembering to take your medicines with your chosen cue, what can you do to remind yourself (set an alarm, have another person help remind you, or leave a sticky note next to the cue)?

FIG. 11.3 Habit worksheet. *Data from Witry, M., Hoehns, J., Phillips, L.A., 2026. Pilot of a pharmacist-delivered habit-based intervention to support medication adherence in primary care. Research in Social and Administrative Pharmacy, 22 (1), 147–151. https://doi.org/10.1016/j.sapharm.2025.09.003.*

2.7 Analysis

Paper surveys were entered into Microsoft Excel, cleaned, and imported into SPSS for analysis. Demographic items were analyzed descriptively. Measure reliability was assessed using Cronbach's alpha, and bivariate correlations were calculated for transparency and potential incorporation into future metaanalyses.

To test the hypothesis that the intervention group would report stronger habits and greater adherence than the control condition at approximately 100 days postbaseline, we conducted independent samples t-tests with control versus intervention groups as the grouping factor (independent variable) and used three different outcome variables at follow-up: MARS-5 score, participants' responses on the number of missed doses in the past week, and habit strength for taking their new medicine. A postonly comparison was used instead of a pre–post analysis because the medication was new to the patients and thus they would have no prior experience.

To evaluate the second hypothesis regarding the relative association of patients' beliefs about medicines and their habit strength for taking medicines with reported adherence, we conducted a multivariate linear regression using stepwise entry of variables. Variables included necessity beliefs, concern beliefs, and reported habit strength for taking the new medicine at follow-up. The two outcomes were self-reported adherence, assessed using MARS-5, and, separately, the single-item measure of missed doses in the previous week.

Lastly, for objective 3, the habit worksheets were analyzed descriptively using conceptualizations of cues and habit formation by Bolman et al. (2011) and Lally et al. (2011) to summarize cue type frequencies and characterize the use of back-up plans. MARS-5 scores and SRBAI scores were described by the three types of cues: meals (e.g., breakfast, coffee), hygiene (e.g., showering, brushing teeth), and location (e.g., nightstand, pillbox).

3 Results

Thirty-three people enrolled in the study, 16 in the control group and 17 in the habit worksheet intervention group (Table 11.1). The two groups had similar demographic characteristics, including a mean age of 59 and similar proportions of men and women. The number of daily doses of the newly prescribed medication was slightly higher in the intervention group. Postresponses were received from 12 control patients (75%) and 16 intervention patients (94%) (Witry et al., 2026).

At baseline, patients reported having a routine for taking their medicines (existing, not the new medicine): the average on this item, which ranged from 1 (definitely no) to 5 (definitely yes), was 4.45 (SD = 1.2) for the control group and 4.73 (SD = 0.55) for the intervention group. Only one participant reported "definitely no" (score = 1) to having a medication-taking routine.

Overall, participants reported relatively high levels of automaticity in taking their medications, which did not differ significantly between groups or across the study period (Table 11.1). The item "I do automatically" had the highest mean score of 4.21 (SD = 0.93), which slightly decreased to 4.00 (SD = 1.31) at follow-up. The statement "I do without having to consciously remember" increased slightly from 3.58 (SD = 1.25) to 3.64 (SD = 1.34) at follow-up. Similarly, "I do without thinking" rose slightly from 3.30 (SD = 1.20) to 3.36 (SD = 1.47). The lowest scores were observed for "I start doing before I realize I'm doing it," which changed little from 2.61 (SD = 1.20) at baseline to 2.67 (SD = 1.21) at follow-up (Witry et al., 2026).

TABLE 11.1 Participant characteristics at baseline.

Variable	Control (n = 16) Mean (SD)	Intervention (n = 17) Mean (SD)	Difference	t	Sig.
Age	57.3 (16.8)	57.7 (16.8)	0.4	−0.07	0.95
Daily medicines	3.3 (1.9)	4.9 (3.3)	1.7	−1.79	0.08
Conditions	3.0 (2.3)	3.6 (1.8)	−0.6	−0.82	0.42
New med daily doses	1.1 (0.34)	1.3 (0.47)	0.17	−1.18	0.25
Women N (%)	7 (44%)	10 (59%)	–	0.85	0.40
Automaticity index	13.8 (3.38)	13.7 (4.62)	0.1	0.07	0.94
Concern beliefs	14.5 (4.03)	13.7 (5.51)	0.8	0.48	0.64
Necessity beliefs	16.1 (4.97)	17.3 (4.58)	−1.23	−0.74	0.46

Data from Witry, M., Hoehns, J., Phillips, L.A., 2026. Pilot of a pharmacist-delivered habit-based intervention to support medication adherence in primary care. Research in Social and Administrative Pharmacy, 22 (1), 147–151. https://doi.org/10.1016/j.sapharm.2025.09.003.

Both groups reported high baseline scores for the five BMQ items related to perceived medication necessity: 16.1 (SD = 5.0) for the control group and 17.3 (SD = 4.6) for the intervention group (Table 11.1). Concern beliefs were also relatively high for both groups: 14.5 (SD = 4.0) and 13.7.5 (SD = 5.0), respectively (Table 11.1). For both groups, scaled responses were significantly correlated at baseline and follow-up (Witry et al., 2026). Scales were found to be reliable, with coefficients >0.8: Automaticity (0.89 pre and 0.87 post), BMQ necessity (0.88 pre and 0.89 post), BMQ concerns (0.82 pre and 0.88 post), and MARS ([post only] 0.85) (Witry et al., 2026). The test of the first hypothesis showed that the intervention group reported lower levels of nonadherence on the MARS-5, but this difference was not statistically significant (Table 11.2). Both groups also reported low frequencies of missed doses in the past week (<1), although the difference was not statistically significant (Witry et al., 2026).

The test of the second hypothesis, regarding the relative association of beliefs and habit with adherence at follow-up (approximately 100 days after baseline), using stepwise linear regression, suggested that greater automaticity scores were the sole significant predictor of lower MARS-5 (lower scores associated with better adherence) at follow-up ($p = 0.017$) (Table 11.3). For the outcome of doses missed in the past week, necessity beliefs were the sole significant predictor ($p = 0.031$) (Table 11.3). Receiving the intervention and other covariates were not statistically significant, although receiving the intervention neared significance for influencing doses missed in the past week ($p = 0.075$) (Table 11.3).

MARS-5 and automaticity index were compared by the type of cue selected in a habit worksheet (Table 11.4). Participants who selected a meal-related cue ($N = 9$) had a mean MARS-5 score of 1.56 (SD = 1.33) and a postintervention automaticity score of 15.50 (SD = 4.75). Those who chose a hygiene-related cue ($N = 3$) reported a slightly better MARS-5 score of 1.00 (SD = 1.00) but a comparable automaticity score of 15.33 (SD = 3.51). In contrast,

TABLE 11.2 Participant self-report at follow-up.

Variable	Intervention ($n = 15$) mean (SD)	Control ($n = 12$) mean (SD)	Difference (intervention-control)	Sig	Effect size estimate	Effect size 95% confidence interval
Automaticity index[a]	14.3 (4.29)	12.7 (4.78)	1.61	0.37	0.324	−0.431–1.138
Concern beliefs[b]	15.0 (4.94)	13.9 (5.14)	1.08	0.58	0.215	−0.548–0.975
Necessity beliefs[c]	17.0 (4.22)	16.3 (5.64)	0.75	0.35	0.153	−0.609–0.912
MARS-5[d]	2.12 (2.18)	2.92 (3.50)	−0.79	0.47	−0.281	−1.03–0.474
Doses missed last week	0.38 (0.62)	0.75 (0.75)	−0.37	0.16	−0.552	−1.31–0.474

[a]*Automaticity index: 0 = low automaticity, 20 = high automaticity.*
[b]*Concern beliefs: 0 = Low concerns, 20 = high concerns.*
[c]*Necessity beliefs: 0 = Low necessity, 20 = high necessity.*
[d]*MARS-5 0 = never misses/modifies doses; 20 = always misses/modifies doses.*
Data from Witry, M., Hoehns, J., Phillips, L.A., 2026. Pilot of a pharmacist-delivered habit-based intervention to support medication adherence in primary care. Research in Social and Administrative Pharmacy, 22 (1), 147–151. https://doi.org/10.1016/j.sapharm.2025.09.003.

TABLE 11.3 Stepwise linear regression for MARS-5 and doses missed last week ($n = 24$).

Dependent variable	MARS-5 Std B	Sig	Dependent variable	Doses missed last week Std B	Sig
Constant		<0.001	**Constant**		0.003
Automaticity index FU	−0.47	0.02	**Necessity FU**	−0.43	0.03
Excluded			**Excluded**		
Age	−0.08	0.66	Age	−0.22	0.24
Gender	0.16	0.38	Gender	−0.25	0.19
Intervention	0.07	0.74	Intervention	−0.34	0.08
Routine at FU	0.28	0.14	Routine at FU	−0.004	0.98
Necessity beliefs at FU	−0.05	0.80	Concerns FU	−0.05	0.79
Concern beliefs at FU	−0.11	0.56	Auto FU	−0.08	0.72

Data from Witry, M., Hoehns, J., Phillips, L.A., 2026. Pilot of a pharmacist-delivered habit-based intervention to support medication adherence in primary care. Research in Social and Administrative Pharmacy, 22 (1), 147–151. https://doi.org/10.1016/j.sapharm.2025.09.003.

TABLE 11.4 Description of MARS-5 and automaticity index scores by habit worksheet cue type.

Cue	MARS-5 Mean (SD)	Automaticity Post Mean (SD)
Meal Cue (*N* = 9)	1.56 (1.33)	15.50 (4.75)
Hygiene cue (*N* = 3)	1.00 (1.00)	15.33 (3.51)
Location cue (*N* = 5)	3.60 (3.13)	13.0 (4.58)

Data from Witry, M., Hoehns, J., Phillips, L.A., 2026. Pilot of a pharmacist-delivered habit-based intervention to support medication adherence in primary care. Research in Social and Administrative Pharmacy, 22(1), 147–151. https://doi.org/10.1016/j.sapharm.2025.09.003.

participants using a location-based cue (*N* = 5) showed the highest MARS-5 score of 3.60 (SD = 3.13), suggesting more missed doses, and a lower automaticity score of 13.00 (SD = 4.58). These results suggest that location cues may be associated with less consistent medication-taking behaviors, while meal and hygiene cues are more conducive to medication-taking automaticity (Witry et al., 2026).

The worksheet had space for participants to specify a backup plan, for which several used a pillbox (*n* = 4), stated a spouse would help remind them (*n* = 2), would use a phone alarm (*n* = 3), keep extra pills in their briefcase in case they missed their usual dose (*n* = 1), or use a sticky note to remind themselves (*n* = 1). Six (35%), however, did not specify a backup plan for their chosen cue (Witry et al., 2026).

4 Discussion

Overall, this study demonstrated that a pharmacist could collaborate with patients to complete a medication-taking habit worksheet that included the selection of cues and affirming commitment to their new regimen. Less established was the role of the patient in selecting a backup plan, which could be related to most patients already having well-established medication-taking routines for the other maintenance medications they take.

Patients in both groups reported high levels of necessity beliefs and lower levels of concern beliefs about medicines, which did not change significantly across the study period. Patient adherence to their newly prescribed medication remained high at the end of the study period, with most patients reporting few, if any, missed doses in the last week and responses to the MARS-5 suggesting that most patients reported never or rarely engaging in behaviors like forgetting medications or taking less of a medication than prescribed.

While the intervention was not significant, potentially due to the participants having well-developed routines at baseline, we did observe some confirmation in the hypothesized direction that both habit (automaticity) and necessity beliefs about medicine were positively associated with self-reported medication-taking behaviors, as measured by the MARS-5 and doses missed in the past week, which provides some additional validity for the salience of the study procedures. These exploratory findings are consistent with the propositions of the extended CSM theoretical model (Phillips et al., 2016b).

The present study used the 4-item automaticity index. This measure is commonly used for studies of habit formation, including those related to diet and exercise. However, it is less frequently used to measure habits related to medication-taking. From an examination of the response frequencies of the individual items, participants reported lower levels of agreement as they progressed through the 4 items, with *"I do automatically"* consistently rated higher than *"I start doing before I realize I'm doing it"*. This difference in automaticity could be desirable for someone's medication-taking practices, as it may be safer for a medication user to engage more deliberately in the behavior of medication-taking once they have started the process. The lower scores on items like *"I do without thinking* and *I start doing before I realize I'm doing it"* may reflect a patient's desire to be careful and deliberate when taking their medicines, rather than engaging in an automatic process, given the potential safety concerns associated with taking medications. Future research could examine whether the 4-items of the automaticity index are ideal for assessing medication-taking habits or if other items or modifications to the existing items may be warranted. Such modifications could better reflect the idea that, while someone may respond to an automatic urge to begin the medication-taking process, the actual act of taking medications may involve deliberate and careful execution rather than *being performed without thinking.*

The study findings suggest that meal and hygiene cues could be more potent facilitators of adherence and habit automaticity than the use of location or the visibility of a medication bottle or pillbox. This warrants further exploration, as little research has examined how different cues influence habit strength (Keller et al., 2021).

The present study had several implementation challenges. While the study was conducted in a primary care clinic with experience recruiting patients for studies, the process of having the patient consult with the pharmacist following a new prescription was challenging to coordinate consistently. In some instances, the patient was consulted after the new prescription encounter over the telephone, which may not have been the most ideal process for collaborative engagement with the habit worksheet. Settings like community pharmacies or pharmacist encounters for medication reviews may be more suitable for discussions of medication-taking habit formation.

Further, most participants recruited for this study had already formed medication-taking routines and reported relatively strong automaticity associated with their medication-taking behaviors. Given this ceiling effect, there was little room for improvement to be demonstrated by using the habit worksheet. Another potential reason for the null effect was that more control patients than intervention patients did not complete the follow-up survey. It is unknown if these patients were potentially less adherent and had less developed medication-taking habits.

4.1 Limitations

This study has several limitations. First, the study used a nonrandomized design, which has the potential for selection bias. The rationale for having control patients recruited first, followed by patients engaging with the habit worksheet, was to avoid the habit intervention being inadvertently applied to control patients. This study is also limited by its generalizability. While there was variation in age and gender, most of the participants were white and had well-developed medication-taking routines. Patients with other demographic characteristics could have different experiences with the habit intervention, and people of other backgrounds may experience the habit intervention differently. This study is also limited by reliance on self-reported data for adherence measures. Using other methods to record doses or prescription refills could provide additional information about medication-taking behaviors. Additionally, the scales asked about medication beliefs and behaviors in general, which could have reduced specificity to the newly prescribed medication, potentially contributing to a misalignment in the unit of analysis (regimen versus specific medication). Lastly, given the small sample, stepwise regression was used, and no adjustments were made for multiple tests. Hence, findings should be considered exploratory.

4.2 Future research

Next steps for this effort should include optimizing the design of the medication-taking habit tool through a codesign process involving both medication users and pharmacists. Such an approach may enhance the usability, acceptability, and relevance of the tool. Future studies should also prioritize patient subgroups most likely to benefit from habit-based interventions, such as patients with documented nonadherence. This could include patients without an established medication-taking routine, patients with complex regimens, and patients experiencing frequent disruptions to their routine. Targeted implementation in these populations could increase the salience of habit-based interventions for medication adherence.

Future research using habit science in pharmacy could also explore the use of habit-based interventions in different settings, with diverse populations, and for other health behaviors, expanding beyond medications to encompass the broader role of pharmacists in supporting healthy habits related to diet, exercise, and behaviors involved in chronic disease management, such as testing blood glucose, checking blood pressure, or creating substitute habits for smoking cessation. It is also important to investigate the long-term effectiveness of these interventions and how and why people may lose their habits and need to redevelop them. Another avenue is to investigate how pharmacists can integrate habit science into routine encounters.

5 Conclusions

Researchers in pharmacy have a long history of working to understand and improve behavior maintenance in areas such as medication adherence. Incorporating habit science provides pharmacy researchers with a new avenue for developing and conceptualizing behavior change interventions. By focusing on how health behaviors become automatic through repeated performance, pharmacists potentially have a new target for their health promotion efforts. The methods and measures reviewed in this chapter, including the automaticity scales and suggested readings on assessing habit measurement, offer tools for researching these mechanisms in medication-taking and other health behaviors.

The pilot pharmacist-delivered habit intervention illustrates how habit principles can be operationalized in pharmacy practice for a health behavior of primary concern to pharmacists—medication adherence. Patients collaborating with a pharmacist were able to identify cues, create action plans, and articulate backup strategies, demonstrating the feasibility of integrating habit-formation techniques into clinical encounters. Although the sample's preexisting routines limited the ability to detect strong intervention effects, the study affirmed the value of assessing both reflective and automatic pathways, as habit strength and necessity beliefs each showed associations with adherence outcomes.

Together, the conceptual foundations, measurement strategies, and example pharmacy intervention presented in this chapter demonstrate how habit science can facilitate mechanistic understanding and intervention design in pharmacy research. The principles described and discussed in this chapter provide researchers with an initial exposure to habit-based approaches, how pharmacists can support cue-driven routines during medication initiation, and how automatic and reflective processes jointly shape sustained health behavior. Habit science offers a promising, mechanism-focused approach for advancing health behavior-focused research in pharmacy and across the health system.

6 Application exercise

6.1 Designing and evaluating a pharmacist-provided habit-based intervention for home blood pressure monitoring

Home blood pressure monitoring is a recommended self-management behavior for hypertension, especially treatment-resistant hypertension, yet adherence is often low. As a pharmacy researcher, you are tasked with designing, developing, and evaluating a pharmacist-delivered habit-based intervention that increases the consistency of daily home blood pressure monitoring. Propose an intervention based on principles of habit science that is feasible for pharmacists to implement, and propose an evaluation plan for the intervention.

1. What theories and behavior change techniques might you consider for guiding the study?
2. What is the primary behavioral target?
3. What protocol elements and consultation components would you implement to help the patient and pharmacist collaborate to consistently measure and report home BP measurements?
4. How might the intervention support patients who initially struggle to test and report their measurements?
5. What is the role of reflective factors in the intervention, and how can these be measured?
6. What behavioral measures could you use, and what are the benefits and downsides of each?
7. How will you measure habit strength?
8. How will you recruit patients who are most likely to benefit from a habit-based intervention?
9. What modifications might be needed for diverse populations?
10. What advantages and limitations might a habit-based intervention design offer compared to an intervention based primarily on education and motivation?

PearlNeurobiological basis for Habit

The neurobiological mechanism for habit formation has been proposed. Studies suggest that the basal ganglia, a group of nuclei associated with procedural learning and habit formation, play a crucial role in this process (Seger and Spiering, 2011). The interaction between the basal ganglia and the dopaminergic systems facilitates the transition from goal-directed actions to habitual behaviors through cues, context, and reward repetition. These brain mechanisms incorporate various regions of the brain, linking the visual, motor, and reward systems. Repetition strengthens these connections, which is how we can perform habitual behaviors like brushing our teeth, tying our shoes, or buckling our seat belts on what feels like autopilot, with our bodies knowing what to do without conscious effort. These nonconscious processes are reflected in how we define and measure habits.

PearlHabit Science and Behavioral Medicine

Habit science connects to two influential movements in the field of behavioral medicine and health psychology: 1) proposing and testing the mechanisms underlying behavior change (Nielsen et al., 2018) and 2) the taxonomy of behavior change techniques (Michie et al., 2013).

The mechanistic movement in behavioral medicine emphasizes identifying and testing the underlying processes that drive changes in health behaviors (Nielsen et al., 2018). This represents a shift from simply testing and reporting which interventions work better than a control condition. Understanding the proposed mechanisms addresses the black box problem of not knowing why some interventions work and others do not by attempting to isolate the specific psychological, social, and neurobiological mechanisms. Habit science has adopted this framework, utilizing measures of automaticity and other tools for assessing how repeated behaviors within consistent contexts shift behavior from goal-directed actions to automatic, cue-driven routines.

Habit science also draws from the taxonomy of behavior change techniques to inform intervention design and evaluation (Michie et al., 2013). This taxonomy provides a structured framework for identifying, categorizing, and implementing the various strategies that can facilitate the formation of new habits and the modification of existing ones. By integrating behavior change techniques—such as cue identification, context-dependent repetition, and action planning—into habit-based interventions, researchers and practitioners are better equipped to understand not only whether an intervention works but also why and how it works. This approach supports a more comprehensive understanding of the connection between automatic and reflective processes in health behavior maintenance, furthering the development of interventions grounded in evidence-based components.

PearlOptions for Measuring Habit Strength

While the SRHI and SRBAI are popular for measuring habit, there are other options (Rebar et al., 2018). Another self-reported measure is to ask, "How often did you pair medication with a chosen cue?" (1 = never, 5 = always) or simply to ask, "How many days did you take your medication last week?" (0–7 days). Habit strength can also be assessed using behavioral measures like MEMS Caps, which infer habit strength from time-of-day consistency (Phillips and More, 2022; Vrijens et al., 2014) and Ecological Momentary Assessment, which captures behavior in real-time via mobile phone prompts (Rebar et al., 2018). Lastly, implicit measures involving reaction time tasks could be used to test the ease of cognitive associations between the cue, context, and behavior (Rebar et al., 2018).

7 Questions for further discussion

- How do habit-based interventions differ from traditional behavior change strategies in promoting medication adherence?
- What are the key mechanisms through which habits influence long-term health behaviors?
- In what ways can healthcare providers integrate habit-formation components into existing practices?
- What are the potential challenges and benefits of habit-based interventions in various pharmacy settings?
- How do we best target habit-based interventions?
- How can habit-based interventions work alongside other patient-centered counseling techniques, such as the Indian Health Method and Motivational Interviewing?
- How can pharmacists expand their roles to support habit formation related to diet, exercise, and chronic disease management?
- What environmental cues and patient commitments are most effective in establishing and maintaining medication habits?

References

Bolman, C., Arwert, T.G., Völlink, T., 2011. Adherence to prophylactic asthma medication: habit strength and cognitions. Heart Lung 40 (1), 63–75. doi:10.1016/j.hrtlng.2010.02.003.

Conn, V.S., Ruppar, T.M., 2017. Medication adherence outcomes of 771 intervention trials: systematic review and meta-analysis. Prev. Med. 99, 269–276. doi:10.1016/j.ypmed.2017.03.008.

Du, Y., Liu, B., Sun, Y., Snetselaar, L.G., Wallace, R.B., 2019. Wei Bao, Trends in Adherence to the Physical Activity Guidelines for Americans for Aerobic Activity and Time Spent on Sedentary Behavior among US Adults, 2007 to 2016. JAMA Netw. Open 2 (7). doi:10.1001/jamanetworkopen.2019.7597.

Fialko, L., Garety, P.A., Kuipers, E., Dunn, G., Bebbington, P.E., Fowler, D., Freeman, D., 2008. A large-scale validation study of the Medication Adherence Rating Scale (Mars). Schizophr. Res. 100 (1-3), 53–59. doi:10.1016/j.schres.2007.10.029.

Fritz, H., Yi-Ling, H., Gahman, K., Almacen, C., Ottolini, J., 2020. Intervention to Modify Habits: a Scoping Review. OTJR Occupation, Participation and Health 40 (2), 99–112. doi:10.1177/1539449219876877.

Gardner, B., 2015. A review and analysis of the use of 'habit' in understanding, predicting and influencing health-related behaviour. Health Psychol. Rev. 9 (3), 277–295. doi:10.1080/17437199.2013.876238.

Gardner, B., Abraham, C., Lally, P., de Bruijn, G.-J., 2012. Towards parsimony in habit measurement: testing the convergent and predictive validity of an automaticity subscale of the Self-Report Habit Index. Int. J. Behav. Nutr. Phys. Act. 9. 10.1186/1479-5868-9-102

Gardner, B., Lally, P., 2013. Does intrinsic motivation strengthen physical activity habit? Modeling relationships between self-determination, past behaviour, and habit strength. J. Behav. Med. 36 (5), 488–497. doi:10.1007/s10865-012-9442-0.

Gardner, B., Lally, P., 2023. Habit and habitual behaviour. Health Psychol. Rev. 17 (3), 490–496. doi:10.1080/17437199.2022.2105249.

Horne, R., Weinman, J., Hankins, M., 1999. The beliefs about medicines questionnaire: the development and evaluation of a new method for assessing the cognitive representation of medication. Psychol. Health 14 (1), 1–24. doi:10.1080/08870449908407311.

Kaushal, N., Nemati, D., Jekauc, D., Luszczynska, A., Hagger, M.S., 2025. Maintaining habitual physical activity by overcoming disruptive competing actions: mechanisms and interventions. J. Behav. Med. 48 (1), 90–98. doi:10.1007/s10865-024-00541-y.

Keller, J., Kwasnicka, D., Klaiber, P., Sichert, L., Lally, P., Fleig, L., 2021. Habit formation following routine-based versus time-based cue planning: a randomized controlled trial. Br. J. Health Psychol. 26 (3), 807–824. doi:10.1111/bjhp.12504.

Labrecque, J.S., Lee, K.M., Wood, W., 2024. Measuring context–response associations that drive habits. J. Exp. Anal. Behav. 121 (1), 62–73. doi:10.1002/jeab.893.

Lally, P., Gardner, B., 2013. Promoting habit formation. Health Psychol. Rev. 7 (SUPPL1). doi:10.1080/17437199.2011.603640.

Lally, P., Van Jaarsveld, C.H.M., Potts, H.W.W., Wardle, J., 2010. How are habits formed: modelling habit formation in the real world. Eur. J. Soc. Psychol. 40 (6), 998–1009. doi:10.1002/ejsp.674.

Lally, P., Wardle, J., Gardner, B., 2011. Experiences of habit formation: a qualitative study. Psychology, Health and Medicine 16 (4), 484–489. doi:10.1080/13548506.2011.555774.

Leventhal, H., Leventhal, E.A., Contrada, R.J., 1998. Self-regulation, health, and behavior: a perceptual-cognitive approach. Psychol. Health 13 (4), 717–733. doi:10.1080/08870449808407425.

Michie, S., Richardson, M., Johnston, M., Abraham, C., Francis, J., Hardeman, W., Eccles, M.P., Cane, J., Wood, C.E., 2013. The behavior change technique taxonomy (v1) of 93 hierarchically clustered techniques: building an international consensus for the reporting of behavior change interventions. Ann. Behav. Med. 46 (1), 81–95. doi:10.1007/s12160-013-9486-6.

Nielsen, L., Riddle, M., King, J.W., Aklin, W.M., Chen, W., Clark, D., Collier, E., Czajkowski, S., Esposito, L., Ferrer, R., Green, P., Hunter, C., Kehl, K., King, R., Onken, L., Simmons, J.M., Stoeckel, L., Stoney, C., Tully, L., Weber, W., 2018. The NIH Science of Behavior Change Program: transforming the science through a focus on mechanisms of change. Behav. Res. Ther. 101, 3–11. doi:10.1016/j.brat.2017.07.002.

Osterberg, L., Blaschke, T., 2005. Adherence to medication. N. Engl. J. Med. 353 (5), 487–497. doi:10.1056/NEJMra050100.

Phillips, L.A., Chamberland, P.-É., Hekler, E.B., Abrams, J., Eisenberg, M.H., 2016a. Intrinsic rewards predict exercise via behavioral intentions for initiators but via habit strength for maintainers. Sport, Exercise, and Performance Psychology 5 (4), 352–364. doi:10.1037/spy0000071.

Phillips, L.A., Cohen, J., Burns, E., Abrams, J., Renninger, S., 2016b. Self-management of chronic illness: the role of 'habit' versus reflective factors in exercise and medication adherence. J. Behav. Med. 39 (6), 1076–1091. doi:10.1007/s10865-016-9732-z.

Phillips, L.A., Leventhal, H., Leventhal, E.A., 2013. Assessing theoretical predictors of long-term medication adherence: patients' treatment-related beliefs, experiential feedback and habit development. Psychol. Health 28 (10), 1135–1151. doi:10.1080/08870446.2013.793798.

Phillips, L.A., More, K.R., 2022. Evaluating behavior change factors over time for a simple vs. complex health behavior. Front. Psychol. 13. 10.3389/fpsyg.2022.962150

Phillips, L.A., Mullan, B.A., 2023a. Practical parsimony and complexity in conceptualising habit. Health Psychol. Rev. 17 (3), 497–504. doi:10.10 80/17437199.2022.2154242.

Phillips, L.A., Mullan, B.A., 2023b. Ramifications of behavioural complexity for habit conceptualisation, promotion, and measurement. Health Psychol. Rev. 17 (3), 402–415. doi:10.1080/17437199.2022.2060849.

Ramachandran, R., 2022. Evidence and opportunity costs of lifestyle interventions in clinical medicine. BMJ Med. 1 (1). doi:10.1136/bmjmed-2022-000336.

Rebar, A.L., Gardner, B., Rhodes, R.E., Verplanken, B., 2018. The Measurement of Habit the Psychology of Habit: Theory, Mechanisms, Change, and Contexts. Springer, Springer, pp. 31–49. doi:10.1007/978-3-319-97529-0_3.

Ryan, R.M., Deci, E.L., 2000. Self-determination theory and the facilitation of intrinsic motivation, social development, and well-being. Am. Psychol. 55 (1), 68–78. doi:10.1037//0003-066X.55.1.68.

Seger, C.A., Spiering, B.J., 2011. A Critical Review of Habit Learning and the Basal Ganglia. Front. Syst. Neurosci. 5, p. 66. doi:10.3389/fnsys.2011.00066.

Shams-White, M.M., Pannucci, T.E., Lerman, J.L., Herrick, K.A., Zimmer, M., Mathieu, K.M., Stoody, E.E., Reedy, J., 2023. Healthy Eating Index-2020: review and Update Process to Reflect the Dietary Guidelines for Americans, 2020-2025. J. Acad. Nutr. Diet. 123 (9), 1280–1288. doi:10.1016/j.jand.2023.05.015.

Singh, B., Murphy, A., Maher, C., Smith, A.E., 2024. Time to Form a Habit: a Systematic Review and Meta-Analysis of Health Behaviour Habit Formation and Its Determinants. Healthcare (Basel) 12 (23). doi:10.3390/healthcare12232488.

Skinner, B.F., 1953. Science and Human Behavior, Macmillan, Macmillan.

Unni, E., Bae, S., 2022. Exploring a New Theoretical Model to Explain the Behavior of Medication Adherence. Pharmacy(MDPI). 10 (2), 1–10. Available from https://www.mdpi.com/2226-4787/10/2/43.

Verplanken, B., Orbell, S., 2003. Reflections on Past Behavior: a Self-Report Index of Habit Strength. J. Appl. Soc. Psychol. 33 (6), 1313–1330. doi:10.1111/j.1559-1816.2003.tb01951.x.

Verplanken, B., Orbell, S., 2022. Attitudes, Habits, and Behavior Change. Annual Reviews Inc., United Kingdom Annual Review of Psychology. 15452085. 73, 327–352. Available from http://www.annualreviews.org/journal/psych. doi:10.1146/annurev-psych-020821-011744.

Vrijens, B., Urquhart, J., White, D., 2014. Electronically monitored dosing histories can be used to develop a medication-taking habit and manage patient adherence. Expert Rev. Clin. Pharmacol. 7 (5), 633–644. doi:10.1586/17512433.2014.940896.

Wiedemann, A.U., Gardner, B., Knoll, N., Burkert, S., 2014. Intrinsic rewards, fruit and vegetable consumption, and habit strength: a three-wave study testing the associative-cybernetic model. Appl. Psychol. Health Well Being 6 (1), 119–134. doi:10.1111/aphw.12020.

Witry, M., Hoehns, J., Phillips, L.A., 2026. Pilot of a pharmacist-delivered habit-based intervention to support medication adherence in primary care. Res. Soc. Adm. Pharm. 22 (1), 147–151. doi:10.1016/j.sapharm.2025.09.003.

Wood, W., 2019. Good Habits, Bad Habits: How to Make Positive Changes that Stick. Macmillan; Farrar, Straus and Giroux, New York.

Wood, W., Neil, D., 2016. Healthy through habit: interventions for initiating & maintaining health behavior change. Behav. Sci. Policy 2 (1), 71–83. Available from https://journals.sagepub.com/doi/abs/10.1177/237946151600200109. doi:10.1177/237946151600200109.

CHAPTER

12

Complexity in pharmacy practice: Methodological insights from a realist evaluation of community pharmacy development in Aotearoa New Zealand

Tara N. Officer[a], *Nora Parore*[b], *Janet McDonald*[b], *Kirsten Smiler*[b], *Lynne Russell*[b], *and Jacqueline Cumming*[b]

[a]Te Puna Hauora - School of Health, Te Herenga Waka - Victoria University of Wellington, Wellington, New Zealand

[b]Te Hikuwai Rangahau Hauora - Health Services Research Centre, Te Herenga Waka - Victoria University of Wellington, Wellington, New Zealand

CHAPTER OBJECTIVES

This chapter introduces realist evaluation principles and suggests practical applications for pharmacy research, drawing on our realist evaluation of the development of community pharmacist roles and services in Aotearoa New Zealand (Aotearoa). The chapter will:

- Outline key realist evaluation features
- Describe how program theories can be developed and refined in relation to complex, system-embedded workforce change
- Show the potential for realist evaluation to inform role development, service delivery, and health workforce planning
- Demonstrate how realist evaluation approaches can contribute to equity-focused research
- Reflect on practical lessons and challenges from conducting realist evaluations in real-world settings

Contemporary Research Methods in Pharmacy and Health Services - Volume 2
https://doi.org/10.1016/B978-0-443-44607-8.00016-9

1 Introduction

The complex nature of health systems, characterized by the interplay between clinicians and patients, organizations, and policy directions, necessitates theory-driven, context-sensitive research approaches. Realist evaluation is one such approach (Pawson, 2013; Pawson and Tilley, 1997). Rather than merely asking whether programs designed to bring about change in a given setting "work", realist evaluation explores how and why particular outcomes occur, for whom, and under what circumstances (Pawson et al., 2004). In this way, realist evaluations can be described as opening a "black box" and moving beyond examining a particular outcome to instead analyzing the internal workings of a program. This is pertinent when considering large-scale programs, such as health workforce change, where new roles intersect with entrenched policy and practice arrangements (such as professional boundaries, service models, and funding). For pharmacy, this complexity might be characterized in part by the multidisciplinary interface, policy constraints, and various workforce models in which pharmacy operates. There is significant complexity in the interplay between the different elements of these arrangements. A realist evaluation approach offers a way to tease out such elements and understand how they influence successful change.

This chapter reports on research we conducted on the development of community pharmacists' roles and extended services in Aotearoa (Morris et al., 2024) to provide tangible lessons about conducting realist evaluations in challenging real-world circumstances. The overarching research questions we sought to answer were:

1. What changes were expected in the delivery of community pharmacy services in Aotearoa over the next five years? How were these changes expected to influence health and health system outcomes?
2. How were current community pharmacy strategies being implemented nationally, at the district level, and locally? What initiatives were community pharmacists involved in to extend the range of services they deliver? How were pharmacists, consumers, and other primary health care practitioners responding? How were different contexts influencing the development of community pharmacy services in Aotearoa?
3. Which initiatives and mechanisms worked well with respect to the development of community pharmacy services, and in which contexts was success occurring? In which contexts were key initiatives and mechanisms not working as well, and what were the barriers to progress?

In this chapter, we outline the foundations underpinning realist evaluation and its use in pharmacy practice research. We begin by offering brief introductions to pharmacy practice and health research in Aotearoa, including how Te Tiriti o Waitangi, the founding document of Aotearoa, shapes these. We then describe the key features of realist evaluation methodology and outline how we designed our realist evaluation research and our choice of research methods. Next, we discuss the implications of realist evaluation approaches for equity, policy, practice, and future research. We conclude by offering reflections for emerging realist researchers and highlighting the strengths and limitations of realist evaluation approaches.

1.1 The pharmacy scene in Aotearoa

Pharmacy practice is transforming, driven by increased health service demand, workforce pressures, and policy shifts toward multidisciplinary care and patient-centered outcomes (Ministry of Health, 2016a; Royal Pharmaceutical Society and The King's Fund, 2022). Responses to these pressures differ globally. In Aotearoa, changes reflect broader efforts to address health inequities and enhance service accessibility, particularly in primary health care (Ministry of Health, 2016a). Against this backdrop, pharmacists operate in an increasing range of roles, including prescribing, extended service delivery, and greater medicines optimization (Mossialos et al., 2015). In community pharmacy, pharmacists have begun delivering extended services, such as point-of-care testing, long-term condition management, and specialized medicine supply. However, prevailing practice models remain anchored in pharmacy services continuing to manage medicine supply (Smith et al., 2018), even as funding and professional drivers emphasize medicines optimization, adherence, and deprescribing.

Role development does not occur in isolation; it is shaped by the complex interplay of policy and practice. In Aotearoa, the Ministry of Health's *Pharmacy Action Plan 2016 to 2020* envisioned that "pharmacist services, as an integrated component of a people-powered, collaborative model of care, will be delivered in innovative ways, across a broad range of settings, so that everyone has equitable access to medicines and health care services" (Ministry of Health, 2016a, p. 1). In July 2012, a new Community Pharmacy Services Agreement (CPSA; now the Integrated Community Pharmacy Services Agreement, or ICPSA) changed the government funding model for community pharmacy. This shifted funding from a fee-per-item-dispensed model to a mixed model that included service fees for people registered with a pharmacy to receive Long Term Conditions and other specified services (Health New Zealand–Te Whatu Ora, 2025; Smith et al., 2018). The new model aimed to improve the use of pharmacists' skills, be more person-focused, and limit dispensing costs (Smith et al., 2018). Under the CPSA/ICPSA, services offered by pharmacists have increased (Smith et al., 2018). Some community pharmacy services are nationally available (such as dispensing and professional advisory services), some are locally commissioned[1], and others are delivered under a user-pays model (Health New Zealand–Te Whatu Ora, 2025).

Although community pharmacy services and roles have grown in Aotearoa, there has been limited research on how new extended services are implemented, what successful outcomes look like, and the barriers to their success. Understanding what works, and how, is vital to inform policy and practice decision-making regarding the ongoing development of effective, accessible, and acceptable pharmacy services in Aotearoa. While comparable insights may exist in other countries, country-specific research is essential given differences in how health systems are funded and organized and differences in population demographics and health needs. In our case, this extends to the role of Te Tiriti o Waitangi in guiding health system policy and practice.

1.2 Te Tiriti o Waitangi and Indigenous rights

Te Tiriti o Waitangi (Te Tiriti) is the founding document of Aotearoa, signed in 1840 between representatives of Māori (the Indigenous peoples) and the British Crown (Manatū Taonga | Ministry for Culture and Heritage, n.d.). Te Tiriti confers rights and obligations between the signing partners and, importantly, affirms the rights of Māori to self-determination, guarantees the protection of taonga (that which is sacred and treasured), including hauora (health, vitality, and wellbeing), and enshrines a mutual commitment to notions of equity and equality (Waitangi Tribunal, 2019; Te Heuheu Tukino and Orange, 2017).

Imperial and colonial agendas exercised since 1840, alongside enduring political, economic, and institutional structures, have entrenched a stratified society where there is unequal wealth and resource distribution, which has had deleterious impacts on Māori (Reid et al., 2019). In 1975, a permanent commission of inquiry, the Waitangi Tribunal, was established so Māori could bring forward claims of Crown actions and omissions (enacted by successive governments) that are alleged to breach Te Tiriti. One of these claims, the Health Services and Outcomes Inquiry (the WAI 2575 claim), considered by the Tribunal in 2019, exposed over a century of institutional racism within the Crown health system and the system's inability to ensure health equity and equitable health outcomes for Māori (Cram et al., 2019; Sheridan et al., 2024; Waitangi Tribunal, 2019). The Tribunal concluded the Crown breached Te Tiriti and recommended principles be adopted to inform future Crown primary health care policy and practice:

- The guarantee of tino rangatiratanga (provides for sovereignty and Māori self-determination; mana motuhake)
- Commitment to achieving equitable health outcomes for Māori
- Active protection to achieve equitable outcomes
- Options for services (providing and resourcing kaupapa Māori primary health services and ensuring all primary health care services are culturally appropriate)
- The Crown and Māori working in partnership in primary health service governance, provision, and monitoring (Waitangi Tribunal, 2019)

Māori scholars have positioned Te Tiriti as an inaugural human rights statement and commitment (Mikaere, 2007). Te Tiriti affirms existing Māori human rights frameworks, including the rights of Māori as an Indigenous population, alongside a commitment to universal human rights (Erueti, 2017). Te Tiriti has also been used as a structural framework for developing pharmacist-led services, such as medicines reviews for Māori older adults, to ensure interventions are culturally safe and pro-equity (Hikaka et al., 2021). Key international human rights conventions ratified (and supported) by Aotearoa in a post-World War II society strengthen the centrality of Te Tiriti and the human right to health and wellbeing in our society (Jones et al., 2014). Te Tiriti-informed health policy with these imperatives is, thus, a legal, ethical, and moral obligation and provides the political context for all Aotearoa health research (Came et al., 2018). Te Tiriti shapes health care delivery in Aotearoa, including how pharmacy services are practised and the approaches taken in health research, including in our realist evaluation research.

[1] Previously by a District Health Board (DHB), the 20 organizations then responsible for providing or funding health services within their geographical district, since replaced by a national organization, Te Whatu Ora | Health New Zealand following health reforms in July 2022.

1.3 What is realist evaluation?

Realist research commonly takes the form of (1) realist synthesis or realist review (including rapid reviews) in which researchers draw on existing literature to develop explanations of how and why programs/ interventions work and (2) realist evaluation where this explanation develops through a process of empirical inquiry. Realist evaluations, guided by Pawson and Tilley (1997) and reporting standards for realist evaluations (Wong et al., 2016), are grounded in a philosophical positioning that asserts external reality exists independent of individual perceptions, but that this reality is mediated through human understanding and reasoning (Wong et al., 2014). For our community pharmacy research example, the health system, pharmacy policy environment, community pharmacy workplaces, and the structural and relational arrangements underpinning them constitute part of this "real" world. While reality is not directly observable or measurable, it can be understood indirectly—through stakeholder reasoning and responses (Wong et al., 2013). Pharmacists and other health professionals, policy actors, and patients and their families operate in this real world and interpret it through their experiences, backgrounds, and social positioning. Programs become "constituted in complex processes of human understanding and interaction" (Vaessen and Leeuw, 2010, p. 13).

Realism shares with positivism a singular external reality. However, unlike positivism, realism acknowledges contingencies—contextual conditions—governing whether and how particular outcomes emerge (Befani et al., 2007). That is, an intervention, such as a medicines use review service, will not have universal effects; rather, its effects are contingent upon service design, resourcing, and experience within pharmacy settings. These contingencies reflect the social nature of change: outcomes are not produced mechanically but arise through actors' responses to the resources available in given contexts.

While realism recognizes the value of subjective experiences, it differs from constructivist paradigms. Constructivism holds that reality is individually constructed and that multiple, equally valid realities exist. Realism, however, asserts that an external social reality exists—and while we can never know it directly, it influences human behavior; understanding of it can improve over time (Wong et al., 2011, 2012). In applied settings, where programs are complex and context-sensitive, constructivist approaches offer rich descriptive insights but lack explanatory leverage to identify causal relationships between program inputs and outcomes. A purely constructivist evaluation of community pharmacist role development might describe perspectives without accounting for why certain implementation patterns consistently appear across different pharmacies. Instead, realist researchers build cumulative knowledge through testing and refining theories.

Realist evaluation research has a slowly growing base in pharmacy practice as the field seeks to unpack the complexity of modern health service delivery. Outside of our own work, this methodology has been applied to studies on pharmacist-led interventions and role development, pharmacist education, and medicines review/deprescribing programs (for example, Astbury et al., 2024; Kaae et al., 2025; Kerr et al., 2021; Martin and Tannenbaum, 2017; McDermott et al., 2025; Stewart et al., 2017). Realist evaluation encourages engagement with research sharing a family resemblance, i.e., having similar underlying characteristics explaining how they change (Pawson, 2002, 2006). This supports future researchers in deepening methodological rigor through identifying, testing, adapting, and strengthening explanatory accounts. In so doing, evaluations move beyond application to a single program and toward more transferable, context-attuned findings. Other earlier articles on realist research approaches in pharmacy research and policy development highlight its potential for influencing policy and practice outcomes (Luetsch et al., 2020, 2021). The rise in realist evaluations and the opportunity to build on extant theory signal gradual moves in pharmacy practice research toward methodologies that account for complexity and, as described earlier, open the "black box" of evaluation. The explanatory leverage provided by realist evaluation can then inform decisions about the likely impacts of future changes.

1.4 Complexity

Realist evaluation is increasingly used when conducting applied health research, particularly for exploring complex system changes (Wong et al., 2013). When considering whether a realist evaluation approach is appropriate, a first step involves understanding what is meant by a complex system. Complexity can be characterized by multiple interacting components—service and function inflows and outflows, nonlinear relationships, and behaviors not fully predicted from individual health system parts. Changes can be dynamic or adaptive and shaped by the interplay between diverse agents and structures. This contrasts with models describing expected linear inputs and consistent, measurable outputs/outcomes. In pharmacy practice research, complexity arises from the interdependence of factors, including human behavior, institutional settings, cultural norms, and shifting environments, making simplistic evaluation models insufficient for understanding how programs work in practice.

TABLE 12.1 Defining complexity (Pawson, 2013).

VICTORE terms	Definition
Volition	Intentions and motivations of people and how they engage with a program
Implementation	Processes and actions taken to deliver a program
Contexts	Circumstances in which a program is implemented; this can relate to individual and interpersonal characteristics, institutional settings, and infrastructure
Time	Temporal aspects of a program, including program duration and timing, as well as variations in these factors
Outcomes	Results and effects produced by a program and how these are monitored. Outcomes can occur at several time points and stages of a program
Rivalry	Presence of competing programs and their impact on the evaluated program. This may be a direct impact or impact those delivering the program for example, through program buy-in
Emergence	The unforeseen and emergent effects arising during a program

Based on Pawson, R., 2013. The Science of Evaluation: A Realist Manifesto. SAGE Publications Ltd https://doi.org/10.4135/9781473913820.

When conducting realist evaluations, unlike controlled trials, complexity is not an obstacle but a feature to be understood. The VICTORE framework (Pawson, 2013)—standing for Volition, Implementation, Contexts, Time, Outcomes, Rivalry, and Emergence—offers a checklist to characterize complexity. These terms are defined in Table 12.1.

Incorporating the VICTORE checklist into an evaluation will facilitate a deeper understanding of what is complex in a program and how it sits within the real-world, that is, not within a vacuum (Pawson, 2013). In this way, researchers begin to understand what could be researched, grounded in the lived realities of program delivery and uptake.

We began our research by recognizing that the extension of pharmacy services represented a complex policy intervention (Skivington et al., 2021) due to several factors. Firstly, multiple organizations and health professional groups were involved, including the Ministry of Health (national policymaking), the then DHBs (district service planning and commissioning), pharmacists (through professional bodies and as individuals), and other primary health care service providers impacted by any changes (particularly general practice). Secondly, the number of outcomes sought in policy documents (for example, Ministry of Health, 2016b), ranging from individual to population-level health outcomes, to be realized at a local pharmacy level through to system-level changes, presented challenges. Thirdly, the degree of flexibility and tailoring likely to occur at district and local levels meant the "same" initiative could be implemented differently in various places. These factors suggested that strategies and initiatives to extend pharmacy services would be successful depending on the environment into which they were introduced, and a theory-based research approach would be appropriate.

1.5 Generative causation

While complexity highlights the health system's dynamic interdependence, generative causation provides a way to understand how outcomes arise within this complexity. Realist evaluation is grounded in realism, which posits that causation is generative rather than linear. This means that contexts "trigger" underlying causal mechanisms, leading to outcomes. Outcomes, therefore, arise not solely from the intervention but from the interaction between the intervention and context that triggers mechanisms (Jagosh et al., 2012). A realist evaluation researcher, therefore, asks not, "*Did it work?*" but rather, "*What works for whom, in what circumstances, in what respects, and how?*" (Pawson et al., 2004, p. 3).

At its core, realist evaluations recognize that programs, such as community pharmacist role development, do not produce uniform effects. Instead, success (and therefore causation) depends on interactions between the intervention and local conditions, so-called *contexts* (Hewitt et al., 2012). In particular contexts, stakeholders (such as pharmacists, consumers, or health professionals) respond in semipredictable ways, activating *mechanisms* (changes in resources or reasoning) that lead to *outcomes*. Key definitions (Pawson and Tilley, 1997) follow:

- **Context (C)** refers to the conditions or structures (organizational, social, cultural, economic) that influence whether mechanisms are triggered.
- **Mechanism (M)** comprises resources offered in programs and the reasoning or response of actors to those resources.

- **Outcome (O)** is the observable result of the mechanism firing in a particular context.

The concept of generative causation becomes clearer when examining how components work in practice. For example, in our evaluation, extended pharmacist services uptake was not simply a function of availability. Rather, outcomes depended on whether pharmacists viewed services as professionally valuable, whether owners could support necessary training, and whether consumers trusted pharmacists as providers (to give three examples). These mechanisms were triggered—or not—depending on context, such as pharmacists' role expectations shaped by their education, business models, and whether pharmacists had culturally safe relationships with consumers. Realist evaluation enabled us to theorize these complex interdependencies and move beyond descriptive or correlational analysis.

Challenges arise in operationalizing generative causation. These often relate to identifying "what counts as a mechanism", particularly in system-embedded programs, such as in our evaluation, where lines between programs and rivals or usual business blur. Mechanisms are explanatory propositions about human action. For example, a funding model is not a mechanism in itself; it becomes one only when interacting with stakeholders' reasoning—such as a pharmacist's sense of legitimacy, value, or capacity to act. This challenge of identifying mechanisms is compounded when working with multiple stakeholder perspectives, each offering differing interpretations and perspectives. Therefore, to avoid producing superficial circular explanations through misidentified mechanisms, adopt iterative approaches to theory development, use careful triangulation across data sources and multimethods, and remain open to uncertainty as explanatory patterns begin to take shape. See Dalkin and colleagues' (2015) work for a discussion on mechanisms.

The foundation of generative causation rests on identifying and refining context-mechanism-outcome (CMO) configurations, where generative causation is established through chains or logic explaining causality. These configurations are described next.

1.6 Context-mechanism-outcome configurations

Realist evaluation researchers explicitly, iteratively, and cumulatively refine theories with the aim of identifying the generative causality of a program. In our evaluation of extended pharmacist roles in community pharmacy, we developed CMO configurations, the backbone of generative causation, to articulate how particular roles and service developments occurred differently across settings. These configurations function as explanatory tools, clarifying how cascades of mechanisms, triggered within specific contexts, produce varying outcomes (Pawson, 2006, 2013; Pawson and Tilley, 2004). They can also be empirically tested.

Many CMO configurations may arise during the research process. An example of one such configuration might be a mechanism, such as a pharmacist's confidence to deliver a new service, being activated in contexts that demonstrate strong professional support and adequate staffing, leading to service expansion. Importantly, outcomes from one configuration may become the context for another configuration, as illustrated by some of our work laid out in Table 12.2. Recognizing these layered and dynamic interdependencies enhances explanatory depth.

This kind of theorizing is particularly valuable in pharmacy practice research, where programs are implemented within open systems because it allows researchers to account for the situational, relational, and adaptive nature of changes. Such accounts then offer practical relevance for policymakers, health service managers, and frontline pharmacy teams, who may identify levers for change from CMO configurations, facilitating adaptive, scalable changes to programs. In this way, a realist evaluation approach supports the development of practically relevant and transferable evidence.

1.7 What is a program theory?

While context, mechanism, outcomes, and their linked configurations are building blocks for realist research, program theories bring these blocks together into coherent accounts of how and why programs are expected to work. Realist evaluation uses a "theory-testing strategy" (Pawson and Tilley, 1997) to unpack CMO configurations. In practice, this involves identifying and proposing initial program theories, usually drawn from existing literature and key strategy and initiative documents. Theories capture core assumptions explaining how programs work (Coryn et al., 2011; Vaessen and Leeuw, 2010), and they account for the fact that programs occur in nonexperimental "real-world" (complex) conditions (Pawson et al., 2004). These theories—termed middle-range theories at the level of CMO configurations, and program theories at the point of bringing CMO configurations together—offer

TABLE 12.2 Examples of cascading configurations.

Configuration one outcomes cascade into context for ...		→	Configuration two, which has outcomes that cascade into...	→	Configuration three	
Context	**Mechanism**	**Outcome**	**Mechanism**	**Outcome**	**Mechanism**	**Outcome**
Increasing expectations suggest that pharmacists will take on more consumer-facing roles.	Pharmacists' willingness to adopt new roles and change existing work patterns. Use of robotics. Utilization of Pharmacy Accuracy Checking Technician (PACT) role.	Development of more extended, consumer-focused services.	Awareness of availability of services. Accessibility of the pharmacist. Timely and convenient access. Acceptability of services; culturally-competent pharmacists.	Consumers access additional services from community pharmacies and gain early access to health services.	Improved medicines management. Public health activities. Improved health literacy and self-management. (In)equitable access to medicines and community pharmacy health services.	Improved health outcomes. Reduced demand for other primary health care and secondary services. (In)equitable health outcomes.
		Development of an evolving and more consumer-focused role for pharmacists.	Full use of existing pharmacists' skills. Full utilization of the early graduate pharmacy workforce, with the capacity to contribute more. Greater professional satisfaction. Improved health outcomes.	Improved workforce retention. Value-for-money from pharmacists' contribution to health care.		

Modified from Morris, C., McDonald, J., Officer, T.N., Fa'asalele Tanuvasa, A., Smiler, K., Parore, N., Dunn, P., McKinlay, E., Kennedy, J., McBride-Henry, K., Cumming, J., 2024. A realist evaluation of the development of extended pharmacist roles and services in community pharmacies. Research in Social and Administrative Pharmacy, 20 (3), 321–334. https://doi.org/10.1016/j.sapharm.2023.11.006.

explanatory models accounting for outcome variation across different settings, capturing typical patterns and important exceptions (Wong et al., 2012). These theories are tested and refined throughout data collection and analysis to examine how well initial theories explain outcomes achieved across different contexts. Further rounds of data collection and analysis facilitate the testing and refinement of increasingly developed theories. In relation to pharmacist role expansion, such theories help policymakers, educators, and professional bodies understand what supports role development and where adaptations are necessary.

1.8 Identifying a program

Identifying program theories presupposes the ability to clearly delineate a program. Consequently, defining what constitutes the program under study is an essential preliminary step. A program is understood as structured, often circumscribed, activities or intentions/interventions designed to cause change in a given setting. Examples include formal interventions, such as introducing services or policies, or more evolutionary health system practice changes.

From a realist perspective, programs are not neutral packages but theories incarnate (Pawson and Tilley, 2005). Every program carries assumptions about how change is expected to occur. For example, assumptions that national contracting models would lead to consistent service delivery across community pharmacies represent a theory—one that requires testing in relation to real-world contexts and mechanisms. In our evaluation, we found that such assumptions often did not hold. Services were variably implemented depending on local business models, workforce capacity, and community demand. Recognizing these as contingent outcomes rather than implementation failures required a realist lens.

Identifying programs can present challenges when considering the system-embedded nature of pharmacy practice programs with multiple moving parts. These are complex processes that may not be singular interventions but rather more widespread changes in processes. Unlike time-bound interventions or projects with discrete end points, health service innovations—such as new services brought in and then delivered through community pharmacy, or pharmacist role development that becomes part of business as usual—may lack clearly defined start and end points for individual practices (or potentially clearly identifiable outcomes); they may evolve in response to policy, funding, and local needs. In our realist evaluation research, our program was not composed of a single intervention but a collection of services and practice changes introduced incrementally and variably across contexts. Yet, as a program, they represented fundamental changes in expectations around what a pharmacy or pharmacist may do. We consequently faced challenges delineating coherent, bounded program theories at the outset.

In addressing this, we undertook a layered approach involving analyzing policy intentions, service specifications, and professional guidance to surface the formal logic behind extended services. We then examined how commissioners and pharmacies locally interpreted and enacted these intentions. Therefore, rather than imposing rigid definitions, we treated the program as a policy-driven reform trajectory with porous boundaries, shaped by professional discretion, organizational will, and patient expectations. This approach enabled the construction of initial program theories reflective of the contingent, negotiated nature of the program and its embeddedness within wider primary health care reforms.

2 Methods

This section provides an instructive account of how we applied realist evaluation methodology to study pharmacist role and extended service development in Aotearoa. Applying realist methodology to data collection and analysis is not prescriptive but is guided by its explanatory purpose. For example, when conducting a realist-informed literature review, it is important to include literature if it helps to identify theories of the topic under study or to test those theories (Pawson et al., 2004). Literature appraisal in this process, therefore, becomes iterative and purposive, with the aim of populating, strengthening, and refining theories (Pawson et al., 2004); i.e., the test of relevance then becomes whether the literature being reviewed makes a "methodologically credible contribution" (Pawson et al., 2005, p. s1:30).

Our study unfolded iteratively, aligned with five overarching stages:

1. Choosing a research team
2. Establishing advisory support
3. Eliciting initial program theories
4. Collecting data
5. Testing and refining theory

2.1 The research team

Realist evaluation crucially enables the incorporation of diverse knowledge systems; realist evaluation approaches accept researchers' roles in positing theories for testing how programs work (Pawson and Tilley, 2005). Engaging with these knowledge systems alongside traditional academic paradigms strengthens realist research and ensures that findings are relevant, respectful, and impactful.

Our team comprised experienced health services researchers with knowledge of pharmacy and clinical practice, Indigenous methods and methodologies, disability, and Pacific health services research. Although our program was not tightly bounded (an acknowledged limitation), our team was collaborative, and theory-building became grounded in empirical insight and system understanding. Program theory identification, therefore, became an exercise in methodological rigor and epistemic inclusivity—laying foundations for a contextually attuned evaluation (led by experts in pharmacy practice and supported by the wider team) and the possibility of developing more actionable insights.

2.2 Advisory support

Acknowledging the foundational context that Te Tiriti provides to our society, we began this project by forming two partnering advisory groups. The first included experts in policy, service commissioning, pharmacy, medicine, nursing, and consumer advocacy, as well as representatives of priority populations experiencing significant health inequities (such as Pacific communities). The second group, Te Rōpū Kaitiaki, comprised Māori experts in Te Tiriti, rongoā Māori (traditional healing systems), Tikanga Māori (Māori custom), Whānau Ora (family-centered services and systems of support), Whānau Hauā and Whaikaha (disability studies), health services and systems research, pharmacy, public policy, and service delivery.

These groups served two primary functions. Firstly, they functioned as sounding boards for proposed CMO configurations and facilitated the refinement of early theories and critical reflection beyond the research team. Secondly, they helped facilitate the placement of research findings within policy and practice and supported culturally responsive data collection and analysis. Te Rōpū Kaitiaki was especially critical to this process since, during the 2017–2021 period of our project, the Aotearoa public health system underwent significant reform, whereby Te Tiriti was being embedded into legislation, policy, and practice to reflect the principles the Waitangi Tribunal recommended in response to the 2019 WAI 2575 Inquiry. In sum, our engagement with advisory support reflected a research approach shaped by the priorities and experiences of those closest to the system and service being evaluated.

2.3 Eliciting program theories

We began our research by developing initial program theories. These were constructed through the analysis of national policy and strategy documents, including the *Pharmacy Action Plan (2016–2020)* and the CPSA/ICPSA (Health New Zealand–Te Whatu Ora, 2025; Ministry of Health, 2016a). We also drew on published international literature and speeches by New Zealand Ministers of Health to identify assumptions about the expected effects of extended pharmacist roles. Our review of these documents continued throughout the evaluation as successive governments and districts released policies, and media statements about extended community pharmacist roles and service delivery. In this way, our work remained responsive to longer-term changes.

In realist evaluation, initial program theories take the form of plausible explanations. In this research (see Table 12.2), initial theories included, for example:

- Changes to the CPSA in 2012 (C) shifted funding (M) from dispensing toward more extended, consumer-focused services (particularly long-term conditions), driving a shift in services offered through community pharmacies (O).
- To offer more extended, consumer-focused services (O), pharmacists needed to change the way they work to free up more time away from dispensing to spend with their customers (C). This required pharmacists' willingness to work in different ways (M). The use of robotics for dispensing and the support of other pharmacy staff (particularly pharmacy accuracy checking technicians—PACT) may have freed up time for pharmacists' patient-facing roles (M).

Although no definitive final theories could be created through this elicitation process, these propositions served as starting hypotheses, which were interrogated and refined through fieldwork.

2.4 Iterative data collection

Policy and strategy reviews supported the development of our knowledge around intended processes and outcomes. Following our initial review, we adopted a multimethod approach to test and refine program theories. Each data collection method was chosen for its contribution to explaining variation and providing details to create richer program theories. Data collection and analysis processes were iterative; subsequent interviews facilitated testing of why extended services were or were not developing as expected. This enabled further CMO configuration and theory refinement but invariably also meant that ethics approval processes were longer than those for a single-method study. Our multimethod study included:

- Key informant interviews (50 participants): Purposefully sampled policymakers, health professionals, commissioners, and consumer representatives. These interviews helped uncover big-picture expectations and constraints.
- A national survey (612 participants): A survey of pharmacists and interns provided broader data on service provision and related enablers and barriers.
- Pharmacist/intern interviews (41 participants): These interviews explored in depth how pharmacists experienced extended roles, what influenced uptake, and how funding, staffing, interprofessional relationships, and local population needs shaped their practice.
- Case studies (119 participants): We undertook ten in-depth case studies of community pharmacies, selected for their diversity in location, business model, service profile, and population mix. In line with Te Tiriti obligations

and commitments to Indigenous rights and equity, this design intentionally included sites serving significant Māori populations, Pacific peoples, and/or low-income communities. Within each case, we interviewed pharmacy staff (pharmacists including owners/managers, interns, technicians, and retail staff), local primary health care professionals (including members of the Māori health workforce), and service users. This approach enabled the examination of contextual variation and supported the refinement of CMO configurations.

Each data collection round served explanatory and confirmatory purposes—adding depth to existing theories and challenging assumptions. For example, key informant interview analysis contributed questions to our pharmacist and intern pharmacist survey. Regression analyses on the survey data relating to enablers and barriers to offering extended services supported the identification of relevant contexts and mechanisms and enabled the team to begin planning case studies by highlighting potential points of context variation (McDonald et al., 2021). Conducting individual pharmacist/intern interviews and separate case studies meant we could engage with program theories at two levels: individual practice and expectations, and translation into practice within a community pharmacy environment. Such approaches were particularly important due to the unexpected pandemic-related disruptions we experienced during our later data collection efforts. Each successive data collection phase and triangulation of the findings consequently provided depth unavailable in extant literature or through one data collection phase alone.

2.5 Teacher-learner cycles

Teacher-learner cycles are foundational to realist evaluations (Pawson, 1996) and occur during data collection. Rather than treating participants solely as data sources, realist evaluators applying a teacher-learner cycle to data collection identify and engage with participants as co-theorists—individuals with valuable contextual and experiential knowledge to refine or refute emerging theories (Manzano, 2016). In teacher-learner cycles, researchers present tentative theories (acting as the "teacher") and invite participants to critique them (with the researcher taking on a "learner" role). As participants respond, offer insights, and reframe theory, researchers use these perspectives to refine theory.

Our first key informant interviews were based initially on the literature we reviewed. Subsequent interviews tested and refined theories formed during this stage. Our approach to identifying health care professionals and consumers via the pharmacist when undertaking case studies enabled us to seek individuals more likely to contribute to theory development. Similarly, our deliberate decision-making when identifying case study sites ensured diversity by including settings that differed in geography, population profile, and services delivered. This purposive approach allowed us to explore how potential mechanisms operate differently depending on context and to test whether emerging theories held explanatory power across cases. Such testing occurred within individual interviews, within cases, between cases, and in advisory group discussions, where participants with system-level perspectives contributed to theory refinement, particularly in areas where the research team sought more certainty around contested theories. Insights generated through teacher-learner cycles in one case were explored and refined in subsequent cases and during data analysis within our team and advisory groups. Throughout data collection and analysis, the research team, therefore, remained responsive to emerging explanations, supporting theory development with empirical depth and context-sensitivity.

2.6 Theory testing and refinement

Having identified CMO configuration cascades through initial program theory elicitation and after commencing data collection, it became apparent that cascades could be further categorized based on distinct groups who triggered a mechanism. We, therefore, identified intermediate (more observable) outcomes around which to frame CMO configurations:

- Development of extended services: Influenced by policy settings, business models, and professional expectations
- Consumer use of extended community pharmacist services: Shaped by awareness, affordability, cultural safety, and trust in pharmacists
- Integrated, collaborative primary health care services: Dependent on interprofessional relationships, access to shared records, and joint clinical priorities
- Fit-for-purpose community pharmacy workforce: Affected by training pathways, role legitimacy, and alignment of services with pharmacists' aspirations

Data analysis involved iterative theory testing. Notably, aligning with the method neutrality of the methodology, realist evaluators apply no singular analysis approach, with much of the extant literature offering scant information on analysis (Gilmore et al., 2019). The analytical mix and sequence should instead depend on the purpose, data, and stage of theory development, ensuring methods match program complexity rather than a fixed template. We applied retroductive thematic coding (in NVivo) with subsequent attention to CMO logic in the analysis of the coded data. Deductive logic begins with theory, which is then tested with empirical research; inductive logic begins with data and draws out theory from it; retroduction uses both deduction and induction, along with "insights or hunches" to search for the hidden causes that sit behind observed patterns (Greenhalgh et al., 2017, p. 1).

As our research team had mixed familiarity with realist evaluation methodology, a thematically guided initial data analysis approach allowed us to work from our research strengths to begin refining and testing theories. Codes were applied deductively (informed by initial theories) and inductively (based on new insights), with the back-and-forth characteristic of the overall retroductive approach. Analysis focused not on theme prevalence but on explanatory power. Emerging patterns were articulated (both aloud in team meetings and interviews, and in writing) in part through so-called *if-then propositions*. Such propositions express the generative logic of developing CMO configurations (Pawson and Manzano-Santaella, 2012). These propositions provided a structured means of testing and refining our developing theories. This process moved us from surface-level patterns to generative explanations and refined theories. It should be noted, however, that thematic approaches may not by themselves be optimal, with some arguing that realist evaluation researchers often lack detail in their analytical processes (Gilmore et al., 2019) and others highlighting the need for abductive research approaches (to develop inferences from the data) and concerns around how thematic analysis is applied to realist research (Griffiths et al., 2025). For further discussion of realist evaluation analysis approaches, we recommend Rees et al. (2025).

Following analysis refinement, and while we were completing case study data collection, we developed configurational maps to display and refine data. Each configuration was mapped diagrammatically (drawing on the styles of Greenhalgh et al. (2009) and Officer (2018), as shown in the example of Fig. 12.1, distinguishing enabling and constraining contexts, activated or suppressed mechanisms, and outcomes. At the top of the diagram are outcomes that will result (either successfully or suboptimally) through the combination of linked mechanisms and contexts. The central column shows mechanisms through which outcomes are achieved. Enabling contexts were placed on the left, and constraining contexts on the right; enablers trigger, and constraining contexts inhibit, mechanism firing, thus supporting or diminishing the likelihood of a successful outcome (Greenhalgh and Manzano, 2022). As context is so influential, the same context may inevitably have appeared within more than one configurational diagram, firing subtly different mechanisms with quite different outcomes. In addition, each pharmacy case study site would have different combinations of enabling and constraining contexts, which interacted to produce outcomes. This is why nuance, not generalization, is the hallmark of realist explanation.

When considering the program theory underlying Fig. 12.1, we described it as follows:

A fit-for-purpose pharmacy workforce, reflecting the principles of Te Tiriti, will develop through the activation of five mechanisms (by the contexts that enable them): 1. The pharmacy workforce reflects the population it serves, particularly by supporting Māori and Pacific Island students to succeed in pharmacy. 2. Pharmacists feel able to fully utilize their clinical skills, with contracting and funding aligned with desired service outcomes. 3. Pharmacists feel valued in their roles, with recognized and valued career pathways, and through having their skills recognized by other health professionals and consumers. 4. Technicians have opportunities to develop their careers, particularly through PACT training. 5. Retail staff also have satisfying roles, working as part of the pharmacy team (Morris et al., 2024).

Together, this program theory and its diagrammatic representation illustrate how context is linked to change: we specify *what* outcomes occurred and *how* they arose (or did not arise) in practice. The theory described above is not in any way stating that all our research participants/cases had a 'final' successful outcome, but rather we highlight the if-thens required for success. In other words, it is at this point that the practical utility of realist evaluation can come to light as a tool for supporting adaptation, implementation, and learning. By making causality explicit in this way, realist evaluation approaches enable researchers to question the plausibility of an expected causal pathway, consider where evidence supports or challenges assumptions, and, in the case of the theory above, reflect on how Te Tiriti principles are embedded in workforce design to inform an Indigenous understanding brought to pharmacy policy and practice to help address inequities. This transparency transforms the diagram from a static representation into an analytical output supporting program evaluation and implementation.

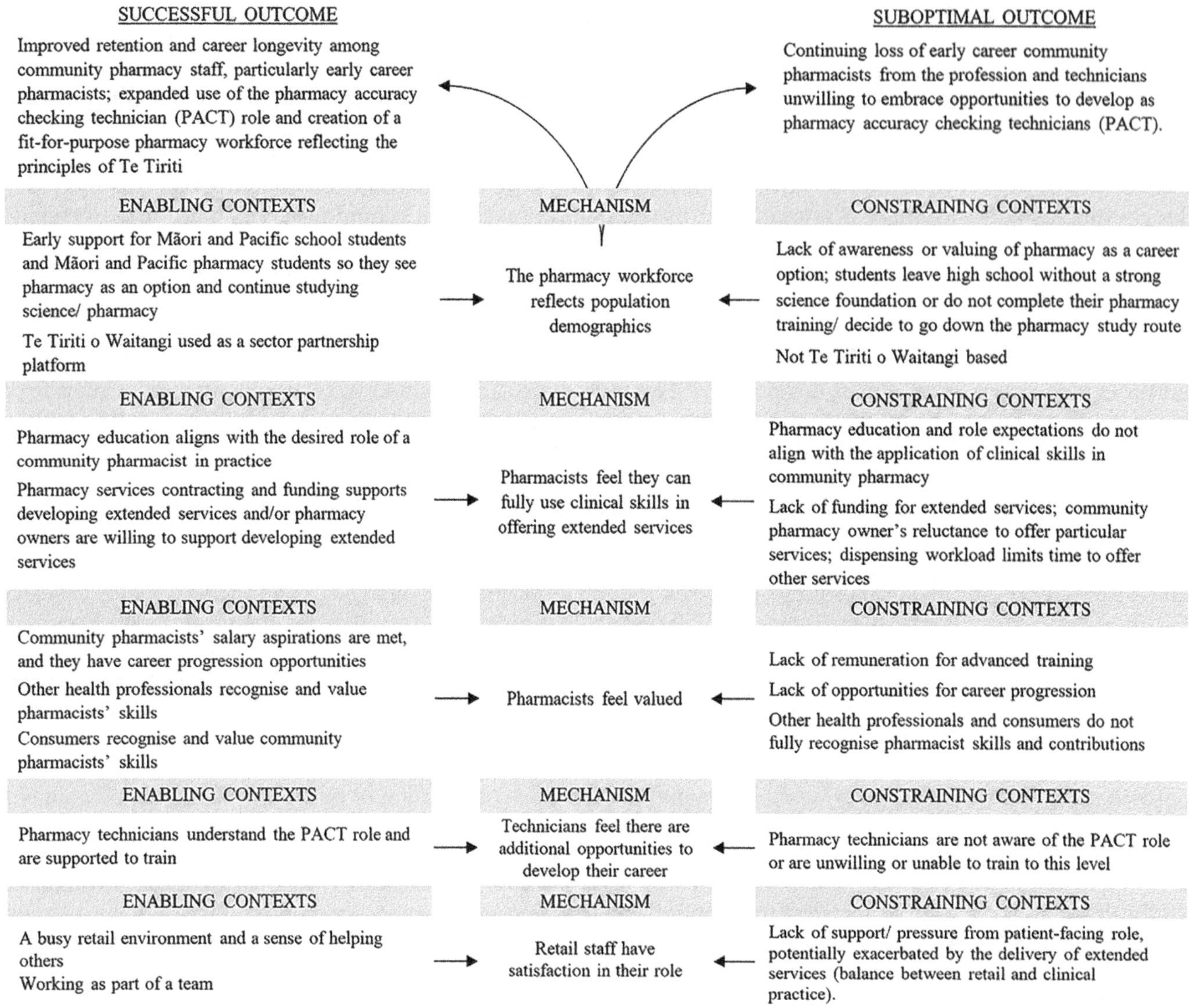

FIG. 12.1 Diagrammatic representation of CMO configurations around the creation of a fit-for-purpose community pharmacy workforce. Context–Mechanism–Outcome (CMO) configurations illustrate the factors that enable or constrain the creation of a fit-for-purpose community pharmacy workforce. The diagram highlights how specific contextual conditions interact with underlying mechanisms to influence workforce development outcomes. *Data from Morris, C., McDonald, J., Officer, T.N., Fa'asalele Tanuvasa, A., Smiler, K., Parore, N., Dunn, P., McKinlay, E., Kennedy, J., McBride-Henry, K., Cumming, J., 2024. A realist evaluation of the development of extended pharmacist roles and services in community pharmacies. Research in Social and Administrative Pharmacy, 20 (3), 321–334. https://doi.org/10.1016/j.sapharm.2023.11.006. CC BY.*

3 Discussion

Traditionally, community pharmacy has focused on dispensing. Globally, community pharmacist roles have expanded with the development of extended services delivered alongside dispensing. Our work explored the development of these extended community pharmacist services and the relevant contexts and mechanisms enabling or constraining outcomes within the community pharmacy environment.

3.1 Equity implications

Our work in evaluating developments in community pharmacist extended services moved beyond interactions at the service delivery end and instead encompassed system-wide equity considerations framed in part around Te Tiriti. We positioned structural conditions—such as colonization, racism, community pharmacy rurality, and patient socioeconomic deprivation—as potential causal contexts that eventually, through mechanisms, influenced resultant outcomes. This perspective moved our evaluation beyond individual-level explanations to interrogating how pharmacy service changes perpetuate or disrupt health system inequities.

Realist evaluation can create space for different knowledge systems rather than treating them as supplementary considerations. At the outset of an evaluation, it is, therefore, important to be deliberate about research team and advisory group compositions, and which potential research participants' perspectives will be gathered. These invariably shape the contexts and mechanisms surfaced and carried forward during the research, and determine whose perspectives are consequently prioritized. In this way, realist evaluation research can guide contextually responsive and culturally grounded pharmacy service development that can advance (or constrain) equity. In turn, this consideration is also important when thinking about how realist evaluation methodologically sits alongside other ways of knowing, priorities, definitions of success, and ways of understanding program processes and outcomes.

3.2 Realist evaluation compared to other health service research methodologies

Realist evaluation offers a generative and theory-driven means of understanding how programs function in complex adaptive systems. While traditional methodologies may quantify change or capture stakeholder perspectives, they often struggle to account for why programs succeed or fail. Realist evaluation, in contrast, foregrounds mechanisms, contexts, and outcomes, enabling deeper interrogation of system-level change. This is particularly relevant in workforce development research, where workforce training and distribution, as well as power, policy, and relational conditions under which work is enacted, shape outcomes.

3.3 Reflections for emerging realist researchers

Despite intentions, our project unfolded nonlinearly and sometimes unpredictably (for example, our pivots due to social distancing during the COVID-19 pandemic). We had moments where boundaries between context and mechanism blurred, where theory refinement lagged behind data collection, and where practicalities constrained fieldwork. We offer the following reflections as practical insights to support emerging researchers in making pragmatic and principled decisions during their own realist research.

1. Embrace complexity: Avoid oversimplifying programs and recognize that they operate in complex real-world settings, as characterized by the VICTORE checklist. Expect program theories to evolve as new data, stakeholder perspectives, and contextual influences emerge.
2. Start with theory, not data: It is vital to identify the program that will be evaluated. This program should ideally be discrete: where does it start and finish? Use theory as a guide for data collection and iterative refinement.
3. Mechanisms are not variables: They are context-sensitive explanations of how actors respond to resources; they may also be hidden and emerge, to some extent, through interpretation of data. They should not be thought of as standing alone but rather as belonging with or working alongside context (Greenhalgh et al., 2009).
4. Context matters: As part of considering "what counts as context or mechanism", realist researchers run the risk of inadvertently seeing CMO configurations as simple linear relationships (Astbury, 2013) and consequently overlooking multimechanism cascades, where outcomes from one program part serve as context for another (Astbury, 2013). The same program works differently in different settings, and not all parts of a setting constitute context (Greenhalgh and Manzano, 2022). Analysis must address this variation, and researchers must identify contexts that trigger mechanisms in these settings. Iterative analysis, team discussion, and advisory group/ stakeholder engagement may help in strengthening conceptual clarity.
5. Attend to power and voice: Ensure the perspectives of marginalized groups—such as non-English speakers, disabled participants, or those without formal diagnoses—are not excluded from your analysis, as this will influence theory formation. Involve different participant groups, which might include policymakers, service users, clinicians, and rivals, in testing and refining program theories to enhance relevance and recommendation uptake. Recognize that people participating in your research, whether in advisory roles or as research participants, influence theory identification, development, and refinement.
6. Data collection is staged and iterative: Realist evaluation is theory-driven and adaptive; be open to revising program theories as insights emerge from the data. Research will evolve as theories develop; having an established advisory group can support identifying next stages and meaning-making. Allow sufficient time for iterative analysis.

7. Reflexivity is essential: How you frame mechanisms, select cases, and interpret findings is influenced by your standpoint and the standpoints of those brought into the research.
8. Document reasoning and rationale: Make assumptions and analytical decisions transparent, particularly if working as part of a large group or within a multistage project. This supports the credibility of the findings and also helps in developing and critically testing emerging theories. For publishing, this documentation also helps others build on your work and explains how theories form. This documentation needs to be initiated at the study's conception, for example, through keeping a field log.
9. Reach out to other realist researchers: Sign up for the RAMESES mailing list (https://www.ramesesproject.org/Mailing_list.php), an active and supportive platform for the realist research community. Follow established reporting and publication standards (Wong et al., 2016) and identify opportunities to attend realist training sessions.

3.4 Strengths and limitations of realist evaluation research

Our evaluation drew on extensive data sources, including gray literature and voices across the continuum of community pharmacy service design, delivery, and reception. We also captured the perspectives of potentially rival service providers by engaging with others in primary health care. Although a wide range of viewpoints was sought, we invariably captured the views of individuals who were more actively engaged and more willing to dedicate their time to our study; participants also had varying levels of involvement in conceptualizing developments in the community pharmacy space. Consequently, this meant that individuals provided differing contributions to theory refinement, which influenced the final theories created. Therefore, as with all realist evaluations (Pawson and Tilley, 2004), the CMO configurations proposed in our research and the resulting program theories remain provisional and open to further refinement. For an international audience, their applicability in other jurisdictions with different elements of program complexity may be limited by varying policies, health systems and service arrangements, and population health needs.

One question often asked within realist evaluation is when to stop data collection and analysis. On the one hand, program theories run the risk of becoming overly simplified—for example, through identifying that where people work alongside each other (context), trust (a mechanism) is built, thereby facilitating good working relationships (outcome). On the other hand, they run the risk of being too abstract to provide recommendations for policy and practice change. A good realist evaluation, therefore, provides a starting point for more questions and a more nuanced understanding of what works. This, in turn, will support subsequent researchers in asking questions such as, "Well, if that works for these populations, what else needs to be understood?" In this way, future evaluations can learn from existing research to make a program's black box less opaque.

Overall, the realist methodology was particularly appropriate for our study of extended community pharmacist roles. It allowed us to unpack how structural and interpersonal dynamics shaped the success or stagnation of service development. It also provided a robust framework for theorizing the role of equity, cultural responsiveness, and professional motivation in sustaining change. In contrast to experimental or purely constructivist approaches, realism enabled us to explain not only *what happened*, but *why it happened as it did, for whom, and under what circumstances.*

4 Questions for further discussion

The following questions may prompt reflection on methodological and practical challenges raised when conducting a realist evaluation. They highlight areas for further dialog when applying realist evaluation theory development to practice change.

- How could realist evaluation inform your pharmacy practice/health workforce study?
- What are the common pitfalls in CMO reasoning, and how can they be addressed?
- How transferable are the findings?
- How does a realist evaluation approach compare to process evaluations in implementation science?

5 Application exercise | scenario

Our research team has applied realist evaluation approaches to pharmacy practice projects, including investigations into community pharmacist role development, practice pharmacist role and service development, and pharmacist prescriber role development in primary health care (McDonald et al., 2024; Morris et al., 2024;

Officer, 2018; Officer et al., 2019, 2021, 2025). The following exercise is designed to help you apply realist evaluation in your thinking.

Scenario: A health authority partners with regional community pharmacies to run a pharmacist-led medicines adherence and engagement service for underserved populations. The service includes funded walk-in patient consultations and follow-ups, as well as a minor ailments scheme. Community representatives led its design to ensure cultural responsiveness and accessibility. Word of mouth suggests inconsistent uptake and engagement across pharmacies. Following training, some pharmacists deliver and promote the service, while others face limited staffing and unclear role expectations.

Exercise: Using the VICTORE checklist, characterize the potential complexity in implementing this program. Next, choose one hypothesized pattern (for example, high or low service uptake) and identify how specific contexts (for example, pharmacy structure, leadership, relationships with local health providers, cultural norms, funding certainty) interact with the reasoning and resources of pharmacists, patients, or teams (mechanisms) to influence the outcome. Express this interaction as a realist program theory. For example: *Where pharmacy teams have longstanding partnerships with local health advocates and have access to shared clinical systems [CONTEXT], pharmacists perceive the new service as aligned with their professional role and community needs [MECHANISM], leading to sustained service delivery [OUTCOME].*

Questions:

- How do these CMO configurations explain differences in service access or outcomes across population groups?
- What data would be helpful when testing your theories?
- If you are based in Aotearoa, how could Te Tiriti be embedded in the design, delivery, and evaluation of this service? If you are working elsewhere, how might Indigenous rights and relationships be recognized in your region?
- How would you apply inclusive and ethically sound research methods to evaluate this research scenario?

6 Te Reo Māori words used in the text

Aotearoa: New Zealand

Hauora: holistic health, vitality, and wellbeing

Kaupapa Māori: by Māori, with Māori, for Māori; a term used to describe traditional Māori ways of doing, being, and thinking, encapsulated in a Māori worldview

Mana motuhake: autonomy, self-determination, sovereignty, and self-government

Māori: the Indigenous people of Aotearoa

Rangatiratanga: chieftainship, authority, the right to exercise authority, chiefly autonomy, and chiefly authority

Rongoā Māori: traditional healing systems

Taonga: prized possession, property, treasured

Te Tiriti o Waitangi (Te Tiriti): the Treaty between Indigenous Māori and the Crown; it is the founding document of Aotearoa

Tikanga Māori: Māori custom

Tino rangatiratanga: self-determination, sovereignty, autonomy, self-government—the fullest expression of rangatiratanga

Whānau Ora: family-centered services and systems of support

Whānau Hauā and Whaikaha: disability studies

Acknowledgements

We gratefully acknowledge our coauthors of the original community pharmacy evaluation, which informed the methodological examples presented in this chapter (Caroline Morris, Ausaga Fa'asalele Tanuvasa, Phoebe Dunn, Eileen McKinlay, Jonathan Kennedy, and Karen McBride-Henry), along with members of the research advisory group and the Te Rōpū Kaitiaki Māori advisory group.

References

Astbury, B., 2013. Some reflections on Pawson's Science of Evaluation: a Realist Manifesto. Evaluation. 19 (4), 383–401. doi:10.1177/1356389013505039.

Astbury, J.L., Jacobs, S., McDermott, I., Willis, S.C., Moss, A., Stearns, S., Fenton, C., Hindi, A.M.K., Seston, E.M., Schafheutle, E.I., 2024. Workforce development in community pharmacies in England: opportunities and tensions for a private sector provider of NHS services. PLoS ONE. 19 (11). doi:10.1371/journal.pone.0310332.

Befani, B., Sager, F., Ledermann, S., 2007. Realistic evaluation and QCA: conceptual parallels and an empirical application. Evaluation 13 (2), 171–192. doi:10.1177/1356389007075222.

Came, H., Cornes, R., McCreanor, T., 2018. Treaty of Waitangi in New Zealand public health strategies and plans 2006–2016. N. Z. Med. J. 131 (1469), 32–37.

Coryn, C.L.S., Noakes, L.A., Westine, C.D., Schröter, D.C., 2011. A systematic review of theory-driven evaluation practice from 1990 to 2009. Am. J. Eval. 32 (2), 199–226. doi:10.1177/1098214010389321.

Cram, F., Huia, B.T., Huia, T.T., Williams, M.M., Williams, N., 2019. Oranga and Māori Health Inequities, 1769-1992 (Prepared for the Ministry of Health in the Wai 2575 - the Health Services and Outcomes Kaupapa Inquiry). Available from https://www.waitangitribunal.govt.nz/en/reports-and-documents?Query=Oranga+and+M%C4%81ori+health+inequities&action_search=Search&WaiNumber=&Roi=&PublishedFrom=&PublishedTo=&Type=.

Dalkin, S.M., Greenhalgh, J., Jones, D., Cunningham, B., Lhussier, M., 2015. What's in a mechanism? Development of a key concept in realist evaluation. Implement. Sci. 10 (1). doi:10.1186/s13012-015-0237-x.

Erueti, A., 2017. International Indigenous Rights in Aotearoa New Zealand, Victoria University Press.

Gilmore, B., McAuliffe, E., Power, J., Vallières, F., 2019. Data analysis and synthesis within a realist evaluation: toward more transparent methodological approaches. Int. J. Qual. Methods. 18. doi:10.1177/1609406919859754.

Greenhalgh, J., Manzano, A., 2022. Understanding 'context' in realist evaluation and synthesis. Int. J. Soc. Res. Methodol. 25 (5), 583–595. doi: 10.1080/13645579.2021.1918484.

Greenhalgh, T., Humphrey, C., Hughes, J., MacFarlane, F., Butler, C., Pawson, R., 2009. How do you modernize a health service? A realist evaluation of whole-scale transformation in London. Milbank Q. 87 (2), 391–416. doi:10.1111/j.1468-0009.2009.00562.x.

Greenhalgh, T., Pawson, R., Wong, G., Westhorp, G., Greenhalgh, J., Manzano, A., Jagosh, J., 2017. Retroduction in realist evaluation (the RAMESES II project). Available from: https://www.ramesesproject.org/pgm-download_media.php?name=RAMESES_II_Retroduction.pdf.

Griffiths, S., Wheat, H., Morgan-Trimmer, S., Weston, L., Gude, A., Oh, T.M., Sheaff, R., Byng, R., 2025. Using a realist informed qualitative approach to elaborate programme theory: experiences from the feasibility phase of the D-PACT project. Int. J. Qual. Methods. 24. doi:10.1177/16094069251370659.

Health New Zealand–Te Whatu Ora, 2025. 2025 Community Pharmacy Agreement. https://www.tewhatuora.govt.nz/health-services-and-programmes/community-pharmacy/community-pharmacy-agreement.

Hewitt, G., Sims, S., Harris, R., 2012. The realist approach to evaluation research: an introduction. Int. J. Ther. Rehabil. 19 (5), 250–259. doi:10.12968/ijtr.2012.19.5.250.

Hikaka, J., Jones, R., Hughes, C., Connolly, M.J., Martini, N., 2021. Utilising te Tiriti o Waitangi to approach health intervention development and research: pharmacist-facilitated medicines review interventions for Māori older adults. J. Prim. Health Care. 13 (2), 124–131. doi:10.1071/HC20114.

Jagosh, J., MacAulay, A.C., Pluye, P., Salsberg, J., Bush, P.L., Henderson, J., Sirett, E., Wong, G., Cargo, M., Herbert, C.P., Seifer, S.D., Green, L.W., Greenhalgh, T., 2012. Uncovering the benefits of participatory research: implications of a realist review for health research and practice. Milbank Q. 90 (2), 311–346. doi:10.1111/j.1468-0009.2012.00665.x.

Jones, R., Bennett, H., Keating, G., Blaiklock, A., 2014. Climate change and the right to health for Māori in Aotearoa/New Zealand. Health Hum. Rights. 16 (1), 54–68.

Kaae, S., Holst, S.S., Hansen, J.M., Vermehren, C., 2025. New program theory in pharmacist-led patient-centered medication review in general practice - a qualitative pilot study. Res. Soc. Adm. Pharm. 21 (12), 1070–1078. doi:10.1016/j.sapharm.2025.07.002

Kerr, A., Strawbridge, J., Kelleher, C., Barlow, J., Sullivan, C., Pawlikowska, T., 2021. A realist evaluation exploring simulated patient role-play in pharmacist undergraduate communication training. BMC Med. Educ. 21 (1). doi:10.1186/s12909-021-02776-8.

Luetsch, K., Maidment, I., Twigg, M., Rowett, D., 2021. Realist research to inform pharmacy practice and policy. Res. Soc. Adm. Pharm. 17 (12), 2075–2081. doi:10.1016/j.sapharm.2021.06.026.

Luetsch, K., Twigg, M., Rowett, D., Wong, G., 2020. In search for gold - The relevance of realist reviews and evaluations to pharmacy research and policy development. Res. Soc. Adm. Pharm. 16 (6), 836–839. doi:10.1016/j.sapharm.2019.07.002.

Manatū Taonga | Ministry for Culture and Heritage, n.d. Treaty of Waitangi. Available from: https://nzhistory.govt.nz/politics/treaty-of-waitangi. (Accessed 30/10/2025).

Manzano, A., 2016. The craft of interviewing in realist evaluation. Evaluation. 22 (3), 342–360. doi:10.1177/1356389016638615.

Martin, P., Tannenbaum, C., 2017. A realist evaluation of patients' decisions to deprescribe in the EMPOWER trial. BMJ Open. 7 (4), e015959. doi:10.1136/bmjopen-2017-015959.

McDermott, I., Spooner, S., Checkland, K., 2025. Employment and deployment of additional staff roles in general practice: a realist evaluation of what works for whom, how, and why. Br. J. Gen. Pract. 75 (752), e153. doi:10.3399/bjgp.2024.0562.

McDonald, J., Morris, C., Officer, T.N., Cumming, J., Kennedy, J., Russell, L., McKinlay, E., Jeffreys, M., 2024. Practice pharmacists in the primary healthcare team in Aotearoa New Zealand: a national survey. J. Prim. Health Care. 16 (4), 332–340. doi:10.1071/HC24049.

McDonald, J., Morris, C., Pledger, M., Dunn, P., Fa'asalele Tanuvasa, A., Smiler, K., Cumming, J., 2021. A national survey of pharmacists and interns in Aotearoa New Zealand: provision and views of extended services in community pharmacies. BMC Health Serv. Res. 21 (1). doi:10.1186/s12913-021-07158-w.

Mikaere, A., 2007. Seeing human rights through Māori eyes. Jurisprudence 10, 53–58.

Ministry of Health, 2016a. Pharmacy Action Plan: 2016 to 2020. https://www.health.govt.nz/publications/pharmacy-action-plan-2016-to-2020.

Ministry of Health, 2016b. Pharmacy Action Plan 2016–2020: Analysis of Submissions. http://www.health.govt.nz/publication/pharmacy-action-plan-2016-2020-analysis-submissions.

Morris, C., McDonald, J., Officer, T.N., Fa'asalele Tanuvasa, A., Smiler, K., Parore, N., Dunn, P., McKinlay, E., Kennedy, J., McBride-Henry, K., Cumming, J., 2024. A realist evaluation of the development of extended pharmacist roles and services in community pharmacies. Res. Soc. Adm. Pharm. 20 (3), 321–334. doi:10.1016/j.sapharm.2023.11.006.

Mossialos, E., Courtin, E., Naci, H., Benrimoj, S., Bouvy, M., Farris, K., Noyce, P., Sketris, I., 2015. From "retailers" to health care providers: transforming the role of community pharmacists in chronic disease management. Health Policy. 119 (5), 628–639. doi:10.1016/j.healthpol.2015.02.007.

Officer, T., 2018. Nurse practitioners and pharmacist prescribers in primary health care: A realist evaluation of the New Zealand experience. Victoria University of Wellington, Wellington, New Zealand. https://openaccess.wgtn.ac.nz/articles/thesis/Nurse_practitioners_and_pharmacist_prescribers_in_primary_health_care_A_realist_evaluation_of_the_New_Zealand_experience/17068688?file=31560839.

Officer, T., Cumming, J., McBride-Henry, K., 2019. Successfully developing advanced practitioner roles: policy and practice mechanisms. J. Health Organ. Manag. 33 (1), 63–77. doi:10.1108/jhom-02-2018-0064.

Officer, T.N., Cumming, J., McBride-Henry, K., 2021. 'She taught me': factors consumers find important in nurse practitioner and pharmacist prescriber services. Hum. Resour. Health. 19 (1). doi:10.1186/s12960-021-00587-y.

Officer, T.N., McDonald, J., Smiler, K., Russell, L., Kennedy, J., McKinlay, E., Churchward, M., Fa'asalele Tanuvasa, A., Cumming, J., Pere, M., Jeffreys, M., Morris, C., 2025. Developing integrated extended pharmacist roles and services for equitable access and outcomes in primary health care: a realist evaluation. Int. J. Health Policy Manag. doi:10.34172/ijhpm.9127.

Pawson, R., 1996. Theorizing the interview. Br. J. Sociol. 47 (2), 295–314. doi:10.2307/591728.

Pawson, R., 2002. Evidence-based policy: the promise of 'realist synthesis'. Evaluation. 8 (3), 340–358. doi:10.1177/135638902401462448.

Pawson, R., 2006. Evidence-based Policy: A Realist Perspective, Sage Publications Ltd.

Pawson, R., 2013. The Science of Evaluation: A Realist Manifesto. SAGE Publications Ltd. doi:10.4135/9781473913820.

Pawson, R., Greenhalgh, T., Harvey, G., Walshe, K., 2004. 2004 ESRC Research Methods Programme. University of Manchester. RMP Methods Paper 2/2004 Realist Synthesis: An Introduction http://www.researchgate.net/publication/228855827_Realist_synthesis_an_introduction.

Pawson, R., Greenhalgh, T., Harvey, G., Walshe, K., 2005. Realist review – a new method of systematic review designed for complex policy interventions. J. Health Serv. Res. Policy 10 (1), 21–34. doi:10.1258/1355819054308530.

Pawson, R., Manzano-Santaella, A., 2012. A realist diagnostic workshop. Evaluation. 18 (2), 176–191. doi:10.1177/1356389012440912.

Pawson, R., Tilley, N., 1997. Realistic Evaluation. Sage Publications Ltd.

Pawson, R., Tilley, N., 2004. Realist Evaluation (Paper for the British Cabinet Office). Available from: https://www.urban-response.org/system/files/content/resource/files/main/pawson—tilley-%282004%29-realist-evaluation.pdf.

Pawson, R., Tilley, N., 2005. Realistic evaluation. In: Mathison, S. (ed.), Encyclopedia of Evaluation. Sage Publications. pp. 363–368. doi:10.4135/9781412950558.n474.

Rees, C.E., Proctor, D.W., Nguyen, V.N.B., Ottrey, E., Mattick, K.L., 2025. Realist analysis of qualitative data in health professions education research. Med. Educ. 59 (5), 503–518. doi:10.1111/medu.15482.

Reid, P., Cormack, D., Paine, S.-J., 2019. Colonial histories, racism and health—The experience of Māori and Indigenous peoples. Public Health. 172, 119–124. doi:10.1016/j.puhe.2019.03.027.

Royal Pharmaceutical Society and The King's Fund, 2022. 2022 Vision for Pharmacy Practice in England. https://www.rpharms.com/england/vision-for-pharmacy-practice-in-england.

Sheridan, N., Jansen, R.M., Harwood, M., Love, T., Kenealy, T., Aguirre-Duarte, N., Arroll, B., Atmore, C., Carryer, J., Crampton, P., Dowell, A., Fishman, T., Gauld, R., Hoare, K., Jackson, G., Kerse, N., Lampshire, D., McBain, L., MacRae, J., Mills, J., Øvretveit, J., Percival, T., Perera, R., Roland, M., Ryan, D., Schmidt-Busby, J., Stokes, T., Stubbe, M., Māori, H., 2024. Hauora Māori – Māori health: a right to equal outcomes in primary care. Int. J. Equity Health. 23 (1). doi:10.1186/s12939-023-02071-6.

Skivington, K., Matthews, L., Simpson, S.A., Craig, P., Baird, J., Blazeby, J.M., Boyd, K.A., Craig, N., French, D.P., McIntosh, E., Petticrew, M., Rycroft-Malone, J., White, M., Moore, L., 2021. A new framework for developing and evaluating complex interventions: update of Medical Research Council guidance. BMJ. 374:n2061. doi:10.1136/bmj.n2061.

Smith, A.J., Scahill, S.L., Harrison, J., Carroll, T., Medlicott, N.J., 2018. Service provision in the wake of a new funding model for community pharmacy. BMC Health Serv. Res. 18 (1). doi:10.1186/s12913-018-3120-z.

Stewart, D., Anthony, B., Morrison, C., MacRae, Y., Dixon, L., Friel, E., Yoong, E., Cunningham, S., MacLure, K., 2017. Evaluating pharmacist input into the pharmaceutical care of patients in dispensing medical practices in remote and rural areas of Scotland. Fam. Pract. 34 (4), 491–499. doi:10.1093/fampra/cmx014.

Te Heuheu Tukino, T., Orange, C., 2017. Te Tiriti o Waitangi: The Treaty of Waitangi, 1840. Bridget Williams Books. doi:10.7810/9780947518981.

Vaessen, J., Leeuw, F.L., 2010. Mind the Gap Perspectives on Policy Evaluation and the Social Sciences. Routledge, New York. doi:10.4324/9781315124537.

Waitangi Tribunal, 2019. Hauora: Report on Stage One of the Health Services and Outcomes Kaupapa Inquiry (Wai 2575). Available from: https://forms.justice.govt.nz/search/Documents/WT/wt_DOC_195476216/Hauora%202023%20W.pdf.

Wong, G., Greenhalgh, T., Westhorp, G., Buckingham, J., Pawson, R., 2013. RAMESES publication standards: realist syntheses. BMC Med. 11 (1). doi:10.1186/1741-7015-11-21.

Wong, G., Greenhalgh, T., Westhorp, G., Pawson, R., 2012. Realist methods in medical education research: what are they and what can they contribute? Medical Education. 46 (1), 89–96. doi:10.1111/j.1365-2923.2011.04045.x.

Wong, G., Greenhalgh, T., Westhorp, G., Pawson, R., 2014. Development of methodological guidance, publication standards and training materials for realist and meta-narrative reviews: the RAMESES (Realist And Meta-narrative Evidence Syntheses – Evolving Standards) project. Health Serv. Deliv. Res. 2 (30), 1–252. doi:10.3310/hsdr02300.

Wong, G., Pawson, R., Owen, L., 2011. Policy guidance on threats to legislative interventions in public health: a realist synthesis. BMC Public Health. 11 (1). doi:10.1186/1471-2458-11-222.

Wong, G., Westhorp, G., Manzano, A., Greenhalgh, J., Jagosh, J., Greenhalgh, T., 2016. RAMESES II reporting standards for realist evaluations. BMC Med. 14 (1). doi:10.1186/s12916-016-0643-1.

CHAPTER

13

Interpretative phenomenological analysis in support of collaboration among healthcare providers

Robin Crunenberg
Department of Pharmacy, ULiège, Liège, Belgium

CHAPTER OBJECTIVES

This chapter

- Describes the use of Interpretative Phenomenological Analysis to explore interprofessional collaboration in nursing homes, with particular attention to the pharmacist's perspective.
- Seeks to illuminate the interpersonal, institutional, and cultural dynamics that either facilitate or inhibit effective teamwork in nursing homes.
- Contributes to a growing body of knowledge aimed at improving patient care in one of the most challenging and critical healthcare environments.

1 Introduction

In the context of aging populations and increasingly complex medication regimens, interprofessional collaboration has become a cornerstone of quality healthcare. This is especially true in nursing home settings. In these environments, patients are often elderly, medically fragile, and reliant on multiple medications to manage chronic conditions. These residents need continuous and coordinated support. Their care depends on the involvement of a wide range of healthcare professionals. Physicians play a central role, but nurses, pharmacists, physiotherapists, and dietitians also contribute essential expertise.

Despite the clear need for collaborative practice, research has consistently shown that such collaboration is often inadequate in long-term care facilities (Babiker et al., 2014). Problems arise from fragmented communication, and a lack of shared documentation also contributes to disorganization. In addition, professional roles are often poorly defined, which creates confusion and delays in decision-making. Unequal power dynamics between professions further complicate collaboration. Altogether, these factors hinder effective teamwork (Busari et al., 2017). The pharmacist's role is particularly affected by this situation. Pharmacists play a crucial part in ensuring medication safety and optimizing treatment; however, their contribution is not always fully integrated into care teams. In many settings, their involvement remains inconsistent and insufficiently recognized.

Contemporary Research Methods in Pharmacy and Health Services - Volume 2
https://doi.org/10.1016/B978-0-443-44607-8.00002-9

The pharmacist is uniquely positioned to identify and address drug-related problems (DRPs). They can manage polypharmacy and educate both staff and patients. Despite this, pharmacists often experience limited access to interdisciplinary meetings. Their contributions are frequently overlooked, and structural barriers prevent them from taking a more proactive role in resident care (Sanchez et al., 2022). This situation undermines the potential of pharmacy services to enhance therapeutic outcomes and prevent adverse events.

The Belgian healthcare system, where this study is situated, is undergoing reforms aimed at reinforcing interprofessional collaboration, particularly in primary care and nursing homes. However, the pace of change is uneven, and empirical evidence about the lived experiences of professionals in these contexts is still emerging. Understanding how collaboration is experienced on the ground is essential for designing interventions that are both effective and contextually relevant.

Qualitative research offers a powerful means of capturing these experiences. In particular, Interpretative Phenomenological Analysis (IPA) (Smith et al., 2009) provides a structured yet flexible approach to exploring how individuals make sense of their work environment, their interactions with others, and their perceived value within a team. By focusing on lived experience, IPA allows for the emergence of nuanced insights into both personal and systemic factors that influence behavior.

2 Theoretical framework

IPA (Smith et al., 2009) is a qualitative research methodology that draws from three philosophical traditions: phenomenology, hermeneutics, and idiography. It is designed to explore how individuals make sense of significant events and experiences in their personal and professional lives. In the context of healthcare, IPA enables researchers to access the deeper meanings behind actions, beliefs, and interactions among professionals.

IPA's foundation in phenomenology allows for an emphasis on the lived experiences of participants. Rather than seeking generalizable truths, IPA focuses on detailed accounts from a small number of individuals to reveal the subjective realities they inhabit. This approach is particularly relevant in the study of interprofessional collaboration in nursing homes, where each professional navigates their role within complex, hierarchical, and emotionally charged environments. In our research (Crunenberg et al., 2024), we employed this method to uncover how professionals, including pharmacists, understand and respond to collaboration challenges in real time.

The hermeneutic component of IPA underscores the interpretative nature of the research process. Researchers engage in a double hermeneutic: participants make sense of their experiences, and researchers, in turn, interpret those interpretations. This layered process is ideal for studying interprofessional collaboration, where meanings are coconstructed in social interactions, often shaped by institutional norms, past experiences, and expectations about professional boundaries.

IPA's idiographic commitment requires in-depth engagement with each participant's narrative before drawing broader thematic conclusions. In our study, pharmacists' accounts revealed not only their expertise in pharmacotherapy but also their feelings of marginalization when excluded from care discussions. The study illuminated the tension between professional knowledge and organizational positioning—insights that might not have emerged through a purely quantitative or general thematic approach.

The use of IPA enabled a nuanced and in-depth exploration of pharmacists' lived experiences within interdisciplinary teams. By examining how pharmacists made sense of their day-to-day interactions, IPA captured the subjective meanings attached to professional identity, access to patient information, and perceived respect from colleagues. These elements emerged not merely as contextual factors but as central determinants of engagement in collaborative practice.

In line with Crunenberg et al. (2024), pharmacists' narratives revealed a dynamic and situational positioning within care teams. Depending on the local collaborative culture, pharmacists described feeling either empowered when their expertise was recognized and integrated into decision-making or marginalized when their role was confined to logistical or dispensing tasks. This oscillation illustrates that interprofessional collaboration is not a fixed condition but a relational process shaped by daily interactions, institutional norms, and informal power dynamics.

As pharmacy services increasingly evolve toward more integrated care models, particularly in long-term care settings, IPA offers a valuable methodological approach to evaluate how these services are experienced in practice. For instance, it can be used to assess how pharmacists perceive their evolving roles in medication reviews, deprescribing initiatives, and participation in interprofessional rounds.

To provide additional structure and explanatory power, the Theory of Planned Behavior (TPB) (Ajzen, 1991) was integrated into the analytical framework. TPB is a psychological theory that explains human behavior as a function of intention, which is itself influenced by three constructs: attitudes toward the behavior, subjective norms, and perceived behavioral control. This framework complements IPA by offering a lens to understand why healthcare professionals might engage in or refrain from engaging in collaborative practices.

For example, in our study, pharmacists expressed a willingness to participate in interdisciplinary meetings but often felt that their input was undervalued. This perception impacted their attitudes and sense of control, ultimately shaping their behavior within the team. Subjective norms also played a role: if the organizational culture did not prioritize or respect the pharmacist's contributions, motivation to engage decreased. TPB thus helps to contextualize the personal reflections gathered through IPA within broader behavioral dynamics.

Combining IPA with TPB enables a richer, multilayered understanding of interprofessional collaboration. IPA provides depth and emotional texture, while TPB offers a structured model for interpreting how cognitive, normative, and contextual factors influence professional behavior. This dual approach allows researchers to explore both what professionals experience and why they act the way they do—an essential duality when seeking to improve collaborative healthcare environments.

3 Methods

This study employed IPA to explore the lived experiences of healthcare professionals involved in interprofessional collaboration in Belgian nursing homes. A total of 19 participants were included in the study, comprising physicians, nurses, and pharmacists. This purposive sampling strategy aimed to capture a diverse range of perspectives across disciplines, seniority levels, and care settings.

The study was conducted between 2022 and 2023. Participants were recruited via professional networks and direct contact with nursing homes. Inclusion criteria required active involvement in direct patient care within a nursing home and experience working as part of an interdisciplinary team. Ethical approval was obtained from the appropriate institutional review board, and all participants provided informed consent.

Semistructured interviews were chosen to allow participants the freedom to describe their experiences in depth while maintaining consistency across interviews. Interviews lasted between 45 and 75 minutes and were conducted either face-to-face or via secure video conferencing platforms, depending on participant availability and pandemic-related restrictions.

Interview questions focused on the nature of collaboration, perceptions of professional roles, communication practices, challenges encountered, and strategies used to enhance teamwork. Special emphasis was placed on understanding the unique contributions of pharmacists, including their involvement in medication review, patient education, and interdisciplinary decision-making.

All interviews were audio-recorded and transcribed verbatim. Transcripts were anonymized and imported into qualitative data analysis software, NVivo 12 (NVivo (Version 12) [Computer software], 2018) to support the coding process. The analysis followed the six-step IPA process outlined by Smith et al. (2009):

1. Reading and rereading the transcripts to ensure immersion in the data is essential.
2. Initial noting to document descriptive, linguistic, and conceptual observations
3. Developing emergent themes by identifying key patterns in the notes
4. Searching for connections across emerging themes within individual cases
5. Moving to the next case and repeating the above steps
6. Looking for patterns across cases allows for the identification of shared experiences and divergences

Particular attention was paid to the narratives of pharmacists. Their contributions shed light on several key issues: limited involvement in strategic care planning, lack of access to shared patient records, and the need for greater recognition of their clinical competencies. As one pharmacist explained, "Sometimes I only find out about a patient's change in condition days later, when I could have helped adjust the medication immediately."

To enhance the interpretative depth, findings were analyzed using the TPB as a sensitizing framework. For instance, pharmacists' intention to participate in collaborative activities was influenced by their perceived usefulness within the team (attitude), perceived expectations from other professionals (subjective norms), and their access to resources or authority to act (perceived behavioral control).

The combined use of IPA and TPB allowed for both a bottom-up exploration of lived experience and a structured interpretation of behavioral drivers. This methodological approach was especially suited to the nursing home context, where complex interpersonal and institutional factors shape collaborative practice.

4 Findings

The analysis of 19 in-depth interviews conducted with physicians, nurses, and pharmacists working in Belgian nursing homes revealed ten interrelated themes (Table 13.1) shaping interprofessional collaboration (Crunenberg et al., 2024). These findings reflect a complex landscape in which collaboration is both facilitated and hindered by structural, relational, and perceptual factors. The study emphasizes the lived experiences of healthcare professionals and how their day-to-day interactions and institutional settings influence team dynamics. Particular attention is given to the role of the pharmacist, whose contributions were both valued and, at times, marginalized.

The themes did not exist in isolation. Leadership support influenced the presence of standardized protocols and technological integration, which, in turn, shaped communication practices and role clarity. This interplay contributed to professionals' perceptions of working as part of a team rather than in isolation.

The TPB was used as an interpretative framework to contextualize these findings. Themes related to recognition of value, trust, and confidence reflected attitudes toward collaboration, while leadership support and mutual familiarity aligned with subjective norms. Communication structures, role clarity, protocols, technology, and physical proximity informed perceived behavioral control, as they shaped professionals' ability to engage in collaborative practice.

Ultimately, interprofessional collaboration in nursing homes emerged as a layered process shaped by interpersonal trust, institutional culture, and professional autonomy. While pharmacists play a key role in medication safety, their contributions remain underleveraged due to fragmented systems and insufficient organizational support.

TABLE 13.1 Themes influencing interprofessional collaboration in nursing homes among physicians, nurses, and pharmacists.

Theme	Description	Illustrative quotation
Communication	Communication was identified as fundamental to collaboration, yet it was often informal, fragmented, and reactive rather than structured. Regular and integrated communication enhanced alignment and professional empowerment.	"There's a lack of real communication with the doctors. We are only contacted when there's an urgent problem." (Pharmacist)
Clarity of roles and responsibilities	Ambiguity regarding professional roles led to inefficiencies and tension. Pharmacists' contributions were frequently reduced to dispensing functions, limiting their involvement in care decisions.	"I feel like I'm just seen as someone who provides drugs, not as someone who can contribute to treatment plans" (Pharmacist)
Recognition of value	Acknowledgment of pharmacists' pharmacological expertise strengthened collaboration and shifted perceptions among other professionals.	"The pharmacist helped resolve a potential medication interaction I had missed. That changed how I view their role." (Physician)
Mutual knowledge and familiarity	Sustained collaboration fostered familiarity with colleagues' competencies and working styles, increasing consultation and trust.	"When you work together regularly, you know whom to contact and what each person can contribute." (physician)
Trust	Trust is developed over time through reliability, openness, and respect. Feeling heard and valued contributes to team cohesion.	"Once I realized how useful the pharmacist's input was, I started involving them more regularly." (Physician)
Confidence in team members	Confidence emerged from consistent performance and shared goals. Pharmacists felt more empowered when their expertise was demonstrated and acted upon.	"When my advice is taken into account, I feel more confident speaking up." (Pharmacist)
Leadership support	Managerial and administrative support enabled collaboration by formalizing roles and encouraging interdisciplinary interactions.	"If management doesn't support collaboration, we are left to push our way into meetings." (Pharmacist)
Standardized protocols	Clear procedures and structured meetings facilitated teamwork. Protocols that formally included pharmacists in medication reviews were particularly effective.	"Having a protocol makes it clear that everyone has a place at the table." (Nurse)
Technology	Electronic health records supported information sharing, but limited access hindered timely interventions and communication.	"It would be ideal if we had a shared space to leave notes. Currently, we depend on emails or calls." (Pharmacist)
Physical proximity	Physical presence in the nursing home enhanced spontaneous interaction and inclusion, while limited on-site presence reduced involvement in decision-making.	"When you're not physically there, you're easily forgotten in discussions." (Pharmacist)

5 Discussion

This study reinforces previous research (Rawlinson et al., 2021) highlighting the foundational role of communication, trust, and role clarity in successful interprofessional collaboration. It also provides new insights by placing pharmacists at the center of the narrative—a group whose involvement in nursing homes remains limited despite their distinct clinical expertise.

When pharmacists are integrated into the healthcare team, they contribute significantly to patient safety, medication optimization, and clinical decision-making. However, these benefits depend on their ability to participate meaningfully in care processes. This participation, in turn, is shaped by institutional structures, leadership support, and team culture. As our findings show, pharmacists expressed a strong desire to be more involved but were frequently constrained by systemic barriers.

This gap between potential and reality reflects a broader challenge in interprofessional care: the disconnect between formal role definitions and lived professional experiences. Although policies often promote collaboration, everyday practice in nursing homes reveals inconsistencies in how these principles are implemented. For pharmacists, in particular, this tension is amplified when they are not physically based on-site.

The TPB helps to contextualize these findings. Pharmacists were more likely to engage proactively when they perceived their role as valued (positive attitudes), felt supported by colleagues and managers (subjective norms), and had sufficient time, tools, and access to information (perceived behavioral control). In contrast, the absence of these enablers often resulted in disengagement, frustration, or passive compliance.

An important contribution of this study lies in the emotional dimension of the narratives. Participants described professional pride when their input was acknowledged, but also discouragement and resignation when their efforts were overlooked. These emotional responses are rarely captured in traditional evaluations, yet they are essential for understanding the sustainability of collaborative practices.

Pharmacist integration should, therefore, be understood as more than physical presence. It requires symbolic and functional inclusion within the care team. This includes visible leadership endorsement, shared decision-making spaces, and regular interdisciplinary meetings. In addition, training programs should incorporate interprofessional education (IPE) that explicitly addresses role expectations, communication skills, and shared accountability.

The findings also highlight the influence of organizational culture. Facilities characterized by openness and mutual respect foster more effective collaboration. Pharmacists working in such environments reported feeling empowered to contribute beyond dispensing roles. By contrast, hierarchical and rigid cultures limited innovation and reinforced siloed practices.

Consistent with these findings, this chapter argues that empowering pharmacists is not optional but essential to high-quality care. Their expertise in pharmacotherapy, detection of DRPs, and patient counseling remains underutilized. To fully leverage these contributions, institutions must address both structural barriers (e.g., protocols, access to records) and cultural factors (e.g., team attitudes, leadership signals).

Finally, the results underscore the value of longitudinal evaluation. Interprofessional collaboration is dynamic and evolves over time. Future research should examine how collaborative practices are sustained, adapted, or weakened in response to policy shifts, staffing models, and professional development initiatives. Such insights are crucial for designing systems that not only initiate collaboration but also support it over the long term.

6 Research implications and future directions

This study underscores the importance of examining interprofessional collaboration in nursing homes through the lens of lived experience, a dimension that remains underexplored in existing research. By focusing on everyday practice, the findings highlight not only structural and procedural barriers but also the emotional and identity-based dimensions of collaboration—elements that are often overlooked in quantitatively driven evaluations.

6.1 Methodological strengths and limitations

A key strength of the IPA approach lies in its capacity to generate rich, person-centered insights from relatively small samples, making it well suited to pilot studies and the exploration of emerging healthcare models. In this study, IPA amplified pharmacists' perspectives—voices that are often underrepresented in institutional or policy-oriented assessments—and provided detailed insight into their professional identity, daily challenges, and contributions to interprofessional collaboration in nursing homes.

Building on the methodological approach described by Crunenberg et al. (2024), the analysis followed a process of interpretative layering. First, interviews were analyzed inductively to identify experiential themes grounded in participants' narratives, with attention to language, emotional expressions, and meaning-making. In the second layer, these themes were examined relationally, focusing on how individual experiences were shaped by interactions with colleagues, organizational structures, and local collaborative cultures. Finally, the themes were interpreted through theTPB, allowing attitudes, subjective norms, and perceived behavioral control to serve as an explanatory framework for pharmacists' engagement in collaborative practices. This layered approach preserved the idiographic depth of IPA while strengthening the analytical coherence of the findings.

Despite these strengths, IPA also presents limitations. The methodology does not aim for statistical generalizability, which may constrain its relevance in policy contexts that prioritize large-scale evidence. Moreover, IPA is inherently time- and resource-intensive, requiring substantial effort for transcription, coding, and interpretation. Given its interpretative nature, researcher reflexivity is essential to ensure credibility and transparency. In this study, reflexive journaling and peer debriefing were employed throughout the analytical process to manage potential bias and support the trustworthiness of the findings.

6.2 Recommendations for future research

Based on these findings, several avenues for future investigation are proposed:

1. Longitudinal studies: Tracking interprofessional dynamics over time, especially in facilities undergoing organizational change, can provide insights into how collaboration evolves and how pharmacists adapt to shifting roles.
2. Implementation research: Studying how specific pharmacist-led initiatives (e.g., medication reconciliation programs, polypharmacy reviews) affect team functioning and patient outcomes could provide concrete evidence for policy advocacy.
3. Mixed-methods approaches: Combining IPA with quantitative methods can enrich understanding while enhancing validity. For example, survey data can be used to identify patterns, while IPA provides depth and context.
4. IPE evaluations: IPA could be used to assess the effectiveness of IPE initiatives, capturing how students from different professions learn to work together and internalize team-based values.
5. Comparative studies: Cross-country or cross-setting comparisons using IPA can uncover cultural and systemic influences on collaboration, such as the regulatory status of pharmacists or institutional openness to shared leadership.
6. Technology and communication: Future research might explore how digital tools, such as shared electronic health records or secure messaging platforms, facilitate or hinder pharmacist integration.

In all these directions, the focus should remain not only on operational outcomes but also on how professionals experience, interpret, and emotionally respond to collaboration. The feelings of pride, frustration, or resignation expressed by pharmacists in this study reveal that professional behavior is inseparable from affective and social dimensions.

By continuing to explore these lived realities, researchers can support the development of collaborative structures that are not only functional but also emotionally and ethically sustainable for all involved.

7 Application exercise

Consider the following two settings and discuss how IPA can be applied to explore the lived experiences of interprofessional collaboration among the healthcare professionals involved. Discuss the likely similarities and differences in the themes compared to the themes identified in the example of nursing homes provided in this chapter.

- General practice—physicians, pharmacists, and nurse practitioners
- Hospital emergency department—emergency physicians, nurses, pharmacists, and paramedics

8 Questions for further discussion

- Why might researchers choose IPA instead of surveys or quantitative methods when studying teamwork experiences?
- What kinds of insights about collaboration can lived-experience interviews reveal that structured questionnaires might overlook?
- What challenges might researchers face when interpreting participants' experiences using IPA?
- How can IPA findings be translated into real-world strategies to foster interprofessional collaboration?

AI disclosure

During the preparation of this work the author(s) used Chat GPT 5 in order to The author used AI in a limited and responsible manner, primarily to refine sentence structure and improve the clarity and accuracy of the English language. AI was also occasionally used to assist with technical tasks such as identifying and formatting academic references in the right style. All scientific content, interpretations, and conclusions remain the author's own. After using this tool/service, the author(s) reviewed and edited the content as needed and take(s) full responsibility for the content of the publication.

References

Ajzen, I., 1991. The theory of planned behavior. Organ. Behav. Hum. Decis. Process. 07495978. 50 (2), 179–211. doi:10.1016/0749-5978(91)90020-t.

Babiker, A., Husseini, M.E., Nemri, A.A., Frayh, A.A., Juryyan, N.A., Faki, M.O., Assiri, A., Saadi, M.A., Shaikh, F., Zamil, F.A., 2014. Health care professional development: working as a team to improve patient care. Sudanese J. Paediatr. 14 (2), 9–16.

Busari, J.O., Moll, F.M., Duits, A.J., 2017. Understanding the impact of interprofessional collaboration on the quality of care: a case report from a small-scale resource limited health care environment. J. Multidiscip. Healthc. 10, 227–234. doi:10.2147/JMDH.S140042.

Crunenberg, R., Charles, C., Lallemand, A., Buret, L., Philippe, G., Ethgen, O., 2024. Interpretative phenomenological analysis of the collaboration among healthcare professionals in the nursing home setting. Explor. Res. Clin. Soc. Pharm. 26672766. 13, 100424. doi:10.1016/j.rcsop.2024.100424.

NVivo (Version 12) [Computer software], 2018. QSR International Pty Ltd. https://www.qsrinternational.com/nvivo-qualitative-data-analysis-software.

Rawlinson, C., Carron, T., Cohidon, C., Arditi, C., Hong, Q.N., Pluye, P., Peytremann-Bridevaux, I., Ingrid, G., 2021. An overview of reviews on interprofessional collaboration in primary care: barriers and facilitators. Int. J. Integr. Care 21 (2). doi:10.5334/ijic.5589.

Sanchez, S., Ecarnot, F., Voilmy, D., Mariam Ndiongue, B., Cormi, C., Letty, A., Hay, P.E., Novella, J.L., 2022. A qualitative study of the perception of nursing home practitioners about the implementation of quality indicators for drug consumption in nursing homes. Aging Clin. Exp. Res. 34 (4), 897–903. doi:10.1007/s40520-021-01989-7.

Smith, J.A., Flowers, P., Larkin, M., 2009. Interpretative Phenomenological Analysis: Theory, Method and Research (London: SAGE Publications).

CHAPTER

14

Designing for health equity: The application of critical Indigenous methodology in health services research

Joanna Hikaka[a,b], *Brendon McIntosh*[a], *Nora Parore*[c], *Anneka Anderson*[b,d], *Rachel Brown*[d], *and Robert Haua*[a]

[a]Ngā Kaitiaki o Te Puna Rongoā o Aotearoa, Taupō, New Zealand
[b]University of Auckland, Te Kupenga Hauora Māori, Auckland, New Zealand
[c]Te Hikuwai Rangahau Hauora - Health Services Research Centre, Te Herenga Waka - Victoria University of Wellington, Wellington, New Zealand
[d]National Hauora Coalition, Auckland, New Zealand

CHAPTER OBJECTIVES

- Introduce the role of critical methodologies in health services research
- Describe the principles and practices of Kaupapa Māori research
- Demonstrate the application of Kaupapa Māori research methodology in pharmacy research
- Discuss the role of critical methodologies in designing for health equity

1 Introduction

Inequities in access to healthcare and health outcomes between different groups and populations are an international phenomenon. Health inequities exist when some groups are privileged while others are disadvantaged or oppressed, leading to inequitable access to the determinants of health, such as education, employment, housing, and healthcare itself (Baciu et al., 2017).

When developing health interventions and services that aim to achieve equity in access and outcomes, it is important to be explicit in addressing equity considerations. Equity considerations and pro-equity action need to occur at all stages of health service development, from deciding which services are important to develop and how the service will be delivered, through to identifying appropriate markers of success, determining how decisions about further implementation and ongoing resourcing will be made, and by whom (Huria et al., 2019; Hikaka et al.,

https://doi.org/10.1016/B978-0-443-44607-8.00015-7

2024). Achieving health equity through design requires a critical examination of the underlying structural barriers embedded within current health systems or services, such as disparities in power, access, and resources. It is essential to deliberately address and challenge these imbalances. Central to this approach is the meaningful involvement of the communities most affected by these inequities, ensuring the design of solutions genuinely reflects their realities and aspirations.

1.1 Critical methodologies

Critical research is grounded in the understanding that all knowledge is shaped by power dynamics that are socially and historically constructed (Morrow and Brown, 1994). Certain groups are recognized as being privileged over others, and mainstream research often, albeit sometimes unintentionally, reinforces the dominant social and historical structures that maintain such systems of oppression (Denzin and Lincoln, 2018). This is due to collective and individual biases, identities, positions of power, and perspectives that shape underlying assumptions, which can inadvertently impact research unless addressed (Ford and Airhihenbuwa, 2010). Critical methodologies focus on liberation against such power differentials and therefore "speak to lived experiences, historical exigencies, and systemic operations of power in both situated and broad scopes" (Baugh-Harris and Wanzer-Serrano, 2018). They are increasingly recognized in health services research as vital for uncovering how hidden power structures, structural inequity, and marginalization shape health systems, outcomes, and access.

1.2 Critical research in Aotearoa New Zealand

1.2.1 Māori and Aotearoa New Zealand

Māori are the Indigenous people of Aotearoa New Zealand (NZ) and comprise 19.6% of the total population (Statistics, 2025). This means that almost every health service and piece of health research in NZ will impact Māori to some extent. Te Tiriti o Waitangi (NZ's founding legal document; the binding and te reo Māori (Māori language) version of the Treaty of Waitangi) guarantees Māori the right to equitable health outcomes, partnership in health care design, delivery, and governance, the right to active protection, and the right to healthcare options, including culturally safe mainstream services and Kaupapa Māori services (Hauora -Report on Stage One of the Health Services and Outcomes Kaupapa Inquiry, 2019). A glossary of terms has been provided to support readers with the use of Māori language throughout this chapter (Table 14.1).

1.2.2 Kaupapa Māori methodology

Kaupapa Māori methodology originated from centuries of Indigenous knowledge and has been developed in academic settings over the last four decades (Smith, 2023). Broadly translated, Kaupapa Māori means a "Māori way," and this methodology centers Māori ways of knowing, being, and doing in the research process and in wider society, addressing issues of power, colonization, and social justice, often with activist and positive transformative intent (Smith, 2023; Pihama, 2010; Curtis, 2016). Within academia, Kaupapa Māori methodology has its foundations in critical Māori education; however, it has developed into one of the key critical methodologies applied in health services research in NZ, with national guidelines recognizing Kaupapa Māori research as best practice when research involves Māori.

1.2.3 Kaupapa Māori principles and practices

Kaupapa Māori methodology is underpinned by principles and practices that reflect Māori values, knowledge systems, and aspirations. These principles guide the research process and are intended to ensure it is culturally grounded and beneficial to Māori. Importantly, they do not form a rigid checklist but instead provide a flexible, relational framework that honors the diverse realities of whānau (families), hapori (communities), hapū (subtribes), and iwi (tribes) while resisting homogenizing assumptions about Māori identity and experience (McKinley and Smith, 2019).

Kaupapa Māori principles

Kaupapa Māori methodology is grounded in interrelated principles guiding Indigenous research in NZ, centering Māori ways of being, knowing, and doing (Smith, 2023). These principles are methodological guidelines that also, importantly, express a philosophical commitment to Māori self-determination, relational ethics, and collective transformation. They are inherently dynamic and are applied contextually in ways that reflect the diverse Māori realities across NZ.

TABLE 14.1 Glossary of terms.

Te Reo Māori	English
ako Māori	Māori ways of teaching/learning
āta	Gently, deliberately, clearly
hapori	Community/ies
hapū	Subtribe/s
iwi	Tribes
kawa	Values
kōhanga reo	Māori immersion early childhood education
kura	Māori immersion schools
mamae	Pain
mana motuhake	Autonomy
marae	Open area in front of a meeting house, often used to describe the collection of buildings around this space as well
mātauranga Māori	Māori knowledge
Pākehā	NZ european
rangatahi	Māori youth
taonga tuku iho	Knowledge, treasures, and heritage passed on by ancestors
te ao Māori	The Māori world
te reo Māori	Māori language
Te Tiriti o Waitangi	The Treaty of Waitangi, although it is to be noted that the te reo Māori and English versions are different in wording and interpretation
tikanga	Protocols/ways of doing/cultural practices
tino rangatiratanga	Māori self-determination
tuakana–teina	Older sibling-younger sibling
wairuatanga	Spirituality
wānanga	To discuss, deliberate, or consider different issues or agendas.
whakamā	Shame
whakapapa	Genealogy
whakawhiti kōrero	Back-and-forth exchange of dialog
whānau	Family
whanaungatanga	Relationships

A core principle of Kaupapa Māori methodology is tino rangatiratanga, or Māori self-determination. It affirms that Māori must lead and define research processes, framing research as a tool to support the political, cultural, and social aspirations of Māori communities (Pihama, 2010). Tino rangatiratanga positions Māori as the rightful authorities in research concerning Māori, rejecting deficit-based framings and privileging Māori-led inquiry (Smith, 2023). This principle is enacted through codesign processes, shared decision-making, and collective governance over data and outcomes, reflecting mana motuhake (autonomy), thus supporting Māori to retain control over how their knowledge is used and interpreted (Smith, 2023). Codesign is widely recognized as good practice in Kaupapa Māori research, aligning with principles such as tino rangatiratanga and whanaungatanga by fostering collective decision-making, relational accountability, and Māori control over research processes (Smith, 2023; Cram and Kennedy, 2010). However, the value of Indigenous-led or Indigenous-partnered research extends beyond Kaupapa Māori contexts and should be recognized as essential across all health services research, where it brings critical cultural, political, and historical knowledge that informs more equitable, culturally safe, and structurally responsive systems (Moewaka Barnes et al., 2021).

Closely aligned with this is the constitutional principle of Te Tiriti o Waitangi, which affirms Māori rights to equity, partnership, and protection. In Kaupapa Māori methodology, Te Tiriti o Waitangi provides a structural and ethical framework for power-sharing, cultural safety, and accountability within research practice. Together, these principles position research as a vehicle for restoring sovereignty and dismantling colonial structures that have historically marginalized Māori.

The principle of taonga tuku iho affirms the validity and centrality of mātauranga Māori (Māori knowledge), te reo Māori (the Māori language), tikanga (protocols), and kawa (values) as legitimate and essential epistemological foundations (Smith, 2011; Royal, 2018). It also acknowledges the emotional and spiritual dimensions of knowledge that are often excluded from Western research paradigms (Royal, 2018). Alongside this, ako Māori emphasizes culturally preferred pedagogies and reciprocal learning (Smith, 2023). It highlights the shared responsibilities of researchers and participants in cocreating knowledge and reinforces the idea that learning is situated within connected relationships and shaped by community. Kaupapa Māori methodology privileges Māori worldviews and positions Māori realities at the center of inquiry. This includes embracing whakapapa (genealogy), whanaungatanga (relationships), and wairuatanga (spirituality) as integral parts of both the research process and outcomes that need to be considered when making choices, such as the type of data collection methods that are most appropriate (Smith, 2023). As Chilisa describes in the broader Indigenous research context, such approaches resist the colonial tendency to compartmentalize knowledge and instead assert its embeddedness in relationships with people, land, and the metaphysical (Chilisa, 2020).

Relationality is not just a principle but an ethical stance. Shawn Wilson notes that "we are the research", meaning the researcher's positionality, obligations, and relationships cannot be separated from the research itself (Wilson, 2020). Relationality is a defining feature of Kaupapa Māori methodology and is reflected in the principles of whānau and āta. Whānau, as a principle, moves beyond the nuclear family to emphasize extended, collective relationships and the responsibilities accompanying them (Bishop, 1999). Whānau values reciprocal, enduring engagement and recognizes that research occurs within webs of connection and social obligation (McIntosh, 2005). The principle of āta deepens the principle of whānau by articulating how relationships should be nurtured with care, respect, reflection, and deliberate intent (Pohatu, 2013). Āta encourages researchers to engage slowly and ethically, maintaining humility and integrity throughout the research process. Understanding one's whakapapa and the values and commitments that guide one's work becomes essential to ensuring research is done *with* and *for* Māori rather than *on* Māori.

Kaupapa Māori also holds positive transformation as a central goal. Research should lead to meaningful outcomes, not just the production of knowledge (Smith, 2023b). At its heart, Kaupapa Māori is about transformation, creating real-world change that uplifts Māori communities. This aligns with Indigenous research traditions globally, which prioritize strengths-based, emancipatory approaches that support Indigenous aspirations and futures (Rigney, 1999).

Finally, Kaupapa Māori resists essentialism. It acknowledges that Māori are not a homogeneous population but a diverse collective of different groupings with distinct histories, dialects, and ways of being. Tracey McIntosh emphasizes that reducing Māori to a single category risks re-inscribing the colonial logic of simplification and control (McIntosh, 2005). Instead, Kaupapa Māori methodology remains deliberately open and responsive to community-specific aspirations, embedding the principle of flexibility within the methodology itself while still providing a framework of principles and practices to undertake robust, critical research (McKinley and Smith, 2019).

Kaupapa Māori practices

Kaupapa Māori principles are upheld by a set of practices that guide the way in which research is operationalized (Smith, 2023; F. Cram, 2009). We introduce Kaupapa Māori practices in Table 14.2.

Together, these principles and practices form a research methodology that is uniquely Indigenous to NZ and yet resonates with other Indigenous movements globally. Kaupapa Māori methodology offers a model for conducting ethical, rigorous, and transformative research that reflects and advances Māori health and wellbeing.

In the next part of this chapter, we discuss how we used Kaupapa Māori methodology in research relating to pharmacists' roles in supporting minor ailment treatment and care in community pharmacy settings. Understanding the context of research is important in critical methodologies, and so we begin by introducing you to pharmacist minor ailments care in NZ and internationally, and by describing inequities in access to medicines and pharmacist care in NZ. We then describe how we applied Kaupapa Māori principles and practices as we undertook the research. Finally, we present the research findings and consider the relevance of these findings in the broader context of national and international literature.

TABLE 14.2 Kaupapa Māori practices.

Practice	Explanation
Kanohi kitea—Being a "seen" face	This practice involves privileging face-to-face engagement and recognizes the importance of being known and present within the communities where research is taking place.
Titiro, whakarongo … kōrero—Look, listen … speak	This practice highlights the need to observe and listen to research communities before centering yourself as a researcher in the conversation. This approach privileges the voices of research participants and empowers them as knowledge holders.
Manaaki ki te tangata—share and host people, be generous, and be caring	This practice signifies the act of caring for, respecting, and nurturing the wellbeing of people involved, emphasizing Māori values of hospitality, support, and reciprocal relationships. Research participants can be considered as guests we value and look after throughout the research process and beyond.
Kia tūpato—Be cautious	This practice emphasizes caution in the researchprocess, ensuring harm is not caused. This could include how research is carried out, how research is reported, and being aware of the expectations of those involved in the research.
Kaua e takahia te mana o te tangata—Do not trample on the mana (honor, authority, prestige, power) of the people	This practice ensures that researchers respect local power and authority within research communities. This may include understanding and abiding by local governance practices.
Kaua e mahaki—Do not flaunt your knowledge	This practice urges researchers to embrace humility, shifting from a position of "all-knowing" to recognizing that multiple knowledge holders and knowledge systems exist.
Aroha ki te tangata—Respect for people	This practice emphasizes the need to have genuine respect for the people involved in research. This can be demonstrated in a number of ways, including being responsive to other people's suggestions, disseminating research findings back to those impacted by them, and being honest and transparent in your dealings with others.

2 Background

2.1 Pharmacists and minor ailments treatment

Pharmacists working in community pharmacies provide minor ailment treatment and care in their everyday practice. Minor ailments can be defined as (often) self-limiting conditions that are easily described and recognized by patients themselves and fall "within the scope of a pharmacist's knowledge and training to treat" (Dineen-Griffin et al., 2019). Examples of minor ailments include sprains, coughs, colds, headaches, fever, and hay fever, and care may or may not include the recommendation and provision of a pharmacological agent. Although pharmacist minor ailments care is common globally, the extent to which these services are private versus publicly funded differs.

In countries with publicly funded Pharmacist Minor Ailments Services (PMAS), such as the United Kingdom, service evaluations have demonstrated that PMAS lead to high rates of symptom resolution (69–94%), trends toward reductions in general practice consultations and prescribing, and save the health system money (Baqir et al., 2011; Paudyal et al., 2013). When comparing minor ailment care outcomes across the different settings of general practice, emergency departments, and community pharmacies, symptom resolution and quality of life improvements were similar, suggesting health outcome equivalence.

2.2 Inequities in access to care and the role of Pharmacist Minor Ailments Services

Inequities in access to, and outcomes from, healthcare exist across the globe, mediated by inequities in access to the determinants of health, such as education, employment, racism, and housing. Factors associated with poorer health access and outcomes include lower income, rural location, and ethnic minority groups, including Indigenous populations. Where access to PMAS is publicly funded internationally, public funding is rarely universal, instead employing eligibility criteria to target access for those experiencing inequities. Examples of such criteria include age, financial need, and comorbidities (Aly et al., 2018).

In NZ, PMAS have not been routinely implemented within community pharmacies, although there are pockets of pilot programs in some areas (2024). Nationally developed and implemented PMAS could help improve equitable access to medicines in NZ, where Māori face lower access to care and poorer health outcomes than non-Māori across many clinical areas, including medicine access (Hauora -Report on Stage One of the Health Services and Outcomes Kaupapa Inquiry, 2019; Metcalfe et al., 2018). Cost is also more frequently reported as a barrier to medicines by Māori than by those of other ethnicities (Jeffreys et al., 2024). When "designing for equity," equity must be considered at all stages, from intervention or service development right through to evaluation of effectiveness and impact, and there are now implementation frameworks available to facilitate the explicit review of equity (Gustafson et al., 2024; Hikaka et al., 2024). Although PMAS are often established with the desire to achieve equity, there is little evidence to support that PMAS improve equity (Hikaka and Haua, 2022).

2.3 Involving end-users in the development of PMAS

The involvement of end-users is an essential step in best practice when developing health services (Skivington et al., 2021). Crucially, this involvement needs to start prior to feasibility testing and implementation to maximize the likelihood of the service delivering a positive impact (Skivington et al., 2021). Although there has been discussion of national PMAS in NZ to improve pharmacists' scope of care, reduce primary care utilization, and improve access to care, there is no national literature on Māori experiences and aspirations for PMAS. In addition, we could not find any literature discussing the incorporation of Indigenous or other marginalized populations into PMAS development.

To address this lack of information, we conducted research with Māori across the country to explore the following:

- What types of minor ailments do Māori access care for?
- Māori experiences of access to medicines for minor ailments
- Māori perceptions of the role pharmacists play in minor ailment care

3 Methods

We undertook a convergent, parallel mixed-methods study, applying Kaupapa Māori methodology. In this chapter, we describe in detail aspects relevant to Kaupapa Māori methodology; additional methods used can be found in an earlier publication (Hikaka et al., 2023).

3.1 Research partnership and team development

3.1.1 Building a research partnership

A partnership was formed between Ngā Kaitiaki o Te Puna Rongoā o Aotearoa—The Māori Pharmacists' Association (MPA) and The National Hauora Coalition (NHC) to develop a research proposal and grant application to explore how pharmacists can better support equitable access to medicines for Māori. Individual members from each organization had worked together previously, although formal collaboration between the organizations was new. Something that supported the partnership was the overlap in organizational visions. The shared vision of both organizations created a strong foundation by aligning a commitment to Māori-led healthcare improvements with the empowerment of individuals and whānau (families) to achieve autonomy, fostering self-determined, culturally grounded success in medicines optimization and overall health outcomes.

3.1.2 Applying the practice of "kanohi kitea" in research team development

The practice of kanohi kitea—the value of being visibly present and engaging face-to-face—was central to how we worked within communities. This approach fostered familiarity, trust, and meaningful connection. As Māori researchers, most of whom were frontline health professionals, we were already well-known within the communities we engaged with, spanning six regions across NZ. Our connection to these communities extended beyond our professional roles; many of us were actively involved in local initiatives such as kura (Māori schools), kōhanga reo (Māori immersion early childhood education), marae committees, and Māori health networks.

This idea of being recognizable and trusted was not limited to individual relationships; it was also reflected at an organizational level. Both the MPA and NHC hold Māori health equity as a core principle across their operations—from vision and strategy to everyday decision-making. These organizations are well-established and respected within Māori communities. Applying the principle of kanohi kitea to organizational involvement was a deliberate and strategic choice. We recognized that working through trusted, Māori-led, and Māori-governed organizations was crucial. In contrast, partnering with larger, mainstream institutions lacking this cultural grounding could have risked undermining the trust and engagement we sought to build with our communities.

3.2 Research team positionality and reflexivity

When developing a research team, we critically considered team membership, thinking about shared values and identities, as well as the unique skills that needed to be brought to the research team, helping to define our collective and individual positionalities (Cayir et al., 2022). Researchers applying Kaupapa Māori methodology are expected to critically examine their own positionality, including their cultural, professional, and institutional affiliations. This involves interrogating the power dynamics inherent in the research relationship and acknowledging how Western research traditions have historically marginalized Māori voices. Reflexivity in Kaupapa Māori research is not performative but ethical; it is a commitment to being accountable to the communities one serves.

During our researcher training session, we discussed our collective positionality. We discussed our shared and unique skills, and then one of the team members drafted our positionality for the rest of the team to review, refine, and approve. Undertaking these discussions prior to starting the research data collection and analysis allowed us to come to a collectively shared vision of what was important to us and to document the epistemological, axiological, and ontological positions that guided our work. Documenting this at the start allowed us to return to it as an anchor throughout our work when we were considering the approaches we would take and as we analyzed and presented data.

3.2.1 *Collective positionality*

Our team consisted of nine Māori researchers who all acknowledged that the way in which current health services are developed and implemented contributes to inequitable health outcomes for Māori and that pharmacists can provide high-quality health care. As a group, we acknowledged the rights of Māori to receive excellent, clinically and culturally safe health care. We believed in the positive, transformative potential of Kaupapa Māori research methods in health service development. We also all had experience receiving publicly funded health care in NZ.

3.2.2 *Diverse and unique aspects of individual positionality*

Within our research team, we had community and hospital pharmacists from six different regions of NZ. Some had experience as pharmacy owners, some had experience in public health, the majority had experience in qualitative and/or quantitative research, and the majority of those with research experience had experience undertaking Kaupapa Māori research, one of whom taught this to graduate students. Some members of the team lived in the communities they worked in, while others traveled across regional borders to deliver care.

3.3 Research team training and capacity building

We undertook research team training, led by the Principal Investigator and supported by different team members who could lead various components within the training. In addition to all the research team members completing the training, three research assistants who supported data collection also participated. The training focused on two key areas: Kaupapa Māori theory and practices, and the study-specific protocol along with related components and practices. We recognized the need to train the team to understand the intention behind the research, ways to undertake strengths-based facilitation, and the theoretical framing of the research—from research questions through to the contextualization of research findings and potential impact. We completed the training online in two two-hour sessions, with informal refreshers and check-ins conducted by the Principal Investigator with team members ahead of each data collection session.

We also facilitated Māori research workforce development by supervising three research studentships (Māori pharmacy students) and one Master's student, while three team members also completed their doctoral studies during the course of the research. These efforts contributed to growing Indigenous research capacity and sustaining Kaupapa-driven approaches, with an enduring impact through the tuakana–teina learning and mentorship model (older sibling-younger sibling; representing a reciprocal relationship between those with varying levels of experience) (Nicholls et al., 2021).

3.4 Recruiting research participants

People were eligible to participate if they were 18 years or older, were Māori, and had obtained at least one medicine (over-the-counter or prescribed) from a pharmacy in the last three years. We took an inclusive approach regarding ethnicity; if family members of Māori participants were eligible but not Māori, they could participate. This facilitated acknowledgment of collective, family-centric approaches to health care that are common within Māori frameworks of wellbeing (Durie, 1998).

We used convenience sampling to recruit eligible participants across seven different regions of NZ, drawing on our personal and professional networks in each area. Our team members were based in both urban and rural locations, which allowed us to engage with a broad cross-section of communities. Recruitment was carried out through various channels, including pharmacy-related social media platforms, face-to-face conversations, and email. Each potential participant received a brief overview of the project, along with a Participant Information Sheet. We also made use of snowball sampling, encouraging participants to refer others who might be interested. Our recruitment approach was deliberately flexible, enabling each researcher to connect with their community using communication styles and methods that were familiar and effective for the communities they served.

3.5 Data collection

3.5.1 *Wānanga—Collaborative knowledge-sharing group discussions*

In te reo Māori, wānanga means to meet to discuss, deliberate, or consider different issues or agendas. Wānanga are seen as a time for knowledge exchange between two or more people or groups, and it would be expected that all involved would walk away having learned something new. When formalizing data collection methods, we chose to use the concept of wānanga to explicitly recognize that the researchers and participants were both knowledge holders and that the sharing of information was a way to build reciprocal relationships. As participants would be sharing their insights during the wānanga, facilitators shared information about pharmacist training and educational background, minor ailments, and PMAS to balance the knowledge transfer.

3.5.2 *The use of te reo māori during data collection*

To enable participants to respond in their language of choice, we ensured that at least one of the two facilitators in each wānanga was able to speak te reo Māori to the level required to actively facilitate a research wānanga. We informed participants prior to the wānanga that they would have the option to speak in either English or te reo Māori, and the transcriptionist was fluent in both te reo Māori and English. Where te reo Māori was spoken, translation occurred at the stage of transcription. When translations occurred, the facilitators of that wānanga confirmed that the translation upheld the context of the data shared. Often, when data collection occurs in a nondominant language, it is useful to analyze the data in the original language to further ensure cultural understandings and nuances are considered. Our team had to make a pragmatic decision to translate prior to data analysis, as those analyzing the data did not have the language abilities to analyze in te reo Māori, and so that findings could be synthesized across the data set.

3.5.3 *In-person and online wānanga*

Our research approach prioritized face-to-face methods for recruitment, obtaining consent, and participation. However, this research was conducted in 2021 during the COVID-19 pandemic, when limits were placed on in-person interactions. For many months during the data collection period, the NZ general public's physical interaction with others was restricted to household contacts. At the same time, we prepared for the possibility of shifting to online engagement if COVID-related restrictions were intensified. COVID-19 restrictions did, in fact, intensify, and for most of the data collection period, large parts of the country were restricted to contact only with those in their household. Unless working in essential jobs, people were unable to drive or move around communities except by walking. The foundation of strong Kaupapa Māori values within our research partnership enabled us to adapt swiftly and confidently from planned in-person wānanga to online formats. Allowing for both in-person and online options enabled us to uphold the practice of manaaki ki te tangata—caring for those involved in research. The feasibility of remote participation was supported by the fact that members of the research team were already familiar to many within the communities, having built relationships through previous in-person interactions, further supporting the concept of kanohi kitea.

While our research initially centered on in-person engagement, we were reassured by examples of Kaupapa Māori research that had successfully used online approaches (Dawes et al., 2021), demonstrating that Kaupapa

Māori practices could still be meaningfully upheld in digital spaces. We recognized the ongoing digital divide in NZ (Grimes and White, 2019), with Māori communities experiencing less access to digital tools and infrastructure compared to non-Māori—an important equity consideration. There are both challenges and opportunities involved with online data collection, and literature and guidance to support safe and effective practices continue to increase (Lobe et al., 2020; Hensen et al., 2021; Salvador et al., 2020; Newman et al., 2021). At the same time, we acknowledged that online participation might offer greater accessibility for some people, particularly those facing barriers to attending in-person gatherings. While these flexible approaches were initially introduced in response to the disruptions caused by COVID-19, our research team believes that such options should be standard practice in all research. Providing participants with choices about how and when to engage respects their circumstances and supports meaningful, culturally safe participation.

We audio-recorded wānanga, transcribed them verbatim through a transcriptionist, and then anonymized the transcripts.

3.6 Data analysis

At the end of each wānanga, facilitators summarized key discussion points and presented them back to participants for consensus building. Participants were given the opportunity to provide feedback, add points, discuss different interpretations, and offer alternative suggestions to the key points that were raised in the wānanga. This process gave participants a role in data analysis.

Our analysis followed a general inductive approach (Thomas, 2006), grounded in Kaupapa Māori theory. Two researchers independently coded an initial set of five transcripts in NVivo (Version 12) before meeting to discuss their coding decisions, refine and consolidate similar codes, and organize them into a structured hierarchy. This collaborative process informed the development of a draft coding framework, which was then shared with the wider research team for feedback and refinement. One researcher then applied the revised framework to re-code the initial five transcripts and to code the remaining eight transcripts. The framework remained flexible, allowing new codes to be added as needed. These codes informed the development of preliminary themes, which we reviewed against the data and refined through team discussions. We agreed on final themes collectively through consensus and supported by a review of relevant codes and participant quotes.

3.7 Researching during a pandemic—Kaupapa māori practices to guide actions

The principle of kia tūpato—acting with caution—guided our decision-making throughout the research process. As a team, we chose to adopt a more cautious approach than that required by government guidelines, recognizing both the historic and ongoing inequities in health outcomes for Māori during pandemics (Steyn et al., 2020a; Gurney et al., 2020). Our decisions were influenced by emerging research highlighting the disproportionate risks Māori communities faced and were grounded in our responsibility to protect those most affected (Pihama and Lipsham, 2020). Of note, the anticipated inequities in COVID-19 outcomes have since been identified in research, whereby Māori were at greater risk of COVID-19 infection, related morbidity and mortality, and reduced access to vaccination compared to non-Māori (Steyn et al., 2020a; Jefferies et al., 2020; Steyn et al., 2020b; Datta et al., 2024; Jefferies et al., 2025).

In line with this approach, we agreed that no interregional travel would occur between regional areas operating under different COVID-19 Alert Levels (Cumming, 2022). Although this meant the Principal Investigator could no longer travel to support less experienced team members or assist with the local dissemination of findings, we prioritized the safety and preferences of communities. Following the government's announcement of a vaccination-led strategy on 4 October 2021, we reached a consensus that face-to-face data collection would only proceed with participants who were fully vaccinated. We submitted an ethics amendment, with subsequent approval, to permit us to ask about vaccination status. Online options remained available for those who were unvaccinated, preferred not to disclose, or simply felt more comfortable participating remotely.

Decisions about holding in-person wānanga, in places where government policy allowed, were left to the discretion of the local researchers, who were embedded within their communities and best placed to assess local readiness, safety protocols, and comfort levels. This localized, cautious approach was also necessary to protect communities where some team members continued to work as front-line health professionals. Our approach aligned with broader Māori-led responses during the pandemic, which have emphasized the importance of iwi- and Māori-driven public health strategies grounded in care and equity (Curtis et al., 2024; Davies et al., 2022; Russell et al., 2023).

4 Results and discussion

4.1 Research participants and settings

Between September 2021 and February 2022, we held 13 wānanga, 10 conducted online and three in person, with a total of 62 participants. The wānanga typically lasted around 95 minutes, with durations ranging from just over an hour to three and a half hours. A high level of engagement was evident, with 94% of participants (n = 58) completing an online or physical questionnaire that included demographic information as well as their experiences with minor ailments.

Participants spanned a broad age range—from 18 to over 75 years—with the median falling in the 35–44 age bracket. Most identified as female (71%), and over a quarter (28%) reported having a physical disability. Those who took part were based in seven different regions across NZ and were collectively affiliated with 37 iwi (tribes). The majority (76%) chose to engage in both te reo Māori and English during the research process.

To support inclusive and culturally safe participation, individuals were encouraged to bring support people if they wished. In two instances, accompanying whānau members who met the study's eligibility criteria also chose to consent and participate.

4.2 Overarching themes

We developed four themes from the qualitative wānanga data (Hikaka et al., 2023) Fig. 14.1) and have presented the overarching concepts in a diagram. Three themes are presented in more detail below.

4.2.1 Designing the right environment for minor ailment care

The healthcare environment played a significant role in shaping participants' experiences and their willingness to seek advice or treatment for minor ailments. This environment encompassed not only the physical setting but also the accessibility and professionalism of healthcare providers. Participants identified a range of environmental factors that either supported or hindered their ability to access effective care, with several insights specific to their experiences in pharmacies.

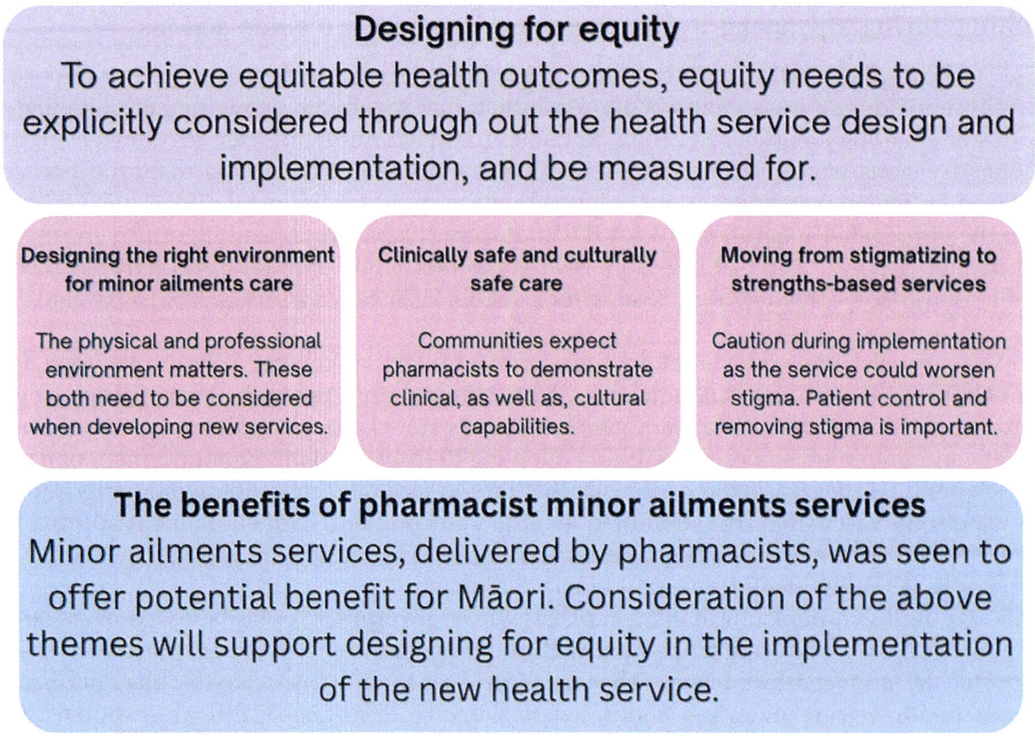

FIG. 14.1 Equitable pharmacist minor ailments service design. Aspects required to design and implement an equitable pharmacist minor ailments service.

The design and layout of pharmacy spaces emerged as particularly influential. Many participants noted that pharmacies often resembled retail stores more than healthcare facilities, which affected how they perceived and engaged with the services offered. Creating spaces that more clearly signal a focus on health care—rather than commercial activity—was seen as important for fostering trust and encouraging people to view pharmacies as reliable sources of clinical advice and treatment.

You walk in the [pharmacy] door, and you're assaulted by the stink of perfume … When you have a pharmacist who goes out into the community and meets you in a comfortable setting, not surrounded by those bright lights and shiny shelves, you're more likely to listen to what they're saying, [and the] advice on products, than someone that kinda looks like a retail salesperson.

In some pharmacies, physical barriers, such as raised dispensary counters, reinforced perceived power imbalances between pharmacists and patients.

[Pharmacists need to remove] perceived power balance between me as the Māori that goes in, versus *that very flash looking Pākehā [NZ European] behind the bench that I think is looking down on me.*

Participants' sense of safety within healthcare settings was shaped not only by their own interactions but also by observing how others were treated. Several described situations where they overheard private conversations or witnessed staff "gossiping" about other individuals. These experiences undermined their trust in the environment and led some to feel reluctant or unwilling to share personal information, even when they needed support.

A couple of times I've been there having to wait for my medication and these three ladies are like gossipers. So, hell no, gee, you tell them nothing.

4.2.2 Clinically safe and culturally safe care

This theme reflects Māori participants' perspectives on the clinical and cultural capabilities they expect from pharmacists delivering care for minor ailments. It also includes suggestions for how care can be designed to be both accessible and culturally safe.

Many participants expressed confidence in pharmacists' clinical knowledge and their ability to provide effective care for minor health concerns. They felt empowered to make informed choices about which health provider—such as a pharmacist, GP, or physiotherapist—would be most appropriate for their minor ailments care. In addition to providing frontline care, pharmacists were seen as competent and professional in recognizing when referral to another health professional was necessary. This trust often stemmed from participants' own positive experiences receiving care in pharmacy settings.

While participants generally expressed trust in the clinical expertise of pharmacists, many also shared experiences of racism and culturally unsafe care within pharmacy settings. For some, these incidents had occurred in the past yet continued to influence their sense of safety and willingness to develop professional relationships with pharmacists. These experiences ranged from subtle disregard to overtly racist encounters. One participant explained that even when the clinical care itself was not in question, the absence of a culturally safe environment was enough to deter them from seeking support. These insights highlight that clinical competence alone is not sufficient—cultural safety is essential for Māori to feel respected, understood, and willing to access care.

You can make it as accessible as you want. But if there's mamae (pain) about going into the pharmacy shop, it'll always be there. I think, in terms of cultural safety, [pharmacists] would score low, but in terms of the ability to give a really good professional advice based on their tenure of their education I wouldn't have an issue with that.

Participants identified several ways to foster culturally safe environments for Māori within pharmacy settings. A key recommendation was to grow the Māori health workforce—both pharmacists and support staff. Increasing the visibility of pharmacists' roles, particularly their capacity to provide minor ailments care within Māori communities, including in places such as te reo Māori immersion schools, was seen as a way to raise awareness of pharmacy services while also encouraging rangatahi (Māori youth) to consider pharmacy as a career pathway.

Participants also emphasized the importance of pharmacists gaining a deeper understanding of Māori culture and the historical and contemporary place of Māori in NZ. This cultural knowledge was viewed as essential for delivering care that is respectful, relevant, and safe. Building strong relationships with local community organizations and health providers was also highlighted as a way to support more holistic, connected approaches to minor ailments care.

When healthcare encounters, providers, or settings were perceived as racist or culturally unsafe, participants described withdrawing from care—an experience echoed in healthcare systems worldwide (Gadsden et al., 2019; Nelson and Wilson, 2018). Pharmacists in NZ are required to demonstrate competency in knowledge of different cultures, cultural safety, and to engage in reflective practices relating to differences between their own and others' cultures (Competence standards for Aotearoa New Zealand Pharmacists, 2023). The concepts of cultural competence and cultural safety are interrelated but distinct. While competence focuses on knowledge of other cultures and a set of skills required to deliver high-quality care, cultural safety goes further by requiring a critical examination of power relationships within clinical engagements (Curtis et al., 2025). In this framework, it is the person receiving care—not the provider—who determines whether an interaction or environment feels culturally safe.

4.2.3 Moving from stigmatizing to strengths-based services

Some minor ailment conditions, such as head lice and scabies, are associated with stigma, which can influence people's likelihood of accessing associated care and treatment (Amoako et al., 2023; Hurst et al., 2020). In our study, participants also identified with the stigma associated with certain conditions.

If you asked for something for nits [in the pharmacy], it was like you knew you were being judged. That's how it felt really. So, to be honest, when I go to a pharmacy, I try keep that time in there ... minimal.

Some participants suggested that enabling people to access minor ailments medicines directly—without needing to consult a health professional, either in the pharmacy or from collection points in schools, for example—could help reduce feelings of stigma and improve access to care. This approach was seen as particularly beneficial for those who may feel uncomfortable or judged when seeking help for certain conditions. Others suggested it could be useful to initiate targeted minor ailments services for those conditions where stigma is not associated—for example, hay fever—as a start, with other conditions being introduced later.

Maybe a drop basket or somewhere [could be used] where whānau [family] don't have to come in and engage, but they can just know that it's there.

Participants were asked whether certain groups should be prioritized for funded access to pharmacist-provided minor ailments care. While many felt this type of care should ideally be available to everyone, they also acknowledged the realities of limited resources. In that context, there was broad support for prioritizing groups more likely to experience barriers to healthcare, such as Māori, Pacific peoples, young people, older adults, and those facing financial hardship. There was a strong emphasis on ensuring eligibility policies avoid reinforcing stigma and instead reflect the lived realities of those the services aim to support.

I think one of the big stigmas for Māori and the lower economic whānau is the stigma of whakamā (shame). With those types of ailments that you spoke to [scabies and head lice], If we're gonna say that we're only going to fund those people that in the lower end of the pay scale, that's immediately gonna drag on a whakamā (shame) over them.

While stigma-related barriers to accessing healthcare have been well-documented in relation to various conditions (Knaak et al., 2017; Nguyen and Li, 2020; Chang and Cataldo, 2014) this has not previously been explored in the context of PMAS. Some participants shared negative experiences that occurred many years ago, yet these memories continued to shape their perceptions of pharmacy care in the present. These insights are important to consider when designing new services, as past experiences—positive or negative—can have a lasting impact on trust and willingness to seek care (Alcalá et al., 2018; Schwei et al., 2017).

5 Additional discussion

5.1 Benefits of critical methodologies in health services research

The application of critical methodological approaches in health services research enables the exploration of root causes of inequities, shines a light on power and marginalization within privileged and oppressed populations, and facilitates the development of service, policy, and political-level solutions designed to achieve equity (Todić et al., 2022; Paradis-Gagné and Pariseau-Legault, 2022). One of the most tangible benefits of using Kaupapa Māori methodology in the context of the research discussed in this chapter was how it enabled us to navigate power dynamics through the strength of our relationships with the communities involved. While some research methodologies might criticize our sampling strategy as introducing bias or limiting generalizability, we deliberately prioritized an approach that allowed us to meaningfully engage with people who might otherwise avoid participating in research due to past negative experiences or a lack of trust. Our team members were not arriving as outsiders, as many of us were already part of these communities or had long-standing connections with the area. That sense of kanohi kitea (being a "seen" and trusted face) helped create a level of comfort that can be difficult to achieve through standard recruitment methods, particularly when working with marginalized communities.

This trust was critical. It allowed participants to speak openly about deeply personal experiences, including racism, feelings of whakamā (shame), and past negative interactions with pharmacy services. The safe, affirming environment we were able to foster meant that the insights shared were not only richer but also grounded in the everyday realities of those we spoke with. This would have been difficult to achieve without the relational foundation that Kaupapa Māori methodology is built upon.

5.2 Broader application of the practices used in Kaupapa Māori research

Kaupapa Māori is distinct from other forms of critical research due to its grounding in te ao Māori (the Māori world), use of te Tiriti o Waitangi as a foundational framework, and focus on tino rangatiratanga and mana motuhake. While self-determination is a concept that may be present in other cultures and critical methodologies, tino rangatiratanga and mana motuhake are forms of political and spiritual authority that are uniquely Māori. However, while Kaupapa Māori methodology is notably grounded in Māori worldviews, values, and tikanga (protocols) and was developed to aid research with Māori, the methodology still holds significant learnings for research outside of this setting.

Practices such as kanohi kitea, manaaki ki te tangata, and kia tūpato are values important for research involving any marginalized community. Moreover, whanaungatanga (connection and relationship development) is central to the research process with all such communities. Relationship-building should not just be a methodological step but a foundational practice to be sustained throughout the life of a project. This includes kanohi-ki-te-kanohi (face-to-face) engagement, reciprocal information sharing, and ongoing feedback loops that reflect the values of trust, respect, and reciprocity (Royal, 2018). Research hui, whakawhiti kōrero (exchanges), and wānanga are all examples of culturally embedded practices that enable deep, respectful engagement with communities.

In addition, sharing results with participants and communities in accessible, culturally appropriate ways is a core requirement of Kaupapa Māori research that is also applicable to other settings. This might include returning to community spaces (halls, churches, clubs, etc.) to disseminate findings, creating bilingual summaries, or engaging in coauthorship with community leaders (F. Cram, 2009) Citation itself becomes a Kaupapa Māori practice, as Hana Burgess et al. suggest; citing Māori scholars and thought leaders is an act of whanaungatanga, recognition, and intellectual sovereignty (Burgess et al., 2021). Likewise, researchers working with other marginalized cultures should also cite scholarship from within those cultures.

A word of caution, though: other cultures and marginalized groups will have their own unique values, concepts, and historical, political, and cultural realities that should be privileged when undertaking critical research with non-Māori. It should not be automatically assumed that the principles outlined in this chapter will fit neatly into these spaces, and engaging in meaningful dialog with communities in the design phase of the research is always encouraged to ensure methods are appropriate and safe. Instead of suggesting that non-Māori researchers should adopt Kaupapa Māori methodology, we are showcasing the value and benefit of applying critical methodological practices that are relevant to the communities and people with whom you are doing research.

5.3 Tools and frameworks to design for equity

Researchers working in the sphere of health equity and equitable health service development use a variety of tools to frame, plan, and evaluate their research. One common tool is the CONSolIDated critERia for strengthening the reporting of health research involving Indigenous Peoples (CONSIDER) statement. The CONSIDER statement is a reporting guideline that aims to strengthen the reporting of health research involving Indigenous Peoples (Huria et al., 2019). It does so by specifying that research papers should report on the following eight domains to ensure the quality, transparency, and ethical standards of research involving Indigenous Peoples: governance, prioritization, relationships, methodologies, participation, capacity, analysis and interpretation, and dissemination. These domains emphasize the importance of partnership, accountability, responsiveness, reciprocity, and cultural safety, thus motivating researchers to move beyond tokenistic engagement toward meaningful collaboration with participants. While it is primarily published as a reporting tool, it can be equally useful for planning purposes when designing health research involving Indigenous Peoples.

Readers interested in additional equity-based frameworks or tools are referred to the Health Equity Assessment Tool (Signal et al., 2008), the Equity-focused Implementation Framework (Gustafson et al., 2024), and the Conceptual Framework of Equity-focused Implementation Research for Health Programs (Eslava-Schmalbach et al., 2019). There are also equity-focused tools developed specifically for certain stages of research, such as the Readiness Assessment for Pragmatic Trials—Indigenous model (Hikaka et al., 2024).

5.4 Inform government policy and evaluate a new service

Too often, government policy in health focuses on winning the support of the majority, given the politicization of health and the pressure on political parties to attract as many voters as possible. Consequently, health services are typically designed to meet the needs of the many, rather than addressing the realities of marginalized communities who face poorer, unjust, and inequitable health outcomes. This pattern is becoming increasingly common as societal divides deepen, with some governments not recognizing the historical, political, social, and cultural contexts that have contributed to these disparities, and therefore refuting the need for targeted action.

It is important to note, however, that critical methodologies, like Kaupapa Māori methodology, are not partisan. Their strength lies in the grounding of lived experience, focus on social change, and ability to challenge the power structures ingrained in the status quo. While health researchers using critical methodologies need to be cognizant of the political context in which they conduct research and how this impacts the design and implementation of health services, it should not detract from the use of critical approaches that aim to improve outcomes for those most often left behind. In fact, it is precisely in these contexts that critical methodologies are most needed. Critical research can help ensure governments and health systems both design and evaluate services that are not only effective but also fair, inclusive, and responsive to the realities experienced by underserved communities. The research presented in this chapter sought to elevate and give power to Māori communities when exploring the topic of minor ailment care, not only by highlighting experiences but also by developing solutions to current inequities. This was only made possible through the intentional use of Kaupapa Māori methodology.

6 Questions for further discussion

1. What are some of the key components of practices in Kaupapa Māori methodology that align with the approaches you use in research?
2. What are some considerations when facilitating data collection events with marginalized groups?
3. What are some of the benefits to health services research when power-sharing research practices are utilized?
4. How might the evaluation of a current health service by Indigenous or marginalized communities inform and shape the design of current or future health services and research practices?

7 Application exercise—scenario

Your research team is developing a research project aimed at addressing inequities in outcomes in pharmacist-led diabetes services in your local health region. You want to understand why inequities are occurring and develop an initiative to achieve equity. How will you build a research team to investigate this issue? What tools would be useful to help you plan for equity from the beginning of your work? How will you involve communities of interest in the design of the initiative, evaluation of success, and translation of research findings into practice?

Pearls/Reflective prompts

What are some important social and cultural contexts relevant to the research project you are currently involved in?

Who are the important groups and partners who should be involved in a research project you are currently working on? How can you foster relationships with these groups?

What is your experience with privilege and oppression in your own life? How might these experiences influence the research you conduct?

Who are some important research mentors in your work? What opportunities and skills do you bring to mentoring others?

Which practices guide the research you conduct, and how do you respond when the research does not go as planned?

How would taking a critical approach to your research be beneficial?

Do you use equity-based frameworks in your research? Do the examples provided align with the research you conduct?

References

Alcalá, H.E., Valdez-Dadia, A., von Ehrenstein, O.S., 2018. Adverse childhood experiences and access and utilization of health care. J. Public Health. 1741-3842. 40 (4), 684–692. doi:10.1093/pubmed/fdx155.

Aly, M., García-Cárdenas, V., Williams, K., Benrimoj, S.I., 2018. A review of international pharmacy-based minor ailment services and proposed service design model. Res. Social Adm. Pharm. 15517411. 14 (11), 989–998. Available from http://www.journals.elsevierhealth.com/periodicals/rsap. doi:10.1016/j.sapharm.2017.12.004.

Amoako, Y.A., van Rietschoten, L.S., Oppong, M.N., Amoako, K.O., Abass, K.M., Anim, B.A., Laryea, D.O., Phillips, R.O., Stienstra, Y., 2023. Beliefs, attitudes and practices towards scabies in central Ghana. PLoS Negl. Trop. Dis. 19352735. 17 (2). Available from https://journals.plos.org/plosntds/article?id=10.1371/journal.pntd.0011175. doi:10.1371/journal.pntd.0011175.

Baciu, A., Negussie, Y., Geller, A., Weinstein, J.N., 2017. Communities in Action: Pathways to Health Equity. National Academies Press, Washington, D.C.

Baqir, W., Learoyd, T., Sim, A., Todd, A., 2011. Cost analysis of a community pharmacy 'minor ailment scheme' across three primary care trusts in the North East of England. J. Public Health. 17413850. 33 (4), 551–555. doi:10.1093/pubmed/fdr012.

Baugh-Harris, S., Wanzer-Serrano, D., 2018. Against canon: engaging the imperative of race in rhetoric. Commun. Crit. Cult. Stud. 14794233. 15 (4), 337–342. Available from http://www.tandfonline.com/toc/rccc20/current. doi:10.1080/14791420.2018.1526386.

Bishop, R., 1999. [Waikato University] Kaupapa Maori Research: An indigenous approach to creating knowledge (Thesis). https://researchcommons.waikato.ac.nz/bitstream/10289/874/1/1999%20Bishop.pdf.

Burgess, H., Cormack, D., Reid, P., 2021. Calling forth our pasts, citing our futures: an envisioning of a kaupapa Māori citational practice. MAI J. 10 (1), 58–68.

Cayir, E., Felder, T.M., Nkwonta, C.A., Jackson, J.R., Dawson, R., 2022. Discovering New Connections: insights From Individual and Collective Reflexivity in a Mixed Methods Study. Int. J. Qual. Methods. 16094069. 21. Available from https://journals.sagepub.com/home/IJQ. doi:10.1177/16094069221105707.

Chang, S.-H., Cataldo, J.K., 2014. A systematic review of global cultural variations in knowledge, attitudes and health responses to tuberculosis stigma. Int. J. Tuberc. Lung Dis. 1027-3719. 18 (2), 168–173. doi:10.5588/ijtld.13.0181.

Chilisa, B., Situating knowledge systems Indigenous research methodologies. (2020), 1–17

Competence standards for Aotearoa New Zealand Pharmacists, 2023.

Cram, F., 2009. Kaupapa Māori evaluation: a culturally grounded approach to evaluation. N.Z. J. Eval. 15 (1), 7–14.

Cram, F., Kennedy, V., 2010. Researching with whānau collectives. Mai Rev. 3 (1), 1–12.

Cram, F., 2009. Maintaining Indigenous Voices. SAGE Publications, pp. 308–322. doi:10.4135/9781483348971.n20.

Cumming, J., 2022. Going hard and early: aotearoa New Zealand's response to Covid-19. Health Economics, Policy and Law. 1744-1331. 17 (1), 107–119. doi:10.1017/s174413312100013x.

Curtis, E., Loring, B., Jones, R., Tipene-Leach, D., Walker, C., Paine, S.J., Reid, P., 2025. Refining the definitions of cultural safety, cultural competency and Indigenous health: lessons from Aotearoa New Zealand. Int. J. Equity Health. 14759276. 24 (1). Available from https://equityhealthj.biomedcentral.com. doi:10.1186/s12939-025-02478-3.

Curtis, E., 2016. Indigenous Positioning in Health Research: the importance of Kaupapa Māori theory-informed practice. AlterNative. 1177-1801. 12 (4), 396–410. doi:10.20507/alternative.2016.12.4.5.

Curtis, E., Loring, B., Latham, K., Jordan, A., Chee, N., Hunia, R., Snowden, K., Tari, K., Murupaenga, P., Tipene, R., Whitcombe, S., Embers, K., Jansen, R.M., 2024. An innovative Indigenous-led model for integrated COVID-19 case management in Auckland, New Zealand: lessons from implementation. Front. Public Health. 2296-2565. 12. doi:10.3389/fpubh.2024.1324239.

Datta, S., Vattiato, G., Maclaren, O.J., Hua, N., Sporle, A., Plank, M.J., 2024. The impact of Covid-19 vaccination in Aotearoa New Zealand: a modelling study. Vaccine. 18732518. 42 (6), 1383–1391. Available from https://www.sciencedirect.com/science/journal/0264410X. doi:10.1016/j.vaccine.2024.01.101.

Davies, C., Timu-Parata, C., Stairmand, J., Robson, B., Kvalsvig, A., Lum, D., Signal, V., 2022. A kia ora, a wave and a smile: an urban marae-led response to COVID-19, a case study in manaakitanga. Int. J. Equity Health. 14759276. 21 (1). Available from http://www.equityhealthj.com/home/. doi:10.1186/s12939-022-01667-8.

Dawes, T., Muru-Lanning, M., Lapsley, H., Hopa, N., Dixon, N., Moore, C., Tukiri, C., Jones, N., Muru-Lanning, C., Moana, O., 2021. Hongi, Harirū and Hau: kaumātua in the time of COVID-19. J. R. Soc. N. Z. 0303-6758. 51 (sup1), S23. doi:10.1080/03036758.2020.1853182.

Denzin, N., Lincoln, Y., The SAGE Handbook of Qualitative Research. (2018),

Dineen-Griffin, S., Garcia-Cardenas, V., Rogers, K., Williams, K., Benrimoj, S.I., 2019. Evaluation of a Collaborative Protocolized Approach by Community Pharmacists and General Medical Practitioners for an Australian Minor Ailments Scheme: protocol for a Cluster Randomized Controlled Trial. JMIR Res. Protoc. 1929-0748. 8 (8), e13973. doi:10.2196/13973.

Durie, M., Whaiora: māori health development. (1998), 68–74

Eslava-Schmalbach, J., Garzón-Orjuela, N., Elias, V., Reveiz, L., Tran, N., Langlois, E.V., 2019. Conceptual framework of equity-focused implementation research for health programs (EquIR). Int. J. Equity Health. 14759276. 18 (1). Available from http://www.equityhealthj.com/home/. doi:10.1186/s12939-019-0984-4.

Ford, C.L., Airhihenbuwa, C.O., 2010. The public health critical race methodology: praxis for antiracism research. Soc. Sci. Med. 02779536. 71 (8), 1390–1398. doi:10.1016/j.socscimed.2010.07.030.

Gadsden, T., Wilson, G., Totterdell, J., Willis, J., Gupta, A., Chong, A., Clarke, A., Winters, M., Donahue, K., Posenelli, S., Maher, L., Stewart, J., Gardiner, H., Passmore, E., Cashmore, A., Milat, A., 2019. Can a continuous quality improvement program create culturally safe emergency departments for Aboriginal people in Australia? A multiple baseline study. BMC Health Serv. Res. 1472-6963. 19 (1). doi:10.1186/s12913-019-4049-6.

Grimes, A., White, D., 2019. Digital Inclusion and Wellbeing in New Zealand. SSRN. 15565068. Available from https://www.ssrn.com/index.cfm/en/. doi:10.2139/ssrn.3492833.

Gurney, J., Stanley, J., Sarfati, D., 2020. The inequity of morbidity: disparities in the prevalence of morbidity between ethnic groups in New Zealand. J. Comorb. 2235-042X. 10, 2235042X2097116. doi:10.1177/2235042x20971168.

Gustafson, P., Lambert, M., Bartholomew, K., Ratima, M., Aziz, Y.A., Kremer, L., Fusheini, A., Carswell, P., Brown, R., Priest, P., Crengle, S., 2024. Adapting an equity-focused implementation process framework with a focus on ethnic health inequities in the Aotearoa New Zealand context. Int. J. Equity Health. 14759276. 23 (1). Available from https://equityhealthj.biomedcentral.com. doi:10.1186/s12939-023-02087-y.

Hauora -Report on Stage One of the Health Services and Outcomes Kaupapa Inquiry, 2019.

Hensen, B., Mackworth-Young, C.R.S., Simwinga, M., Abdelmagid, N., Banda, J., Mavodza, C., Doyle, A.M., Bonell, C., Weiss, H.A., 2021. Remote data collection for public health research in a COVID-19 era: ethical implications, challenges and opportunities. Health Policy Plan. 1460-2237. 36 (3), 360–368. doi:10.1093/heapol/czaa158.

Hikaka, J., McCreedy, E.M., Jutkowitz, E., McCarthy, E.P., Baier, R.R., 2024. Modifications of the readiness assessment for pragmatic trials tool for appropriate use with Indigenous populations. BMC Med. Res. Methodol. 14712288. 24 (1). Available from https://bmcmedresmethodol.biomedcentral.com/. doi:10.1186/s12874-024-02244-z.

Hikaka, J., Haua, R., Parore, N., McIntosh, B., Anderson, A., Pewhairangi, K., Brown, R., 2023. Designing for health equity: a mixed method study exploring community experiences and perceptions of pharmacists' role in minor ailment care. Res. Social Adm. Pharm. 15517411. 19 (4), 643–652. doi:10.1016/j.sapharm.2022.12.011.

Hikaka, J., Haua, R., 2022. Examining equity in a void of evidence - Pharmacist minor ailments services and the role of systematic reviews. Explor. Res. Clin. Soc. Pharm. 26672766. 7, 100174. doi:10.1016/j.rcsop.2022.100174.

Huria, T., Palmer, S.C., Pitama, S., Beckert, L., Lacey, C., Ewen, S., Smith, L.T., 2019. Consolidated criteria for strengthening reporting of health research involving indigenous peoples: the CONSIDER statement. BMC Med. Res. Methodol. 14712288. 19 (1). Available from http://www.biomedcentral.com/bmcmedresmethodol/. doi:10.1186/s12874-019-0815-8.

Hurst, S.K., Dotson, J.A.W., Butterfield, P., Corbett, C.F., Oneal, G., 2020. Stigma resulting from head lice infestation: a concept analysis and implications for public health. Nurs. Forum. 17446198. 55 (2), 252–258. Available from http://onlinelibrary.wiley.com/journal/10.1111/(ISSN)1744-6198. doi:10.1111/nuf.12423.

Jefferies, S., French, N., Gilkison, C., Graham, G., Hope, V., Marshall, J., McElnay, C., McNeill, A., Muellner, P., Paine, S., Prasad, N., Scott, J., Sherwood, J., Yang, L., Priest, P., 2020. COVID-19 in New Zealand and the impact of the national response: a descriptive epidemiological study. Lancet Public Health. 24682667. 5 (11), e612. Available from http://thelancet.com/journals/lanpub/issue/vol1no2/PIIS2468-2667(16)X0003-5. doi:10.1016/S2468-2667(20)30225-5.

Jefferies, S., Gilkison, C., Duff, P., Grey, C., French, N., Carr, H., Priest, P., Crengle, S., 2025. Ethnic equity in Aotearoa New Zealand's COVID-19 response: a descriptive epidemiological study. Public Health. 00333506. 244, 105732. doi:10.1016/j.puhe.2025.105732.

Jeffreys, M., Pledger, M., McKenzie, F., Ellison-Loschmann, L., Lopez, M.I., Cumming, J., 2024. Consequences of cost barriers to prescriptions: cohort study in Aotearoa New Zealand. N. Z. Med. J. 11758716. 137 (1595), 48–63. Available from https://nzmj.org.nz/media/pages/journal/vol-137-no-1595/consequences-of-cost-barriers-to-prescriptions-cohort-study-in-aotearoa-new-zealand/10418895de-1715896898/6431.pdf. doi:10.26635/6965.6431.

Knaak, S., Mantler, E., Szeto, A., 2017. Mental illness-related stigma in healthcare: barriers to access and care and evidence-based solutions. Healthc. Manage. Forum. 23523883. 30 (2), 111–116. Available from https://journals.sagepub.com/home/HMF. doi:10.1177/0840470416679413.

Lobe, B., Morgan, D., Hoffman, K.A., 2020. Qualitative Data Collection in an Era of Social Distancing. Int. J. Qual. Methods. 16094069. 19. Available from http://ijq.sagepub.com/content/by/year. doi:10.1177/1609406920937875.

McIntosh, T., Māori identities: fixed, fluid, forced New Zealand identities: departures and destinations. (2005), 38–51

McKinley, E., Smith, L.T., 2019. Towards Self-Determination in Indigenous Education Research: An Introduction. Springer Science and Business Media LLC, pp. 1–15. doi:10.1007/978-981-10-1839-8_77-2.

McKinley, L.S., 2019. Handbook of Indigenous Education. Springer, pp. 413–432.

Metcalfe, S., Beyene, K., Urlich, J., Jones, R., Proffitt, C., Harrison, J., Andrews, Ā., 2018. Te wero tonu—the challenge continues: māori access to medicines 2006/07–2012/13 update. N. Z. Med. J. 11758716. 131 (1485), 27–47. Available from http://www.nzma.org.nz/__data/assets/pdf_file/0004/86008/Metcalfe-FINAL.pdf.

Moewaka Barnes, H., Harmsworth, G., Tipa, G., Henwood, W., McCreanor, T., 2021. Indigenous-led environmental research in Aotearoa New Zealand: beyond a transdisciplinary model for best practice, empowerment and action. AlterNative. 1177-1801. 17 (2), 306–316. doi:10.1177/11771801211019397.

Morrow, R.A., Brown, D.D., 1994. Critical theory and methodology. Sage 3.

Nelson, S.E., Wilson, K., 2018. Understanding barriers to health care access through cultural safety and ethical space: indigenous people's experiences in Prince George, Canada. Soc Sci Med. 02779536. 218, 21–27. doi:10.1016/j.socscimed.2018.09.017.

Newman, A., Bavik, Y.L., Mount, M., Shao, B., 2021. Data Collection via Online Platforms: challenges and Recommendations for Future Research. Appl Psychol. 14640597. 70 (3), 1380–1402. Available from http://onlinelibrary.wiley.com/journal/10.1111/(ISSN)1464-0597. doi:10.1111/apps.12302.

Nguyen, T., Li, X., 2020. Understanding public-stigma and self-stigma in the context of dementia: a systematic review of the global literature. Dementia. 17412684. 19 (2), 148–181. Available from http://www.sagepub.com/journalsProdDesc.nav?prodId=Journal201266. doi:10.1177/1471301218800122.

Nicholls, L., Parore, N., Buckthought, L., 2021. He Wānanga Whakarite: preparing Māori for surgical selection interviews. ANZ J. Surg. 14452197. 91 (6), 1143–1147. Available from http://onlinelibrary.wiley.com/journal/10.1111/(ISSN)1445-2197. doi:10.1111/ans.16864.

Ora, T.W., 2024. 2023 Minor Health Conditions Service Pilot Evaluation Report.

Paradis-Gagné, E., Pariseau-Legault, P., 2022. Critical Research and Qualitative Methodologies: theoretical Foundations and Contribution to Nursing Research. Res. Theory Nurs. Pract. 15416577. 36 (2), 119–138. Available from http://www.ingentaconnect.com/content/springer/rtnp. doi:10.1891/RTNP-2021-0014.

Paudyal, V., Watson, M.C., Sach, T., Porteous, T., Bond, C.M., Wright, D.J., Cleland, J., Barton, G., Holland, R., 2013. Are pharmacy-based minor ailment schemes a substitute for other service providers? A systematic review. Br. J. Gen. Pract. 09601643. 63 (612), e472. Available from: http://docserver.ingentaconnect.com/deliver/connect/rcgp/09601643/v63n612/s26.pdf?expires=1374213874&id=74911465&titleid=30000031&accname=Elsevier+BV&checksum=E58CD179A4D75143A71DAC885C20CBD2. doi:10.3399/bjgp13X669194.

Pihama, L., 2010. Kaupapa Māori theory: transforming theory in Aotearoa. He Pukenga Korero 9 (2), 5–14.

Pihama, L., Lipsham, M., 2020. Noho haumaru: reflecting on Māori approaches to staying safe during Covid-19 in Aotearoa (New Zealand). J. Indig. Soc. Dev. 9 (3), 92–101.

Pohatu, T.W., 2013. Āta. Ata J. Psychother. Aotearoa N. Z. 2253-5853. 17 (1), 13–26. doi:10.9791/ajpanz.2013.02.

Rigney, L.-I., 1999. Internationalization of an Indigenous Anticolonial Cultural Critique of Research Methodologies: a Guide to Indigenist Research Methodology and Its Principles. Wicazo Sa Rev. 07496427 14 (2), 109. doi:10.2307/1409555.

Royal, T., Politics and knowledge: kaupapa Māori and mātauranga Māori Handbook of Indigenous Education. (2018), 437–450

Russell, L., Levy, M., Barnao, E., Parore, N., Smiler, K., Boulton, A., 2023. Enacting Mana Māori Motuhake during COVID-19 in Aotearoa (New Zealand): "We Weren't Waiting to Be Told What to Do". Int. J. Environ. Res. Public Health. 1660-4601. 20 (8), 5581. doi:10.3390/ijerph20085581.

Salvador, P.T.C.D.O., Alves, K.Y.A., Rodrigues, C.C.F.M., Oliveira, L.V.E., 2020. Online data collection strategies used in qualitative research of the health field: a scoping review. Revista Gaucha de Enfermagem. 19831447. 41. Available from https://www.scielo.br/j/rgenf/a/ZTDgnm7Y8f8KhKr6jbCKddK/?format=pdf&lang=en. doi:10.1590/1983-1447.2020.20190297.

Schwei, R.J., Johnson, T.P., Matthews, A.K., Jacobs, E.A., 2017. Perceptions of negative health-care experiences and self-reported health behavior change in three racial and ethnic groups. Ethn Health. 14653419. 22 (2), 156–168. Available from www.tandf.co.uk/journals/titles/13557858.asp. doi:10.1080/13557858.2016.1244621.

Signal, J.M., Cram, B.R., 2008. The health equity assessment tool: a user's guide. Ministry of Health.

Skivington, K., Matthews, L., Simpson, S.A., Craig, P., Baird, J., Blazeby, J.M., Boyd, K.A., Craig, N., French, D.P., McIntosh, E., Petticrew, M., Rycroft-Malone, J., White, M., Moore, L., 2021. A new framework for developing and evaluating complex interventions: update of Medical Research Council guidance. BMJ. 374:n2061. Available from http://www.bmj.com/. doi:10.1136/bmj.n2061.

Smith, L., Opening keynote: story-ing the development of Kaupapa Māori - A review of sorts. Kei Tua o Te Pae Hui Proceedings. (2011),

Smith, L.T., 2023. Decolonizing methodologies: research and indigenous peoples Foundational Concepts of Decolonial and Southern Epistemologies. Channel View Publications, pp. 159–181.

Statistics, 2025. 2023 Census population counts (by ethnic group, age, and Māori descent) and dwelling counts [Internet]. Available from: https://www.stats.govt.nz/information-releases/2023-census-population-counts-by-ethnic-group-age-and-maori-descent-and-dwelling-counts/.

Steyn, N., Binny, R.N., Hannah, K., Hendy, S.C., James, A., Kukutai, T., Lustig, A., McLeod, M., Plank, M.J., Ridings, K., Sporle, A., 2020a. Estimated inequities in COVID-19 infection fatality rates by ethnicity for Aotearoa New Zealand. N. Z. Med. J. 11758716. 133 (1521), 28–39. Available from https://journal.nzma.org.nz/journal-articles/estimated-inequities-in-covid-19-infection-fatality-rates-by-ethnicity-for-aotearoa-new-zealand.

Steyn, N., Binny, R.N., Hannah, K., Hendy, S.C., James, A., Lustig, A., Ridings, K., Plank, M.J., Sporle, A., 2020b. Māori and Pacific people in New Zealand have higher risk of hospitalisation for COVID-19. medRxiv. Available from https://www.medrxiv.org/. doi:10.1101/2020.12.25.20248427.

Thomas, D.R., 2006. A General Inductive Approach for Analyzing Qualitative Evaluation Data. Am. J. Eval. 10982140. 27 (2), 237–246. doi:10.1177/1098214005283748.

Todić, J., Cook, S.C., Spitzer-Shohat, S., Williams, J.S., Battle, B.A., Jackson, J., Chin, M.H., 2022. Critical Theory, Culture Change, and Achieving Health Equity in Health Care Settings. Acad. Med. 1938808X. 7, 977–988. https://journals.lww.com/academicmedicine/pages/default.aspx. doi:10.1097/ACM.0000000000004680.

Wilson, S., 2020. Research Is Ceremony: Indigenous Research Methods [Internet], Fenwood Publishing.

CHAPTER

15

Scoping reviews in pharmacy and health services research

Cathal Cadogan[a], *Nátalia Stollárová*[a,b], *Michelle Cleary*[c], *Carmel Doyle*[c], *and Cristín Ryan*[a]

[a]School of Pharmacy and Pharmaceutical Sciences, Trinity College Dublin, Dublin, Ireland
[b]Department of Pharmacology and Toxicology, Faculty of Pharmacy, Comenius University Bratislava, Bratislava, Slovakia
[c]School of Nursing and Midwifery, Trinity College Dublin, Dublin, Ireland

CHAPTER OBJECTIVES

- Discuss the role of scoping reviews in evidence-based practice
- Differentiate between scoping reviews and systematic reviews
- Outline the key stages of a scoping review
- Describe the key components of a scoping review protocol
- Discuss key considerations for data extraction and analysis

1 Introduction

Evidence-based healthcare in pharmacy, medicine, and other healthcare disciplines integrates healthcare professionals' practical experience with the best available evidence, as well as patients' preferences and values, to achieve optimal patient outcomes (Alexa et al., 2025). A key challenge for healthcare professionals is that the evidence base underpinning modern science is growing at such a pace that it can be difficult to keep abreast. For example, a previous analysis of scientific publications estimated that the number of publications is growing exponentially and doubling approximately every seventeen years (Bornmann et al., 2021). Consequently, evidence synthesis methods have an increasingly important role in evidence-based healthcare.

The systematic review has a long-standing and established history in healthcare in terms of its role in developing clinical guidelines, setting policy, and informing decision-making at governmental and organizational levels (Moher et al., 2012). Systematic reviews involve the use of systematic methods and explicit eligibility criteria to identify, appraise, and summarize results from all the available studies that meet inclusion criteria, using reproducible methods that minimize bias and errors (Brignardello-Petersen et al., 2025). However, scoping reviews are also now recognized as an important part of evidence synthesis (Moher et al., 2015) and are increasingly used in pharmacy

Contemporary Research Methods in Pharmacy and Health Services - Volume 2
https://doi.org/10.1016/B978-0-443-44607-8.00001-7

and the wider field of health services research (Ní Sheachnasaigh et al., 2022; Johnson et al., 2025; Brandt et al., 2024; Jeffares et al., 2025; Cadogan et al., 2020). A scoping review is defined as "a type of evidence synthesis that aims to systematically identify and map the breadth of evidence available on a particular topic, field, concept, or issue, often irrespective of source (i.e., primary research, reviews, nonempirical evidence) within or across particular contexts" (Munn et al., 2022). Scoping reviews can be used to provide comprehensive overviews of existing research and policy, highlight knowledge gaps that need to be addressed, and identify areas for future evidence synthesis (Peters et al., 2021).

A seminal paper by Munn et al. has compared key defining characteristics between scoping and systematic reviews (Table 15.1) and provided guidance on when a scoping review is considered appropriate (Munn et al., 2018). Systematic reviews seek to identify evidence relating to specific questions and to appraise and synthesize the search results with a view to informing healthcare policy, clinical practice, and, in some cases, future research. A systematic review is the most suitable approach when researchers want to address questions regarding the feasibility or effectiveness of a specified intervention (Peters et al., 2021). For example, a previous systematic review examined the efficacy of pharmacist-led interventions on health outcomes for patients with severe mental illness (i.e., schizophrenia or bipolar affective disorder) (Pimenta Netto et al., 2026). Based on a metaanalysis involving statistical synthesis of data from four of the seven included randomized controlled trials (RCTs), the interventions were found to have had a positive effect on patients' quality of life. However, the review also highlighted that the identified studies had a high risk of bias, which led the authors to conclude that additional high-quality RCTs were needed.

Scoping reviews, on the other hand, are conducted to provide a comprehensive overview of existing research and can help clarify key concepts and definitions in the literature. They can also help identify knowledge gaps and act as a precursor to systematic reviews by identifying the evidence that exists on a particular topic (Pollock et al., 2024). Scoping reviews are considered the correct approach for addressing review questions that focus on identifying, exploring, mapping, or reporting key characteristics or concepts in a field of research and can also incorporate evidence from a range of sources (Peters et al., 2021). For example, a scoping review by Rodriguez et al. examined a much broader question, which sought to classify the mental health services for severe mental illness that have been evaluated using RCTs (Rodriguez et al., 2025). The review included 233 studies and classified services into eight categories. In contrast to the previously discussed systematic review by Pimenta Netto et al., the scoping review did not pool outcome data using a metaanalysis, nor did it report on the effectiveness of the services or conduct a critical appraisal of the identified studies (Rodriguez et al., 2025). Instead, it focused on providing a comprehensive overview of existing research and highlighted the need for better quality reporting of interventions in future study reports. These examples serve to illustrate key differences between the types of questions that can be answered by systematic reviews and scoping reviews, respectively.

Several methodological frameworks and reporting guidelines have been developed to promote transparency and consistency in the methods and terminology used in relation to scoping reviews. The first methodological framework for scoping reviews was published by Arksey and O'Malley in 2005 and outlined five stages: (1) identifying the research question; (2) identifying relevant studies; (3) selecting studies for inclusion; (4) charting the data; and (5) collating, summarizing, and reporting the results (Arksey and O'Malley, 2005). The methodological framework for scoping reviews has evolved over subsequent years, primarily led by the Joanna Briggs Institute (JBI), which published a seminal guidance paper in 2015 (Peters et al., 2015). This guidance was subsequently updated in 2020 (Peters et al., 2020). The Preferred Reporting Items for Systematic Reviews extension for Scoping Reviews (PRISMA-ScR) checklist was published in 2018 to promote a greater understanding of relevant scoping review concepts and terminology and to outline key items to ensure consistency in the reporting of scoping reviews (Tricco et al., 2018).

TABLE 15.1 Comparison of key defining characteristics between scoping reviews and systematic reviews.

	Scoping review	Systematic review
Review protocol	Yes	Yes
Detailed search strategy	Yes	Yes
Standardised data extraction forms	Yes	Yes
Mandatory critical appraisal	No	Yes
Synthesis of outcome data/results from individual studies using metaanalysis or metasynthesis	No	Yes

Adapted from Munn, Z., Peters, M.D.J., Stern, C., Tufanaru, C., McArthur, A., Aromataris, E., 2018. Systematic review or scoping review? Guidance for authors when choosing between a systematic or scoping review approach. BMC Med. Res. Methodol. 14712288. 18 (1). Available from http://www.biomedcentral.com/bmcmedresmethodol/, used under Creative Commons Attribution (CC BY) license.

This chapter provides guidance on how to conduct a scoping review, using a previous scoping review to illustrate the key steps and highlight lessons learned. The chapter draws primarily from the experience of conducting a scoping review that formed an important component of a prior research project on potentially inappropriate prescribing in older adults with cancer receiving palliative care (Cadogan et al., 2021a; Cadogan et al., 2021b). This project employed a Delphi consensus exercise to develop criteria for identifying potentially inappropriate prescribing of medications for symptom relief in older adults (≥65 years) with cancer who were receiving palliative care (Cadogan et al., 2021a) . Before the Delphi exercise, a scoping review was conducted to inform the development of a draft list of criteria, which were subsequently presented to an expert panel over two rounds of an online Delphi questionnaire (Cadogan et al., 2021b). The scoping review provided a broad overview of existing research by characterizing prescribing practices in patients receiving palliative care and examining the methods used to evaluate these practices. A scoping review was deemed the most appropriate approach because it offered a descriptive overview of existing research and helped identify relevant knowledge gaps. A systematic review was not undertaken, as the authors were not aiming to perform any statistical synthesis of data from the included studies or appraise their methodological quality.

2 Methods

The scoping review by Cadogan et al., presented in this chapter, was conducted in accordance with JBI guidance published in 2015 (Peters et al., 2015). As previously noted, this guidance was subsequently updated in 2020 (Peters et al., 2020). Therefore, the methods below describe what was done in the original review and emphasize what has changed in terms of the latest available guidance.

The key stages of a scoping review are presented in Table 15.2. The PRISMA-ScR checklist details key information that should be reported in scoping reviews (Tricco et al., 2018) and a PRISMA-ScR checklist can be included as an appendix for a completed scoping review. It is important to note that the PRISMA-ScR checklist is not a methodological guideline for conducting a scoping review. Instead, it is intended to be used as a complementary checklist alongside relevant methodological guidance (e.g., as published by JBI) to support the comprehensive and transparent reporting of a scoping review's methods and findings (Peters et al., 2021).

2.1 Developing a protocol

Developing a protocol is a vital first step when undertaking a scoping review. As with a systematic review, a protocol can help to improve transparency, reduce the potential for bias, and ultimately enhance the trustworthiness of the final review findings by specifying the scoping review's aims and proposed methods at the outset (Peters et al., 2022). As was recognized in the guidance paper by Peters et al. (2015), deviations from the original protocol may be necessary with a scoping review due to its iterative nature. However, where any deviations occur, they should be documented and justified in the final review.

The updated guidance by Peters et al. (2020) includes additional discussion points on options for registering and publishing scoping review protocols. These include open-access platforms such as Open Science Framework, Research Square, and Figshare. It should be noted that the PROSPERO database is dedicated exclusively to systematic reviews and does not currently accept scoping reviews for registration. There is also a JBI journal called JBI Evidence Synthesis that publishes scoping review protocols and subsequent reviews conducted in accordance with the JBI methodology. In order for a scoping review protocol to be published in JBI Evidence Synthesis, authors must

TABLE 15.2 Key stages of a scoping review as outlined by the Joanna Briggs Institute (Peters et al., 2020).

(1) Develop a protocol
(2) Specify the scoping review title and questions
(3) Define the inclusion criteria
(4) Develop the search strategy
(5) Screen and select evidence
(6) Data extraction
(7) Data analysis
(8) Present the results

pay a publication fee unless they qualify for an exemption (e.g., affiliation with a JBI Center or Group). The journal operates a hybrid publishing model for completed reviews, whereby authors can elect to make the article open access upon payment of a publication fee. If authors do not pay a publication fee, access to the article will be restricted to journal subscribers.

Since the publication of the updated guidance on scoping reviews by Peters et al. (2020), separate dedicated guidance has been published on developing and reporting protocols for scoping reviews (Peters et al., 2022). This guidance includes recommended items for inclusion in a protocol under each of the relevant stages (Stages 2.2–2.8 below).

The scoping review by Cadogan et al. (2021b) presented in this chapter had a protocol developed a priori, which is available from the authors upon request. Subsequent scoping reviews that the authors have been involved in have registered and/or published their protocols on various open-access platforms (Murphy et al., 2020; Boland et al., 2022; Cole et al., 2023; Cleary et al., 2026).

2.2 Specify the scoping review title and questions

The scoping review title and review question should be clear, aligned with the topic, and incorporate key elements of the inclusion criteria. The population, concept, context (PCC) framework, which is discussed in more detail under Stage 2.3 below, can also help ensure the clarity of the review title and its alignment with the review question.

For example, the review presented in this chapter was titled: "Prescribing practices, patterns, and potential harms in patients receiving palliative care: A systematic scoping review" (Cadogan et al., 2021b). The review question was centered around the aim of providing an overview of observational research on prescribing practices, patterns, and potential harms (concept) in adult patients with life-limiting illnesses (population) who were receiving palliative care (context). Stemming from the main review question and aim was a series of subquestions, which were framed as review objectives:

1. To examine the number and types of medications prescribed (i.e., preventive and symptom-specific medications) for patients receiving palliative care
2. To investigate the methods used to assess the appropriateness of medication prescribing for patients receiving palliative care
3. To examine the risk factors and determinants of potentially inappropriate prescribing for patients receiving palliative care
4. To establish the types of potential harms (i.e., adverse drug events, drug interactions) associated with prescribing for patients receiving palliative care
5. To examine changes in medication prescribing for patients receiving palliative care over time

2.3 Define the inclusion criteria

The PCC framework, as previously mentioned, is not only helpful in specifying the review title and question, but it can also help define the inclusion criteria for the review. The PCC framework provides a much broader scope compared to the Population, Intervention, Comparison, Outcome framework, which is often used in systematic reviews that typically focus on examining the outcomes of a particular intervention in a population of interest using RCT designs (Cochrane Library—What is PICO?, 2025).

In defining the population of interest, the inclusion criteria should specify key characteristics of the review's participants. For example, in the scoping review by Cadogan et al. (2021b), the population of interest was adult patients (≥18 years) receiving palliative care for any life-limiting illness. Palliative care was defined using the World Health Organization's definition (*WHO definition of palliative care, 2025).* On reflection, the title of this review could have specified adults to ensure greater clarity for readers. However, this additional detail was included in the abstract and main body of the review. It is also important to recognize that not all scoping reviews necessarily focus on a specific population of interest. For example, some reviews may focus on other parameters or phenomena of interest, such as the terminology or research methods used in a particular field of research (Pollock et al., 2025; Patel et al., 2025).

In defining the concept, the inclusion criteria should describe aspects relating to the intervention, phenomena of interest, or outcomes. For example, in the scoping review by Cadogan et al. (2021b), the concept of interest was medication prescribing. The scope of this concept was defined in terms of one or more of the following: (1)

assessments of prescribed medications; (2) assessments of the appropriateness of medication prescribing and/or associated risk factors for potential harms; (3) assessments of changes in medication prescribing over time. Any assessment of the appropriateness of prescribing was considered acceptable and within scope, including clinicians' professional judgment and validated assessment criteria (e.g., Beers Criteria for older adults) (By the American Geriatrics Society Beers Criteria Update Expert P, 2019) In addition to this, studies were also required to have reported a summary statistic regarding the number of medications that patients were receiving and information on the types of medication prescribed. Studies that focused on single medication types, medication classes, or clinical indications were excluded from the review as they were not considered to provide a holistic overview of prescribing practices for the sample population.

In defining the context, the inclusion criteria should provide relevant contextual information in relation to the clinical setting, geographical location, or other relevant factors (e.g., social, cultural). In the scoping review by (Cadogan et al., 2021b), studies were eligible for inclusion in any setting where patients received palliative care for a life-limiting illness. This enabled studies to be identified across both traditional hospice and palliative care centers, as well as other settings, including general practice, hospitals, nursing homes, and long-term care facilities.

In addition to the key elements of the PCC framework as described above, scoping reviews also need to specify the information sources that are eligible for inclusion. These can include a range of research designs (e.g., quantitative, qualitative, mixed methods), as well as nonresearch sources (e.g., websites, policy documents). However, reviewers may wish to specify some restrictions on the eligibility criteria relating to information sources to ensure that they are directly relevant to addressing the review question. In the scoping review by Cadogan et al. (2021b), eligible study designs consisted of observational studies involving cross-sectional, case-control, and cohort designs. Published conference abstracts were excluded due to a lack of sufficient information.

The use of the PCC framework helps to ensure alignment between the scoping review title, question, and inclusion criteria, which can, in turn, facilitate the search process (Stage 2.4).

2.4 Develop the search strategy

In developing the search strategy, it is recommended that reviewers aim to be as comprehensive as practically possible in order to identify all relevant literature. An information retrieval specialist or research librarian can provide valuable insights into developing and refining the search strategy. In the scoping review by Cadogan et al. (2021b), preliminary searches of the selected electronic databases were undertaken to identify keywords and index terms for articles relating to the review topic. This informed the development of a comprehensive search strategy, which was developed with the assistance of a research librarian using all identified keywords and index terms for each electronic database.

The search strategy should be documented in sufficient detail to enable searches to be replicated. This includes information on the databases searched, search terms, and dates of searches, as well as any other sources that were used (e.g., reference lists of studies meeting inclusion criteria). A complete search strategy for at least one key database should be included in the review protocol and final review. Any restrictions on the search strategy should be documented and justified. For example, in the scoping review by Cadogan et al. (2021b), only English-language publications were eligible for inclusion due to resource limitations.

2.5 Screen and select evidence

All titles and abstracts of studies identified from the searches must be screened against the inclusion criteria. Where a study appears to meet the inclusion criteria or cannot be excluded based on the title or abstract alone, the full-text article should be retrieved and assessed for inclusion. Ideally, this process should be conducted by at least two reviewers working independently to minimize the potential for errors. In the scoping review by Cadogan et al. (2021b), all titles and abstracts were screened for inclusion by one author, and a 20% sample of abstracts was double-screened by a second author. This was due to resource limitations. However, all full-text articles that were subsequently retrieved were assessed for inclusion by two authors working independently. Any disagreements were resolved by discussion with other members of the research team.

As with the search strategy, key information relating to the screening process should be recorded and reported using a PRISMA flow diagram. This diagram captures the flow of information through each phase of the search process, including the number of references identified, included, and excluded at both the initial stage of title/abstract screening and following full-text review. The reasons for excluding any retrieved full-text articles should be documented and included as an appendix in the final review.

In contrast to systematic reviews, formal critical appraisal or assessment of risk of bias is typically not recommended in scoping reviews, as the aim is to map the available evidence as opposed to providing a definitive answer to a review question.

2.6 Data extraction

Data extraction (also referred to as data charting) involves recording key information from the included studies or information sources. This information should align with the review objectives and help address the review question. The JBI provides standardized data extraction forms that can be adapted by reviewers to their specific scoping review. The data extraction form may also need to be iteratively refined if additional information of interest to the review is identified during the data extraction process. It is generally recommended that data extraction be undertaken by at least two reviewers to minimize the potential for error and bias.

Again, owing to resource limitations, data extraction in the scoping review by Cadogan et al. (2021b) was performed by one author using a data extraction form that was developed in accordance with the methodological guidance. The data extraction form was piloted on a sample of three included studies and refined accordingly. Data were extracted relating to each of the following key headings, which were aligned with the review question and objectives:

1. *Study*: Authors, year of publication, country, study design, study setting, and study outcomes.
2. *Patients*: Sample size, age, gender, life-limiting illness, and other medical conditions.
3. *Prescribing*: Assessment time points, medication burden (number of medicines), preventive medications, medications for symptomatic relief, potentially inappropriate prescriptions and criteria used to assess them (if any), and medication changes (new and/or discontinued prescriptions).
4. *Potential harms:* Assessment methods and time points, types of adverse drug events or drug interactions, and associated risk factors.

The data extraction process was intended to enable a logical and descriptive summary of the review findings to be presented, aligning with the review objectives.

2.7 Data analysis

Plans for data analysis should be prespecified in the scoping review protocol to ensure that the process is explicit and transparent. In contrast to systematic reviews, the synthesis of outcome data from included studies using metaanalysis of quantitative data or metasynthesis of qualitative data is not undertaken with scoping reviews. The focus of data analysis is typically on basic descriptive analysis using frequency counts relating to key parameters and findings of interest. Summary tables and figures can be used to visually map the results.

The findings of the scoping review by Cadogan et al. (2021b) were described using narrative synthesis, which involved the following key steps.

1. A preliminary synthesis of the findings of the included studies was developed, in which study characteristics and findings were tabulated to summarize key information.
2. Extracted study data was reviewed to explore any relationships in the data.
3. The findings of the synthesis process were critically reviewed by the review team in terms of the available evidence, potential limitations of the evidence sources, and any discrepancies or uncertainties identified in relation to the review question.

Given the sizable number of studies included in the scoping review, a decision was made to use NVivo QSR 12 (*QSR* International; Burlington, Massachusetts) to manage the extracted data. This involved coding the extracted data under key headings from the data extraction form (outlined above) and performing a content analysis of this data to identify key similarities and differences across included studies.

2.8 Present the results

As with data analysis, plans for the presentation of results should also be prespecified in the scoping review protocol. Key results from the scoping review typically relate to both the search process and the information extracted from included studies. Search-related results can be described narratively in text format and accompanied by a visual summary using the PRISMA flow diagram (Tricco et al., 2018). Information extracted from included studies can be summarized using narrative synthesis with accompanying tables and figures that address the review objectives.

3 Discussion

Scoping reviews provide a robust and structured methodology to address specific review questions that often involve a diverse body of literature, while also allowing for flexibility and iterative refinement of key stages within the review process. These reviews enable the existing literature to be mapped to clearly defined review questions and objectives. The scoping review presented in this chapter played an important role in developing criteria for identifying potentially inappropriate prescribing of medications for symptom relief in older adults (≥65 years) with cancer who were receiving palliative care (Cadogan et al., 2021b). For example, it helped to identify the tools that had been used in the existing literature to assess the appropriateness of medication for the population of interest. The scoping review findings identified important gaps in the available literature. Of particular note, none of the included studies applied tools that specifically focused on the prescribing of medication for symptomatic relief. This finding highlighted the need for the criteria that were subsequently developed. In terms of limitations of the scoping review approach, because they typically focus on broader research questions compared to systematic reviews and involve descriptively mapping the existing literature on a particular topic, scoping reviews often lack depth (Khalil et al., 2021). The absence of formal critical appraisal of the methodological quality or risk of bias of identified studies, as well as statistical synthesis of outcome data, also means that scoping reviews should not be used to make recommendations to inform clinical practice. However, scoping reviews can help to identify knowledge gaps and highlight areas for future research.

Conducting high-quality scoping reviews is not without challenges. Several key challenges have been outlined by Khalil et al. (2021) and include difficulties related to the conduct of the review itself and issues associated with publishing the final scoping review. For example, a lack of adequate training in scoping review methodology among the research community can pose challenges in undertaking high-quality scoping reviews, from the initial stage of protocol development through to data extraction, analysis, and reporting of the final review. Since the publication of the scoping review by Cadogan et al. (2021b), not only has the guidance on scoping reviews been updated (Peters et al., 2020) but several additional useful resources have also been published by the JBI. These include best practice guidance for developing and reporting scoping review protocols (Peters et al., 2022) guidance on planning and conducting large scoping reviews (>100 studies) (Alexander et al., 2024) as well as recommendations for the processes of data extraction, analysis, and presentation of results (Pollock et al., 2022). As this emerging methodology continues to evolve, it will be important for researchers, including journal editors and peer reviewers, to keep up to date with the latest methodological guidance. The authors have had the unfortunate experience of submitting completed scoping reviews to journals for publication and receiving peer reviewer comments that assessed the submissions using criteria intended for systematic reviews. A greater awareness of the distinction between scoping reviews and other review types could help avoid unnecessary delays and inefficiencies in the peer-reviewed publication process.

In reflecting on the lessons learned from the previous scoping review and approaches used in subsequent scoping reviews, a key challenge experienced by the authors of the review presented in this chapter was the fact that it was relatively large, with over 50 included studies. This posed particular challenges with the processes of data extraction and analysis. With the benefit of hindsight, the data extraction process could have been made easier by focusing more on high-level data. This would have, in turn, aided the process of data analysis. Based on experience with other scoping reviews, developing the data extraction template in Microsoft Excel could have made for a more efficient data extraction process than extracting data into individual Microsoft Word documents and uploading these to NVivo to facilitate data management.

4 Questions for further discussion

4.1 How to navigate the terminology related to evidence synthesis approaches?

Scoping reviews are one of a range of evidence synthesis approaches that can help address specific questions of interest to a variety of stakeholders, including researchers, clinicians, and policymakers (Trapé et al., 2025). However, the plethora of review types and the lack of clear distinctions between individual methodologies can create difficulties for researchers in ensuring that they select and operationalize the most appropriate evidence synthesis method. For example, a recent scoping review identified over 1000 terms in the literature relating to evidence synthesis methods

(Pollock et al., 2025). It is imperative that researchers familiarize themselves with the methodological guidance of the relevant evidence synthesis approaches and ensure that they select the methodology best matched to their review question. The "Right Review" tool is a free online decision-support tool that has been developed to assist researchers in selecting the most appropriate evidence synthesis approach for a particular research question (Amog et al., 2022). The tool allows researchers to choose fixed responses to a range of questions, enabling them to select the most appropriate evidence synthesis approach.

Going forward, it has been suggested that there is a need for the development of a living taxonomy of evidence synthesis approaches to ensure that the most appropriate review methods are selected to address a particular purpose (Pollock et al., 2025). The development of such a taxonomy would be of immense value to the evidence synthesis field in terms of promoting greater consistency in the use of key terminology among both those who conduct and those who use the findings of various types of evidence synthesis approaches.

4.2 Is there a role for automation and artificial intelligence in scoping reviews?

As described at the beginning of this chapter, the scientific literature is growing at a rapid pace. It is now common for scoping reviews to include hundreds or even thousands of studies (Alexander et al., 2024). This rapid increase in available evidence creates challenges for healthcare professionals in keeping up to date with the latest available evidence, as well as for researchers undertaking reviews, particularly in terms of time demands, resource requirements, and workflow efficiency. There is growing interest in the potential to integrate automation tools and generative artificial intelligence (GenAI) into the scoping review process (Khalil et al., 2024; Clark et al., 2025).

Automation tools in the context of evidence synthesis can be defined as computerized systems that use algorithm-based solutions to assist, expedite, or replace manual reviewer tasks requiring human judgment while aiming to achieve results comparable to human reviewers (Tóth et al., 2024). Specialized software platforms, such as JBI SUMARI and Covidence, support key stages of the review process, from protocol development to article screening, appraisal, data extraction, and reporting (Tóth et al., 2024). JBI SUMARI's main automation features involve pre-populated templates for the development of the protocol and writing up the final review. Covidence, which is endorsed by the Cochrane Collaboration, is used primarily during the stages of screening and data extraction. Covidence can automate the removal of duplicate references during the initial screening process. It also integrates a machine learning classifier that facilitates the identification of RCTs from retrieved articles (Thomas et al., 2021). A previous case study compared the performance of automation tools against manual procedures in completing key parts of the evidence synthesis process and found that these tools could complete most tasks more quickly and with the same quality as human researchers (Clark et al., 2021). However, a key limitation with existing automation tools is their ability to integrate with one another, which can make the review process more fragmented (Khalil et al., 2024). For example, JBI SUMARI does not currently automate the identification and removal of duplicate references, meaning that an alternative tool needs to be used for this step of the review process.

GenAI refers to a more advanced form of AI that is capable of generating content, synthesizing data, and developing innovative solutions to complex problems (Fleurence et al., 2025). There is immense interest in the use of GenAI to expedite the evidence synthesis process and reduce the resource input required from reviewers. However, the evidence base supporting the use of GenAI is still evolving (Clark et al., 2025; Blaizot et al., 2022). For example, a recent systematic review highlighted serious deficiencies in GenAI's ability to complete tasks such as screening, data extraction, and critical appraisal, as well as a lack of robustness in existing evidence (Clark et al., 2025). This led the authors to conclude that the use of GenAI in evidence synthesis is not supported by current evidence and requires caution and human oversight due to its propensity for errors.

4.2.1 Ethical considerations for the use of AI

The widespread availability of GenAI also poses important ethical considerations for researchers whereby it has never been easier to produce written text. It is increasingly challenging to differentiate between AI-generated text and human-authored content. To ensure research integrity, it is important that where AI is used in research that it complements, but never replaces, human expertise and judgment. Many scientific publishers now provide explicit policies on the appropriate use of AI, including requirements for transparent reporting of how and why AI tools were used (Nature Portfolio, n.d.; Elsevier, n.d.). However, breaches of such policies have been identified in the scientific literature which have resulted in retraction of published articles (Teixeira da Silva and Daly, 2025). These fraudulent practices not only have a negative impact on the quality of the scientific literature, but the articles in question also end up being used by large language models for source material which is also an important consideration for researchers using GenAI tools (Gu et al., 2025).

While GenAI offers immense potential to facilitate various stages of the review process and improve workflow efficiency, the use of these tools also has a considerable impact on the environment. The training and deployment of AI models require enormous amounts of energy, which subsequently use substantial volumes of water for electricity generation and to cool data servers in data centers. For example, it has been estimated that GenAI tools consume the equivalent of a 500 ml bottle of water in generating 10–50 medium-length responses to user queries (Li et al., 2025). The environmental impact and long-term sustainability of using these tools need to be considered carefully by researchers before deploying them in research.

4.2.2 The "centaur" model: Human-AI collaboration as a future role of AI

The future of AI in healthcare and research is likely to be based on human–AI collaboration, where AI supports human expertise instead of replacing it (Topol, 2019). A useful analogy to illustrate this point can be derived from *"centaur chess"*, in which human players partner with AI. In the late 1990s, the first major milestone was reached when an AI system defeated the world's best human chess player. Since the mid-2000s, chess grandmasters have no longer been able to consistently outperform modern chess computers. However, in the so-called "centaur chess" teams, comprising amateur human players working with computers, it has been shown that these teams outperform not only the strongest standalone chess computers but also grandmasters using computers, achieving what has been described as the highest standard of chess ever observed. The key factor in the success of the "centaur chess" teams was the humans' ability to effectively "coach" the machines in terms of guiding what data to analyze and synthesize into a coherent and effective overall strategy (Epstein, 2019).

This principle directly translates to clinical research and evidence synthesis. AI systems show immense potential to aid with key stages of evidence synthesis in terms of evidence screening, data extraction, pattern detection, and predictive modeling. However, these systems still require human supervision for final decision-making (Clark et al., 2025). A collaborative human–AI model, therefore, represents what is likely to be the best way forward, with humans guiding AI and integrating its outputs into a coherent and ethically responsible overall strategy that promotes high-quality evidence synthesis.

5 Conclusion

High-quality scoping reviews are an important part of evidence synthesis and can help to advance knowledge and understanding of the existing evidence base in pharmacy and the wider field of health services research. The chapter has outlined the role of scoping reviews in evidence-based practice and explained how scoping reviews are distinct from systematic reviews. The chapter has also provided guidance on all key stages of a scoping review, from initial protocol development through to data extraction, analysis, and final write-up. The role of automation and GenAI, which are areas of intense interest for evidence synthesis, was also discussed. It is imperative for researchers to use any such tools responsibly so that they have oversight of all stages of the scoping review process, are mindful of the quality issues and potential for errors that exist with their use, and ultimately remain accountable for final decision-making in the research outputs that they produce.

6 Questions for further discussion

- How does the choice between a scoping review and a systematic review affect the resources, timeline, and expertise needed across the research team?
- What steps can researchers take to reduce the risk of scope creep during a scoping review, given its iterative nature?
- In which circumstances might a two-reviewer process for title/abstract screening and data extraction be feasible versus impractical, and how should resource limitations be documented and justified?
- How might the growing number of terms used to describe evidence synthesis approaches (over 1000, per Pollock et al., 2025) create challenges for researchers, editors, and readers?
- What safeguards should be in place before incorporating automation tools or generative AI into any stage of a scoping review?
- How can findings from a scoping review be used to justify and inform the design of a subsequent systematic review or primary research study?

7 Application exercise/scenario

Scenario: A hospital pharmacy department is exploring the introduction of pharmacist-led transitions-of-care services for older adults being discharged from an acute medical ward. Before designing a pilot service, the department director wants a comprehensive overview of the existing evidence on pharmacist-led transitions-of-care interventions, including the range of intervention components used, the settings in which they have been studied, and the outcomes that have been measured. The director is not yet ready to commission a systematic review, as it is unclear how broad or narrow the existing evidence base is.

Exercise:

1. **Choosing the review type**
   - Using the comparison in Table 15.1, justify why a scoping review (rather than a systematic review) is the appropriate approach for this question at this stage.
   - Identify at least one follow-up question that could subsequently be addressed using a systematic review.
2. **Define the review using the PCC framework**
   - Draft a population, concept, and context (PCC) statement for this review.
   - Draft a review title and 3–5 review objectives consistent with the PCC framework.
3. **Inclusion criteria and search strategy**
   - Propose inclusion and exclusion criteria for study designs, publication types, and language.
   - Identify at least three electronic databases that you would search, and describe one additional source of grey literature you might consult.
   - Describe how you would document restrictions on your search strategy (e.g., language, date limits) for transparency and reproducibility.
4. **Screening, extraction, and analysis**
   - Describe how you would structure the screening process (e.g., single vs. dual reviewer) given the resources available to your team, and how you would justify any deviations from best practice.
   - Draft 4–5 key headings for a data extraction form aligned with your review objectives.
   - Describe how you would analyze and present your findings (e.g., narrative synthesis, summary tables, PRISMA flow diagram).
5. **Reflection**
   - Discuss the limitations of a scoping review approach for informing a clinical decision about whether to implement the pilot service.
   - Identify at least one part of the review process that could benefit from the use of dedicated software to improve efficiency, based on the broader literature discussed in this chapter.

References

Alexa, J.M., Suter-Zimmermann, K., Bertsche, T., Allemann, S.S., 2025. What Is Evidence-Based Pharmacy? J. Eval. Clin. Pract. 13652753. 31 (4). Available from http://onlinelibrary.wiley.com/journal/10.1111/(ISSN)1365-2753. doi:10.1111/jep.70114.

Alexander, L., Cooper, K., Peters, M.D.J., Tricco, A.C., Khalil, H., Evans, C., Munn, Z., Pieper, D., Godfrey, C.M., McInerney, P., Pollock, D., 2024. Large scoping reviews: managing volume and potential chaos in a pool of evidence sources. J. Clin. Epidemiol. 08954356. 170, 111343. doi:10.1016/j.jclinepi.2024.111343.

Amog, K., Pham, B., Courvoisier, M., Mak, M., Booth, A., Godfrey, C., Hwee, J., Straus, S.E., 2022. Andrea C Tricco, The web-based "Right Review" tool asks reviewers simple questions to suggest methods from 41 knowledge synthesis methods. J. Clin. Epidemiol. 147, 42–51.

Arksey, H., O'Malley, L., 2005. Scoping studies: towards a methodological framework. Int. J. Soc. Res. Methodol. 1364-5579. 8 (1), 19–32. doi:10.1080/1364557032000119616.

Blaizot, A., Veettil, S.K., Saidoung, P., Moreno-Garcia, C.F., Wiratunga, N., Aceves-Martins, M., Lai, N.M., Chaiyakunapruk, N., 2022. Using artificial intelligence methods for systematic review in health sciences: a systematic review. Res. Synth. Methods. 17592887. 13 (3), 353–362. Available from http://onlinelibrary.wiley.com/journal/10.1002/(ISSN)1759-2887. doi:10.1002/jrsm.1553.

Boland, M., Higgins, A., Doherty, G., Sheaf, G., Framer, A., Cadogan, C., 2022. Mobile phone applications to support psychotropic tapering: a scoping review protocol. HRB Open Res. 2515-4826. 5, 18. doi:10.12688/hrbopenres.13501.1.

Bornmann, L., Haunschild, R., Mutz, R., 2021. Growth rates of modern science: a latent piecewise growth curve approach to model publication numbers from established and new literature databases. Humanit. Soc. Sci. Commun. 2662-9992. 8 (1). doi:10.1057/s41599-021-00903-w.

Brandt, J., Bressi, J., Lê, M.-L., Neal, D., Cadogan, C., Witt-Doerring, J., Witt-Doerring, M., Wright, S., 2024. Prescribing and deprescribing guidance for benzodiazepine and benzodiazepine receptor agonist use in adults with depression, anxiety, and insomnia: an international scoping review. eClinicalMedicine. 25895370. 70, 102507. doi:10.1016/j.eclinm.2024.102507.

Brignardello-Petersen, R., Santesso, N., Guyatt, G.H., 2025. Systematic reviews of the literature: an introduction to current methods. Am. J. Epidemiol. 14766256. 194 (2), 536–542. Available from http://aje.oxfordjournals.org/. doi:10.1093/aje/kwae232.

By the American Geriatrics Society Beers Criteria Update Expert P, 2019. American geriatrics society 2019 updated ags beers criteria(r) for potentially inappropriate medication use in older adults. J. Am. Geriatr. Soc. 67 (4), 674–694.

Cadogan, C.A., Dharamshi, R., Fitzgerald, S., Corish, C.A., Castro, P.D., Ryan, C., 2020. A systematic scoping review of interventions to improve appropriate prescribing of oral nutritional supplements in primary care. Clin. Nutr. 15321983. 39 (3), 654–663. Available from http://www.elsevier-international.com/journals/clnu/. doi:10.1016/j.clnu.2019.03.003.

Cadogan, C.A., Murphy, M., Boland, M., Bennett, K., McLean, S., Hughes, C., 2021b. Prescribing practices, patterns, and potential harms in patients receiving palliative care: a systematic scoping review. Explor. Res. Clin. Soc. Pharm. 26672766. 3, 100050. doi:10.1016/j.rcsop.2021.100050.

Cadogan, C.A., Murphy, M., McLean, S., Bennett, K., Hughes, C.M., 2021a. Development of criteria for identifying potentially inappropriate prescribing in older adults with cancer receiving palliative care (PIP-CPC). J. Geriatr. Oncol. 18794068. 12 (8), 1193–1199. Available from http://www.elsevier.com/wps/find/journaldescription.cws_home/723463/description#description. doi:10.1016/j.jgo.2021.06.003.

Clark, J., Barton, B., Albarqouni, L., Byambasuren, O., Jowsey, T., Keogh, J., Liang, T., Moro, C., O'Neill, H., Jones, M., 2025. Generative artificial intelligence use in evidence synthesis: a systematic review. Res. Synth. Methods. 1759-2879. 16 (4), 601–619. doi:10.1017/rsm.2025.16.

Clark, J., McFarlane, C., Cleo, G., Ramos, C.I., Marshall, S., 2021. The Impact of Systematic Review Automation Tools on Methodological Quality and Time Taken to Complete Systematic Review Tasks: case Study. JMIR Med. Educ. 2369-3762. 7 (2), e24418. doi:10.2196/24418.

Cleary, M., Cadogan, C., Doyle, C., 2026. Mapping the use of covert medication administration: a scoping review protocol. JBI Evid. Synth. doi:10.11124/JBIES-25-00229.

Cochrane Library - What is PICO?, 2025. https://www.cochranelibrary.com/about-pico.

Cole, J., Hughes, C., Cadogan, C., Vellinga, A., Molloy, G., Fahey, T., Sheaf, G., Maher, A., Ryan, C., 2023. Evidence for using point-of-care diagnostics in the management of respiratory tract infections in primary care: a scoping review protocol. HRB Open Res. 2515-4826. 6, 59. doi:10.12688/hrbopenres.13770.1.

Elsevier, n.d. The use of generative ai and ai-assisted technologies in writing for Elsevier.

Epstein, D., 2019. Range: Why Generalists Triumph in a Specialized World. Riverhead Books, New York.

Fleurence, R.L., Wang, X., Bian, J., Higashi, M.K., Ayer, T., Xu, H., Dawoud, D., Chhatwal, J., 2025. A Taxonomy of Generative Artificial Intelligence in Health Economics and Outcomes Research: an ISPOR Working Group Report. Value Health. 15244733. 28 (11), 1601–1610. Available from https://www.sciencedirect.com/science/journal/10983015. doi:10.1016/j.jval.2025.04.2167.

Gu, T., Feng, H., Minghui, L., Weikuan, G., Wang, G., 2025. Alarm: retracted articles on cancer imaging are not only continuously cited by publications but also used by ChatGPT to answer questions. J. Adv. Res. 20901232. 71, 1–3. doi:10.1016/j.jare.2025.03.020.

Jeffares, I., Friars, D., Plapp, H., Allott, K., Cadogan, C., Keating, D., Mooney, C., O'Connor, K., 2025. Brian O'Donoghue, A Scoping Review of Methods, Guidelines, and Protocols Used for Dose Reduction or Discontinuation of Antipsychotic Medication in People Affected by Psychotic Disorders. Schizophr. Bull. 0586–7614. doi:10.1093/schbul/sbaf181.

Johnson, L., Khattab, S., Strawbridge, J., Cadogan, C., Stewart, D., De Frein, A.M., Eustace-Cook, J., Lowrey, M.A., Brady, A.M., Harding, S., O'Connell, J., Ryan, C., 2025. Pharmacist prescribing in cancer services: a scoping review. Res. Soc. Adm. Pharm. 15517411. 21 (12), 951–974. doi:10.1016/j.sapharm.2025.05.004.

Khalil, H., Peters, M.D., Tricco, A.C., Pollock, D., Alexander, L., McInerney, P., Godfrey, C.M., Munn, Z., 2021. Conducting high quality scoping reviews-challenges and solutions. J. Clin. Epidemiol. 18785921. 130, 156–160. Available from www.elsevier.com/locate/jclinepi. doi:10.1016/j.jclinepi.2020.10.009.

Khalil, H., Pollock, D., McInerney, P., Evans, C., Moraes, E.B., Godfrey, C.M., Alexander, L., Tricco, A., Peters, M.D.J., Pieper, D., Saran, A., Ameen, D., Taneri, P.E., Munn, Z., 2024. Automation tools to support undertaking scoping reviews. Res. Synth. Methods. 17592887. 15 (6), 839–850. Available from http://onlinelibrary.wiley.com/journal/10.1002/(ISSN)1759-2887. doi:10.1002/jrsm.1731.

Li, P., Yang, J., Islam, M.A., Ren, S., 2025. Making AI Less 'Thirsty'. Commun. ACM. 0001-0782. 68 (7), 54–61. doi:10.1145/3724499.

Moher, D., Stewart, L., Shekelle, P., 2012. Establishing a new journal for systematic review products. Syst. Rev. 2046-4053. 1 (1). doi:10.1186/2046-4053-1-1.

Moher, D., Stewart, L., Shekelle, P., 2015. All in the Family: systematic reviews, rapid reviews, scoping reviews, realist reviews, and more. Syst. Rev. 2046-4053. 4 (1). doi:10.1186/s13643-015-0163-7.

Munn, Z., Peters, M.D.J., Stern, C., Tufanaru, C., McArthur, A., Aromataris, E., 2018. Systematic review or scoping review? Guidance for authors when choosing between a systematic or scoping review approach. BMC Med. Res. Methodol. 14712288. 18 (1). Available from http://www.biomedcentral.com/bmcmedresmethodol/. doi:10.1186/s12874-018-0611-x.

Munn, Z., Pollock, D., Khalil, H., Alexander, L., McLnerney, P., Godfrey, C.M., Peters, M., Tricco, A.C., 2022. What are scoping reviews? Providing a formal definition of scoping reviews as a type of evidence synthesis. JBI Evid. Synth. 26898381. 20 (4), 950–952. Available from https://journals.lww.com/jbisrir/Pages/issuelist.aspx. doi:10.11124/JBIES-21-00483.

Murphy, M., Bennett, K., Hughes, C.M., Lavan, A., Cadogan, C.A., 2020. Interventions to optimise medication prescribing and adherence in older people with cancer: a systematic scoping review. Res. Soc. Adm. Pharm. 15517411. 16 (12), 1627–1631. Available from http://www.journals.elsevierhealth.com/periodicals/rsap. doi:10.1016/j.sapharm.2020.02.021.

Who definition of palliative care, n.d. http://www.Who.int/cancer/palliative/definition/en/. (Accessed 1 December 2017).

Nature Portfolio, n.d. Artificial Intelligence (AI). Available from https://www.Nature.com/nature-portfolio/editorial-policies/ai. (Accessed 8 December 2025).

Ní Sheachnasaigh, E., Cadogan, C., Strawbridge, J., Sahm, L.J., Ryan, C., 2022. A scoping review of the methods and processes used by regulatory bodies to determine pharmacists' readiness for practice. Res. Soc. Adm. Pharm. 15517411. 18 (12), 4028–4037. Available from http://www.journals.elsevierhealth.com/periodicals/rsap. doi:10.1016/j.sapharm.2022.06.010.

Patel, Y.P., Ghaddar, L., Lin, Y., Karim, N., Chan, K., Dupuis, L., Tadrous, M., Heybati, K., 2025. Application of observational research methods to real-world studies for rare disease drugs: a scoping review protocol. PLoS One. 1932-6203. 20 (3), e0304540. doi:10.1371/journal.pone.0304540.

Peters, M.D.J., Godfrey, C.M., Khalil, H., McInerney, P., Parker, D., Soares, C.B., 2015. Guidance for conducting systematic scoping reviews. Int. J. Evid. Based Healthc. 1744-1609. 13 (3), 141–146. doi:10.1097/xeb.0000000000000050.
Peters, M.D.J., Godfrey, C., McInerney, P., Khalil, H., Larsen, P., Marnie, C., Pollock, D., Tricco, A.C., Munn, Z., 2022. Best practice guidance and reporting items for the development of scoping review protocols. JBI Evid. Synth. 26898381. 20 (4), 953–968. Available from https://journals.lww.com/jbisrir/Pages/issuelist.aspx. doi:10.11124/JBIES-21-00242.
Peters, M.D.J., Marnie, C., Colquhoun, H., Garritty, C.M., Hempel, S., Horsley, T., Langlois, E.V., Lillie, E., O'Brien, K.K., Tunçalp, ö., Wilson, M.G., Zarin, W., 2021. Andrea C Tricco, Scoping reviews: reinforcing and advancing the methodology and application. Syst. Rev. 10 (1). doi:10.1186/s13643-021-01821-3.
Peters, M.D.J., Marnie, C., Tricco, A.C., Pollock, D., Munn, Z., Alexander, L., McInerney, P., Godfrey, C.M., Khalil, H., 2020. Updated methodological guidance for the conduct of scoping reviews. JBI Evid. Synth. 26898381. 18 (10), 2119–2126. Available from https://journals.lww.com/jbisrir/Pages/issuelist.aspx. doi:10.11124/JBIES-20-00167.
Pimenta Netto, J., Barbosa, A.V., Dias Fernandes, B., Rotta, I., Aguiar, P.M., 2026. Pharmacist interventions in schizophrenia and bipolar affective disorder: a systematic review and meta-analysis. Res. Soc. Adm. Pharm. 22 (1), 44–53.
Pollock, D., Evans, C., Jia, R.M., Alexander, L., Pieper, D., de Moraes, É.B., Peters, M.D.J., Tricco, A.C., Khalil, H., Godfrey, C.M., Saran, A., Campbell, F., Munn, Z., 2024. "How-to": scoping review? J. Clin. Epidemiol. 08954356. 176, 111572. doi:10.1016/j.jclinepi.2024.111572.
Pollock, D., Hasanoff, S., Barker, T.H., Clyne, B., Tricco, A.C., Booth, A., Godfrey, C., Khalil, H., Jia, R.M., Taneri, P.E., Saif-Ur-Rahman, K., Conway, T., Konstantinidis, M., Stratton, C., Edwards, D., Alexander, L., Carrier, J., Habibi, N., Zaccagnini, M., Stern, C., Valenzuela, C., Price, C., Stone, J.C., Aromataris, E., Jordan, Z., Dias, M., McBride, G., Kanukula, R., Schuenemann, H.J., Mustafa, R.A., Pearson, A., Klugar, M., Rojas, M.X., Alonso-Coello, P., Whaley, P., Langendam, M., Merlin, T., Straus, S., Moola, S., Alper, B.S., Munn, Z., 2025. Over 1000 terms have been used to describe evidence synthesis: a scoping review. BMJ Evid. Based Med. 25154478. Available from http://ebm.bmj.com/. doi:10.1136/bmjebm-2024-113391.
Pollock, D., Peters, M.D.J., Khalil, H., McInerney, P., Alexander, L., Tricco, A.C., Evans, C., De Moraes, É.B., Godfrey, C.M., Pieper, D., Saran, A., Stern, C., Munn, Z., 2022. Recommendations for the extraction, analysis, and presentation of results in scoping reviews. JBI Evid. Synth. 26898381. 21 (3), 520–532. Available from https://journals.lww.com/jbisrir/Pages/issuelist.aspx. doi:10.11124/JBIES-22-00123.
Rodriguez, P.R., Chen, X., Arancibia, M., Madrid, E., Shokraneh, F., Adams, C.E., Víctor Ariel Franco, J., 2025. Mental Health Services for Serious Mental Illness: scoping Review of Randomised Controlled Trials. Nurs. Open. 12 (1). doi:10.1002/nop2.70100.
Teixeira da Silva, J.A., Daly, T., 2025. Letters to the editor generated by AI in neuroscience: the role of neuroethics. Neuroscience. 18737544. 573, 244–246. Available from https://www.sciencedirect.com/science/journal/03064522. doi:10.1016/j.neuroscience.2025.03.040.
Thomas, J., McDonald, S., Noel-Storr, A., Shemilt, I., Elliott, J., Mavergames, C., Marshall, I.J., 2021. Machine learning reduced workload with minimal risk of missing studies: development and evaluation of a randomized controlled trial classifier for Cochrane Reviews. J. Clin. Epidemiol. 18785921. 133, 140–151. Available from www.elsevier.com/locate/jclinepi. doi:10.1016/j.jclinepi.2020.11.003.
Topol, E.J., 2019. High-performance medicine: the convergence of human and artificial intelligence. Nat. Med. 1546170X. 25 (1), 44–56. Available from http://www.nature.com/nm/index.html. doi:10.1038/s41591-018-0300-7.
Tóth, B., Berek, L., Gulácsi, L., Péntek, M., Zrubka, Z., 2024. Automation of systematic reviews of biomedical literature: a scoping review of studies indexed in PubMed. Syst. Rev. 2046-4053. 13 (1). doi:10.1186/s13643-024-02592-3.
Trapé, C.A., Maria Sivalli Campos, C., de Freitas Oliveira, C., da Silva, J.G.S.T., Uchimura, L.Y.T., Figueiró, M.F., de Bortoli, M.C., Domingues, S.M., Yonekura, T., Luis C Ramalho, A., 2025. Scoping review of evidence synthesis: concepts, types and methods. PLoS One. 1932-6203. 20 (5), e0323555. doi:10.1371/journal.pone.0323555.
Tricco, A.C., Lillie, E., Zarin, W., O'Brien, K.K., Colquhoun, H., Levac, D., Moher, D., Peters, M.D.J., Horsley, T., Weeks, L., Hempel, S., Akl, E.A., Chang, C., McGowan, J., Stewart, L., Hartling, L., Aldcroft, A., Wilson, M.G., Garritty, C., Lewin, S., Godfrey, C.M., MacDonald, M.T., Langlois, E.V., Soares-Weiser, K., Moriarty, J., Clifford, T., Tunçalp, Ö., Straus, S.E., 2018. PRISMA extension for scoping reviews (PRISMA-ScR): checklist and explanation. Ann. Intern. Med. 15393704. 169 (7), 467–473. Available from http://annals.org/aim/fullarticle/2700389/prisma-extension-scoping-reviews-prisma-scr-checklist-explanation. doi:10.7326/M18-0850.

CHAPTER

16

Development of a complex medication review intervention in a cross-sector setting

Sara Sommer Holst[a], *Susanne Kaae*[c], *and Charlotte Vermehren*[a,b]

[a]Capital Region Pharmacy, Copenhagen University Hospital Bispebjerg, Copenhagen, Denmark
[b]Department of Drug Design and Pharmacology, Faculty of Health and Medical Sciences, University of Copenhagen, Copenhagen, Denmark
[c]Department of Pharmacy, Faculty of Health and Medical Sciences, University of Copenhagen, Copenhagen, Denmark

CHAPTER OBJECTIVES

- Discuss the meaning of, and sometimes the necessity for, implementing a "complex intervention" versus more "simple" ones
- Identify points of attention in complex intervention development research
- Describe the United Kingdom Medical Research Council (MRC) framework for developing complex interventions
- Describe how the MRC framework can be applied to a clinical study setting
- Illustrate the utility and drawbacks of the MRC framework in a clinical study setting

1 Introduction

This chapter provides an overview of key considerations in the development of complex interventions within healthcare research. It begins by characterizing the core features that define a complex intervention and highlights critical points of attention in the research and development process. The chapter introduces the United Kingdom Medical Research Council (MRC) framework as a guiding structure for developing complex interventions and explores its practical application within a clinical study context. Finally, the chapter discusses the utility and limitations of the MRC framework when applied in real-world clinical settings, offering insights into its strengths, challenges, and implications for research and practice.

Contemporary Research Methods in Pharmacy and Health Services - Volume 2
https://doi.org/10.1016/B978-0-443-44607-8.00012-1

2 Background

2.1 Public health interventions

In public health research, new services or practices are often the focus of interest. Such research is typically intervention-based, examining how a new health service or practice can be applied in an existing health care setting to improve health outcomes in a large population group (Rehfuess and Akl, 2013). Such health care interventions often consist of several interacting components, e.g., involving different healthcare professions, coordination across different sectors of care (e.g., primary, secondary, and community healthcare), and changes to professional roles. Due to this complexity, they are often referred to as complex interventions.

2.2 Medication reviews in intervention studies

Medication reviews (MRs) are an intervention targeting rational and appropriate prescribing, conducted by healthcare professionals with the objective of enhancing medication use and improving health outcomes—namely, by maximizing therapeutic effectiveness and minimizing potential harms without compromising the intended benefits of the prescribed treatment (Bülow et al., n.d.). MRs encompass a spectrum of activities, ranging from straightforward point-of-care updates to medication lists to more comprehensive interventions that require full access to clinical records and multidisciplinary collaboration prior to engaging in shared decision-making with the patient (Bülow et al., n.d.). Given the diverse nature of MRs, the optimal approach to conducting them remains a subject of ongoing discussion. A recent Cochrane metaanalysis investigating the effect of MR interventions in hospitalized adult patients identified three components that exhibited considerable variability across the included studies:

1. Who performed the MRs,
2. The content of the MRs, and
3. The implementation of the MRs.

In most cases, MRs were conducted solely by pharmacists. However, alternative configurations were also observed, including interdisciplinary teams comprising pharmacists alongside other healthcare professionals, such as pharmacy technicians, clinical pharmacologists, physicians, or nurses. In some instances, reviews were performed independently by physicians without pharmacist involvement (Bülow et al., n.d.).

The content of the MR also varied significantly depending on the underlying criteria used to assess the medication lists. Some studies used published and validated tools, such as the Screening Tool of Older Persons' Potentially Inappropriate Prescriptions criteria or the Screening Tool to Alert to Right Treatment criteria (Gallagher et al., 2008). Other studies employed web-based clinical decision support systems, while some did not rely on any predefined criteria for conducting MRs. Furthermore, MR interventions differed in whether they were delivered as standalone interventions or accompanied by additional measures, such as discharge counseling or written communication to the primary care physician (Bülow et al., n.d.).

How the suggested medication changes from the MRs were implemented was also a varying component in the MR intervention studies. In the majority of cases, MRs were discussed directly with the prescribing physicians. Nonetheless, alternative approaches were employed in some instances, such as communicating recommendations in writing or combining both verbal and written formats (Bülow et al., n.d.).

Due to this considerable variability in MR intervention studies, it has been difficult to gather sufficient evidence of clinically relevant outcomes such as mortality, hospital readmissions, emergency department (ED) contacts, adverse drug events, and health-related quality of life. Although the evidence regarding the efficacy of MRs is still emerging, there is broad consensus that they play a valuable role in enhancing therapeutic effectiveness and reducing potential harm associated with prescribed medications.

Due to substantial variations in both the content delivered by MRs and the implementation of MRs across studies, interventions involving MRs are frequently classified as complex interventions.

2.3 What are complex interventions?

Although there is no universally agreed-upon definition for the term "complex intervention" (Blackwood, 2006; Kühne et al., 2015), the United Kingdom MRC guidance on developing and evaluating complex interventions (Craig et al., 2013; Skivington et al., 2024) is arguably the most influential document conceptualizing sources of complexity arising from the interventions themselves (Tanner-Smith and Grant, 2018).

TABLE 16.1 Overview of what makes an intervention complex.

What makes an intervention complex?
• Number of interacting components within the experimental and control interventions.
• Number and complexity of behaviors required from those delivering or receiving the intervention
• Number of groups or organizational levels targeted by the intervention
• Number and variability of outcomes being measured
• The extent to which the intervention allows for flexibility or individual tailoring (Craig et al., 2013)

Complex interventions are typically characterized by the presence of multiple interacting components that influence outcomes in dynamic and context-dependent ways (Craig et al., 2013). However, they also possess additional characteristics that should be considered during evaluation (see Table 16.1).

The distinction between simple and complex interventions is not always clear-cut, as few interventions are entirely simple. Instead, the degree of complexity may vary substantially in terms of the number of components involved and the diversity of their potential effects (Craig et al., 2013).

While the classification of an intervention as simple or complex is not the primary concern in itself, it provides researchers with important insights into the likely challenges associated with its evaluation. Generally, the more complex an intervention is, the more demanding and resource-intensive its development and evaluation processes tend to be.

2.4 Why complex intervention development research?

Randomized controlled trials (RCTs) are widely regarded as the gold standard for assessing intervention effectiveness; however, the majority of such trials have focused on evaluating the impact of single-component interventions, typically pharmacological treatments (Campbell et al., 2000). A recent Cochrane metaanalysis examined interventions aimed at improving the appropriateness of polypharmacy and reducing medication-related problems in older adults (Cole et al., 2023). Of the 38 studies included, 36 focused on complex, multifaceted pharmaceutical care interventions—defined as the responsible provision of pharmacotherapy to achieve optimal patient outcomes—across diverse healthcare settings. These findings underscore the inherent challenges in designing genuinely simple interventions within the context of pharmaceutical care.

Challenges in evaluating complex interventions frequently stem from the insufficient definition and development of the intervention prior to its assessment (Campbell et al., 2000). Therefore, placing particular emphasis on the systematic development and rigorous evaluation of complex interventions is essential.

Research on complex interventions extends beyond determining whether an intervention achieves its intended outcomes. It encompasses a broader set of questions, such as evaluating additional impacts, assessing the intervention's value in relation to the resources required for its delivery, theorizing the underlying mechanisms of action, examining its interaction with the implementation context, exploring its contribution to system-level change, and considering how the resulting evidence can inform real-world decision-making (Skivington et al., 2024).

Complex intervention research that is primarily focused on determining effectiveness may fall short in producing interventions that are feasible, cost-effective, transferable, and scalable in real-world settings. To generate solutions that are applicable in practice, such research must involve early and meaningful engagement with patients, practitioners, and policy makers. This approach shifts the emphasis from simply asking whether an intervention is effective to exploring whether and how it can be accepted, implemented, sustained, scaled, and adapted across diverse contexts (Skivington et al., 2024).

Therefore, attention is directed not only toward the design of the intervention itself but also toward the contextual conditions necessary to activate its mechanisms of change, as well as the resources required to ensure its reach and impact in real-world implementation (Skivington et al., 2024).

There is an inherent trade-off between generating precise, unbiased answers to narrowly defined questions and producing more uncertain, yet potentially more informative, answers to broader and more complex inquiries. Researchers should prioritize addressing the questions that are most relevant and useful to decision-makers, even if these cannot be answered with the same level of certainty as more narrow questions (Skivington et al., 2024).

When developing complex interventions, it is crucial to provide a clear and detailed account of each stage of the development process in the research study setting. This transparency helps to enhance reproducibility, supports informed decision-making, and minimizes research waste arising from developing interventions that ultimately fail to translate into a real-world healthcare setting (Hoddinott, 2015; Chalmers et al., 2014). The development phase of a study plays a critical role in enhancing the likelihood of successful implementation of a new complex intervention. A comprehensive and systematic approach during this phase increases the potential for identifying facilitators and barriers to adoption and contributes to a deeper understanding of the intervention development process (May et al., 2007; Hølmkjær et al., 2022; Duncan et al., 2020).

3 Methods—The Medical Research Council framework

In this section, we describe the United Kingdom MRC framework for developing complex interventions and illustrate how the MRC framework can be applied to a clinical study setting.

3.1 A framework for developing complex interventions

The United Kingdom MRC has published a framework for developing and evaluating complex interventions (Craig et al., 2013; Skivington et al., 2024). This framework provides researchers with a tool to plan and conduct complex intervention development research. The framework divides complex intervention research into four distinct phases:

- **Development** or identification of an intervention
- Assessment of the **feasibility** of the intervention and evaluation design
- **Evaluation** of the intervention
- Impactful **implementation** (Skivington et al., 2024)

These phases are not restricted to a specific order and can be repeated several times if uncertainties remain unresolved. At each phase, six core elements should be considered to answer the following questions:

- How does the intervention interact with its **context**?
- What is the underlying **program theory**?
- How can diverse **stakeholders'** perspectives be included in the research?
- What are the **key uncertainties**?
- How can the intervention be **refined**?
- What are the **economic considerations** of the intervention?

The answers to these questions should be used to decide whether the research should proceed to the next phase, return to a previous phase, repeat a phase, or stop (Skivington et al., 2024). An overview of the purpose, key questions, typical methods, and expected outputs of each MRC phase is provided in Table 16.2.

3.2 Application to a clinical study setting

The MRC framework provides a robust foundation for planning intervention studies involving multiple stakeholders across diverse health sectors. Accordingly, we adopted this framework to guide the development and evaluation of a complex intervention. Prior to outlining the study design and the various phases of intervention development, we will first describe the clinical study setting in Denmark.

3.2.1 National context: Polypharmacy in Denmark

In Denmark, more than half of the population aged 75 or older is categorized as polypharmacy patients, i.e., individuals undergoing treatment with five or more different concurrent prescription drugs daily (Kornholt and Christensen, 2020), and this is likely to be the case in many other countries. This development presents a considerable challenge for the healthcare system, particularly considering the emerging evidence suggesting the benefits of MRs for patients experiencing polypharmacy. Moreover, general practitioner (GP) clinics within the primary healthcare sector are increasingly regarded as the central point of contact for health services targeting patients with multimorbidity and polypharmacy. However, recent reports from Denmark indicate a rising incidence of professional burnout among GPs, which appears to be associated with the level of multimorbidity among their patient populations (Pedersen et al., 2020). With the growing proportion of elderly patients managing multiple medications, the burden on clinicians is anticipated to escalate. Consequently, there is an urgent need to explore strategies that support clinicians—particularly those aimed at alleviating the workload associated with multimorbid patients

TABLE 16.2 Overview of the MRC framework for developing complex interventions.

MRC phase	Purpose	Key questions	Typical methods	Expected outputs
1. Development/ Identification	To develop or identify an intervention based on existing evidence, theory, and stakeholder input.	• What is the underlying program theory? • What evidence supports the intervention components? • How will the intervention interact with its context? • How can stakeholders' perspectives be integrated?	• Literature reviews and evidence synthesis • Theoretical modelling • Stakeholder and expert consultations • Logic model or program theory development.	• Refined intervention model • Defined theoretical framework • Initial program theory • Identified contextual factors
2. Feasibility/ Piloting	To assess the feasibility and acceptability of the intervention and its evaluation design.	• Is the intervention acceptable and feasible for stakeholders? • What are the key uncertainties or barriers? • How can the intervention be refined? • What are the preliminary economic considerations?	• Pilot studies or small-scale trials • Focus groups and interviews • Process evaluation • Feasibility testing of recruitment, delivery, and data collection	• Feasibility data (e.g., recruitment, adherence) • Acceptability assessment • Refined intervention components • Updated program theory
3. Evaluation	To determine the effectiveness and mechanisms of action of the intervention under controlled or real-world conditions.	• Does the intervention produce the intended outcomes? • How and why does it work? • What contextual factors influence outcomes? • What are the cost-effectiveness implications?	• Randomized controlled trials (RCTs) or quasiexperimental studies • Process evaluation • Mixed-methods studies • Economic evaluation	• Evidence of effectiveness • Insights into mechanisms of action • Contextual understanding • Economic evaluation results
4. Implementation	To promote sustainable and effective implementation in both practice and policy.	• How can the intervention be scaled up and sustained? • What factors facilitate or hinder implementation? • How does it adapt to different contexts? • What are the long-term economic impacts?	• Implementation research • Real-world evaluations • Stakeholder engagement • Continuous monitoring and feedback	• Implementation strategy • Evidence of scalability and sustainability • Policy and practice recommendations • Long-term impact data

undergoing polypharmacy, such as redistributing responsibilities to other healthcare professionals, including clinical pharmacists (CP) (Holst et al., 2024).

Conducting MRs is a complex and time-intensive endeavor, which poses challenges in the context of busy clinical settings. CPs, with specialized training in rational pharmacotherapy and clinical pharmacology, are well-positioned to contribute meaningfully to MR initiatives. Their extensive and comprehensive expertise in medication enables them to:

- Design and coordinate the implementation of MRI interventions
- Identify patients with complex polypharmacy profiles
- Perform MRs independently or in collaboration with clinicians, clinical staff, and patients
- Foster patient engagement through shared decision-making processes
- Support the consistent adoption of medication adjustments by providing supplementary clinical resources
- Serve as intermediaries across healthcare sectors to enhance the continuity of care

To alleviate GPs' workload and leverage the specialized competencies of CPs, a new MR initiative was designed involving the secondment of a hospital-based CP from a Department of Clinical Pharmacology, with access to support from medical doctors in the field of clinical pharmacology. Clinical pharmacology is a paraclinical discipline that provides expert support in pharmacotherapy without direct patient care responsibility. The secondment of the CP was planned to facilitate continuity of care across sectoral transitions by serving as a direct liaison to prescribing hospital physicians and CPs at the hospital wards, thereby enabling access to hospital records for patient data collection. The intervention encompassed both a pharmacological component—focused on MRs aimed at optimizing medication use and improving health outcomes—an organizational component, whereby the reviews were conducted collaboratively between hospital-based CPs seconded to general practice clinics, and a patient-engaging component emphasizing individual preferences and treatment wishes through patient conversations and consultations (Fig. 16.1). Such interventions, consisting of multiple interacting components, are considered a complex intervention.

We used the MRC framework for developing complex interventions to create an MR intervention in a sector transition setting, where different healthcare professions collaborated across sectors. The present study aimed to develop an interdisciplinary, collaborative, and clinically feasible MR intervention model that bridges primary and secondary healthcare in Denmark, while transparently describing the steps taken to tailor the intervention for general practice and polypharmacy patients, thereby supporting transferability to similar international settings. The study was structured according to the MRC framework, beginning with the development phase, followed by pilot testing the intervention during the feasibility phase, and culminating in the evaluation phase to further refine the existing program theory. The development and feasibility phases were each presented in a dedicated publication (Holst et al., 2024), followed by a separate publication detailing the evaluation phase (Kaae et al., 2025). The core

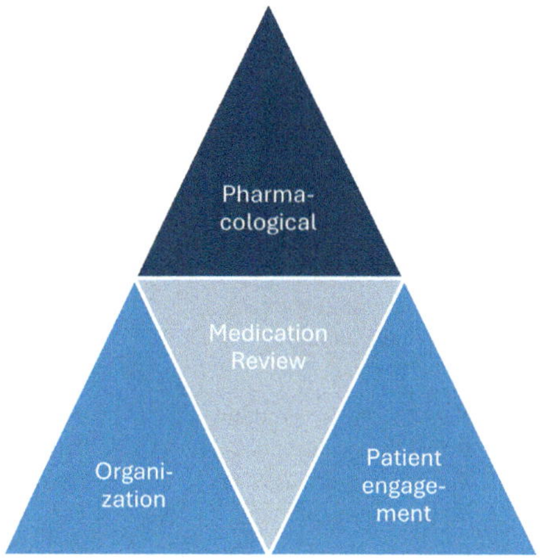

FIG. 16.1 Components of the medication review intervention. The medication review intervention encompassed both a pharmacological component—focused on MRs aimed at optimizing medication use and improving health outcomes—an organizational component, whereby the reviews were conducted collaboratively between hospital-based CPs seconded to general practice clinics, and a patient-engaging component emphasizing individual preferences and treatment wishes through patient conversations and consultations.

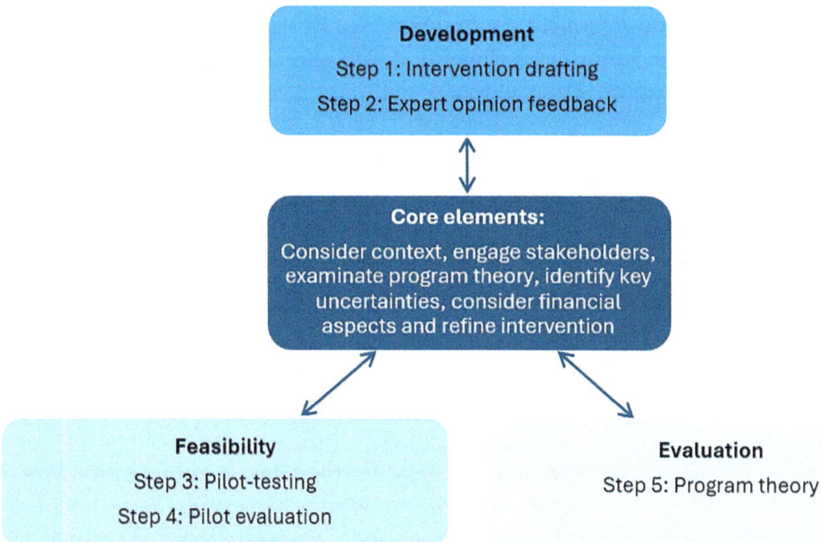

FIG. 16.2 The study design of the two following studies inspired by the MRC framework. Overview of the study design inspired by the MRC framework containing three phases: development, feasibility, and evaluation, and 5 steps: intervention drafting, expert opinion feedback, pilot-testing, pilot evaluation, and program theory. In all phases and steps, the core elements—context consideration, stakeholder engagement, program theory examination, key uncertainty identification, economic consideration, and intervention refinement—were included.

elements consisted of context consideration, program theory examination, stakeholder engagement, key uncertainties identification, economic consideration, and intervention refinement. Figure 16.2 illustrates the study designs of the two interrelated studies, both guided by the MRC framework.

To investigate the two-phase development and feasibility, we included four steps in our study design:

1. Intervention drafting
2. Expert opinion
3. Pilot testing
4. Pilot evaluation

In each step, the MR intervention was adjusted based on the findings from the previous step.

The existing program theory about successful patient-centered, pharmacist-led MR interventions in primary care was evaluated during the evaluation phase in step 5. The purpose was to investigate how the new MR model in Denmark was enacted in daily practice as the basis for understanding how it worked and how it was perceived by the involved participants (Kaae et al., 2025).

An overview of methods, main findings, and adjustments made to the MR intervention in each study step is presented in Table 16.3.

3.2.2 *Development phase*

Step 1: intervention drafting

In Step 1, the intervention context was considered by reviewing MR interventions from the authors' previous experiences, as well as relevant literature. The literature was analyzed to inspire the first draft of the MR intervention.

Literature was identified by searching databases for original research on MR intervention studies conducted in a primary care setting, including the utilization of CPs and a focus on patient involvement.

The intervention draft consisted of several elements, including medication reconciliation and a MR.

Medication reconciliation procedure: A medication reconciliation conversation with the patient was conducted by the CP to explore the patient's medication use prior to the formal MR. Patients were asked to bring all current medications to the appointment at the GP clinic. Each medication was discussed individually, covering aspects such as administration time, indication, method of intake (e.g., crushed, with food), perceived effectiveness, adverse effects, and unmet symptom management needs. The use of over-the-counter drugs, supplements, and herbal remedies was also assessed. Patient preferences regarding potential changes—such as reducing pill burden or dosing frequency—were explored, along with attitudes toward discontinuation of specific medications. The medication

TABLE 16.3 Development and evaluation steps of the medication review intervention, inspired by the MRC framework.

Step	Method	Main findings	Adjustments made
1. Intervention drafting	Review of literature and prior MR interventions; drafting the initial model, including medication reconciliation and medication review procedures	Identified key elements for MR intervention (e.g., medication reconciliation conversation, structured review framework)	Draft intervention compiled for expert review
2. Expert feedback	Review by a panel of specialists in clinical pharmacology, toxicology, clinical pharmacy, and GP quality consultants	Feedback on clinical feasibility, resource distribution, subelement sequence, and optimization needs	Draft adjusted according to expert recommendations
3. Pilot testing	Implementation in two GP clinics with ongoing opportunities for adjustments	Identified practical challenges and clinic-specific concerns	Adaptations were made based on GP staff and patient feedback during testing
4. Pilot evaluation	Quantitative analysis of MR data: patient characteristics, medication change suggestions, GP acceptance/implementation	Provided insight into the acceptability and uptake of the MR intervention in practice	Refinements informed by evaluation findings
5. Evaluation phase (program theory)	Qualitative nonparticipatory observations and semistructured interviews with GPs, patients, and CPs	Developed a new program theory emphasizing "shared mental models" and relational work between GPs and CPs	No direct refinements; insights informed the theoretical understanding of intervention mechanisms

reconciliation conversation was concluded with a summary of findings written down for the purpose of including it in the MR.

MR Procedure: Insights from the medication reconciliation conversation were used to compile an updated medication list, which subsequently formed the basis for a comprehensive MR. The MR process was guided by a structured clinical framework divided into two key components: evaluative alignment with clinical indications (Part A) and pharmacotherapeutic optimization (Part B).

Part A: Clinical relevance and indication mapping Initial assessments focused on establishing the rationale for each prescribed medication in relation to the patient's diagnoses and clinical indications. The review sought to determine:

- Whether all prescriptions have valid therapeutic indications.
- If any indications remain untreated or undertreated.
- Whether preventive treatments were absent or clinically relevant, given the patient's prognosis.

This step aimed to ensure a coherent and indication-based rationale behind the entirety of the patient's pharmacological treatment.

Part B: Pharmacological appropriateness and optimization The subsequent evaluation centered on pharmacotherapeutic optimization across multiple domains:

- Drug selection: Appropriateness was assessed based on national and regional guidelines.
- Dosing: Prescribed doses were compared with evidence-based recommendations to ensure accuracy and suitability.
- Dosing intervals and timing: Evaluated for appropriateness based on clinical guidance, drug-specific information, and patient preferences.
- Treatment duration: The treatment duration was evaluated for clinical justification.
- Formulation and administration: Examined for alignment with patient needs and rational use.
- Duplicate prescriptions: Checked to avoid unnecessary therapeutic redundancy.
- Interactions and contraindications: Screened for clinically significant drug-drug interactions and contraindications using validated sources.
- Adverse effects: Symptoms suggestive of side effects were explored.
- Compliance: Patient compliance was assessed based on a patient conversation and reimbursement data.
- Monitoring: Identified whether relevant monitoring practices (e.g., blood pressure, laboratory tests) were planned or in place.

This comprehensive MR approach provided a foundation for informed clinical decisions aimed at optimizing therapy and minimizing risk. The CP compiled the information and, in collaboration with the GP, evaluated whether adjustments were warranted. If changes required monitoring or gradual tapering, the CP conducted follow-ups via telephone consultations to assess progress and support adherence.

Inclusion and exclusion criteria: This study included polypharmacy patients, defined as individuals prescribed five or more daily prescription drugs. The following exclusion criteria were subsequently applied:

- Immobility
- Medication dispensed in automated unit doses
- Terminal diagnosis
- Active malignant disease
- Known dementia
- Conditions deemed unsuitable for inclusion by the GP clinics

Step 2: Feedback from the expert opinion panel

In step 2, the first draft of the intervention was reviewed by an expert opinion panel consisting of specialists in clinical pharmacology and clinical toxicology, CPs from the Department of Clinical Pharmacology at Copenhagen University Hospital Bispebjerg experienced in MR, and consultants affiliated with the organization "Quality in General Practice in the Capital Region", which is a collaboration between the GPs' Organization in Denmark and the Capital Region of Denmark promoting quality in general practice. The expert opinion panel was presented with the first draft of the MR intervention and was asked to provide feedback on clinical feasibility, resource and responsibility distribution between different healthcare professions in the clinic, the sequence and content of the subelements in the MR intervention, method optimization, and improvement proposals. The intervention draft was adjusted accordingly.

3.2.3 *Feasibility phase*

Step 3: Pilot testing

In step 3, the intervention was tested in two general practice clinics. The MR intervention was open to adjustments if the clinic found it necessary at any time during the testing phase. Adjustments could be made if the GP clinic staff or the patients verbally expressed concerns or wishes for alternative procedures. Therefore, the GP clinic staff had a high degree of influence. Any adjustments to the MR intervention were recorded to analyze the types of changes.

Step 4: Pilot evaluation

In step 4, the pilot test of the MR intervention was evaluated based on an analysis of quantitative MR data, including characteristics of enrolled patients, medication change suggestions from the CP, and the degree of acceptance and implementation rates of these by the GP.

3.2.4 *Intervention model*

From the four steps of the development process inspired by the MRC framework, a new MR intervention was presented (Fig. 16.3). The comprehensive development phase provided relevant inputs for intervention refinements. These refinements guided the tailoring process, resulting in a patient-centered MR intervention with an increased focus on collaboration between GPs and CPs, as well as patient involvement in decision-making (Holst et al., 2024).

3.2.5 *Evaluation phase*

Step 5: Program theory

In step 5, qualitative descriptive nonparticipatory observations of the MR model were carried out in two general practices in Denmark to identify context elements and determine how the intervention was enacted. Semistructured interviews with GPs, patients, and the pharmacist were conducted to establish outcomes. Through principles of realist evaluation, mechanisms, i.e., links connecting context, intervention, and outcomes, were inferred (Kaae et al., 2025).

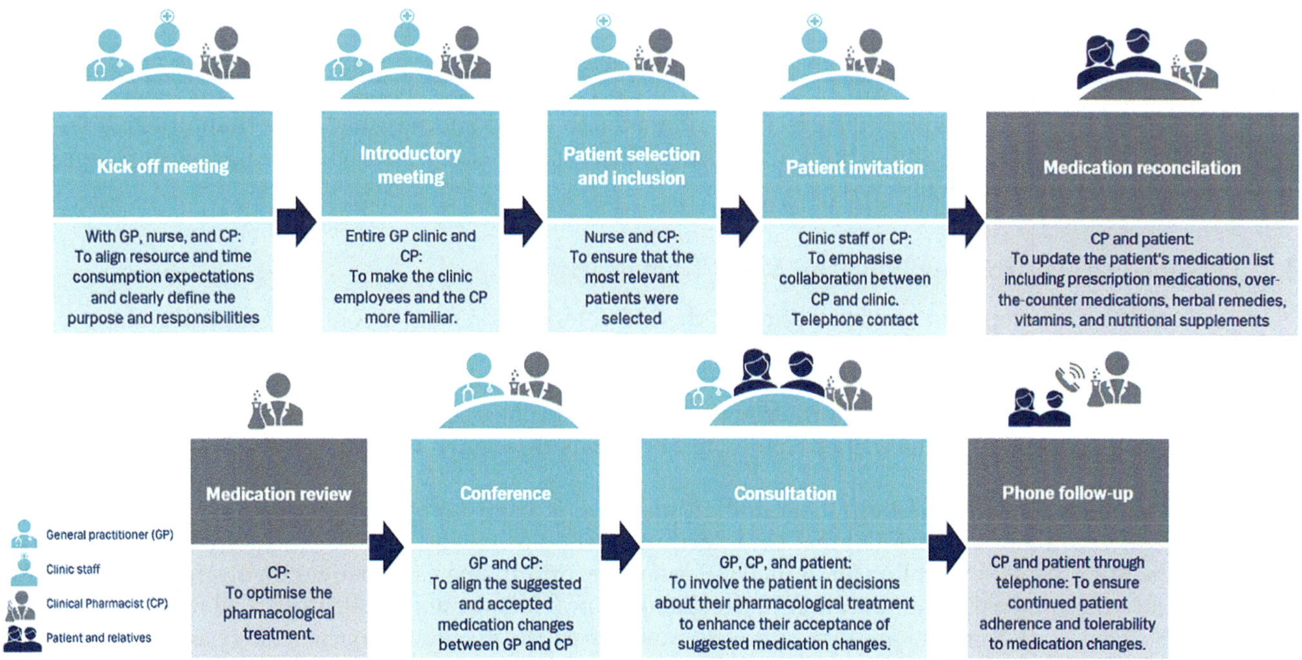

FIG. 16.3 Overview of the patient-centered, pharmacist-led MR intervention (Kaae et al., 2025). The patient-centered, pharmacist-led MR intervention is divided into nine consecutive steps. Green color indicates that the general practitioner (GP) and clinic staff are involved in the step. Gray color indicates that the clinical pharmacist (CP) is involved. Blue color indicates that the patient and/or relatives are involved in the step.

TABLE 16.4 Program Theory (Context/Intervention—Outcomes—Mechanisms) for the Pharmacist-Led, Patient-Centered Medication Review in General Practice. The model illustrates how contextual and intervention-related factors (C/I) lead to observable outcomes (O), from which underlying mechanisms (M) are inferred. These mechanisms explain how the intervention functions in real-world practice and how sustainability can be achieved through cross-sector collaboration.

C/IOM No.	Context & intervention	Outcomes	Mechanisms
1	The pharmacist-led, patient-centered medication review (MR) is conducted in the GP clinic	Improved communication between sectors, clearer medication lists, and enhanced patient understanding of their treatment	Activation of shared mental models between the GP and CP regarding appropriate polypharmacy management
2	Local organizational conditions: variation in GP engagement, workflow, time, and existing trust relationships	Acceptance of CP input and greater satisfaction among GPs occur when collaboration aligns with existing routines	Relational work builds trust and mutual respect, enabling effective knowledge exchange and joint decision-making
3	Patient inclusion in MR conversations and flexible adaptation to patient complexity and preferences	Patients experience empowerment and greater involvement in medication decisions, as well as improved adherence and confidence	Patient engagement mechanisms are triggered through open dialog and shared decision-making
4	Intervention flexibility allows adaptation to GP clinic structures and resources	Better integration of MR intervention into daily practice, promoting sustainability and continuity of collaboration	Adaptive learning among pharmacists and GPs reinforces feasibility and long-term integration
5	Established collaboration and observed benefits encourage the continued presence of CP in primary care	Sustained motivation among GPs and pharmacists to maintain the intervention beyond the pilot phase	Institutionalization of the MR model across sectors, embedding it into existing workflows and organizational routines

The evaluation phase yielded new insights into the new program theory regarding the importance of compatible perspectives between pharmacists and GPs on appropriate polypharmacy work, i.e., "shared mental models", the ways GPs can develop their mental models when interacting with pharmacists, and the usefulness of relational work when the models clash (Kaae et al., 2025) (Table 16.4).

4 Discussion

In this section, we discuss some of the practical and methodological findings that arose from utilizing the MRC framework in a clinical study setting, with a view to informing how other researchers might wish to apply this methodology in a similar setting.

4.1 Lessons learned from applying the MRC framework

We initiated the development and evaluation of the MR intervention with a comprehensive development and feasibility phase, guided by the United Kingdom MRC framework for complex interventions. This approach was chosen due to the novel and inherently complex nature of the MR intervention, which lacked an existing evidence- or theory-based model to build upon. Furthermore, starting with these phases allowed for an open, exploratory process aimed at designing an intervention that would be optimally aligned with the needs and realities of clinical practice.

Our development phase, consisting of the initial intervention draft and an expert opinion feedback session, highlighted important key uncertainties that the intervention should consider, such as including a medicine reconciliation in the MR process, accounting for limited GP resources, prioritizing early patient involvement, and securing productive interdisciplinary communication and collaboration (Holst et al., 2024). It also allowed us to engage stakeholders such as GPs from the primary care sector and specialists in clinical pharmacology and clinical toxicology, as well as CPs from the secondary hospital sector. This provided us with crucial information about relevant inclusion and exclusion criteria and ways to incorporate the MR intervention into existing workflows in GP clinics.

Our feasibility phases, consisting of a pilot-test and pilot-evaluation of quantitative MR data, provided essential insights into the acceptability of the MR intervention in the clinical setting. The pilot-testing in step 3 resulted in several refinements to the MR intervention, including the addition of training in the general practitioner clinics electronic medical record system, the inclusion of exclusion criteria, and changes to the workflow surrounding patient record-keeping. This was not surprising, as pilot testing is a fundamental method for establishing a foundation for future studies, and feasibility explorations are crucial for assessing optimal content and delivery (Hoddinott, 2015; Lee et al., 2019).

After the development and feasibility phases, we proceeded to the evaluation phase to further refine the complex MR intervention. Conducting a process evaluation during a pilot study offers valuable benefits before embarking on large-scale implementation research, as it can provide critical insights into:

- The credibility and quality of the intervention—e.g., what is implemented and how it is delivered.
- The mechanisms of change—e.g., how the delivered intervention induces change in participants
- Accounts for context—e.g., how environmental factors influence both implementation and outcomes
- Causal factors—e.g., why the intervention was effective or ineffective
- Recommendations for refinement—e.g., how the intervention could be further developed (Skivington et al., 2024)

The evaluation phase, consisting of a program theory examination, comprising qualitative observations and semistructured interviews of the MR intervention, provided a deeper understanding of how CPs can effectively support GPs. It also elucidated how the nature of relationships and collaboration among key stakeholders influenced the acceptability of the MR intervention. These findings contributed to the development of a novel program theory emphasizing the significance of aligned perspectives between pharmacists and GPs regarding appropriate polypharmacy management—referred to as "shared mental models". Furthermore, the theory delineates the mechanisms through which GPs adapt their mental models in response to interactions with pharmacists, as well as the role of relational work in resolving conflicts when discrepancies between these models arise (Kaae et al., 2025). The evaluation phase did not yield additional recommendations for the refinement of the MR intervention. However, the collaborative dynamic between GPs and CPs—specifically their shared mental models, relational interactions, and the processes involved in trust-building—was identified as a critical factor in successful implementation and acceptability. To support this, the MR intervention incorporated dedicated time for introductory activities, designed to foster a constructive and trust-based working relationship. Additionally, the strategic secondment of CPs to GP clinics was intended to promote deeper collaboration. These findings highlight the inherent challenges in establishing and sustaining meaningful, trustful professional relationships within the constrained timeframe of a research study.

In future applications of this model, there is strong potential to further involve CPs based in clinical hospital departments with direct patient care responsibilities to create an even more cohesive and enduring model. Their engagement would enhance communication between secondary and primary care and ensure that insights from hospital-based medication management are effectively integrated into the general practice setting through collaboration with the seconded CP. Embedding such cross-sector collaboration would strengthen continuity of care and reinforce the role of the seconded CP in general practice as a bridge-builder between healthcare sectors.

According to the MRC framework, questions about acceptability found through program theory evaluation should be considered in a feasibility phase, examining the optimal delivery (Skivington et al., 2024). Therefore, it could be suggested to revisit the feasibility phase to investigate how the collaboration between GPs and CPs influences the optimal delivery of the complex MR intervention. Additionally, an implementation phase could be planned to focus on prioritizing strategies that facilitate and enhance collaborative trust between CPs and GPs. Such further development of the MR intervention may enhance its clinical relevance and facilitate more seamless implementation.

In addressing the core elements from the MRC framework, we elucidated the complex dynamics of the intervention within its contextual environment, revealing the multifaceted ways in which local organizational structures in the GP clinics, the different professional roles of GPs and CPs, and interprofessional relationships influenced the development of the MR intervention. We also highlighted the importance of including diverse stakeholder perspectives to ensure a comprehensive representation of relevant viewpoints, guiding the development process and enhancing the intervention's contextual relevance. By integrating insights from the previous analyses, we refined the MR intervention several times. This iterative process facilitated the development of targeted recommendations for optimizing intervention components, strengthening interprofessional collaboration, and tailoring implementation strategies to better fit the diverse settings of the GP clinics.

In the complex MR intervention, the CP was responsible for engaging patients through medication reconciliation conversations and MR consultations. Multiple studies indicate that patient involvement in shared decision-making about their medication should be considered an essential component of MRs, as it may enhance both quality of life and compliance with treatment (Stacey et al., 2017; Wilson et al., 2010; Linsky et al., 2019; Elwyn et al., 2017). Enhancing patient involvement during medication consultations has been shown to boost information retention, support adherence to clinical advice, and contribute to better health outcomes (Harrington et al., 2004; Turner et al., 2018). That is why patient involvement was planned to be included in several elements of the MR intervention. However, after carrying out a stepwise approach to develop a complex MR intervention inspired by the MRC framework, it could be suggested that patients should have been involved in the intervention development process from step 1, rather than only in steps 3–4. It has been posited that patients possess a fundamental right to actively participate in and contribute to research pertaining to their health conditions, thereby warranting their inclusion in the developmental stages of patient-centered initiatives (Madden and Speed, 2017). Furthermore, fostering meaningful patient engagement is recognized as a critical factor in enhancing both the rigor and translational value of research. By incorporating patients' lived experiences and real-world perspectives, clinical investigations are rendered more relevant and aligned with patient needs, ultimately facilitating the development of more effective and patient-centric interventions (Esmail et al., 2015). It cannot be ruled out that early patient involvement would have led to more refinements, resulting in a more sustainable MR intervention (e.g., with inclusion criteria that better fit the frail, polypharmacy patients' needs and an increased patient acceptance of medication changes) (Holst et al., 2024).

4.2 Benefits and limitations of the MRC framework

The MRC framework for developing complex interventions has several implications for clinical practice (Table 16.5).

The MRC framework provided a valuable structure for organizing our development process and for identifying the key considerations to address at each stage. The nonlinear structure of the MRC framework allowed us to conduct a more flexible and comprehensive evaluation of our intervention development, as it enabled us to revisit and refine earlier phases in response to emerging insights and contextual factors.

Early-stage considerations in intervention research are often underrepresented in final published outcomes. The growing emphasis on systematic development processes—rather than solely evaluating the impact of interventions based on researchers' assumptions about what might work—has the potential to yield more clinically relevant, feasible, and implementable interventions.

Ultimately, addressing the six core elements outlined in the MRC framework provides substantial benefits for research projects by ensuring a comprehensive and nuanced understanding of complex interventions. Exploring how the intervention interacts with its context reveals critical contextual factors that influence implementation and outcomes. Defining the underpinning program theory clarifies the mechanisms of change and guides hypothesis testing. Including diverse stakeholder perspectives enriches the relevance and acceptability of the intervention. Identifying key uncertainties focuses research efforts on addressing gaps and potential challenges. Refining the intervention based on iterative feedback enhances its effectiveness and feasibility. Finally, integrating economic considerations ensures that resource implications and cost-effectiveness are factored into decision-making, supporting sustainable healthcare solutions. Collectively, these elements foster more robust, relevant, and implementable interventions.

However, the iterative and cyclical nature of the MRC framework necessitates substantial research resources, which are not always readily available, potentially limiting its full implementation in practice. Determining when an intervention has been sufficiently refined for implementation in clinical practice can be challenging. There is a risk of continually modifying the intervention without ever reaching definitive conclusions regarding outcomes such as efficacy or effectiveness. However, it can be argued that assessing these outcomes may not be the primary

TABLE 16.5 Implications of using the MRC framework in clinical practice.

Benefits	Limitations
• Provides a **structured approach** to intervention development, ensuring that key considerations are addressed throughout each stage • Its **nonlinear and flexible design** allows researchers to revisit and refine earlier phases as new insights or contextual factors emerge•Encourages **systematic early-stage development**, moving beyond assumptions to create more relevant, feasible, and implementable interventions	• The iterative and cyclical nature demands significant research **resources**, which may hinder full application in practice • It can be **difficult to determine** the point at which an intervention is sufficiently refined for clinical implementation • There's a risk of **continuous refinement without resolution**, potentially delaying clinical implementation • **Effectiveness and efficacy** assessments are difficult to evaluate and may be better suited to later-stage evaluation methods, such as randomized controlled trials (RCTs)

focus during the intervention development phase and that questions of efficacy and effectiveness are more appropriately addressed through a traditional RCT later.

Compounding the challenges of researching the development and evaluation of complex interventions, designing an RCT for such interventions poses significant methodological difficulties. A strictly quantitative, experimental design is often insufficient for researching complex interventions. To address questions beyond mere effectiveness, qualitative or mixed-methods approaches are frequently necessary. Factors such as the nature of the intervention, its underlying program theory, and stakeholder priorities may shift the emphasis toward refining theories of change. In this context, effect estimates are inherently shaped by local conditions, making average effects less informative for decision-makers operating in diverse settings. Instead, nuanced insights into how interventions produce change—alongside the identification of key facilitators and barriers to implementation—can be more valuable across varied environments (Skivington et al., 2024).

Nonetheless, RCTs have been successfully employed in certain studies to evaluate the efficacy of complex interventions. A randomized clinical multicenter study investigated whether a multifaceted pharmacist intervention, based on MR, patient interviews, and follow-up, could reduce the number of readmissions and ED visits (Ravn-Nielsen et al., 2018). The study found that the multifaceted pharmacist intervention had a significant effect on the number of patients who were readmitted within 30 days (hazard ratio [HR], 0.62; 95% CI, 0.46–0.84) or within 180 days (HR, 0.75; 95% CI, 0.62–0.90). This is an example of how the efficacy of an established complex intervention can be assessed based on predefined outcomes, such as the number of readmissions, in an RCT. However, when the aim is to explore the mechanisms behind the development or evaluation of a multifaceted pharmacist intervention or to identify factors influencing its implementation, alternative study designs may be more appropriate.

It is evident from our study that a comprehensive development phase can provide relevant inputs for intervention refinements. These refinements can guide the tailoring process, resulting in an intervention that entails greater patient satisfaction and adherence. The transparency and transferability in the development of this intervention are hoped to inspire others to apply these findings to other settings concerning complex MR intervention development. Therefore, it is our strongest recommendation to consider the MRC framework for your next intervention development and evaluation project, so that we can build on the increasing amount of research on how to develop complex interventions in public health research.

5 Questions for further discussion

1. Having your local MR services in mind, can you think of an element in the process that could be improved?
2. Could your suggested improvement be achieved by implementing a new intervention, such as adopting a different work approach or expanding cooperation?
3. How could you evaluate this new intervention by utilizing the MRC framework? Consider which phases might be a good starting point and in what order the phases could be planned.

6 Application exercise | Scenario

Consider the present study, where we implemented a complex MR intervention in various general practitioner clinics. The general practitioners' acceptance of the medication changes suggested by the clinical pharmacists varied across the different clinics.

1. What contextual factors could influence this variation?
2. Could you suggest modifications to the intervention design that take these contextual factors into account?
3. How can stakeholder input affect intervention refinement? Think of both positive and negative impacts.
4. How would you manage conflicts of interest among stakeholders?

Learner discussion—Diversity of medication review interventions	
Contributor	Reflect on the role of health care professionals in contributing to medication reviews: • How might the outcomes of medication reviews differ when performed by pharmacists, nurses, or physicians? • What implications does this hold for interprofessional collaboration in your own clinical setting?
Content	Reflect on the content of medication reviews: • How do contextual factors (e.g., health care setting, patient demographics, health literacy, prescribing culture) influence what gets emphasized during medication reviews? • What implications does this have for the outcomes of a medication review?

Learner discussion—Diversity of medication review interventions	
Implementation	Reflect on the implementation of suggested medication changes from medication reviews: • How might the format, tone, and clarity of recommended changes, as well as how they are communicated, influence their uptake and implementation by healthcare professionals? • What implications does this have for the outcomes of a medication review?

Learner discussion—Complex Interventions, Complex Decisions
Reflect on evaluating complex interventions in a research setting: • How do we decide which outcomes and contextual factors matter most for real-world impact—and how do we balance the need for scientific precision with the urgency of practical relevance? • Have you encountered an intervention in your field or experience that seemed effective in theory but struggled in practice? What factors might have influenced that outcome?

AI disclosure

During the preparation of this work, the author(s) used Co-pilot to enhance the language in the chapter. After using this tool/service, the author(s) reviewed and edited the content as needed and take(s) full responsibility for the content of the publication.

References

Blackwood, B., 2006. Methodological issues in evaluating complex healthcare interventions. J. Adv. Nurs. 13652648. 54 (5), 612–622. doi:10.1111/j.1365-2648.2006.03869.x.

Bülow, Clausen, S.S., Lundh, Christensen, M., n.d. Medication review in hospitalised patients to reduce morbidity and mortality - Bülow, C - 2023 | cochrane Library. Available from https://www.cochranelibrary.com/cdsr/doi/10.1002/14651858.CD008986.pub4/abstract?cookiesEnabled.

Campbell, M., Fitzpatrick, R., Haines, A., Kinmonth, A.L., Sandercock, P., Spiegelhalter, D., Tyrer, P., 2000. Framework for design and evaluation of complex interventions to improve health. Br. Med. J. 09598146. 321 (7262), 694–696. Available from http://www.bmj.com/. doi:10.1136/bmj.321.7262.694.

Chalmers, I., Bracken, M.B., Djulbegovic, B., Garattini, S., Grant, J., Gülmezoglu, A.M., Howells, D.W., Ioannidis, J.P.A., Oliver, S., 2014. How to increase value and reduce waste when research priorities are set. Lancet. 01406736. 383 (9912), 156–165. doi:10.1016/s0140-6736(13)62229-1.

Cole, J.A., Gonçalves-Bradley, D.C., Alqahtani, M., Barry, H.E., Cadogan, C., Rankin, A., Patterson, S.M., Kerse, N., Cardwell, C.R., Ryan, C., Hughes, C., 2023. Interventions to improve the appropriate use of polypharmacy for older people. Cochrane Database Syst. Rev. 14651858. 2023 (10). Available from https://www.cochranelibrary.com/cdsr/table-of-contents. doi:10.1002/14651858.CD008165.pub5.

Craig, P., Dieppe, P., Macintyre, S., Michie, S., Nazareth, I., Petticrew, M., 2013. Developing and evaluating complex interventions: the new Medical Research Council guidance. Int. J. Nurs. Stud. 00207489. 50 (5), 587–592. doi:10.1016/j.ijnurstu.2012.09.010.

Duncan, E., O'Cathain, A., Rousseau, N., Croot, L., Sworn, K., Turner, K.M., Yardley, L., Hoddinott, P., 2020. Guidance for reporting intervention development studies in health research (GUIDED): an evidence-based consensus study. BMJ Open. 2044-6055. 10 (4), e033516. doi:10.1136/bmjopen-2019-033516.

Elwyn, G., Cochran, N., Pignone, M., 2017. Shared decision making-The importance of diagnosing preferences. JAMA Intern. Med. 21686106. 177 (9), 1239–1240. Available from http://jamanetwork.com/journals/jamainternalmedicine/data/journals/intemed/936446/jamainternal_elwyn_2017_vp_170011.pdf. doi:10.1001/jamainternmed.2017.1923.

Esmail, L., Moore, E., Rein, A., 2015. Evaluating patient and stakeholder engagement in research: moving from theory to practice. J. Comp. Eff. Res. 20426313. 4 (2), 133–145. Available from https://becarispublishing.com/loi/cer. doi:10.2217/cer.14.79.

Gallagher, P., Ryan, C., Byrne, S., Kennedy, J., O'Mahony, D., 2008. STOPP (Screening Tool of Older Person's Prescriptions) and START (Screening Tool to Alert doctors to Right Treatment). Consensus validation. Int. J. Clin. Pharmacol. Ther. 0946-1965. 46 (02), 72–83. doi:10.5414/CPP46072.

Harrington, J., Noble, L.M., Newman, S.P., 2004. Improving patients' communication with doctors: a systematic review of intervention studies. Patient Educ. Couns. 07383991. 52 (1), 7–16. Available from www.elsevier.com/locate/pateducou. doi:10.1016/S0738-3991(03)00017-X.

Hoddinott, P., 2015. A new era for intervention development studies. Pilot Feasibility Stud. 2055-5784. 1 (1). doi:10.1186/s40814-015-0032-0.

Hølmkjær, P., Vermehren, C., Holm, A., Rozing, M.P., Høj, K., Overbeck, G., 2022. Tailoring a complex intervention to reduce antidepressants in institutionalized older persons with dementia. BMC Health Serv. Res. 14726963. 22 (1). Available from https://bmchealthservres.biomedcentral.com/. doi:10.1186/s12913-022-08961-9.

Holst, S.S., Hansen, J.M., Kaae, S., Vermehren, C., 2024. Development of a medication review intervention by seconding a hospital pharmacist to primary care. Explor. Res. Clin. Soc. Pharm. 26672766. 16. Available from https://www.sciencedirect.com/science/journal/26672766. doi:10.1016/j.rcsop.2024.100505.

Kaae, S., Holst, S.S., Hansen, J.M., Vermehren, C., 2025. New program theory in pharmacist-led patient-centered medication review in general practice - a qualitative pilot study. Res. Soc. Adm. Pharm. 15517411. Available from https://www.sciencedirect.com/science/journal/15517411. doi:10.1016/j.sapharm.2025.07.002.

Kornholt, J., Christensen, M.B., 2020. Prevalence of polypharmacy in Denmark. Dan. Med. J. 22451919. 67 (6), 1–5. Available from https://ugeskriftet.dk/files/scientific_article_files/2020-05/a12190680.pdf.

Kühne, F., Ehmcke, R., Härter, M., Kriston, L., 2015. Conceptual decomposition of complex health care interventions for evidence synthesis: a literature review. J. Eval. Clin. Pract. 13652753. 21 (5), 817–823. Available from http://onlinelibrary.wiley.com/journal/10.1111/(ISSN)1365-2753. doi:10.1111/jep.12384.

Lee, C.Y., Goeman, D., Beanland, C., Elliott, R.A., 2019. Challenges and barriers associated with medication management for home nursing clients in Australia: a qualitative study combining the perspectives of community nurses, community pharmacists and GPs. Fam. Pract. 1460-2229. 36 (3), 332–342. doi:10.1093/fampra/cmy073.

Linsky, A., Gellad, W.F., Linder, J.A., Friedberg, M.W., 2019. Advancing the Science of Deprescribing: a Novel Comprehensive Conceptual Framework. J. Am. Geriatr. Soc. 15325415. 67 (10), 2018–2022. Available from http://onlinelibrary.wiley.com/journal/10.1111/(ISSN)1532-5415. doi:10.1111/jgs.16136.

Madden, M., Speed, E., 2017. Beware Zombies and Unicorns: toward Critical Patient and Public Involvement in Health Research in a Neoliberal Context. Front. Sociol. 22977775. 2. Available from www.frontiersin.org/journals/sociology. doi:10.3389/fsoc.2017.00007.

May, C., Finch, T., Mair, F., Ballini, L., Dowrick, C., Eccles, M., Gask, L., MacFarlane, A., Murray, E., Rapley, T., Rogers, A., Treweek, S., Wallace, P., Anderson, G., Burns, J., Heaven, B., 2007. Understanding the implementation of complex interventions in health care: the normalization process model. BMC Health Serv. Res. 1472-6963. 7 (1). doi:10.1186/1472-6963-7-148.

Pedersen, A.F., Vedsted, P., Nørøxe, K.B., 2020. Influence of patient multimorbidity on GP burnout: a survey and register-based study in Danish general practice. Br. J. Gen. Pract. 14785242. 70 (691), E95. Available from https://bjgp.org/content/bjgp/70/691/e95full.pdf. doi:10.3399/bjgp20X707837.

Ravn-Nielsen, L.V., Duckert, M.L., Lund, M.L., Henriksen, J.P., Nielsen, M.L., Eriksen, C.S., Buck, T.C., Pottegård, A., Hansen, M.R., Hallas, J., 2018. Effect of an in-hospital multifaceted clinical pharmacist intervention on the risk of readmission a randomized clinical trial. JAMA Intern. Med. 21686106. 178 (3), 375–382. Available from https://jamanetwork.com/journals/jamainternalmedicine/currentissue. doi:10.1001/jamainternmed.2017.8274.

Rehfuess, E.A., Akl, E.A., 2013. Current experience with applying the GRADE approach to public health interventions: an empirical study. BMC Public Health. 14712458. 13 (1). doi:10.1186/1471-2458-13-9.

Skivington, K., Matthews, L., Simpson, S.A., Craig, P., Baird, J., Blazeby, J.M., Boyd, K.A., Craig, N., French, D.P., McIntosh, E., Petticrew, M., Rycroft-Malone, J., White, M., Moore, L., 2024. A new framework for developing and evaluating complex interventions: update of Medical Research Council guidance. Int. J. Nurs. Stud. 00207489. 154, 104705. doi:10.1016/j.ijnurstu.2024.104705.

Stacey, D., Légaré, F., Lewis, K., Barry, M.J., Bennett, C.L., Eden, K.B., Holmes-Rovner, M., Llewellyn-Thomas, H., Lyddiatt, A., Thomson, R., Trevena, L., 2017. Decision aids for people facing health treatment or screening decisions. Cochrane Database Syst. Rev. 4. Available from http://as.wiley.com/WileyCDA/Brand/id-6.html. doi:10.1002/14651858.CD001431.pub5.

Tanner-Smith, E.E., Grant, S., 2018. Meta-Analysis of Complex Interventions. Annu. Rev. Public Health. 15452093. 39, 135–151. Available from http://www.annualreviews.org/journal/publhealth. doi:10.1146/annurev-publhealth-040617-014112.

Turner, J.P., Richard, C., Lussier, M.T., Lavoie, M.E., Farrell, B., Roberge, D., Tannenbaum, C., 2018. Deprescribing conversations: a closer look at prescriber patient communication. Ther. Adv. Drug Saf. 20420994. 9 (12), 687–698. Available from http://www.uk.sagepub.com/journals/Journal201944. doi:10.1177/2042098618804490.

Wilson, S.R., Strub, P., Buist, A.S., Knowles, S.B., Lavori, P.W., Lapidus, J., Vollmer, W.M., Bocobo, F., German, D., Poon, A., Nguyen, M., Hoehne, J., Brown, N., Fukui, C., Holup, J., 2010. Shared treatment decision making improves adherence and outcomes in poorly controlled asthma. Am. J. Respir. Crit. Care Med. 15354970. 181 (6), 566–577. Available from http://ajrccm.atsjournals.org/cgi/reprint/181/6/566. doi:10.1164/rccm.200906-0907OC.

CHAPTER

17

Risk indicators and risk groups in register-based medicine use research

Leena Saastamoinen[a] *and Jouko Verho*[b]

[a]Research and Development Unit, Helsinki, Finland

[b]VATT Institute for Economic Research, Helsinki, Finland

CHAPTER OBJECTIVES

This chapter provides an introduction to medicine use research based on comprehensive register data. It discusses the advantages and limitations of administrative registers, their application in measuring medicine use and identifying risks in medication, and considers processes for research permissions and empirical methods. Our overarching perspective is on promoting rational pharmacotherapy and enhancing the use of rich databases for patient benefit.

The objectives to learn:

- Basic concepts, types of registers, and their applicability in medicine use research
- Data protection and research permissions in register-based studies
- Methods for measuring medicine use and associated risks
- How to identify and define risk groups using register data

1 Introduction

Rational pharmacotherapy refers to the safe, effective, economical, and appropriate use of medicine. As defined by the World Health Organization (WHO), medicine use is rational when "patients receive medications appropriate to their clinical needs, in doses that meet their own individual requirements, for an adequate period of time, and at the lowest cost to them and their community" (WHO, 2002). However, this is not always achieved in practice. Problems with medication use are common, and a major concern is the use of potentially inappropriate medications (PIMs), meaning drugs whose risks may outweigh their benefits (Beers et al., 1991).

Promoting rational pharmacotherapy first requires acknowledging the shortcomings of current medical care. This includes conducting systematic research on drug-related problems, developing and applying risk indicators, and

Contemporary Research Methods in Pharmacy and Health Services - Volume 2
https://doi.org/10.1016/B978-0-443-44607-8.00023-6

identifying patients at risk. It is equally important to have a broad understanding of prescribing and medicine use at the individual and population levels, including variations across regions, communities, and healthcare providers.

Pharmaceutical cost containment is often the responsibility of regional authorities and institutions, yet substantial regional variation in prescribing quality has been consistently documented (e.g., Henriksen et al., 2015; Di Martino et al., 2017; Calara et al., 2017). Understanding this variation provides authorities with the necessary tools to guide prescribing practices and improve the quality of care. By identifying regions with high levels of inappropriate prescribing, authorities can target interventions more effectively and improve outcomes in a cost-effective way. Moreover, determining the factors that drive prescribing variation is crucial for developing targeted measures to reduce inappropriate medicine use.

Next, this chapter provides an overview of methods used in register research and their application to PIM analysis. In Section 2, we first introduce the key concepts and measures used to study medicine use through register data. Then, we examine the role of administrative registers in research. In countries with comprehensive health registers, such as the Nordic countries, these data enable population-wide studies with individual-level data (Furu et al., 2010; Laugesen et al., 2021). While registers offer clear advantages in scale and representativeness, they also have limitations, such as complex research permission processes and variable suitability for research purposes.

We then turn to risk indicators as tools for detecting inappropriate prescribing, such as unsuitable medicines or harmful drug combinations (Fastbom and Johnell, 2015; Dimitrow et al., 2011; Paulamäki et al., 2023b; American Geriatrics Society, 2023; Similä et al., 2025). These indicators are based on medication lists that identify the patients, patient groups, and populations at risk of developing adverse outcomes from medical care. Targeting the right patient groups is essential for interventions aimed at improving medication quality. Furthermore, regional analyses offer opportunities to direct measures through health authorities or key opinion leaders in medicine.

In the final part of Section 2, we outline statistical approaches for analyzing regional variation in PIM use. We illustrate how the choice of outcome variable guides model selection, key aspects of hypothesis testing, and the use of model selection techniques to identify influential factors. Using a study of Finnish PIM use as an example, we demonstrate how regression models can quantify regional differences and assess the extent to which regional characteristics explain observed variation.

Section 3 presents a case study on regional variation in PIM use among older adults in Finland. Using nationwide data from the Finnish Prescription Register, the study examined all residents aged 75 years and older who purchased reimbursed medicines in 2011. The results revealed marked regional differences, with higher rates in more urban areas and in regions where private physician visits were common. The findings suggest that physician-related factors may explain much of the variation, emphasizing the value of register-based data for identifying prescribing patterns and the need for richer data on prescriber behavior.

Section 4 begins by discussing why inappropriate pharmacotherapy remains a significant challenge, affecting patient safety, treatment effectiveness, and healthcare costs. It explores factors driving variation in prescribing practices and highlights strategies to reduce inappropriate prescribing. Register data on medicine use provide valuable opportunities to analyze prescribing patterns, identify potential issues, and inform guideline development, although they are limited in capturing actual consumption.

The section then expands the discussion to international comparisons, which can offer valuable insights into systemic factors that influence inappropriate prescribing, ultimately leading to the development of policy measures that promote rational pharmacotherapy. Differences in reimbursement systems, generic substitution, and eligibility restrictions are shown to influence prescribing behavior.

Section 4 concludes by emphasizing the importance of multidisciplinary collaboration and calling for the broader use of quasiexperimental methods from health economics. We highlight Difference-in-Differences (DiD) and Regression Discontinuity Design (RDD), which allow robust causal inference when carefully implemented. Although these methods have limitations, they offer opportunities to generate novel evidence that can inform safer and more effective pharmacotherapy.

Finally, Sections 5 and 6 provide discussion questions and a practical application exercise, inviting readers to apply the methods introduced in this chapter to evaluate the appropriateness of medicine use in their own country using registry data.

2 Methods

2.1 Basic concepts

In this chapter, we use the term "medicine use research" to cover studies on drug utilization, drug consumption, and prescribing research. The WHO defined drug utilization in 1977 as “the marketing, distribution, prescription, and use of drugs in a society, with special emphasis on the resulting medical, social, and economic consequences”

(WHO, 2003). *Drug consumption* can refer to the movement of drugs across different levels of the supply chain, such as between manufacturer, wholesaler, pharmacy, and patient, or the actual intake of drugs by the patient. *Medicine use*, in contrast, specifically focuses on the patient level.

The most commonly used measures of medicine use in register research are defined daily doses (DDDs) and prevalence. The DDD is a standardized unit developed for statistical purposes and is defined as "the assumed average maintenance dose per day for a drug used for its main indication in adults" (*ATC/DDD Index*, 2025). Relating the number of DDDs to the population size and the number of days observed enables comparisons of medicine use across regions and time periods. One commonly used metric is DDDs per 1000 inhabitants per day (DDD/1000 inhabitants/day).

Prevalence of medicine use refers to the proportion of patients using a specific medicine or group of medicines within a given time period, most often a calendar year (Tenny and Hoffman, 2023). *Incidence of medicine use* is a related concept that captures the proportion of new users of a medicine within a given period. *Medicine cost* is also an important measure of medicine use because it is necessary for understanding resource allocation in healthcare and health system planning.

Each of these measures provides a different perspective on medicine use and is essential for accurately interpreting medicine use patterns from registers and for informing policy, practice, and research.

2.2 Register data

Data sources for measuring medicine use are an essential part of medicine use research. In many cases, administrative registers can be used as data sources for research, constructing study samples, and planning and development purposes (Strom, 2006). The main data sources considered here are different registers that include individual-level information on prescriptions and/or medicine purchases at pharmacies (Furu et al., 2010; Laugesen et al., 2021). Other commonly used registers in medical research include those covering hospitalizations, other types of healthcare use, diagnoses, and causes of death (Laugesen et al., 2021).

These registers typically contain large volumes of data and, in the case of national registers, cover the entire population. They are usually updated regularly, sometimes daily. However, since most registers are intended for administrative purposes rather than research, their proper use must be carefully considered. Prescription registers store data as incidents (e.g., prescriptions or purchases) and include information on the amount of medicine prescribed or purchased within a given period.

Using registers in medical research offers several major advantages (Thygesen and Ersbøll, 2014; Laugesen et al., 2021). They provide access to large, population-based datasets in electronic format, often covering long time periods that allow for retrospective analyses. Administrative data are generally representative of the target population and, unlike survey data, are not subject to recall bias.

Registers also have limitations (Thygesen and Ersbøll, 2014; Laugesen et al., 2021). Researchers cannot decide which variables are collected, as they can when designing surveys. Accessing data can be difficult and requires extensive research permission processes that incur high costs. Data may also be stored in challenging formats, requiring extensive data work. Register quality can vary, and documentation may be insufficient for research purposes. Many observed measures are proxies rather than direct outcomes. For example, pharmacy purchases only approximate actual medicine intake. Furthermore, many important health-related variables, such as smoking, body mass index, and alcohol use, are typically not included.

Examples of widely used registers for medicine use research include the Danish National Prescription Registry; Kela Prescription Register and Kanta Prescription Center in Finland; the Norwegian Prescription Database; the National Prescribed Drug Register in Sweden; the Clinical Practice Research Datalink in the UK; and Fair PharmaCare in British Columbia, to mention a few (Laugesen et al., 2021; *Clinical Practice Research Datalink*, 2025; PopulationDataBC, 2025). In the United States., there are various databases for conducting medicine use policy, patient behavior, and/or pharmacovigilance studies, such as the National Ambulatory Medical Care Survey and the Medical Expenditure Panel Survey, though none represent a national register of prescription drug users. Medicare Part D databases are based on administrative data covering most older adults and certain other insured populations (Centers for Medicare & Medicaid Services, 2025). Many of the registers classify the prescription data by the Anatomical Therapeutic Chemical (ATC) classification system developed by the WHO (*ATC/DDD Index*, 2025).

Our specific example register, the Finnish Dispensations reimbursable under the National Health Insurance Scheme register (previously: Kela Prescription Register), includes all prescription drugs reimbursed by the National Health Insurance program which covers all the residents in Finland (*Data resources catalogue: Medicines*, 2025). The register provides information on each purchased drug, basic patient characteristics, as well as the prescriber identification code and specialty. Key information on drug items includes the purchase date, ATC classification code, product number, package size, prescriber identification code, drug cost, and reimbursement details. The data have been available since 1994, which enables long-term studies.

Because these data are based on pharmacy transactions and reimbursement decisions, they are highly reliable and do not require extensive data cleaning. However, some data fields, such as ATC classes, package numbers, and purchase dates, may contain invalid values or typing errors, and standard data validity checks are in order. In addition, dispensations occurring with untypical frequencies, e.g., weekly or two-weekly dose dispensing, may introduce irregularities which have to be taken into account. Furthermore, purchases that are reimbursed retrospectively must be considered, as patients can claim reimbursements six months later. This is uncommon, though, as patients are usually reimbursed directly at the pharmacy.

Pharmacy transactions provide daily data on drug purchases, resulting in datasets with tens of millions of observations per year, even in small countries. This event-level data offers rich opportunities to analyze individual drug consumption, for example, by defining the duration of drug-use using consecutive purchases. However, most research relies on individual data aggregated over longer time spans, such as months or years. In these cases, item-level observations are summed over the period of interest. In our study, we used individual-level data at a yearly level to identify patients who met the risk-use indicators.

2.3 Medicine use risk indicators

Risk indicators for medicine use are developed to identify inappropriate prescribing practices, such as unsuitable medicines or harmful medicine combinations, and to mitigate the risks associated with them. These indicators are typically defined using explicit criteria compiled into structured lists. Most of the lists focus on older adults (Dimitrow et al., 2011; Masnoon et al., 2018; J. Paulamäki et al., 2023a; Vukoja and Mimica, 2024; Jyrkkä et al., 2024). The degree of validation and the suitability of these lists for register-based research vary considerably.

Lists primarily designed for clinical settings often rely on patient-specific clinical information. Consequently, some of these criteria cannot be directly applied in register-based studies, either due to missing variables or because the data are not available in a structured format. However, many risk indicators can be adapted to register data, making them valuable for large-scale register-based research (e.g., Jyrkkä et al., 2024; Rättö et al., 2024). It is also always beneficial for researchers if the list is readily available as open data.

Whenever possible, previously validated lists of risk indicators should be used. If a suitable validated list is unavailable, it is important to invest in validating a new list of criteria. At present, there is a shortage of validated lists, highlighting the need for new validation efforts, which would significantly advance rational pharmacotherapy (Masnoon et al., 2018; J. Paulamäki et al., 2023a).

Because new drugs are continuously introduced and research on inappropriate prescribing evolves rapidly, risk indicator lists require regular updating. Research frequently uncovers emerging safety concerns, and outdated criteria may fail to capture current risks. Therefore, it is essential to ensure that the chosen list reflects current clinical practice and is actively maintained (Jyrkkä et al., 2024).

The context of the study plays a key role in applying risk indicators. First, the selected list must match the relevant clinical subgroup, such as children, working-age adults, or older people, since this determines which inappropriate medication indicators are most meaningful. Second, the list should ideally be tailored to the local healthcare system, either developed within or adapted to the country of study. However, if the primary goal is international comparability, a more general list that is suitable for such settings is preferable.

2.4 Defining risk groups

Identifying the appropriate patient groups is essential for targeting interventions and improving pharmacotherapy. Patient selection can be approached in different ways, for example, by focusing on:

1. Those most likely to benefit from interventions, according to previous evidence,
2. Those with the most severe drug-related problems,
3. Those generating the highest costs,
4. Those with problems that are most feasible to address, or combinations of these criteria.

Alternatively, patient groups may be defined using socioeconomic factors, often guided by health policy priorities. Examples include young women, older adults, men, children with low income, or immigrant populations. Such characteristics are typically available in national registers, making them practical for research.

Evidence shows that a relatively small proportion of patients often accounts for a large share of pharmaceutical costs. In our previous study, the 5% of patients with the highest medicine expenditures accounted for half of the total pharmaceutical spending. Almost half of these high-cost patients had excessive polypharmacy, defined as the use of more than 10 drugs during a year (Saastamoinen and Verho, 2013). In addition, a considerable share of these high-cost polypharmacy patients also used PIMs (Saastamoinen and Verho, 2015).

Importantly, the data needed to identify these groups, such as cost and prescription records, are usually available in registers.

A useful strategy is to cross-tabulate medicine data with patient characteristics, e.g., high costs with demographic background, and, when possible, information on inappropriate medication use. This enables the identification of the most relevant target groups for interventions aimed at reducing inappropriate prescribing.

Regional variation is a specific feature of prescribing practices and offers new opportunities to address inappropriate medication use. Prescribing patterns differ substantially between regions such as countries, health districts, or municipalities (Henriksen et al., 2015; Di Martino et al., 2017; Calara et al., 2017; Selke Krulichová et al., 2025). Importantly, the patient's and prescriber's regions are typically recorded in registers, making regional comparisons feasible.

In areas where inappropriate prescribing is most prevalent, it is important to identify the local channels through which prescribing practices can be influenced. These may include regional health authorities or so-called key evidence leaders. In the context of prescribing, key evidence leaders are physicians who are leading experts in their specialty and region and can influence the prescribing behavior of their peers (Fernández et al., 2025). Reaching and convincing such individuals about appropriate prescribing can, therefore, be a highly effective strategy for improving prescribing.

Physician-related factors are generally the most difficult to find in registry data. Key determinants of prescribing behavior, such as participation in continuing medical education or exposure to pharmaceutical marketing, are rarely recorded. However, basic demographic data, such as physician age, sex, or region, are sometimes available and help to identify relevant target groups.

2.5 Statistical methods for analyzing regional variation

The first steps in the statistical analysis of medicine use register data involve defining one or more outcome variables of interest and the variables used to explain the variation in outcomes. The type of outcome variable (continuous, discrete, categorical) is important, as it dictates the statistical methods suitable for the analysis. In the example analysis shown in this chapter, the outcome of interest is the prevalence of PIM use, which is a continuous fractional variable with values well within the interval (0, 1) and away from the boundaries. To investigate factors that may explain regional variation in PIM use, we employed ordinary least squares (OLS) regression, which provides a simple and interpretable analysis framework.

Statistical analysis requires sufficiently large data sets so that the parameters can be estimated precisely, and statistical testing has the power to reject hypotheses. We compared hospital districts in Finland, which provide a general overview of regional variation in PIM use. However, the number of districts is limited and therefore not sufficient for analyzing variation or conducting statistical testing. Instead, we focus on the municipal level, where primary care is organized. This allows us to take a closer look at geographical differences in PIM use and perform statistical inference with a larger number of observations.

Statistical inference is typically based on hypothesis testing. For instance, the null hypothesis could be that there are no regional differences in PIM use after controlling for observed regional characteristics, and a regression model would be estimated to test if the parameters for the regional differences are zero. In our case, the regional differences were so large that testing this null hypothesis did not appear insightful, and we chose a different approach in the analysis.

Our primary aim was to assess the extent to which municipal-level characteristics can explain variation in PIM use. We first estimated a full model that included all selected characteristics. In the OLS framework, the coefficient of determination (R^2) quantifies the proportion of variance in PIM use explained by these predictors. We then applied a model selection procedure to identify the most influential characteristics. Several methods are available for this purpose, including penalized regression (e.g., Lasso) and approaches based on information criteria. We chose to use the Akaike Information Criterion (AIC) to exclude statistically irrelevant characteristics from the model.

Our approach provides an indirect assessment of how well the studied characteristics explain variation in PIM use. High explanatory power (R^2) means that most of the variation can be attributed to the observed regional characteristics, whereas low explanatory power suggests that important factors remain unobserved. While our dataset was relatively rich in variables describing patient, health system, and economic characteristics of the regions, it lacked information on physicians' prescribing practices and other institutional aspects of health care organizations. Since these factors are known to influence PIM use, we infer that they are the most likely candidates to account for the remaining regional differences.

3 Case study: Regional variation in potentially inappropriate medicine use in older adults

In our example study[a] (Saastamoinen and Verho, 2021), we aimed to explore regional variation in PIM use among older adults and the association with regional health-system-related, patient-related, and economic characteristics and the frequency of PIM use.

We used data from the Finnish Prescription Register, a national database that records all reimbursed prescription drug purchases in Finland. The study included all residents aged 75 years and older (n = 404,034) who purchased medicines covered by the National Health Insurance at community pharmacies in 2011.

During the study period, Finnish health care was organized by local municipalities with government support (Finland: health system review, 2019) (Ministry of Social Affairs and Health Pharmacotherapy, 2026). Municipal health centers provided primary care, while hospitals organized by hospital districts delivered specialized care. Services were publicly funded, with private care supplementing the system. Outpatient prescriptions from health centers and hospital polyclinics were dispensed through community pharmacies. Physicians were not directed by local prescribing budgets or academic detailing but were responsible for rational prescribing and adherence to national guidelines. The universal reimbursement system guided costs toward severe diseases, cost-effective treatments, and generic medicines. The Social Insurance Institution of Finland also provided annual prescribing feedback to prescribers (Ahomäki, 2025).

The Finnish Meds75+ criteria were applied to identify PIM users (Bell et al., 2013). Specifically, drugs classified in category D ("Avoid use in older persons") of the Meds75+ database were used as the indicator of PIM use. A PIM user was defined as any individual who purchased at least one prescribed medicine from category D during 2011.

PIM use was compared between Finnish hospital districts (n = 21) and municipalities (n = 267). A linear regression model was used to explain the variation in PIM use between municipalities. The AIC was used to determine a parsimonious model specification. The municipality-level explanatory variables were obtained from the Sotkanet Indicator Bank, maintained by the Finnish National Institute for Health and Welfare (Table 17.1). The variables were chosen based on their availability in the Sotkanet Indicator Bank, and only one variable was selected from each subcategory to avoid excessive multicollinearity. The variables included health-system-related factors (outpatient physician visits, private physician visits, specialized care outpatient visits, specialized somatic health care days, share of population over 64 years), economic factors (health care net expenditure, at-risk-of-poverty rate), and patient-related factors (population size, population density, share of Swedish-speaking population, share of women, general morbidity index, cancer index, coronary heart disease index, musculoskeletal disorder index, mental health index, accidental injury index).

3.1 Results

Prevalence variation of PIM prescribing in individuals aged 75 and older at the hospital district level was substantial, as the difference between the districts with the least and most PIM prescribing was 45.2% (Fig. 17.1). The prevalence was highest at 39.0%, in the hospital district of South-West Finland and lowest at 26.9% in the hospital district of the Åland Islands. More densely populated areas tended to have higher rates of PIM prescribing, while areas with the largest Swedish-speaking populations had lower rates.

In the municipal-level analysis (Fig. 17.2), an age and gender-adjusted PIM indicator was used to account for differences in population structures and to normalize the city of Helsinki to 0. The adjusted PIM indicator was highest at 8.4%, in the municipality of Aura (South-West Finland) and lowest at −14.8%, in Jomala (The Åland Islands).

The correlation between the size of the population in the municipality and PIM use (Fig. 17.2) showed an association toward greater PIM use in larger municipalities (corr. = 0.145, P = 0.018).

Both the full and parsimonious models, incorporating a set of economic, health system-related, and patient-related factors, provided nearly similar results (Table 17.2). The studied factors were able to explain approximately 23% of municipal-level variation in PIM use. The large population size of the municipality did not appear to be a key factor once the use of private physicians was accounted for in the model. In fact, the association between the log population size and PIM use is negative in the models.

Other significant factors in the models were the higher share of women and higher health care expenditure, which became significant only in the parsimonious specification. When comparing the magnitudes of the coefficients, the significant factors have a relatively similar impact. Private physician visits have the largest impact in the parsimonious model, as one standard deviation change in visits is associated with a 1.2 percentage point increase in PIM use. The higher share of the Swedish-speaking population was strongly associated with lower PIM use.

[a] This section is based on our article Saastamoinen L, Verho J. Regional variation in potentially inappropriate medicine use in older adults.—A national register-based cross-sectional study on economic, health system-related and patient-related characteristics. Res Social Adm Pharm. 2021 Jun;17(6):1223–1227. doi: 10.1016/j.sapharm.2020.08.018. Epub 2020 Oct 15. PMID: 33071213.

TABLE 17.1 Descriptive statistics for the municipality-level explanatory variables.

	Mean	S.D.	Min.	Max.
Health-system related factors				
Outpatient physician visits (per 1000)	1836	898.5	0.00	14,066
Private physician visits (per 1000)	0.51	0.21	0.20	1.30
Specialized care outpatient visits (per 1000)	1408	374.4	781.0	4219
Specialized somatic health care days (per 1000)	681.0	151.6	384.0	1413
Share of population over 64 (%)	20.82	4.95	7.90	34.10
Economic factors				
Health care net expenditure (€ per capita)	1671	421.5	−36.70	2574
At-risk-of-poverty rate (%)	15.46	4.37	4.40	27.10
Patient-related factors				
Population size	19,916	47,393	1994	588,549
Population density (per km2)	65.84	235.7	0.50	2755
Share of Swedish-speaking population (%)	6.84	20.43	0.00	92.90
Share of women (%)	49.84	1.08	46.71	53.04
General morbidity index	117.7	20.70	62.40	180.30
Cancer index	94.38	13.45	54.50	132.80
Coronary heart disease index	127.4	36.47	62.00	280.00
Musculoskeletal disorder index	146.8	41.42	29.30	255.10
Mental health index	113.9	34.39	32.50	252.40
Accidental injury index	112.9	20.27	62.80	174.50
Number of observations				267

Note: Sotkanet data used in defining the explanatory variables are accessible at https://sotkanet.fi/sotkanet/en. Explanatory variables are not available for 11 small municipalities. After excluding these regions, our data included 267 municipalities with at least 1994 inhabitants.

3.2 Interpretation of findings

Regional variation in potentially inappropriate prescribing at both hospital district and municipal levels was significant. PIM prescribing tended to be more common in municipalities with a larger proportion of women, higher health expenditure, and a greater number of private doctor visits, and less common in municipalities with a higher proportion of Swedish-speaking residents.

In line with our study, there is relatively large regional or between-practice variation in PIM prescribing (Beuscart et al., 2017; Stocks et al., 2015). However, only a limited number of studies address the reasons for this variation. It has been shown that regional variation in PIM use still exists, but the prevalence of PIM use has decreased markedly since 2011 (*Use of Avoidable Medications in the Elderly*, 2025). The decreasing trend may be due to an increased focus on rational medicine use in older adults and the promotion of various improvement tools (Fimea, 2020; Ministry of Social Affairs and Health Rational Pharmacotherapy, 2020) and, therefore, improved prescribing practices (Leikola, 2012; Colla et al., 2015). The decreasing trend may also be influenced by changes in the reimbursement system, such as the removal of amitriptyline, nitrazepam, and vaginal estrogen from reimbursement, which means that they do not appear in the prescription register even though they may still be used. However, the prevalence figures greatly depend on the criteria and data used, as has been shown (Paulamäki et al., 2023a).

In this study, the rate of population at risk of poverty showed no association with PIM prescribing. In several studies, social deprivation has been associated with high PIM prescribing or high prescribing of certain drug groups (Colla et al., 2015; Klein et al., 2015; Beuscart et al., 2017; Mordecai et al., 2018). In Finland, the health care system ensures care for the whole population on a national social insurance basis, which may reduce the difference between poor and wealthy regions. We also found an inverse association in PIM prescribing with the areas that have the largest population of the Swedish-speaking minority, which has earlier been associated with lower mortality and slightly better health than the ethnic majority in Finland (Suominen, 2014).

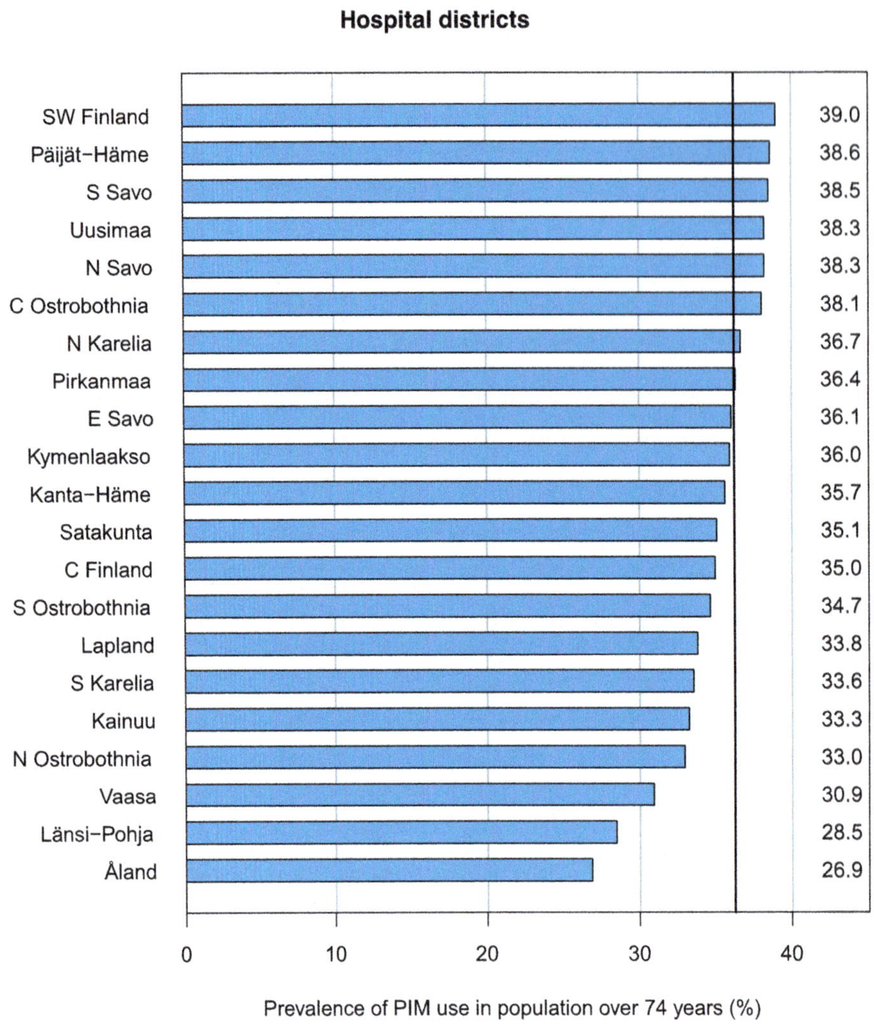

FIG. 17.1 Prevalence of PIM use in the population over 74 years (%).

In line with this study, the female gender (Hyttinen, 2018; Leikola, 2012) and a high number of private doctor visits (Colla et al., 2015) have been shown to be associated with high PIM prescribing. The latter may be partly explained by increased access to medication (Colla et al., 2015). In municipalities with many opportunities for visiting doctors, patient follow-up may fail more easily than in small municipalities with no private doctors.

These results indicate that substantial regional differences in prescribing may contribute to regional inequality and the uneven distribution of pharmaceutical costs. Since patient- and system-related factors explained only a small portion of the observed variation, the underlying causes may relate to physicians' characteristics and prescribing behaviors. Such information is not typically available in administrative registers. Therefore, studies like this are useful for ruling out health system, economic, and patient-related factors as primary explanations for regional variation. However, richer data on physician behavior are needed to establish a clearer link with PIM prescribing. For instance, interactions between the pharmaceutical industry and physicians have been shown to influence PIM prescribing (Fickweiler et al., 2017).

4 Discussion

4.1 Addressing problems in pharmacotherapy

Inappropriate pharmacotherapy remains a persistent challenge in healthcare, with consequences for patient safety, treatment effectiveness, and healthcare costs. Prescribing practices often vary due to organizational culture.

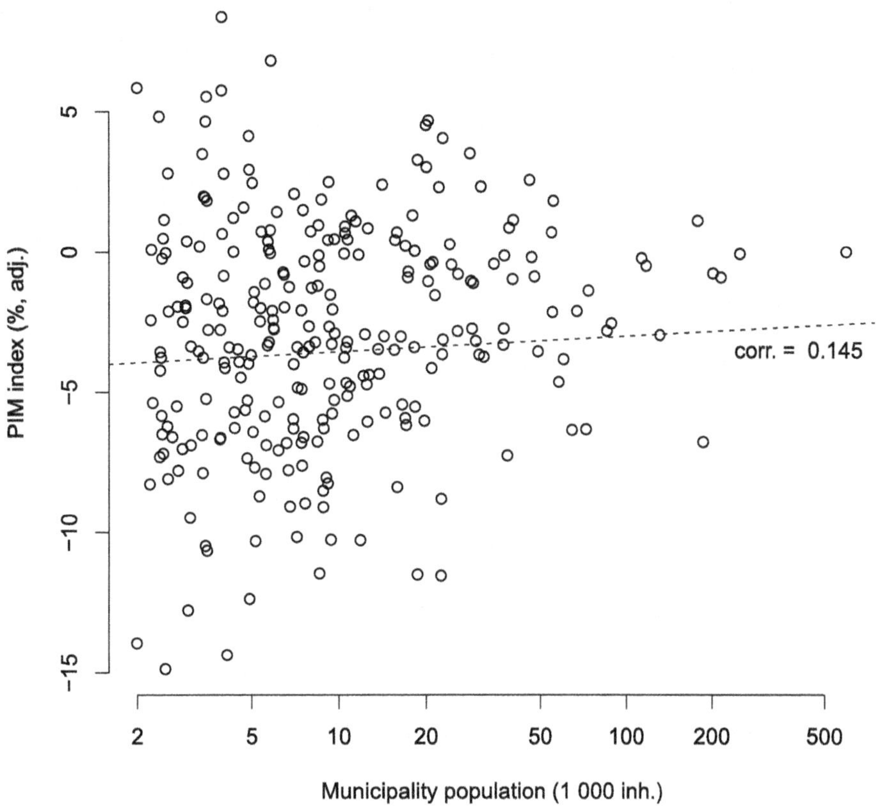

FIG. 17.2 Variation in municipality-level PIM index by municipality population size. The PIM index is age and gender-adjusted (the reference municipality is Helsinki). Population size is presented on a logarithmic scale.

Large variations can indicate suboptimal medication use in certain regions, endangering patient safety. Reducing suboptimal medicine use is therefore essential for mitigating adverse effects and containing costs. One promising strategy is to increase physicians' awareness of medicine costs and inappropriate prescribing. Although behavior change in this area is difficult, well-designed mailed information interventions, particularly those incorporating peer comparisons, have shown some success in influencing prescribing decisions (Doctor et al., 2018; Sacarny et al., 2018; Ahomäki et al., 2020; Navathe et al., 2022; Ahomäki et al., 2023; Hallett et al., 2024).

Register data on medicine use provides valuable opportunities to analyze prescribing patterns and detect potential problems in pharmacotherapy. Such research can highlight areas of concern, stimulate professional debate, and ultimately contribute to guideline development. At the same time, register studies have important limitations: institutional medicine use may not be fully captured, and purchases do not always correspond to actual consumption (Furu et al., 2010). Furthermore, the inappropriate prescribing shown in register research cannot usually be addressed by contacting the actual patients involved due to data protection concerns, so interventions need to be undertaken separately.

Interventions to address potentially inappropriate prescribing have been widely studied, particularly in older adults. Several systematic reviews have demonstrated that such interventions can reduce the number of PIMs prescribed to older adults (Dos Santos et al., 2019; Rodrigues et al., 2022). Combined interventions are especially effective, even though many types of interventions may work (Dos Santos et al., 2019). Successful approaches include medication reviews by health professionals (alone or in teams), pharmacist-led interventions to resolve or prevent medication-related problems, computerized alert systems at prescribing or dispensing, and educational initiatives targeting both clinicians and patients (Dos Santos et al., 2019).

Collaboration among pharmacists, physicians, and statisticians is essential for successful medicine use register studies. Combining clinical, methodological, and pharmacotherapy expertise can lead to more comprehensive and impactful research. Including health economists on the team has the potential to uncover new methodological solutions and address the cost aspect, an enduring concern in resource-constrained healthcare.

Institutional settings also play a central role in shaping prescribing practices. Reimbursement systems, for example, are powerful tools for promoting rational drug use. Measures such as excluding inappropriate medications

TABLE 17.2 Regression models for municipality-level potentially inappropriate medicine (PIM) index (%).

	Model A					Model B				
	Estimate	Std. Error	*t*-value	*P*-value		Estimate	Std. Error	*t*-value	*P*-value	
Intercept	−53.787	14.508	−3.707	<0.001	***	−54.724	12.424	−4.405	<0.001	***
Health-system related factors										
Outpatient physician visits (per 1000 inhabitants)	0.000	0.000	0.500	0.618						
Private physician visits (per 1000 inhabitants)	5.910	1.618	3.653	<0.001	***	6.565	1.369	4.794	<0.001	***
Specialized care outpatient visits (per 1000 inhabitants)	0.000	0.001	−0.285	0.776						
Spec. somatic health care days (per 1000 inh.).	0.001	0.002	0.581	0.562						
Share of population over 64 (%)	0.010	0.081	0.122	0.903						
Economic factors										
Health care net expenditure (€ per capita)	0.001	0.001	1.432	0.154		0.001	0.001	1.986	0.048	**
At-risk-of-poverty rate (%)	−0.087	0.103	−0.847	0.398						
Patient-related factors										
Population size (log)	−0.658	0.352	−1.872	0.062	*	−0.660	0.284	−2.325	0.021	**
Population density (per km^2)	0.000	0.001	−0.030	0.976						
Share of Swedish-speaking population (%)	−0.030	0.014	−2.108	0.036	**	−0.030	0.012	−2.466	0.014	**
Share of women (%)	1.014	0.318	3.190	0.002	***	1.033	0.274	3.770	<0.001	***
General morbidity index	0.041	0.083	0.489	0.625						
Cancer index	−0.003	0.023	−0.112	0.911						
Coronary heart disease index	−0.008	0.012	−0.676	0.500						
Musculoskeletal disorder index	−0.009	0.019	−0.459	0.647						
Mental health index	0.006	0.026	0.213	0.832		0.012	0.008	1.538	0.125	
Accidental injury index	−0.004	0.016	−0.262	0.794						
R^2				0.233					0.228	
Number of observations				267					267	

*Note: The specification for Model B was selected using the AIC. * denotes P < .1, ** denotes P < .05, *** denotes P < .01. Sotkanet data used in defining the explanatory variables are accessible at https://sotkanet.fi/sotkanet/en. Explanatory variables are not available for 44 small municipalities. After excluding these regions, our data included 267 municipalities with at least 1994 inhabitants.*

from reimbursement lists, prioritizing generics, or restricting reimbursement to specific conditions can substantially reduce inappropriate or unwanted prescribing (King and Roberts, 2007; Martikainen et al., 2010).

Despite the challenges, it is imperative to continue developing new methodologies and promoting cooperation among healthcare professionals. Targeting specific groups, such as older adults, children, and regions with high rates of inappropriate medicine use, can make interventions more effective. Ultimately, the goal is to promote rational medicine use, improve patient outcomes, and enhance the overall quality of healthcare.

4.2 International comparisons

Above, we discussed regional comparisons in medicine use. From a broader perspective, it is essential to look beyond local or national contexts and extend research to international comparisons. Cross-country studies can provide valuable insights into differences in medicine use and patterns of inappropriate pharmacotherapy.

Including a larger number of countries allows for a richer understanding of underlying determinants. Equally important is the opportunity to explore within-country variation in multicountry studies, as well as to compare strategies aimed at improving pharmacotherapy across diverse health systems.

Multicountry comparisons, however, present both opportunities and challenges. On one hand, the outcomes selected must be simple and clearly defined to allow for efficient and comparable data collection. In some cases, outcomes can even be aggregated statistics, avoiding the need for individual-level data and the extensive permission processes they require. The versatility and complexity of these studies come from the possibility of comparing the outcomes in different contexts and health care systems.

On the other hand, these studies demand substantial coordination, particularly from the lead author. Identifying suitable collaborators with timely access to data may require persistence. Even with simple outcome measures, the number of datasets is ideally large, making data harmonization a considerable task. Moreover, manuscripts involving many coauthors can face lengthy processes during the writing and review phases. In such cases, the lead author may need to prioritize and manage feedback selectively to keep the process efficient. Despite these challenges, the benefits of diverse collaboration are substantial: discussing results across multiple settings enriches interpretation and often generates new, innovative ideas for improving pharmacotherapy.

4.3 Multidisciplinary collaboration and quasiexperimental research designs

Collaboration among pharmacists, physicians, and statisticians is essential for successful medicine use register studies. Combining clinical, methodological, and pharmacotherapy expertise can lead to more comprehensive and impactful research. Including health economists on the team has the potential to uncover new methodological solutions and address the cost aspect, an enduring concern in resource-constrained healthcare. We believe that medicine research would benefit from a broader application of modern empirical methods used in health economics.

Quasiexperimental research designs make it possible to assess the causal impacts of natural experiments, policy reforms, and intervention discontinuities. When randomized controlled trials are unfeasible, these methods can yield robust evidence to guide improvements in pharmacotherapy, provided they are applied carefully. Next, we discuss two prominent quasiexperimental methods. Other widely used quasiexperimental approaches include instrumental variables, matching, and interrupted time series design (Kim and Steiner, 2016).

DiD can be used when a natural experiment or a policy reform affects one group of individuals (the treatment group) but not another comparable group (the control group). By comparing outcome changes over time between the two, researchers can isolate the causal effect of the intervention (Dimick and Ryan, 2014; Baker, n.d.). In addition to policy reforms, other examples of natural experiments include geographic variation (e.g., distance to hospitals), environmental shocks (e.g., pollution episodes, pandemics), and market shocks (e.g., drug shortages). Overall, the DiD is useful when policies or external events generate treatment and control conditions in ways that mimic random assignment, even if unintended.

Examples of DiD designs include analyses of Medicaid expansions to study the impact of insurance on prescription drug use (Ghosh et al., 2019), regulatory letters on opioid prescribing (Ahomäki et al., 2020), electronic prescription system rollouts on prescribing quality (Böckerman et al., 2025), and liability immunity for military physicians on defensive medicine (Frakes and Gruber, 2019). These studies leverage policy changes and institutional shifts to credibly identify causal effects in medical practice and prescription behavior.

RDD exploits variation in treatment assignment at a predefined cutoff. Individuals or units just above the cutoff are considered treated, while those just below serve as controls (Calonico et al., 2024). When subjects cannot precisely manipulate their position relative to the cutoff, the resulting variation is effectively random, allowing credible causal inference. Examples of RDD designs include age-based eligibility rules, insurance or subsidy cutoffs, and clinical guideline thresholds.

While RDD is highly valuable because it does not depend on a major policy change or external shock to generate variation, it also has important limitations. Reliable estimates usually require a large number of observations near the cutoff. Moreover, the findings are local by design and may not generalize to individuals farther away from the cutoff threshold.

Examples of RDD designs include analyses of Medicare Part D's coverage threshold to study how price salience influences drug purchasing (Dalton et al., 2020), the same discontinuity to assess the effect of drug insurance on inappropriate prescribing (Lee et al., 2024), copayment thresholds to examine demand responses to out-of-pocket drug prices (Verho and Harju, 2025), and guideline-based LDL cholesterol cutoffs to evaluate the impact of statins on myocardial infarction (Odden et al., 2023). These studies illustrate how RDD exploits sharp thresholds in policies or clinical guidelines to credibly estimate causal effects.

4.4 Concluding remarks

Despite the challenges, it is imperative to continue developing new methodologies and promoting cooperation among healthcare professionals. Advancing register-based research to improve pharmacotherapy requires new and innovative ideas. Future generations of researchers have the important task of iteratively refining and building upon earlier work. Targeting specific groups, such as older adults, children, and regions with high rates of inappropriate medicine use, can make interventions more effective. Ultimately, the goal is to promote rational medicine use, improve patient outcomes, and enhance the overall quality of healthcare.

5 Questions for further discussion

1. What are the key advantages of register-based studies? What insights can registers provide into patterns of medicine use?
2. What data protection and ethical considerations must be addressed when planning a register-based study?
3. Which populations are at an increased risk of inappropriate medicine use, and how can these groups be identified using registry data?
4. Which empirical methods can be applied to analyze the factors associated with inappropriate medicine use?

6 The application exercise

You have been commissioned by your country's Medicines Agency to evaluate the appropriateness of medicine use in older adults using national register data. The agency initially suggests applying the Beers Criteria. Your task is to assess which PIM list is most suitable for use with register data. This involves comparing their compatibility with local drug coding systems, data availability, and clinical relevance.

- Besides the Beers Criteria, what other PIM lists, local risk indicators, or tools could be applied in your country to assess inappropriate medicine use?
- Have these indicators been validated, and what evidence supports their reliability and relevance?
- Which medicine use registers are available in your country, and what type of data do they contain?
- Are the available registers suitable for analyzing the selected risk indicators and identifying PIM use?
- Give examples of specific risk groups among older adults relevant to your research question. How can they be identified using registry data?
- What specific variables from the registers are required to conduct your analysis?
- What research permissions and ethical approvals are required to access and use the registry data for this study?

AI disclosure

During the preparation of this work, the author(s) used ChatGPT to proofread and summarize text. After using this tool/service, the author(s) reviewed and edited the content as needed and take full responsibility for the content of the publication.

References

Finnish Medicines Agency Fimea Use of Avoidable Medications in the Elderly, 2025. https://fimea.fi/en/use-of-avoidable-medications-in-the-elderly

Medicines and Health Care Products Regulatory Agency Clinical Practice Research Datalink, 2025. https://www.cprd.com/

The Social Insurance Institution of Finland Data resources catalogue: medicines, 2025. https://aineistokatalogi.fi/catalog/studies/ff551f4e-6842-4732-962d-74499a339c46

WHO Collaborating Centre for Drug Statistics ATC/DDD Index, 2025. https://atcddd.fhi.no/atc_ddd_index/

Ahomäki, I., 2025. Information Interventions and Physician Prescribing Behavior. JYU Dissertations 923, Jyväskylä University School of Business and Economics. https://jyx.jyu.fi/jyx/Record/jyx_123456789_101708.

Ahomäki, I., Böckerman, P., Pehkonen, J., Saastamoinen, L., 2023. Effect of information intervention on prescribing practice for neuropathic pain in older patients: a nationwide register-based study. Adis Finland Drugs Aging. 11791969. 40 (1), 81–88. Available from: https://www.springer.com/journal/40266. doi:10.1007/s40266-022-00993-4.

Ahomäki, I., Pitkänen, V., Soppi, A., Saastamoinen, L., 2020. Impact of a physician targeted letter on opioid prescribing. J. Health Econ. 72, 102344. doi:10.1016/j.jhealeco.2020.

American Geriatrics Society, 2023. American Geriatrics Society 2023 updated AGS Beers Criteria® for potentially inappropriate medication use in older adults. J. Am. Geriatr. Soc. 0002-8614. 71 (7), 2052–2081. doi:10.1111/jgs.18372.

Baker, A., Difference-in-differences designs: a practitioner's guide. J. Econ. Literat. doi:10.1257/jel.20251650.

Beers, M.H., Ouslander, J.G., Rollingher, I., Reuben, D.B., Brooks, J., Beck, J.C., 1991. Explicit criteria for determining inappropriate medication use in nursing home residents. Arch. Intern. Med. 15383679. 151 (9), 1825–1832. doi:10.1001/archinte.1991.00400090107019.

Bell, J.S., Ahonen, J., Lavikainen, P., Hartikainen, S., 2013. Potentially inappropriate drug use among older persons in Finland: application of a new national categorization. Eur. J. Clin. Pharmacol. 69 (3), 657–664.

Beuscart, J.B., Genin, M., Dupont, C., Verloop, D., Duhamel, A., Defebvre, M.M., Puisieux, F., 2017. Potentially inappropriate medication prescribing is associated with socioeconomic factors: a spatial analysis in the French Nord-Pas-de-Calais Region. Age Ageing. 14682834. 46 (4), 607–613. Available from: http://ageing.oxfordjournals.org/. doi:10.1093/ageing/afw245.

Böckerman, P., Laine, L.T., Nurminen, M., Saxell, T., 2025. Information integration, coordination failures, and quality of prescribing. J. Hum. Resour. 0022-166X. 60 (3), 1054–1092. doi:10.3368/jhr.0921-11910r2.

Calara, P.S., Althin, R., Carlsson, K.S., Schmitt-Egenolf, M., 2017. Regional differences in the prescription of biologics for psoriasis in Sweden: a register-based study of 4168 patients. BioDrugs. 1179190X. 31 (1), 75–82. Available from: http://rd.springer.com/journal/40259. doi:10.1007/s40259-016-0209-y.

Calonico, S., Jawadekar, N., Kezios, K., Hazzouri, A.Z.A., 2024. Regression discontinuity design studies: a guide for health researchers. BMJ. 1756-1833. 384, e072254. doi:10.1136/bmj-2022-072254.

Centers for Medicare & Medicaid Services, 2025. Part D Claims Data https://www.cms.gov/medicare/coverage/prescription-drug-coverage/part-d-claims-data

Colla, C.H., Morden, N.E., Sequist, T.D., Schpero, W.L., Rosenthal, M.B., 2015. Choosing wisely: prevalence and correlates of low-value health care services in the United States. J. Gen. Intern. Med. 15251497. 30 (2), 221–228. Available from: http://www.springerlink.com/content/120414/. doi:10.1007/s11606-014-3070-z.

Dalton, C.M., Gowrisankaran, G., Town, R.J., 2020. Salience, myopia, and complex dynamic incentives: evidence from medicare part D. Rev. Econ. Stud. 1467937X. 87 (2), 822–869. Available from: www.oxfordjournals.org/our_journals/restud. doi:10.1093/restud/rdz023.

Di Martino, M., Lallo, A., Kirchmayer, U., Davoli, M., Fusco, D., 2017. Prevalence of antibiotic prescription in pediatric outpatients in Italy: the role of local health districts and primary care physicians in determining variation. A multilevel design for healthcare decision support. BMC Public Health. 1471-2458. 17 (1). doi:10.1186/s12889-017-4905-4.

Dimick, J.B., Ryan, A.M., 2014. Methods for evaluating changes in health care policy: the difference-in-differences approach. JAMA. 15383598. 312 (22), 2401–2402. Available from: http://jama.jamanetwork.com/article.aspx?articleid=2020357. doi:10.1001/jama.2014.16153.

Dimitrow, M.S., Airaksinen, M.S.A., Kivelä, S.L., Lyles, A., Leikola, S.N.S., 2011. Comparison of prescribing criteria to evaluate the appropriateness of drug treatment in individuals aged 65 and older: a systematic review. J. Am. Geriatr. Soc. 15325415. 59 (8), 1521–1530. doi:10.1111/j.1532-5415.2011.03497.x.

Doctor, J.N., Nguyen, A., Lev, R., Lucas, J., Knight, T., Zhao, H., Menchine, M., 2018. Opioid prescribing decreases after learning of a patient's fatal overdose. Science. 10959203. 361 (6402), 588–590. Available from: http://science.sciencemag.org/content/361/6402/588/tab-pdf. doi:10.1126/science.aat4595.

Dos Santos, N.S., Marengo, L.L., Moraes, F.D.S., Barberato-Filho, S., 2019. Interventions to reduce the prescription of inappropriate medicines in older patients. Revista de Saude Publica. 00348910. 53 (1). Available from: http://www.scielo.br/pdf/rsp/v53/1518-8787-rsp-53-07.pdf. doi:10.11606/S1518-8787.2019053000781.

Fastbom, J., Johnell, K., 2015. National indicators for quality of drug therapy in older persons: the Swedish experience from the first 10 years. Drugs Aging. 11791969. 32 (3), 189–199. Available from: http://rd.springer.com/journal/40266. doi:10.1007/s40266-015-0242-4.

Fernández, J., Ribeiro, F., Dick, H.B., Kohnen, T., Rocha-de-Lossada, C., Rodríguez-Vallejo, M., 2025. The conceptualization of 'key evidence leaders' from 'opinion leaders': a review also applicable in ophthalmology. Archivos de la Sociedad Española de Oftalmología (English Edition. 21735794. doi:10.1016/j.oftale.2025.07.016.

Fickweiler, F., Fickweiler, W., Urbach, E., 2017. Interactions between physicians and the pharmaceutical industry generally and sales representatives specifically and their association with physicians' attitudes and prescribing habits: a systematic review. BMJ Open 7, e016408. doi:10.1136/bmjopen-2017-016408.

Fimea, 2020. Finnish Medicines Agency Fimea Meds75+ https://fimea.fi/en/databases_and_registeries/medicines_information/database_of_medication_for_older_persons

Finland: health system review, 2019. Health Systems in Transition 21 (2). https://eurohealthobservatory.who.int/publications/i/finland-health-system-review-2019.

Frakes, M., Gruber, J., 2019. Defensive medicine: evidence from military immunity. Am. Econ. J. Econ. Policy. 1945-7731. 11 (3), 197–231. doi:10.1257/pol.20180167.

Furu, K., Wettermark, B., Andersen, M., Martikainen, J.E., Almarsdottir, A.B., Sørensen, H.T., 2010. The nordic countries as a cohort for pharmacoepidemiological research. Basic Clin. Pharmacol. Toxicol. 17427843. 106 (2), 86–94. doi:10.1111/j.1742-7843.2009.00494.x.

Ghosh, A., Simon, K., Sommers, B.D., 2019. The effect of health insurance on prescription drug use among low-income adults: evidence from recent medicaid expansions. J. Health Econ. 01676296. 63, 64–80. doi:10.1016/j.jhealeco.2018.11.002.

Hallett, M.F., Kjær, T., Bjørnskov Pedersen, L., 2024. The use of nudge strategies in improving physicians' prescribing behavior: a systematic review and meta-analysis. Med. Decis. Making. 0272-989X. 44 (8), 986–1011. doi:10.1177/0272989x241270001.

Henriksen, D.P., Rasmussen, L., Hansen, M.R., Hallas, J., Pottegård, A., Dalal, K., 2015. Comparison of the five Danish Regions regarding demographic characteristics, healthcare utilization, and medication use—a descriptive cross-sectional study. PLOS ONE. 1932-6203. 10 (10), e0140197. doi:10.1371/journal.pone.0140197.

Hyttinen, V., Health and economic aspects of potentially inappropriate medications in older people. Publications of the University of Eastern Finland (2018), Available from: http://urn.fi/URN:ISBN:978-952-61-2955-6.

Jyrkkä, J., Paulamäki, J., Hartikainen, S., Ahonen, J., Antikainen, R., Jauhonen, H.M., Jämsen, E., Kössi, A., Laurila, J., Roitto, H.M., Söderling, R., Tiihonen, M., Huupponen, R., 2024. Prescribing appropriate medicines to older adults: a Finnish experience with the web-based Meds75+ database. Adis Finland Drugs Aging. 11791969. 41 (8), 665–674. Available from: https://www.springer.com/journal/40266. doi:10.1007/s40266-024-01131-y.

Kim, Y., Steiner, P., 2016. Quasi-experimental designs for causal inference. Educ. Psychol. 0046-1520. 51 (3–4), 395–405. doi:10.1080/00461520.2016.1207177.

King, M.A., Roberts, M.S., 2007. The influence of the Pharmaceutical Benefits Scheme (PBS) on inappropriate prescribing in Australian nursing homes. Pharm. World Sci. 09281231. 29 (1), 39–42. doi:10.1007/s11096-005-5618-9.

Klein, E.Y., Makowsky, M., Orlando, M., Hatna, E., Braykov, N.P., Laxminarayan, R., 2015. Influence of provider and urgent care density across different socioeconomic strata on outpatient antibiotic prescribing in the USA. J. Antimicrob. Chemother. 1460-2091. 70 (5), 1580–1587. doi:10.1093/jac/dku563.

Laugesen, K., Ludvigsson, J.F., Schmidt, M., Gissler, M., Valdimarsdottir, U.A., Lunde, A., Sørensen, H.T., 2021. Nordic health registry-based research: a review of health care systems and key registries. Clin. Epidemiol. 11791349. 13, 533–554. Available from: http://www.dovepress.com/clinical-epidemiology-journal. doi:10.2147/CLEP.S314959.

Lee, D., Kim, S., Dugan, J.A., 2024. The effect of prescription drug insurance on the incidence of potentially inappropriate prescribing: evidence from medicare part D. Health Econ. 1057-9230. 33 (1), 137–152. doi:10.1002/hec.4766.

Leikola, S., Development and application of comprehensive medication review procedure to community-dwelling elderly. University of Helsinki (2012), Available from: http://urn.fi/URN:ISBN:978-952-10-7698-5.

Martikainen, J.E., Saastamoinen, L.K., Korhonen, M.J., Enlund, H., Helin-Salmivaara, A., 2010. Impact of restricted reimbursement on the use of statins in Finland: a register-based study. Med. Care. 00257079. 48 (9), 761–766. doi:10.1097/MLR.0b013e3181e41bcb.

Masnoon, N., Shakib, S., Kalisch-Ellett, L., Caughey, G.E., 2018. Tools for assessment of the appropriateness of prescribing and association with patient-related outcomes: a systematic review. Drugs Aging. 1170-229X. 35 (1), 43–60. doi:10.1007/s40266-018-0516-8.

Ministry of Social Affairs and Health Rational Pharmacotherapy, 2020. https://stm.fi/en/rational-pharmacotherapy

Mordecai, L., Reynolds, C., Donaldson, L.J., Williams, A.C.D., 2018. Patterns of regional variation of opioid prescribing in primary care in England: a retrospective observational study. Br. J. Gen. Pract. 14785242. 68 (668), e225. Available from: http://bjgp.org/content/68/668/e225/tab-pdf. doi:10.3399/bjgp18X695057.

Navathe, A.S., Liao, J.M., Yan, X.S., Delgado, M.K., Isenberg, W.M., Landa, H.M., Bond, B.L., Small, D.S., Rareshide, C.A.L., Shen, Z., Pepe, R.S., Refai, F., Lei, V.J., Volpp, K.G., Patel, M.S., 2022. The effect of clinician feedback interventions on opioid prescribing. Health Aff. 15445208. 41 (3), 424–433. Available from: https://www.healthaffairs.org/doi/epdf/10.1377/hlthaff.2021.01407. doi:10.1377/hlthaff.2021.01407.

Odden, M.C., Zhang, A., Jawadekar, N., Tan, A., Moran, A.E., Glymour, M.M., Brayne, C., Hazzouri, A.Z.A., Calonico, S., 2023. Regression discontinuity design to evaluate the effect of statins on myocardial infarction in electronic health records. Eur. J. Epidemiol. 0393-2990. 38 (4), 393–402. doi:10.1007/s10654-023-00982-w.

Paulamäki, J., Jyrkkä, J., Hyttinen, V., Huhtala, H., Jämsen, E., 2023a. Regional variation of potentially inappropriate medication use and associated factors among older adults: a nationwide register study. Res. Soc. Adminis. Pharm. 15517411. 19 (10), 1372–1379. Available from: http://www.journals.elsevierhealth.com/periodicals/rsap. doi:10.1016/j.sapharm.2023.06.005.

Paulamäki, J., Jyrkkä, J., Hyttinen, V., Jämsen, E., 2023b. Prevalence of potentially inappropriate medication use in older population: comparison of the Finnish Meds75+ database with eight published criteria. BMC Geriatr. 1471-2318. 23 (1). doi:10.1186/s12877-022-03706-z.

PopulationDataBC, 2025. PharmaCare data set https://www.popdata.bc.ca/data/health/pharmacare

Rättö, H., Wettermark, B., Saastamoinen, L., Rannanheimo, P., Laukkonen, M.-L., Kälvemark-Sporrong, S., Aaltonen, K., 2024. Protocol Regional variation in prescribing in Finland and Sweden: a register study. https://doi.org/10.17605/OSF.IO/TQ5SN

Rodrigues, D.A., Plácido, A.I., Mateos-Campos, R., Figueiras, A., Herdeiro, M.T., Roque, F., 2022. Effectiveness of interventions to reduce potentially inappropriate medication in older patients: a systematic review. Front. Pharmacol. 16639812. 12. Available from: http://www.frontiersin.org/Pharmacology. doi:10.3389/fphar.2021.777655.

Saastamoinen, L.K., Verho, J., 2013. Drug expenditure of high-cost patients and their characteristics in Finland. Eur. J. Health Econ. 16187601. 14 (3), 495–502. doi:10.1007/s10198-012-0393-8.

Saastamoinen, L.K., Verho, J., 2015. Register-based indicators for potentially inappropriate medication in high-cost patients with excessive polypharmacy. Pharmacoepidemiol. Drug Saf. 10991557. 24 (6), 610–618. Available from: http://onlinelibrary.wiley.com/journal/10.1002/(ISSN)1099-1557. doi:10.1002/pds.3764.

Saastamoinen, L., Verho, J., 2021. Regional variation in potentially inappropriate medicine use in older adults—a national register-based cross-sectional study on economic, health system-related and patient-related characteristics. Res. Soc. Adminis. Pharm. 17 (6), 1223–1227. doi:10.1016/j.sapharm.2020.08.018.

Sacarny, A., Barnett, M.L., Le, J., Tetkoski, F., Yokum, D., Agrawal, S., 2018. Effect of peer comparison letters for high-volume primary care prescribers of quetiapine in older and disabled adults: a randomized clinical trial. JAMA Psychiatr. 2168622X. 75 (10), 1003–1011. Available from: http://archpsyc.jamanetwork.com/issues.aspx. doi:10.1001/jamapsychiatry.2018.1867.

Selke Krulichová, I., Hallberg, A., Selke, G.W., Aaltonen, K., Casula, M., Fürst, J., Gvozdanović, K., Hajiebrahimi, M., Kurdi, A., Nyberg, F., Olmastroni, E., Rättö, H., Slabý, J., Wettermark, B., Mueller, T., 2025. Impact of the COVID-19 pandemic on antidepressant use in eleven European regions: a comparative time series analysis 2018–2022. Soc. Psychiatr. Psychiatr. Epidemiol. 14339285. Available from: https://www.springer.com/journal/127. doi:10.1007/s00127-025-02962-9.

Similä, E., Jyrkkä, J., Airaksinen, M., Toivo, T., 2025. Development and validation of the national high-risk medicine classification using the delphi method. Res. Soc. Adminis. Pharm. 15517411. 21 (5), 371–391. doi:10.1016/j.sapharm.2025.01.016.

Stocks, S.J., Kontopantelis, E., Akbarov, A., Rodgers, S., Avery, A.J., Ashcroft, D.M., 2015. Examining variations in prescribing safety in UK general practice: cross sectional study using the Clinical Practice Research Datalink. BMJ. 1756-1833. 351, h5501. doi:10.1136/bmj.h5501.

Strom, B.L., 2006. Pharmacoepidemiology. John Wiley & Sons. doi:10.1002/9780470059876.

Suominen, S., 2014. The health differences between Swedish and Finnish speakers in Finland [In Finnish]. Duodecim. 130 (2), 161–167. Available from: https://www.duodecimlehti.fi/lehti/2014/2/duo11446.

Tenny, S., Hoffman, M.R., 2023. Prevalence, StatPearls Publishing LLC. https://www.ncbi.nlm.nih.gov/books/NBK430867/.

Thygesen, L.C., Ersbøll, A.K., 2014. When the entire population is the sample: strengths and limitations in register-based epidemiology. Eur. J. Epidemiol. 15737284. 29 (8), 551–558. doi:10.1007/s10654-013-9873-0.

Verho, J., Harju, J., 2025. Copayments for prescription drugs: the drivers of demand responses. Health Econ. 1057-9230. 34 (6), 1160–1170. doi:10.1002/hec.4955.

Vukoja, M., Mimica, S., 2024. Comparison of explicit criteria for potentially inappropriate drug prescribing among the elderly: a narrative review. Discov. Health Syst. 2731-7501. 3 (1). doi:10.1007/s44250-024-00102-9.

WHO, 2002. World Health Organization Promoting rational use of medicines: core components https://iris.who.int/bitstream/handle/10665/67438/WHO_EDM_2002.3.pdf

WHO, 2003. Introduction to Drug Utilization Research. World Health Organization, Oslo. Available from: https://www.who.int/publications/i/item/8280820396924156234X.pdf?sequence=1.

Further Reading Section

Ministry of Social Affairs and Health Pharmacotherapy, 2026. https://stm.fi/en/pharmacotherapy.

SECTION III

Innovative methods and tools in pharmacy research

CHAPTER

18

Implementation frameworks for evaluation in pharmacy and other health services with a focus on the Consolidated Framework for Implementation Research 2.0

Marissa Ryan[a,b] *and Centaine L. Snoswell*[a]

[a]School of Pharmacy and Pharmaceutical Sciences, The University of Queensland, Brisbane, QLD, Australia

[b]Pharmacy Department, Princess Alexandra Hospital, Brisbane, QLD, Australia

CHAPTER OBJECTIVES

1. To describe how implementation science is useful for tailoring implementation strategies, explaining outcomes, and adjusting service models.
2. To become familiar with implementation frameworks that can be used to guide the systematic assessment of potential enablers and barriers in pharmacy service implementation.
3. To describe how the Consolidated Framework for Implementation Research can be used for the evaluation of a pharmacy service model.

1 Introduction

1.1 What is implementation science, and why is it used?

Implementation science is the study of methods and strategies to promote the uptake of evidence-based practices (EBPs). In professional practice, we are always improving both our services and our research skills, but our implementation and translation skills are still developing. Only a small fraction of clinical research is translated into lasting practice change (Kilbourne et al., 2020). By systematically studying how interventions are adopted and sustained, implementation science helps ensure that effective practices reach the people who need them.

https://doi.org/10.1016/B978-0-443-44607-8.00021-2

Learnings from the field of implementation science can support us in using methodological approaches for evaluating our implementation practices and/or our new services, and, most importantly, it can provide language for us to communicate to the broader community the process we use to implement new services in our local context. These benefits can ensure that clinical evidence from research is translated into practice in a way that is scalable and sustainable, with the end goal of improving patient outcomes, organizational outcomes, and staff satisfaction (Kilbourne et al., 2020; Albers et al., 2020; Sarkies et al., 2022).

1.2 Key components of implementation science

Early implementation science research often lacked a strong theoretical foundation, relying instead on trial-and-error methods that limited its overall effectiveness and generalizability. To address this, many theories, models, and frameworks (TMFs) have been developed and utilized to bring structure to assessments and improve the replicability of evaluations (Nilsen, 2015; Wang et al., 2023). However, the growing number of available frameworks has introduced complexity and confusion to the field, making it challenging for researchers and practitioners to determine which framework is most appropriate for a given context. In response to these challenges, there is an increasing emphasis on adapting implementation strategies to specific settings and actively involving stakeholders throughout the process (Nilsen, 2015). This shift aims to enhance the relevance, acceptability, and long-term sustainability of implementation efforts (Wang et al., 2023).

"Poor theoretical underpinning makes it hard to understand and explain how and why implementation succeeds or fails, thus restraining opportunities to identify factors that predict the likelihood of implementation success and to develop better strategies to achieve more successful implementation" (Nilsen, 2015).

Implementation science is dedicated to promoting the systematic integration of evidence-based interventions into everyday practice. This can be achieved through systematic planning of new programs, systematic implementation processes, or systematic postservice evaluation. Some of the core components of implementation science include advocacy for evidence-based interventions, systematic implementation strategies to improve replication and scalability, assessment of outcomes and contextual factors, stakeholder engagement, and program postimplementation adaptation and de-implementation where necessary. To achieve this in a systematic way, TMFs are used to guide research and clinical practice efforts.

In addition, TMFs serve to promote sustainable services so that advancements in health services last beyond the short term. Very often, we observe well-meaning programs that aim to fix an issue in the short term without considering whether these improvements or advancements will stand the test of time. In pharmacy and other health services, implementation science can stimulate and facilitate medium- and long-term thinking, and it plays a critical role in bridging the gap between research and practice. This helps innovations to be adopted, scaled, and sustained over time.

1.3 How can implementation science influence health care professions?

For pharmacy and other health professions, implementation science can improve service effectiveness and the long-term sustainability of services for staff when it is used to assess roles and services. Collecting implementation data and scaffolding analysis with TMFs provides evidence of health care staff effectiveness, which can influence business cases, funding, policy, and expand the scope of practice. In turn, this can contribute to better patient care and outcomes for patients.

1.4 Methodological approach: Theories, models, and frameworks

In implementation science, the methodological approach often revolves around the use of TMFs to guide the design, execution, and evaluation of implementation efforts (Albers et al., 2020; Nilsen, 2015). Theories explain why implementation efforts succeed or fail, often drawing from disciplines such as psychology, sociology, and organizational science. Models typically outline the stages or processes of implementation, usually presented in a linear or cyclical format. Frameworks, on the other hand, provide a structured way to organize and categorize the factors that influence implementation, though they do not necessarily explain the causal relationships between those factors. In addition, frameworks often improve the quality of implementation science assessments and unify methodologies and techniques for comparison with other studies (Pan American Health Organization (PAHO) (2016)).

These tools are all used by researchers and practitioners to understand why implementation has succeeded or failed, to identify barriers and facilitators, and to develop strategies to improve the uptake of EBPs. Practically, they are used to guide research design and data collection, facilitate the interpretation of results in a structured way, and, hopefully, ensure that the findings lead to the successful replication and scaling of EBPs.

In their 2015 paper, Nilsen provides a useful schema to categorize the implementation science TMFs into five groups based on their purpose (Nilsen, 2015). Here, we present an adapted version of the schema with examples; however, the list of examples is not exhaustive. While there is overlap between the groups, these characterizations are helpful for selecting the most relevant TMF for research or practice.

The selection of the most appropriate TMF should be guided by the aim of the research being conducted. For instance, if the aim of your plan is to guide the process of introducing a new pharmacy service, it would be reasonable to choose a process model, such as the four-phased Replicating Effective Programs framework (Graham et al., 2006) or the Knowledge to Action model (Graham et al., 2006). Alternatively, if your aim is to explain or understand why clinicians or patients engage with the new pharmacy service, it would be reasonable to choose a determinant framework, such as the integrated Promoting Action on Research Implementation in Health Services framework (Harvey and Kitson, 2016) or the Consolidated Framework for Implementation Research (CFIR) (Damschroder et al., 2009). Similarly, if the aim is to evaluate an implementation process and measure its success, an evaluation framework would be selected, such as Reach, Effectiveness, Adoption, Implementation, and Maintenance (RE-AIM) (Williams et al., 2017). For a further article not specifically in the telehealth context that provides a comprehensive, instructional case study of how implementation science can be used for program evaluation, we recommend Arora et al. (2017). Another useful article by Sarkies et al. outlines how implementation science can be used to improve clinical practice guidelines (Sarkies et al., 2022). It shows how different implementation science methods can be employed across the guideline development stage as well as the local implementation stage.

1.5 What are some of the implementation frameworks used to evaluate pharmacy service implementation?

Any of the TMFs described above can be used to guide implementation science work examining pharmacy services; however, there are more commonly used TMFs that should be considered. Here, we will describe the two most commonly used frameworks as per the 2024 scoping review by Wohlgemut: RE-AIM, which is used to evaluate service implementation, and the CFIR, which is used to determine the factors leading to either a successful or failed service implementation (Damschroder et al., 2009; Williams et al., 2017; Wohlgemut et al., 2024). There are also examples of the CFIR framework being used to complement RE-AIM, in particular where CFIR is used to expand upon the implementation domain of RE-AIM (Williams et al., 2017).

1.6 Reach, effectiveness, adoption, implementation, and maintenance

The RE-AIM framework was developed by Glasgow et al. in 1999, and its five dimensions are included to address different aspects of evaluating and scaling interventions in real-world settings (Glasgow et al., 1999). As previously mentioned, it is a widely used model in implementation science designed to enhance the translation of research into practice. Although RE-AIM was initially intended to improve the reporting and evaluation of public health interventions, over time, it has evolved into a comprehensive planning and evaluation tool used across diverse settings, including healthcare, education, and community programs (*RE-AIM for Program Planning and Evaluation: Overview and Applications*, 2007).

The dimensions are described as follows (adapted from RE-AIM online content) (Glasgow et al., 1999; *RE-AIM for Program Planning: What It Is and How to Use It*, n.d.).

- Reach: the target population for the intervention. Who is affected by the intervention, and how representative are they?
- Effectiveness: assessing whether the intervention is effective. This involves evaluating the impact of the intervention on important outcomes, including potential negative effects.
- Adoption: The proportion and representativeness of the target staff in the target settings who adopt the intervention.
- Implementation: How well the intervention is delivered as intended, including consistency, service adaptations during delivery, and costs.
- Maintenance: The extent to which the intervention's effects are sustained over time at both the individual and organizational levels.

The RE-AIM framework is particularly beneficial for evaluating the real-world applicability, scalability, and sustainability of evidence-based interventions. It encourages stakeholders to consider external validity and contextual factors, making it a pragmatic tool for program planners, funders, and policymakers.

Like any evaluation, the RE-AIM tool will produce the best results if the intervention is clearly defined, the setting is well understood, and the study outcomes for each domain are carefully planned in advance of data collection (Glasgow et al., 1999; *RE-AIM for Program Planning and Evaluation: Overview and Applications*, 2007; Holtrop et al., 2021). Stakeholders should be engaged to ensure that all of this information is appropriately articulated in a way that provides a helpful evaluation for the organization. RE-AIM does provide online tools to support its use, such as the RE-AIM planning tool, which can assist with guiding reflection and decision-making during study planning.

An example of RE-AIM being applied to a pharmacy service is the Opioid and Naloxone Education (ONE) Program, which focused on community pharmacy-based patient screening and interventions to improve population health with regard to opioid use (Strand and Frenzel, 2024). This article also demonstrates the utility of an evaluation framework and how it can be used at different time points of service maturity, with findings compared. In this example, the purpose was to reevaluate the ONE Program's performance using the RE-AIM model, in comparison to the review performed in 2019 (Strand et al., 2020).

1.7 Consolidated Framework for Implementation Research

The CFIR organizes implementation into five domains, which include intervention characteristics, outer setting, inner setting, characteristics of individuals, and process. CFIR is a comprehensive and flexible framework designed to help researchers systematically assess and understand the factors that influence implementation success or failure across diverse settings. Developed by Damschroder et al. in 2009, CFIR integrates constructs from multiple implementation theories into a single, coherent structure.

CFIR 2.0 organizes 67 constructs across five domains:

1. Innovation, which describes the characteristics of the intervention being implemented.
2. Outer setting, which seeks to describe the external influences such as policies, incentives, and patient needs that impact the intervention.
3. Inner setting is a domain that seeks to describe organizational culture, climate, and readiness for the implementation being planned or assessed.
4. Individuals, which involves describing the roles, beliefs, and capabilities of the stakeholders involved in implementation.
5. Implementation process, which describes planning, engaging, executing, and reflecting on the implementation of the intervention.

CFIR is used both prospectively (planning) and retrospectively (evaluation), making it versatile across the implementation lifecycle. It is used in healthcare, public health, education, and community settings because it helps users systematically identify contextual factors that affect implementation outcomes, enabling tailored strategies and more effective interventions. A limitation of the CFIR is that, due to the number of domains and constructs, it can be complex to apply. Users can struggle with differentiating between constructs, especially when distinguishing between inner and outer settings. In addition, the framework's comprehensiveness can be overwhelming, so its application often requires careful planning and methodological expertise.

An example of using the CFIR 2.0 (Damschroder et al., 2022)—the second version after the original CFIR—to evaluate the implementation of a pharmacy service is provided in the next section, which was novel at the time of publication. The original version of CFIR, comprising 39 constructs, has been used in pharmacy implementation studies previously (Sanchez et al., 2014; Muluneh et al., 2023; James et al., 2023). These studies have applied the CFIR to improve the likelihood of successful planning and implementation for medicines reconciliation (Sanchez et al., 2014), seek recommendations for an oral anticancer adherence intervention (Muluneh et al., 2023), and improve hospital engagement for discharge medicines review referrals (James et al., 2023).

Since the publication of the example implementation evaluation in the next section, two examples of CFIR being used in pharmacy research include a study that explored systemic and procedural factors influencing the development and implementation of a pharmacist-led anticoagulation service in a primary care setting (Alshihab et al., 2025) and another study that used CFIR to describe the ritonavir prescribing process in community pharmacies, along with associated barriers and facilitators (AlMahasis et al., 2025). These examples further demonstrate the application of CFIR across different clinical areas and settings in pharmacy.

Specific influencing factors that have been identified in telehealth studies applying the CFIR framework include the value of a patient's support person to assist in the consult (Thomas et al., 2022), staffing resources (Muluneh et al., 2023; Ward et al., 2021), and the advantages of the innovation over the usual model of care (Ward et al., 2021; Taubert et al., 2022). By determining the potential enablers and barriers from key stakeholders involved in the service, it can assist in the design, adjustment, and evaluation of services (Damschroder et al., 2022).

CFIR can be used in many ways to elicit information from stakeholders, for instance, to develop a survey or an interview guide. Data can then be analyzed descriptively, inductively, or deductively. Descriptive analysis aims solely to summarize data without interpretation and focuses on reporting what was said or observed. Inductive analysis begins with no agenda and seeks to build patterns or themes from the data itself, with the aim of allowing new insights to emerge without predefined categories, as compared to deductive analysis, which applies existing theories or frameworks to the data with the aim of testing or categorizing findings based on prior knowledge. These analyses can be extended by using a *valence rating* as the analytical method, which is the method used in the example presented below in the Methods section (Bauer et al., 2018; Haverhals et al., 2015; Interian et al., 2018; Stevenson et al., 2018; Varsi et al., 2015). All such studies used CFIR as the underpinning framework. Valence rating was used to identify constructs where a negative rating was associated with low implementation success and a high rating was associated with high implementation success. Valence rating analysis involves starting with deductive content analysis of the interview data using the CFIR constructs. Interview responses were then classified for valence (i.e., positive or negative influence on the implementation) and the strength of their influence using a standard five-point rating scale (−2, −1, 0, +1, +2). This scale is described in detail below and in other published literature (Haverhals et al., 2015; Varsi et al., 2015).

Using CFIR in research has several benefits. It offers a standardized vocabulary and structure to build on findings across different implementation studies in pharmacy. For example, with respect to barriers and facilitators of a pharmacy service, findings can be compared across pharmacy service contexts. In addition, CFIR informs intervention design, as it can guide the development and refinement of implementation strategies due to its utility in analyzing factors at different levels.

2 Methods

This CFIR example has been curated from a paper published in 2024 (Damschroder et al., 2022). Here, we have included excerpts to assist with understanding how the implementation TMFs can be applied in pharmacy and other health service evaluations. The CFIR 2.0 was chosen as the most appropriate implementation evaluation framework to provide an example since it contains a comprehensive list of different constructs (or potential factors) to consider that may influence successful implementation, and it was updated in 2022 (Damschroder et al., 2022). In addition, as mentioned above, the CFIR framework has been used in many studies previously (Sanchez et al., 2014; Muluneh et al., 2023; James et al., 2023; AlMahasis et al., 2025) and for telehealth more broadly (Taubert et al., 2022; McHugh et al., 2024; Haun et al., 2024).

2.1 Context for this example of the method

A cancer pharmacist must complete a pretreatment medication history prior to a patient commencing a cancer therapy protocol (*COSA guidelines for the safe prescribing, dispensing and administration of systemic cancer therapy*, 2017; Coutsouvelis et al., 2020). With an accurate medication history completed, any medication-related issues can be resolved by the treating team prior to the patient's first treatment day. Hence, the pretreatment medication history is a crucial step in ensuring the safe, quality, and efficacious use of cancer medicines (Coutsouvelis et al., 2020).

At the institution from which this example comes, and in many services, the current way of obtaining medication histories using telepharmacy is via an unscheduled telephone consult model (Ryan et al., 2021). However, there are challenges associated with this model. At the institution from which this example comes from, and in many services, the current way of obtaining medication histories using telepharmacy, is via an unscheduled telephone consult model (Ryan et al., 2021). However, there are challenges associated with this model (Ryan et al., 2021). Pharmacists often report issues reaching the patient, requiring them to make repeated telephone calls. At the institution from which this example comes from, and in many services, the current way of obtaining medication histories using telepharmacy is via an unscheduled telephone consult model (Ryan et al., 2021). Pharmacists often report issues reaching the patient, requiring them to make repeated telephone calls. In addition, due to the unplanned or unexpected nature of the call, some patients are unable to confirm all details of their medicines at the time of the call.

Via telephone, the pharmacist is also unable to visually verify the medication details. Such challenges can result in medication-related issues not being resolved prior to the first day of treatment. This can cause service inefficiencies, as it then requires an in-person pharmacy consult to occur on the first treatment day, which can create delays in preparing a patient's medication list and potentially impact the commencement of treatment (Ryan et al., 2021). To address these challenges, a scheduled video consultation telepharmacy service model was established (Ryan et al., 2021).

Using the CFIR 2.0 (Damschroder et al., 2022), staff perceptions of the factors that influence implementation, including enablers and barriers for video consultations compared to telephone consultations, were determined. This was carried out with the aim of supporting ongoing sustainability within the current service. More detailed information about the example study has been reported elsewhere (Ryan et al., 2024).

2.2 The use of the CFIR in other implementation evaluation studies

CFIR 2.0 has been used in prior implementation evaluation studies of telepharmacy (Sanchez et al., 2014; Muluneh et al., 2023; James et al., 2023) to examine the potential enablers and barriers to implementing a specific innovation (Damschroder et al., 2022, 2009). These studies have utilized CFIR to identify implementation strategies for medication reconciliation (Sanchez et al., 2014), support an oral anticancer medication adherence intervention (Muluneh et al., 2023), and develop recommendations to improve hospital engagement for discharge medicines review referrals (James et al., 2023). In each of these studies, the benefits of using an implementation framework to identify positive drivers, as well as challenges to service implementation, were reported. Understanding these features can be both value-adding for the institution using the framework to enhance their existing services, while also beneficial to other services seeking to adopt similar models by using implementation strategies to optimize service success (Kirk et al., 2016; Oche et al., 2024).

The application of the CFIR in real-world settings facilitates refinement of the framework itself, contributing to the ongoing growth of implementation science. This growth is encouraged by the original authors of the CFIR (Damschroder et al., 2009). In the telepharmacy example in this chapter, the authors revised the wording of a few constructs so that all were framed in a favorable sense, for ease of data interpretation (Ryan et al., 2024). Such suggestions may help to inform a future version of the CFIR or provide an option for other researchers to consider in their application of the framework.

2.3 Using CFIR to assess pharmacy and health care services— The importance of planning

Researchers may find the following points helpful when considering the use of the CFIR as a determinant framework within their research.

- Prior to commencing the evaluation, ensure that the setting and service options in the local context where the implementation has occurred are well understood. This understanding is essential, as it will guide the selection of the CFIR domains for your study, which ultimately impacts the questions that you will ask your stakeholders for your study. The Additional File 1: CFIR Construct Example Questions can be used to provide guidance on the types of questions you may ask (Alshihab et al., 2025).
- Consider how to most meaningfully use the CFIR across different phases of implementation, particularly if resources are scarce. If resources are not a barrier to the depth of evaluation, think about how the CFIR can be integrated throughout the entire research process—from developing research questions and semistructured interview questions, to refining constructs to make them fit for purpose in the local context, and finally, to promoting theoretical development (Kirk et al., 2016; Shoemaker-Hunt et al., 2022).
- Ensure you provide justification for the CFIR domains and constructs that were selected for your evaluation.
- It is very important to clearly define the domains; e.g., for the inner setting domain, what setting(s) does this include? This is vital to ensure that the data collection accurately represents the context. In addition, ensure there is no overlap with the outer setting domain.
- Identifying the relevant stakeholders is crucial, as you want to ensure, as much as possible, that perspectives are included from a variety of people. It may be useful to consider all the touch points in the particular service you are evaluating by drawing out a flowchart or journey map. This helps to produce data collection that is meaningful.
- To eliminate the possibility of participants feeling that they cannot respond freely, it is recommended that the interviewer be independent of the pharmacy service.

- Consider the relationship between CFIR constructs and the outcomes you are assessing for your pilot or implementation project (Kirk et al., 2016; Shoemaker-Hunt et al., 2022).

2.4 Example methods for participant identification

Staff were recruited over four weeks to participate in semistructured interviews using purposive sampling. Purposive sampling involves the intentional selection of participants with specific knowledge, experiences, or characteristics relevant to the study. Inclusion criteria included staff from four professions: pharmacists, nursing staff, medical officers, and telehealth coordinators. Pharmacists were required to have delivered video consultations and telephone consultations to be eligible for inclusion. Nursing staff and medical officers were eligible if they cared for patients in the clinic who had either pharmacist telephone consultations or video consultations, had knowledge of the pharmacist video consultation model of care, and had themselves delivered telephone consultations and possibly video consultations. Finally, telehealth coordinators were eligible if they organized and provided technical support for the video consultations and had knowledge of the telephone consultation workflow.

2.5 Example methods for data collection tool development and data collection

An independent research assistant conducted the semistructured interviews to ensure all participants felt free to discuss their perceptions of the telepharmacy models. Interviews were held over a 12-week period from May to September 2022. The CFIR interview guide (*The Consolidated Framework for Implementation Research Tools and Templates: Rating Rules*, n.d.) was used to develop the questions for the semistructured interviews. The semistructured interview guide included a short section of closed-ended demographic questions, followed by a series of open-ended questions. The open-ended questions were used to elucidate staff perceptions of the implementation of the usual care telephone consult and video consultation models. Participants were able to speak freely on aspects deemed important to them (Damschroder et al., 2022). Some questions were omitted during the interview if they were deemed irrelevant to the role of the staff member. All interviews were conducted in person, recorded, transcribed, and then checked for accuracy against the recorded interview. Subsequent to the 2024 publication of the example application of CFIR to the telepharmacy model of care, The CFIR User Guide: a five-step guide for conducting implementation research using the framework, includes construct example questions (see supplementary file from publication for question set (Ryan et al., 2024)) that can be used as a starting point for putting together interview questions relevant to your context.

2.6 Example methods for deductive data analysis with valence rating

The four CFIR 2.0 domains of Innovation, Outer Setting, Inner Setting, and Individuals were considered against the transcripts from the semistructured interviews (Shoemaker-Hunt et al., 2022). The Implementation Process Domain was not considered in this study, as this was a pilot of the service and was not fully implemented. Telephone consults are the current model of service delivery, but for the purpose of comparison, constructs from all four of the domains, including the Innovation Domain, were applied to both the telephone consultation and video consultation models. In this study, the Inner Setting related to the locations where the telepharmacy service was carried out, as well as associated areas such as cancer services, while the Outer Setting related to the hospital, state, and country.

To ensure that the perspective for each domain and construct was accurately described, some modifications were made to make constructs more specific, to adjust how constructs were worded positively or negatively, and to ensure they were rated accordingly. Regarding making constructs more specific, four constructs were separated into two categories (two separate constructs) (see Table 18.1). The constructs of structural characteristics—information technology infrastructure, materials and equipment, and access to knowledge and information were divided into patient and staff perspectives, while innovation cost was separated into patient and health service categories (two separate constructs).

Modification of constructs pertaining to how they were described and rated included the construct of complexity, which was renamed to simplicity so that favorable responses indicating simplicity were scored positively (rather than negatively, as would have been the case if the scoring were against complexity), following the example of previous CFIR analyses (Damschroder and Lowery, 2013). In addition, the critical incidents construct descriptor was edited to flip it from a negative score to a positive score by adapting the question language (adding "do not") so the construct would score positively if critical incidents did not impact the innovation. Applying reverse ratings to these two constructs ensured consistency with other constructs, where positive scoring indicates favorability (AlMahasis et al., 2025).

Initially, two authors independently analyzed three blinded interview transcripts and then compared findings to confirm consistency in the coding of content against the CFIR 2.0 domains and constructs (Shoemaker-Hunt et al., 2022). The coding was completed separately for both the unscheduled telephone model and the innovation (scheduled video consultation model). Four of the authors met to discuss the coding of the three transcripts, identify any coding disagreements, and ensure a consistent coding approach. The remaining transcripts were then coded by a single author. To ensure consistency and reliability of coding were maintained, randomly selected paragraphs from across the participant transcripts were checked and coded by a second rater, with any disagreements reconciled through discussion with a third author.

Interview statements pertaining to CFIR 2.0 constructs were identified for each participant, then rated for direction (positive or negative manifestation) and strength (influence = 1, or strong influence = 2). A score of X indicated a mix of both positive and negative manifestations for the construct, and 0 indicated that the construct was noted to be an important consideration but was found to be neutral (Damschroder et al., 2022; *The Consolidated Framework for Implementation Research Tools and Templates: Rating Rules*, n.d.). An overall score was then determined from a review of all individual participant scores against any identified constructs for the unscheduled telephone model and the scheduled video consultation model. Positive scoring constructs (identified as a positive influence [+1] or strong positive influence [+2]) were considered enablers, while negative scoring constructs (identified as a negative influence [−1] or strong negative influence [−2]) were considered barriers (see Table 18.1 below). Following a separate analysis of each model, the construct scores for both models were compared, and any strongly distinguishing scores were identified. A strongly distinguishing score was determined as one where the scores for the two models differed by three or more places from each other, e.g., −1 and +2, or with a −2 or +2 and X (X = mixed influence) for any one construct. Example quotations have been included in the results to illustrate discussions of key constructs, with the participant number indicated in parentheses beside the quote.

2.7 Example results for deductive CFIR analysis with valence ratings

2.7.1 *Perceived enablers*

Positive influencing constructs (or enablers) identified for both the telephone and video consultation service included: critical incidents not disrupting telepharmacy implementation and delivery, local attitudes supporting the innovation implementation, relational connections among staff, communications between telepharmacy-related environments, culture relating to human equality for centredness (which is the shared belief in the equal worth of individuals), and innovation recipients for need (relating to a requirement a patient has that will be addressed by the telepharmacy models, as shown in Table 18.1). A higher number of positive influencing constructs were identified for the video consultation model ($n = 25$) compared to the telephone consultation service ($n = 10$). The strongest enablers among the 25 positively influencing constructs identified for the video consultation service were innovation relative advantage, critical incidents, structural characteristics for support persons assisting with the consultations, financing (referring to funding reimbursement availability), and other implementation support for capability and motivation to deliver the telepharmacy model, which are discussed below.

2.7.2 *Outer setting domain*

Regarding the outer setting, two constructs were positive enablers (Table 18.1). The Critical Incidents construct was strong for video consultations, which provided “a safe way to deliver care infection risk-wise; patients could communicate without wearing a mask” (P1) during the COVID-19 pandemic. Video consultations also facilitated greater support person involvement. In addition, Financing was a strong construct, with many participants reporting the revenue advantage of video consultations over telephone consults: “For video consultations, there’s higher funding potential” (P1).

2.7.3 *Inner setting domain*

The structural characteristics relating to the Support Persons construct were used to code the advantage of having support persons assist in the video consultation (Table 18.1), as opposed to a telephone consultation, which was discussed several times: “The support person helped the patient with their medication list” (P4).

TABLE 18.1 Example results table of CFIR constructs identified and overall rating for telepharmacy consult type.

CFIR domain and constructs with shortened description (Damshroder et al., 2022)	Overall rating	
	Telephone consultation	Video consultation
Outer setting domain (e.g., **hospital, state, country)**		
Critical incidents^		
Large-scale and/or unanticipated events do not disrupt implementation and/or delivery of the innovation.	+1	**+2**
Local attitudes		
Sociocultural values/beliefs encourage outer setting to support innovation implementation and/or delivery.	+1	+1
Local conditions		
Economic, technological, etc. conditions enable outer setting to support innovation implementation and/or delivery.	–1	+1
Financing*		
Funding from external entities (e.g., grants, reimbursement) is available to implement/deliver the innovation	–1	**+2**
Inner setting domain (e.g., **cancer pharmacy, telehealth center, cancer services)**		
Structural characteristics—other (ability of support persons to assist in the consult)*		
Infrastructure components support functional performance of the inner setting	X	**+2**
Structural characteristics—physical infrastructure		
Layout/configuration of space/other tangible material features support inner setting functional performance	–1	X
Structural characteristics—information technology infrastructure~		
Technological systems for telecommunication, documentation, etc. support inner setting performance.		
Staff member	–1	X
Patient	–1	–1
Structural characteristics—work infrastructure		
Organization of tasks and responsibilities and general staffing levels, support inner setting performance.	X	–1
Relational connections		
High quality relationships, networks, and teams within and across inner setting	+1	+1
Communications		
High quality information sharing practices within and across inner setting	+1	+1
Culture—human equality-centeredness		
Shared values, beliefs, and norms about the inherent equal worth and value of all human beings.	+1	+1
Culture—recipient-centeredness		
Shared values, beliefs, and norms around caring, supporting, and addressing recipient needs and welfare.	–1	+1
Culture—deliverer-centeredness		
Shared values, beliefs, and norms around caring, supporting, and addressing deliverer needs and welfare.	–1	+1
Compatibility		
The innovation fits with workflows, systems, and processes.	+1	–1
Incentive systems		
Tangible/intangible incentives and rewards/disincentives support innovation implementation and delivery	–	+1

Continued

TABLE 18.1 Example results table of CFIR constructs identified and overall rating for telepharmacy consult type—cont'd

CFIR domain and constructs with shortened description (Damshroder et al., 2022)	Overall rating	
	Telephone consultation	Video consultation
Available resources—funding		
Funding is available to implement and deliver the innovation.	−1	−1
Available resources- space		
Physical space is available to implement and deliver the innovation.	−1	−1
Materials & equipment~		
Supplies are available to implement and deliver the innovation.		
Staff member	−1	+1
Patient	X	X
Access to knowledge & information~		
Guidance/training is accessible to implement/deliver innovation.		
Staff member	X	+1
Patient	–	+1

Note: Strength of influence: (—) not discussed, (0) neutral, (1) influence, (2) strong influence, (X) mixed influences. Direction of influence: (-) negative, (0) neutral, (+) positive. Bold indicates a score that was a strong positive or negative influence construct. CFIR = Consolidated Framework for Implementation Research.

[#]Reverse rated; innovation "simplicity" used rather than "complexity".
^Reverse rated; the words "do not" were added to the construct.
~Construct has been further separated out to distinguish between individuals/organization.
**Construct has a strongly distinguishable influence between telephone consultations and video consultations.*

From Ryan, M., Ward, E.C., Burns, C., Carrington, C., Cuff, K., Mackinnon, M., Snoswell, C.L., 2024. Telepharmacy for outpatients with cancer: An implementation evaluation of videoconsults compared to telephone consults using the CFIR 2.0. Explor. Res. Clin. Soc. Pharm. 16. https://doi.org/10.1016/j.rcsop.2024.100501.

3 Discussion

3.1 Application of the CFIR

Using implementation science tools like the TMFs discussed here is an excellent way to approach health services research, as their systematic approach improves rigor. As demonstrated by our example, the CFIR framework can be applied to an existing service after implementation to inform service adaptations, methods for scaling the services, and ensuring sustainability. Our example successfully demonstrated that video consultations should be used where possible, and there are certain patient groups that may benefit most from this model. However, due to both models having multiple enablers and barriers, further research into other models, including the potential of a hybrid service using both telephone consults and video consultations, may best meet the needs of patients and the organization. External to this service, health services leaders can consider the many factors that may influence the implementation success of each telepharmacy model when designing and implementing telepharmacy services. These were results that were not highlighted by the standard evaluation methods applied in previous studies of this service, demonstrating the benefit of using an implementation science framework as a method in this research project [refs to other studies]. The strength of this approach was its structured yet unique method for guided data collection and analysis. The use of valences for reporting improved the clarity with which results could be reported.

3.2 Caveats and advice for use of CFIR 2.0

It should be noted that while CFIR 2.0 is used widely, its complexity and comprehensiveness present a challenge for many users who seek to apply it. With 67 constructs across five domains, CFIR can be overwhelming for researchers, especially those new to implementation science. This complexity often leads to inconsistent application, where users may selectively apply constructs without clear justification, which results in inconsistent reporting and a reduction in directly comparable results. A systematic review by Kirk et al. in 2016 found that most studies reporting the use of CFIR applied it primarily as a data analysis tool but did not provide a justification for their selection of the framework or individually selected constructs. This application method limits the framework's ability to support comprehensive and comparable evaluations across studies (Kirk et al., 2016). Our example study, however, was able to demonstrate results in line with other pharmacy implementation studies that have applied the CFIR framework (Sanchez et al., 2014; Muluneh et al., 2023), highlighting the elements that affect the success of telepharmacy service implementation.

Another limitation is that CFIR is not designed to guide the development of innovations or specify implementation processes. It is best used to assess determinants that influence implementation success, not to prescribe specific strategies (Reardon et al., 2025). Reardon et al. noted in 2025 that CFIR is sometimes misapplied in grant reviews and published manuscripts, leading to inconsistent findings and reduced comparability with other results in the field (Reardon et al., 2025).

In addition, CFIR has historically lacked explicit guidance on equity and the role of innovation recipients, which were only addressed in its 2022 update. Even with these improvements, applying CFIR effectively requires methodological expertise and careful planning to avoid oversimplification or misinterpretation of constructs. Researchers are encouraged to integrate CFIR throughout the research process, from study design to dissemination, and to use available tools and templates provided by CFIR to ensure rigorous and meaningful application (Damschroder et al., 2022).

3.3 Strengths and limitations of using CFIR for the example study

Optimal representation of key stakeholders involved in the video consultation service was achieved through a purposive sampling approach, and the number of respondents interviewed was deemed ideal by the authors. Coding the perceptions of 14 staff members allowed for in-depth analysis across the four CFIR 2.0 domains considered. The coders noted that, at times, direct objective experiences by respondents, their perceptions, or a combination of the two were communicated in the transcripts. This challenge of "what is being measured" was also noted by users of CFIR in the CFIR 2.0 update (Damschroder et al., 2022). The authors of this study accepted that direct objective experience was most important, but they also acknowledged that perceptions were significant and that, at times, respondents provided a blend of both. The ability to apply strength analysis to the CFIR constructs was used to demonstrate the degree to which each construct manifested, including its validity, with direct objective experiences carrying more strength. For example, coding of −2 or +2 demonstrates a higher degree of influence strength compared to −1 or +1. With approximately half of the CFIR 2.0 constructs identified across the constructs considered in this study, the value of carrying out such an analysis is demonstrated, as many influential factors need to be considered for successful implementation. Using the menu of constructs approach, as other CFIR users have done, facilitates comparison with other relevant telehealth, pharmacy, and/or cancer studies using the CFIR.

Another strength of the example study was the reframing of negative language constructs into positive ones to ensure uniform reporting of results. For example, instead of the construct "complexity," the authors suggest renaming this construct "simplicity," such that the "favorable" scores have positive valence, rather than in its current form, which is negative for "not complex" and positive if "complex." In addition, for critical incidents, the authors reverse-rated this construct, such that the words "do not" were added to the construct (as seen in Table 18.2) to read: "large-scale and/or unanticipated events do not disrupt implementation and/or delivery of the innovation." This reverse rating of some of the constructs was also carried out by the authors of another study (Damschroder and Lowery, 2013), further strengthening the recommendation we propose to the CFIR authors to rename any negatively stated constructs in a favorable light in their next iteration. This would result in a favorable influence being reflected with a positive valence, a recommendation that could be considered for future CFIR versions (Damschroder et al., 2022, 2009).

The flexibility in the use of CFIR was also apparent, with the authors separating out a construct further to distinguish between patients and staff members. This construct was Structural Characteristics—Information Technology Infrastructure, including technological systems for telecommunication, documentation, etc., which support inner setting performance. Since it was important to elucidate perspectives from both patients and staff members, separating out the construct facilitated more granular data.

While the CFIR 2.0 framework was used to design the semistructured interview questions, it is possible that not all implementation issues related to some constructs were explored in the interview questions. All responses to questions and comments made by interviewees were able to be mapped to relevant constructs, suggesting the questions were appropriately related to the constructs. As noted earlier, the domain of implementation process was not considered, meaning we did not use the CFIR 2.0 framework in its full form and therefore did not elucidate how implementation constructs interact with the other domains. However, as stated earlier, the decision not to include implementation process was intentional, since this study did not focus on the Implementation Process, as the video consultation innovation has neither undergone nor completed an implementation process, largely due to

TABLE 18.2 Theoretical approaches used in implementation science.

Purpose of study	Group of TMFs	Description	Examples
Describing and/or guiding the process of translating research into practice	Process models	These outline the steps required to implement evidence-based practices, serving as a guide for translating research findings into practical applications.	• Replicating Effective Programs (Graham et al., 2006) • Knowledge-to-Action Model (Graham et al., 2006) • Iowa Model (Titler et al., 1994; Titler et al., 2001) • Ottawa Model (Logan and Graham, 1998)
Understanding and/or explaining what influences implementation outcomes	Determinant frameworks	These aim to identify and explain the factors that affect implementation outcomes, emphasizing both barriers and facilitators. However, they often provide limited practical guidance for application.	• CFIR (Damschroder et al., 2009) • iPARIHS (Harvey and Kitson, 2016) • Active Implementation Frameworks (Blase et al., 2014; Holmes et al., 2012)
	Classic theories	These are well-established theoretical models from a range of disciplines (e.g., psychology or sociology) that contribute to understanding and guiding implementation processes.	• Theory of Diffusion (Rogers et al., 2014) • Other theories from various disciplines include, for example, social cognitive theories, theories concerning decision-making, social network theories, professional theories, and organizational theories
	Implementation theories	These are purpose-built theories developed specifically to explain and support implementation processes and outcomes	• Implementation Climate (Klein and Sorra, 1996) • Absorptive Capacity (Zahra and George, 2002) • Organizational Readiness (Weiner, 2009)
Evaluating implementation	Evaluation frameworks	These are used to measure the success of implementation efforts, helping determine whether the desired changes have been effectively carried out	• RE-AIM (Williams et al., 2017) • PRECEDE-PROCEED (Crosby and Noar, 2011)

Adapted from Nilsen, P., 2015. Making sense of implementation theories, models and frameworks. Implement. Sci. 1748-5908. 10 (1). https://doi.org/10.1186/s13012-015-0242-0.

the clinical need for the service and the rapid changes caused by the coronavirus pandemic. It is, however, a useful domain that may be applied in the future for the video consultation service.

Another limitation of the study is that patients and support people who were involved in the consultations were not invited to participate in the study; however, their valuable perceptions about the video consultation service have been explored elsewhere, and we did ask respondents if they had received any feedback from patients about the video consultation service (Ryan et al., 2022). Future research should seek to include patients and support people in interview cohorts.

Although the transcripts were blinded for analysis, there was a theoretical risk that one of the authors analyzing and coding might have been able to identify respondents based on their responses to the demographic questions and professional experience with the respondents. To reduce bias and ensure the integrity of the analysis, the other two authors who analyzed and coded do not work in the department with the respondents and did not have access to unblinded transcripts.

3.4 Use of implementation science in resource-limited countries

It can be argued that implementation science in resource-limited countries and communities is more important than implementation science in resource-rich settings because of the desire to reduce disparities in care between countries, geographical areas, and services (Gustafson et al., 2023), as well as the desire to translate research results into practice to benefit the greatest number of people possible (Yapa and Bärnighausen, 2018). The CFIR is useful in resource-limited countries because of its adaptability, focus on contextual determinants, and comprehensive structure, which includes considerations for both system-level and individual-level factors.

A study by Ojo and colleagues demonstrated the application of CFIR to three case studies conducted in low- and middle-income countries (LMICs) (Zambia, Zimbabwe, and Madagascar) (Ojo et al., 2021). In these case studies, resources were generated or maximized to facilitate ongoing health services. The CFIR was used to identify and map contextual factors that are reported to influence implementation feasibility in LMIC settings. CFIR also allows for flexible data collection, such as interviews, observations, or focus groups, which can be beneficial when countries have limited resources. In addition, its comprehensive website provides tools and guides for users that are freely accessible. The ease of access, free nature of resources, and lack of need for a legal agreement prior to using resources mean that CFIR is a simple tool for any healthcare clinician or researcher in an LMIC to use in a low-resource environment or project. It is also adaptable and can be used with other frameworks, such as RE-AIM, to provide a fuller picture of implementation, notably scalability and sustainability, which are essential for long-term success, even more so in low-resource countries where resources are likely more limited and optimal use of existing resources is required. This applicability was demonstrated by Means et al. in their 2020 article reviewing CFIR use in 34 studies from 21 LMICs and engaging with the authors to gather feedback on the use of CFIR for their projects (Means et al., 2020). This study highlighted which domains were most applicable and suggested that users also ensure they describe the characteristics of their healthcare systems for context alongside their analysis, as this was not covered by a CFIR domain at the time but has been added in the 2022 updated version (Damschroder et al., 2022; Means et al., 2020).

The feasibility of these interventions was influenced by contextual factors such as leadership engagement, local capacity building, readiness for research and implementing EBPs, infrastructural support for multilevel scale-up, and cultural and contextual adaptations. These findings are important as they demonstrate the application of CFIR to evaluate, guide, and execute feasible public health interventions and projects in resource-limited settings. It should be noted that there were previous critiques regarding the lack of equity considerations, which the 2022 update sought to address by adding constructs related to equity and centering innovation recipients in CFIR 2.0 (Damschroder et al., 2022). In addition, strategic selection of constructs is also possible; for example, in many health care services, the domains of intervention characteristics and inner setting may provide the most useful data. Finally, with the 2025 publication of the CFIR User Guide—a five-step guide for conducting implementation research using the framework—this can greatly assist in understanding how to conduct an evaluation using CFIR and improve efficiency by leveraging available resources (Reardon et al., 2025).

4 Questions for further discussion

1. How or why might CFIR 2.0 be used in conjunction with other implementation science frameworks?
2. Why might CFIR 2.0 be a more useful implementation framework for resource-limited countries or regions compared to other implementation frameworks?
3. How can strength analysis be applied to the CFIR? Explain the coding system used, and use Table 18.1 to provide three examples of overall ratings for a construct, and explain what the results mean for that construct.
4. What might be the advantages of incorporating CFIR 2.0 into a research project of yours? Please consider the advantages for patients, the organization, and the health care profession you work in.

5 Application exercise

Think about a pharmacy or health care service you would like to enhance or make more successful.

1. List the key stakeholders you could interview to elucidate their perspectives, and describe how you determined who would be interviewed.
2. Select among the CFIR 2.0 domains of intervention, outer setting, inner setting, individuals, and implementation process that you would emphasize, including potentially all of them (refer to https://cfirguide.org/constructs/). Explain your rationale.
3. Imagine you are preparing questions for semistructured interviews. For the Intervention domain, list some of the questions your key stakeholders could be asked. Please also include some example prompts that the interviewer may need to use when interviewing the interviewee to further elucidate information.
4. Choose one or two other domains you would use, and examine the constructs within those domains. Please elaborate on which constructs you have chosen and why.

References

RE-AIM for Program Planning and Evaluation: overview and Applications, 2007.

COSA guidelines for the safe prescribing, dispensing and administration of systemic cancer therapy, 2017. Available from: https://app.magicapp.org/#/guideline/n3QAOj.

Albers, B., Shlonsky, A., Mildon, R., 2020. Implementation Science 3.0. Springer International Publishing. doi:10.1007/978-3-030-03874-8.

AlMahasis, S.O., Qudah, B., Ford, J.H., Mott, D., 2025. Inside the pharmacy: a qualitative study uncovering community pharmacists' experiences with Paxlovid prescribing. J. Am. Pharm. Assoc. 15443450. 65 (4). Available from: https://www.sciencedirect.com/science/journal/15443191. doi:10.1016/j.japh.2025.102390.

Alshihab, S., Ibrahim, M.I.M., Al-Zaidan, M., Hadi, M.A., 2025. A consolidated framework for implementation research (CFIR) guided exploration of key informant perspectives on establishing a pharmacist-led anticoagulation service in primary care: a qualitative study. Int. J. Clin. Pharm. 22107711. 47 (2), 335–344. Available from: https://www.springer.com/journal/11096. doi:10.1007/s11096-024-01830-x.

Arora, P.G., Connors, E.H., Blizzard, A., Coble, K., Gloff, N., Pruitt, D., 2017. Dissemination and implementation science in program evaluation: a telemental health clinical consultation case example. Eval. Program Plann. 01497189. 60, 56–63. Available from: www.elsevier.com/inca/publications/store/5/9/3/. doi:10.1016/j.evalprogplan.2016.09.003.

Bauer, M.S., Krawczyk, L., Tuozzo, K., Frigand, C., Holmes, S., Miller, C.J., Abel, E., Osser, D.N., Franz, A., Brandt, C., Rooney, M., Fleming, J., Smith, E., Godleski, L., 2018. Implementing and sustaining team-based telecare for bipolar disorder: lessons learned from a model-guided, mixed methods analysis. Telemed. e-Health. 15563669. 24 (1), 45–53. Available from: http://www.liebertpub.com/publication.aspx?pub_id=54. doi:10.1089/tmj.2017.0017.

Blase, Van Dyke, M., Fixsen, D.L., Wallace Bailey, F., 2014. Implementation science: key concepts, themes and evidence for practitioners in education psychology. In: Kelly, B., Perkins, D.F. (Eds.), Handbook of Implementation Science for Psychology in Education. Cambridge: Cambridge University Press.

Coutsouvelis, J., Adams, J., Bortz, H., Chau, M., Chiang, K., Foo, J., Ibrahim, K., Kerr, K., O'Connor, S., Powell, M., Rowan, G., Siderov, J., Tey, A., Tran, J., Vasileff, H., Munro, C., 2020. Standard of practice in oncology and haematology for pharmacy services. J. Pharm. Pract. Res. 1445-937X. 50 (6), 528–545. doi:10.1002/jppr.1686.

Crosby, R., Noar, S.M., 2011. What is a planning model? An introduction to precede-proceed. J. Public Health Dent. 17527325. 71 (1), 7. doi:10.1111/j.1752-7325.2011.00235.x.

Damschroder, L.J., Aron, D.C., Keith, R.E., Kirsh, S.R., Alexander, J.A., Lowery, J.C., 2009. Fostering implementation of health services research findings into practice: a consolidated framework for advancing implementation science. Implement. Sci. 17485908. 4 (1). doi:10.1186/1748-5908-4-50.

Damschroder, L.J., Lowery, J.C., 2013. Evaluation of a large-scale weight management program using the consolidated framework for implementation research (CFIR). Implement. Sci. 17485908. 8 (1). Available from: http://www.implementationscience.com/content/8/1/51. doi:10.1186/1748-5908-8-51.

Damschroder, L.J., Reardon, C.M., Widerquist, M.A.O., Lowery, J., 2022. The updated consolidated framework for implementation research based on user feedback. Implement. Sci. 17485908. 17 (1). Available from: https://implementationscience.biomedcentral.com. doi:10.1186/s13012-022-01245-0.

Glasgow, R.E., Vogt, T.M., Boles, S.M., 1999. Evaluating the public health impact of health promotion interventions: the RE-AIM framework. Am. J. Public Health. 00900036. 89 (9), 1322–1327. Available from: http://ajph.aphapublications.org/loi/ajph. doi:10.2105/AJPH.89.9.1322.

Graham, I.D., Logan, J., Harrison, M.B., Straus, S.E., Tetroe, J., Caswell, W., Robinson, N., 2006. Lost in knowledge translation: time for a map? J. Contin. Educ. Health Prof. 08941912. 26 (1), 13–24. doi:10.1002/chp.47.

Gustafson, P., Aziz, Y.A., Lambert, M., Bartholomew, K., Rankin, N., Fusheini, A., Brown, R., Carswell, P., Ratima, M., Priest, P., Crengle, S., 2023. A scoping review of equity-focused implementation theories, models and frameworks in healthcare and their application in addressing ethnicity-related health inequities. Implement. Sci. 1748-5908. 18 (1). doi:10.1186/s13012-023-01304-0.

Harvey, G., Kitson, A., 2016. PARIHS revisited: from heuristic to integrated framework for the successful implementation of knowledge into practice. Implement. Sci. 17485908. 11 (1). Available from: http://www.implementationscience.com/. doi:10.1186/s13012-016-0398-2.

Haun, J., Philbin, S., McHugh, M., Ballistrea, L., Schneider, T., Angelina Klanchar, S., Smith, B., Saenger, M., 2024. Leveraging a qualitative evaluation of a telehealth pain management program. Arch. Phys. Med. Rehabil. 00039993. 105 (4), e100. doi:10.1016/j.apmr.2024.02.282.

Haverhals, L.M., Sayre, G., Helfrich, C.D., Battaglia, C., Aron, D., Stevenson, L.D., Kirsh, S., Ho, P.M., Lowery, J., 2015. E-consult implementation: lessons learned using consolidated framework for implementation research. Am. J. Manag. Care. 10880224. 21 (12). Available from: http://www.ajmc.com/journals/issue/2015/2015-vol21-n12/E-Consult-Implementation-Lessons-Learned- Using-Consolidated-Framework-for-Implementation-Research.

Holmes, B.J., Finegood, D.T., Riley, B.L., Best, A., 2012. Systems thinking in dissemination and implementation research. In: Brownson, R.C., Colditz, G.A., Proctor, E.K. (Eds.), Dissemination and Implementation Research in Health: Translating Science to Practice. 1st edn. (Oxford: Oxford University Press).

Holtrop, J.S., Estabrooks, P.A., Gaglio, B., Harden, S.M., Kessler, R.S., King, D.K., Kwan, B.M., Ory, M.G., Rabin, B.A., Shelton, R.C., Glasgow, R.E., 2021. Understanding and applying the RE-AIM framework: clarifications and resources. J. Clin. Transl. Sci. 20598661. 5 (1). Available from: https://www.cambridge.org/core/journals/journal-of-clinical-and-translational-science. doi:10.1017/cts.2021.789.

Interian, A., King, A.R., Hill, L.M.S., Robinson, C.H., Damschroder, L.J., 2018. Evaluating the implementation of home-based videoconferencing for providing mental health services. Psychiatr. Serv. 15579700. 69 (1), 69–75. Available from: https://ps.psychiatryonline.org/doi/pdfplus/10.1176/appi.ps.201700004. doi:10.1176/appi.ps.201700004.

James, R., Hodson, K., Mantzourani, E., Davies, D., 2023. Exploring the implementation of discharge medicines review referrals by hospital pharmacy professionals: a qualitative study using the consolidated framework for implementation research. Res. Social Adm. Pharm. 15517411. 19 (12), 1558–1569. doi:10.1016/j.sapharm.2023.08.006.

Kilbourne, A.M., Glasgow, R.E., Chambers, D.A., 2020. What can implementation science do for you? Key success stories from the field. J. Gen. Intern. Med. 15251497. 35, 783–787. Available from: http://www.springerlink.com/content/120414/. doi:10.1007/s11606-020-06174-6.

Kirk, M.A., Kelley, C., Yankey, N., Birken, S.A., Abadie, B., Damschroder, L., 2016. A systematic review of the use of the Consolidated Framework for Implementation Research. Implement. Sci. 17485908. 11 (1). Available from: http://www.implementationscience.com/. doi:10.1186/s13012-016-0437-z.

Klein, K.J., Sorra, J.S., 1996. The challenge of innovation implementation. Acad. Manag. Rev. 03637425. 21 (4), 1055–1080. Available from: http://amr.aom.org/content/by/year. doi:10.5465/AMR.1996.9704071863.

Logan, J., Graham, I.D., 1998. Toward a comprehensive interdisciplinary model of health care research use. Sci. Commun. 10755470. 20 (2), 227–246. Available from: http://www.sagepub.com. doi:10.1177/1075547098020002004.

McHugh, M.C., Fowler, C.A., Philbin, S., Schneider, T., Ballistrea, L.M., Klanchar, S.A., Smith, B.M., Benzinger, R.C., French, D.D., Saenger, M.S., Haun, J.N., 2024. Qualitative evaluation informs the implementation of a telehealth program to manage chronic pain. J. Pain. 15265900. 25 (7), 104493. doi:10.1016/j.jpain.2024.02.007.

Means, A.R., Kemp, C.G., Gwayi-Chore, M.C., Gimbel, S., Soi, C., Sherr, K., Wagenaar, B.H., Wasserheit, J.N., Weiner, B.J., 2020. Evaluating and optimizing the consolidated framework for implementation research (CFIR) for use in low- and middle-income countries: a systematic review. Implement. Sci. 17485908. 15 (1). Available from: http://www.implementationscience.com/. doi:10.1186/s13012-020-0977-0.

Muluneh, B., Muir, M.A., Collins, J.B., Proco, D., Mackler, E., Bryant, A.L., Wood, W.A., Tilkens, M., Reichard, J.S., Foster, M., Gatwood, J., Wheeler, S.B., Zullig, L.L., Lafata, J.E., 2023. Barriers and facilitators associated with implementing interventions to support oral anticancer agent adherence in academic and community cancer center settings. PLoS ONE. 19326203. 18 (7). Available from: https://journals.plos.org/plosone/article/file?id=10.1371/journal.pone.0286630&type=printable. doi:10.1371/journal.pone.0286630.

Nilsen, P., 2015. Making sense of implementation theories, models and frameworks. Implement. Sci. 1748-5908. 10 (1). doi:10.1186/s13012-015-0242-0.

Oche, O., Murry, L.T., Keller, M.S., Pevnick, J.M., Schnipper, J.L., Nguyen, A.T., Ko, E.J.M., Kennelty, K.A., 2024. Pharmacist, nurse, and physician perspectives on the implementation of the pharmacist discharge care (pharm-dc) intervention: a qualitative study. Res. Social Adm. Pharm. 15517411. 20 (8), 740–746. Available from: https://www.sciencedirect.com/science/journal/15517411. doi:10.1016/j.sapharm.2024.04.009.

Ojo, T., Kabasele, L., Boyd, B., Enechukwu, S., Ryan, N., Gyamfi, J., Peprah, E., 2021. The role of implementation science in advancing resource generation for health interventions in low- and middle-income countries. Health Serv. Insights. 1178-6329. 14. doi:10.1177/1178632921999652.

Pan American Health Organization (PAHO)2016. Framework for the Implementation of a Telemedicine Service. Washington: PAHO, https://docslib.org/doc/1632364/framework-for-the-implementation-of-a-telemedicine-service. (Accessed 6 June 2025).

RE-AIM for Program Planning: What It Is and How to Use It. Available from: https://www.ncoa.org/article/re-aim-for-program-planning-what-it-is-and-how-to-use-it/.

Reardon, C.M., Damschroder, L.J., Ashcraft, L.E., Kerins, C., Bachrach, R.L., Nevedal, A.L., Domlyn, A.M., Dodge, J., Chinman, M., Rogal, S., 2025. The Consolidated Framework for Implementation Research (CFIR) user guide: a five-step guide for conducting implementation research using the framework. Implement. Sci. 17485908. 20 (1). Available from: https://implementationscience.biomedcentral.com. doi:10.1186/s13012-025-01450-7.

Rogers, E.M., Singhal, A., Quinlan, M.M., 2014. Diffusion of Innovations an Integrated Approach to Communication Theory and Research, pp. 432–448.

Ryan, M., Carrington, C., Ward, E.C., Burns, C.L., Cuff, K., Mackinnon, M., Snoswell, C.L., 2021. Changing from telephone to videoconference for pre-treatment pharmacist consults in cancer services: impacts to funding and time efficiency. J. Telemed. Telecare. 17581109. 27 (10), 680–684. Available from: http://www.uk.sagepub.com/journals/Journal202189. doi:10.1177/1357633X211048393.

Ryan, M., Ward, E.C., Burns, C., Carrington, C., Cuff, K., Mackinnon, M., Snoswell, C.L., 2024. Telepharmacy for outpatients with cancer: an implementation evaluation of videoconsults compared to telephone consults using the CFIR 2.0. Explor. Res. Clin. Soc. Pharm. 26672766. 16, 100501. doi:10.1016/j.rcsop.2024.100501.

Ryan, M., Ward, E.C., Burns, C.L., Carrington, C., Cuff, K., Mackinnon, M., Snoswell, C.L., 2022. An evaluation of telephone versus videoconference consults for pre-treatment medication history taking by cancer pharmacists. J. Telemed. Telecare. 17581109. 28 (10), 750–756. Available from: https://journals.sagepub.com/home/JTT. doi:10.1177/1357633X221122140.

Sanchez, S.H., Sethi, S.S., Santos, S.L., Boockvar, K., 2014. Implementing medication reconciliation from the planner's perspective: a qualitative study. BMC Health Serv. Res. 14726963. 14 (1). Available from: http://www.biomedcentral.com/bmchealthservres/. doi:10.1186/1472-6963-14-290.

Sarkies, M.N., Jones, L.K., Gidding, S.S., Watts, G.F., 2022. Improving clinical practice guidelines with implementation science. Nat. Rev. Cardiol. 17595010. 19 (1), 3–4. Available from: http://www.nature.com/nrcardio/archive/index.html. doi:10.1038/s41569-021-00645-x.

Shoemaker-Hunt, S.J., Childs, E., Swan, H., Curran, G., 2022. CFIR framework in pharmacy and health services research. In: Contemporary Research Methods in Pharmacy and Health Services. Elsevier, United States, pp. 57–72. Available from: https://www.sciencedirect.com/book/9780323918886. doi:10.1016/B978-0-323-91888-6.00045-4.

Stevenson, L., Ball, S., Haverhals, L.M., Aron, D.C., Lowery, J., 2018. Evaluation of a national telemedicine initiative in the Veterans Health Administration: factors associated with successful implementation. J. Telemed. Telecare. 17581109. 24 (3), 168–178. Available from: http://www.uk.sagepub.com/journals/Journal202189. doi:10.1177/1357633X16677676.

Strand, M.A., Eukel, H., Frenzel, O., Skoy, E., Steig, J., Werremeyer, A., 2020. Program evaluation of the Opioid and Naloxone Education (ONE Rx) program using the RE-AIM model. Res. Social Adm. Pharm. 15517411. 16 (9), 1248–1254. Available from: http://www.journals.elsevierhealth.com/periodicals/rsap. doi:10.1016/j.sapharm.2019.11.016.

Strand, M.A., Frenzel, O., 2024. Revisiting the opioid and naloxone education (ONE) program: program evaluation using the RE-AIM model four years later. Res. Social Adm. Pharm. 15517411. 20 (7), 648–653. Available from: https://www.sciencedirect.com/science/journal/15517411. doi:10.1016/j.sapharm.2024.04.005.

Taubert, S.T., Burns, C.L., Ward, E.C., Bassett, L., 2022. Evaluation of the implementation of a speech and language therapist-led referring model for VFSS using the Consolidated Framework for Implementation Research (CFIR). Int. J. Lang. Commun. Disord. 14606984. 57 (5), 977–989. Available from: http://onlinelibrary.wiley.com/journal/10.1111/(ISSN)1460-6984. doi:10.1111/1460-6984.12733.

The Consolidated Framework for Implementation Research Tools and Templates: rating Rules. Available from: https://cfirguide.org/tools/tools-and-templates/.

Thomas, E.E., de Camargo Catapan, S., Haydon, H.M., Barras, M., Snoswell, C., 2022. Exploring factors of uneven use of telehealth among outpatient pharmacy clinics during COVID-19: a multi-method study. Res. Social Adm. Pharm. 15517411. 18 (9), 3602–3611. Available from: http://www.journals.elsevierhealth.com/periodicals/rsap. doi:10.1016/j.sapharm.2022.02.003.

Titler, M.G., Kleiber, C., Steelman, V., Goode, C., Rakel, B., Barry-Walker, J., Small, S., Buckwalter, K., 1994. Infusing research into practice to promote quality care. Nurs. Res. 15389847. 43 (5), 307–313. doi:10.1097/00006199-199409000-00009.

Titler, M.G., Kleiber, C., Steelman, V.J., Rakel, B.A., Budreau, G., Everett, L.Q., Buckwalter, K.C., Tripp-Reimer, T., Goode, C.J., 2001. The Iowa model of evidence-based practice to promote quality care. Crit. Care Nurs. Clin. North Am. 08995885. 13 (4), 497–509. doi:10.1016/s0899-5885(18)30017-0.

Varsi, C., Ekstedt, M., Gammon, D., Ruland, C.M., 2015. Using the consolidated framework for implementation research to identify barriers and facilitators for the implementation of an internet-based patient-provider communication service in five settings: a qualitative study. J. Med. Internet Res. 14388871. 17 (11). Available from: http://www.jmir.org/article/viewFile/jmir_v17i11e262/2. doi:10.2196/jmir.5091.

Wang, Y., Wong, E.L.Y., Nilsen, P., Chung, V.C.H., Tian, Y., Yeoh, E.K., 2023. A scoping review of implementation science theories, models, and frameworks — an appraisal of purpose, characteristics, usability, applicability, and testability. Implement. Sci. 17485908. 18 (1). Available from: https://implementationscience.biomedcentral.com. doi:10.1186/s13012-023-01296-x.

Ward, E.C., Burns, C.L., Gray, A., Baker, L., Cowie, B., Winter, N., Rusch, R., Saxon, R., Barnes, S., Turvey, J., 2021. Establishing clinical swallowing assessment services via telepractice: a multisite implementation evaluation. Am. J. Speech Lang. Pathol. 15589110. 30 (6), 2456–2464. Available from: https://pubs.asha.org/doi/pdf/10.1044/2021_AJSLP-21-00109. doi:10.1044/2021_AJSLP-21-00109.

Weiner, B.J., 2009. A theory of organizational readiness for change. Implement. Sci. 17485908. 4 (1). doi:10.1186/1748-5908-4-67.

Williams, K.M., Kirsh, S., Aron, D., Au, D., Helfrich, C., Lambert-Kerzner, A., Lowery, J., Battaglia, C., Graham, G.D., Doukas, M., Jain, R., Ho, P.M., 2017. Evaluation of the veterans health administration's specialty care transformational initiatives to promote patient-centered delivery of specialty care: a mixed-methods approach. Telemed. e-Health. 15563669. 23 (7), 577–589. Available from: http://www.liebertpub.com/publication.aspx?pub_id=54. doi:10.1089/tmj.2016.0166.

Wohlgemut, J.M., Pisirir, E., Stoner, R.S., Perkins, Z.B., Marsh, W., Tai, N.R.M., Kyrimi, E., 2024. A scoping review, novel taxonomy and catalogue of implementation frameworks for clinical decision support systems. BMC Med. Inform. Decis. Mak. 14726947. 24 (1). Available from: https://bmcmedinformdecismak.biomedcentral.com/. doi:10.1186/s12911-024-02739-1.

Yapa, H.M., Bärnighausen, T., 2018. Implementation science in resource-poor countries and communities. Implement. Sci. 17485908. 13 (1). Available from: http://www.implementationscience.com/. doi:10.1186/s13012-018-0847-1.

Zahra, S.A., George, G., 2002. Absorptive capacity: a review, reconceptualization, and extension. Acad. Manag. Rev. 03637425. 27 (2), 185–203. Available from: http://amr.aom.org/content/by/year. doi:10.5465/AMR.2002.6587995.

CHAPTER

19

An evidence-based approach to disseminating research

Debi Bhattacharya, Sion Scott, and Bethany Atkins

School of Health Sciences, University of East Anglia, Norwich, Norfolk, United Kingdom

CHAPTER OBJECTIVES

- Explain the concept of knowledge translation and its relevance to health services research
- Distinguish between dissemination, adoption, and implementation within the knowledge translation continuum
- Describe the steps and associated activities required for effective dissemination
- Apply a structured, evidence-informed approach to planning and executing dissemination activities
- Evaluate dissemination strategies using SMART goals and metrics to assess reach, engagement, and impact

1 Introduction

1.1 Why is knowledge translation necessary?

An estimated $200 billion is spent globally on health care research, which consistently generates evidence that new treatments and ways of working have the potential to significantly improve outcomes for patients (Glasziou and Chalmers, n.d.). Evidence generated from health services research can only initiate change if the learning reaches the right people at the right time ("Disseminate research | NIHR. Accessed April 20, 2023. https://www.nihr.ac.uk/partners-and-industry/charities/disseminate-research.htm," n.d.). "Knowledge translation" is the field of research that has emerged to understand the process of utilizing the learning from research to influence policy and/or practice (Government of Canada CI of HR. Knowledge mobilization—CIHR. October 27, 2005. Accessed April 20, 2023. https://cihr-irsc.gc.ca/e/29529.html, n.d.). The field (also interchangeably known as "knowledge transfer", "knowledge exchange", "knowledge mobilization" and "knowledge utilization") (Straus et al., 2009) has grown exponentially over the years and has yielded over 100 theories, models, and frameworks (L. Strifler et al., 2018a, 2018b) to guide researchers, healthcare professionals, and policy makers in their efforts to put new evidence (knowledge) to use in practice.

Contemporary Research Methods in Pharmacy and Health Services - Volume 2
https://doi.org/10.1016/B978-0-443-44607-8.00006-6

Despite a burgeoning scientific field dedicated to knowledge translation across a range of health systems, less than a third of research evidence is translated into policy or practice, and the failure to effectively disseminate this evidence is a core contributor ("Disseminate research | NIHR. Accessed April 20, 2023. https://www.nihr.ac.uk/partners-and-industry/charities/disseminate-research.htm," n.d.). In complex systems like the UK National Health Service, practice is dictated by policy. This is because policy-driven frameworks provide the essential infrastructure for funding, performance monitoring, and medico-legal defense (Lorenc et al., 2024; Doran et al., 2006). A change in practice may therefore be achieved by a change in policy. This requires messages to reach policy makers in formats that they can use, such as policy briefs, and within timelines that align with decision-making cycles to enable policy makers to act for a future financial year (Oliver et al., 2014). However, current dissemination practices are dominated by formats that are inaccessible to policymakers, such as publications in scientific journals (Nieuwland et al., 2024). This failure to translate the knowledge generated from research evidence into practice remains a significant public health burden (Grol and Grimshaw, 2003).

1.2 What does knowledge translation involve?

Knowledge translation encompasses dissemination, adoption, and implementation (Fig. 19.1). These three stages are equally important for successful knowledge translation. Effective dissemination is the process of spreading evidence "to the target audience via determined channels using planned strategies" (Rabin et al., 2008). Dissemination is a core component of knowledge translation in advance of, and alongside, adoption and implementation (Per P. Nilsen, 2015). Adoption is the decision of an organization or a community to commit to implementing new practices (Allen et al., 2017a, 2017b), whereas implementation is the subsequent process of putting to use or integrating new practices within a setting (Rabin et al., 2008; P. Nilsen, 2015). Therefore, effective dissemination is key to successful adoption and, ultimately, implementation (Seaton, 2017).

1.3 What is dissemination?

The goal of dissemination is to reach the people who will use, be impacted by, or influence the use of the evidence. The target audiences of dissemination are, therefore, varied and include patients, healthcare practitioners, commissioners, and policymakers. Dissemination should span the entire lifetime of a research project. This process involves establishing partnerships with key stakeholders before empirical work begins and developing targeted messages that raise awareness of the problem the research seeks to address. Rather than reserving findings for a "big reveal" at the conclusion of a project, early and ongoing dissemination helps to create a receptive environment in which new evidence can be understood, valued, and ultimately used.

There are numerous knowledge translation models and frameworks that incorporate elements of dissemination. However, scoping reviews of these models and frameworks (Esmail et al., 2020) and reported dissemination activities (Baumann et al., 2022) indicate that dissemination is generally only recognized as a single step undertaken toward the end of a project's life. The preparatory stages to support effective dissemination prior to any empirical work (e.g., working with dissemination partners to identify barriers and enablers to dissemination) are largely absent. It is unsurprising, then, that researchers understand dissemination to be an activity undertaken once a project is complete to coincide with adoption and implementation (Scott et al., 2024). This misconception contributes to the translational gap between evidence generation and policy/practice impact and represents a potentially poor return

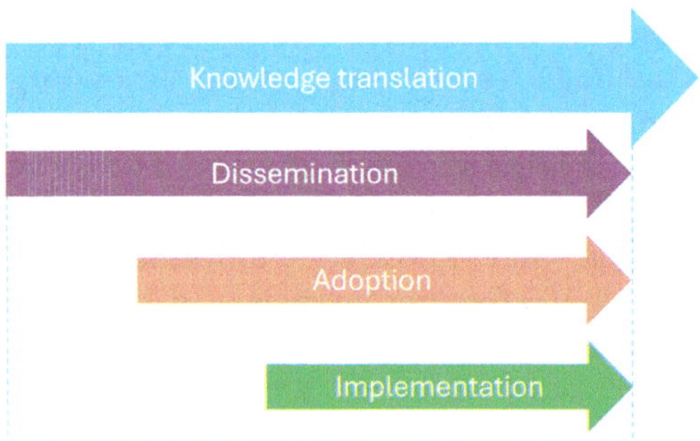

FIG. 19.1 The knowledge translation process.

on research funders' investment ("Paul Glasziou and Iain Chalmers: Is 85% of health research really 'wasted'?—The BMJ. Accessed April 20, 2023. https://blogs.bmj.com/bmj/2016/01/14/paul-glasziou-and-iain-chalmers-is-85-of-health-research-really-wasted/," n.d.).

1.4 Embedding dissemination from the outset of research conduct

The presence of numerous knowledge translation models and frameworks is a welcome indicator that research is being devoted to addressing the gap between research evidence generation and policy and/or practice impact. However, this presents a challenge for researchers attempting to select the most appropriate resource to underpin their dissemination strategy. Furthermore, while these resources may provide some steps for disseminating research, they do not necessarily guide researchers regarding the specific activities to undertake at each step in the process of dissemination. Dissemination strategies underpinned by evidence remain largely absent from programs of research (F. Davidoff et al., 2015a, 2015b; Davies et al., 2010), suggesting that the field of knowledge translation and the guidance buried within it are inaccessible to researchers who are not experts in dissemination. There is, therefore, a need to work with the target audience to develop a framework that unifies the numerous dissemination steps and activities reported in the literature into one consolidated and accessible framework.

Addressing barriers to researchers undertaking activities to facilitate effective implementation of new practices has received significant attention. For example, the Consolidated Framework for Implementation Research (CFIR) combines 19 existing theories and frameworks, providing researchers with a single resource to guide implementation (Damschroder et al., 2022). It is widely accepted that implementation research is evidence-based, with the CFIR at the forefront of enabling researchers to take this approach. Applying a similar concept to the field of knowledge dissemination represents a significant advancement in addressing the translational gap.

1.5 The guide to disseminating research

The Guide to Disseminating Research (GuiDiR) is a consolidated framework of evidence-based steps and activities for disseminating research evidence. The framework is aimed at researchers, research funders, and practitioners and facilitates planning, executing, and evaluating a dissemination strategy. GuiDiR provides a step-by-step approach to planning, executing, evaluating, and refining a dissemination strategy. Its purpose is to enable the research team to generate awareness of the problem that their research intends to address, prompt critical reflection on the limitations of current practices or approaches, and thereby create an environment that is receptive to new insights and recommendations generated from their research. The goal is to ensure that research does not just "sit" in journals but also reaches the people who can use it. This chapter details what is included in GuiDiR and how to apply it to a research study.

The methods used to develop GuiDiR are detailed in a separate publication (Scott et al., 2024). To summarize here, GuiDiR was developed using "coapproach" principles with end users to optimize usability (Grindell et al., 2022; Cowdell et al., 2022). Firstly, the GuiDiR research team identified existing knowledge translation models and frameworks and synthesized them into a prototype dissemination framework. Four authors of the included models and frameworks (dissemination experts) and five health service researchers (end users) from Canada, Belgium, the UK, the Netherlands, Australia, and the USA were then invited to test and refine the prototype framework at a workshop. Dissemination experts were invited to collaborate to ensure that the dissemination framework retained fidelity with the underpinning evidence and reflected any emerging evidence. Health service researchers were invited to collaborate to ensure the acceptability of the new framework among end users without expertise in knowledge translation research or dissemination (Raynor et al., 2011; Jones et al., 2021).

2 Methods

The GuiDiR framework comprises five core steps to help you plan and execute a dissemination strategy:

Step 1: Identify target audiences and dissemination partners
Step 2: Engage with dissemination partners
Step 3: Identify barriers and enablers to dissemination
Step 4: Create dissemination messages
Step 5: Disseminate and evaluate

GuiDiR also details the activities that need to be undertaken at each step. We discuss each step and its associated activities below.

2.1 Step 1: Identify target audiences and dissemination partners

At this step, you need to undertake the following activities:

- Use stakeholder mapping to identify and characterize the target audiences. These will include the end users of the evidence, those who may be impacted by the evidence, and those who may be influenced by the evidence.
- Identify and characterize dissemination partners who can facilitate channels of communication with the target audiences.

2.1.1 What is stakeholder mapping?

Stakeholder mapping (sometimes called stakeholder analysis) is the process of identifying your target audiences. In the context of health services research dissemination, you will identify:

- The "end users" of the evidence (the individuals who will make use of it)
- Those who may be impacted by the evidence (e.g., patients, families, practitioners, membership organizations health services, policymakers, and decision-makers)
- Those who may be influenced by or may influence the use of the evidence (e.g., membership organizations, policymakers, and commissioners)

This process will allow you to prioritize which target audiences (stakeholders) you need to engage with at critical points during your program of research. You should review and refine your stakeholder mapping throughout the research to respond to emerging evidence and changing contexts, e.g., new health policies.

2.1.2 Who are dissemination partners?

Dissemination partners are individuals and organizations who will guide and facilitate you in reaching your target audiences. They are opinion leaders who support credibility and trustworthiness and can act as gatekeepers between you and your target audiences. These may include:

- Organizations representing people with lived experience (e.g., charities/patient groups)
- Key community partners (e.g., religious leaders)
- Membership organizations (e.g., professional bodies and unions)

In addition to working with opinion leaders, you may also partner with "knowledge mobilizers," who are experts in sharing knowledge. They possess key insights into relevant networks and the skills to develop creative knowledge products such as infographics, newsletters, fact-sheets, lay summaries, presentations, and/or video stories.

You will work with your dissemination partners throughout the dissemination process (Steps 2–5) to reach your target audiences.

2.2 Step 2: Engage with dissemination partners

At this step, you need to undertake the following activity:

Form relationships with your dissemination partners at the appropriate stage in the research, as informed by the stakeholder mapping.

You need to engage with dissemination partners to develop and nurture a shared interest in the evidence that requires dissemination. The intention is to inspire and generate commitment from them to support you in your dissemination activities and to problem-solve if necessary. In order to form an effective working relationship with your dissemination partners, it is vital that you:

- Build trust (e.g., by being transparent, empathetic, and consistent in your thoughts and actions)
- Understand how they perceive your evidence
- Foster a shared understanding of each other's goals and expectations related to disseminating the evidence

How do you reach them? Identify members of your research team to engage with the identified dissemination partners. Consider who has existing contacts or is most appropriate—for instance, patient and public representative members of your research team may be most appropriate for organizations representing people with lived experience (e.g., charities) and key community partners (e.g., religious leaders), while clinical members of the research team will be appropriate for membership organizations (e.g., professional bodies and unions).

2.3 Step 3: Identify barriers and enablers to dissemination

At this step, you need to undertake the following activity:

- Work with your dissemination partners to identify the barriers and enablers to effectively disseminating your evidence to the target audiences

Before you can formulate your (active and passive) dissemination strategies, you need to consider which factors may act as barriers or enablers to your evidence reaching the target audiences.

2.3.1 What does identifying and addressing barriers and enablers involve?

It is important to understand how factors such as environmental contexts, socioeconomic circumstances, attitudes, beliefs, and cultural norms might impact your dissemination efforts.

Your dissemination partners will know the target audiences and can help you understand the barriers and enablers that need to be addressed, as well as how these might be addressed. This will be achieved by their sharing of existing knowledge and/or helping you design approaches to generate this knowledge.

For example, you may wish to convene a focus group with patients (members of the target audience) who tell you that they trust information disseminated via a particular charity (enabler). You may also survey the membership of a professional body, with the results indicating that practitioners do not have sufficient capacity to engage with new sources of knowledge during work time (barrier).

Identifying the barriers and enablers to dissemination at this stage will help you formulate your passive and active dissemination strategies at Step 5. It is, therefore, important that you understand what we mean by passive and active dissemination.

- **Passive dissemination** is one-way communication from the research team to the target audiences. This method is intended to generate awareness across a wide range of target audiences, for example, through posters, social media, and letters.
- **Active dissemination** is a two-way communication process between the research team and the target audiences. This method is intended to generate an understanding of the key messages (Step 4) among very specific target audiences, for example, through webinars, workshops, and meetings with individuals and groups.

Examples of dissemination strategies that are informed by potential barriers and enablers are illustrated in Fig. 19.2.

Barriers and enablers	Passive dissemination strategy	Active dissemination strategy
Patients trust information that is disseminated via a particular charity (enabler)	Article in monthly newsletter distributed by the charity	Present evidence followed by a question and answer session at a meeting facilitated by the charity
Practitioners do not have sufficient capacity to engage with new sources of knowledge in work time (barrier)	Disseminate via routes that practitioners are already engaging with outside of work time, e.g. Twitter	Convene an interactive webinar outside of work time and incentivise attendance by awarding continuing professional development points

FIG. 19.2 Example of passive and active dissemination strategies informed by potential barriers and enablers.

2.4 Step 4: Create dissemination messages

At this step, you need to undertake the following activity:

- Work with your dissemination partners to develop and refine key messages for the target audiences

2.4.1 What does creating dissemination messages involve?

You need to work with your dissemination partners to agree on what the key messages about the evidence are and how to frame them so that they are engaging and accessible to the specific target audiences. For example, the key messages and how you frame them may differ for practitioners, patients, and policymakers. Your dissemination messages need to:

- Convey the gap in practice, knowledge, or needs relevant to your target audience that the research evidence is addressing
- Be as specific as possible, and include only the essential information presented in an accessible and attractive format
- Convey the credibility and provenance of the evidence to the end user
- Provide enough detail for the target audience to make informed decisions

Once you have created your dissemination messages, you can refer back to them throughout the duration of your research program and incorporate them into your dissemination strategies (Step 5).

2.5 Step 5: Disseminate and evaluate

At this step, you need to undertake the following activities:

- Set goal(s) to raise awareness at local and broader levels of the gap in practice or evidence that the dissemination strategies aim to fulfill
- Formulate dissemination strategies (that address the Step 3 barriers and enablers) to fulfill the goals set
- Evaluate and refine your dissemination strategies

Your passive and active dissemination strategies should aim to address the barriers and enablers identified in Step 3 and have a clear goal they are trying to achieve. Typically, passive dissemination is undertaken first to prepare the target audiences for subsequent active dissemination strategies.

2.5.1 Examples of passive dissemination strategies

Websites, newsletters, scientific publications, radio, posters, social media, newspapers, letters, brochures, and podcasts.

2.5.2 Examples of active dissemination strategies

Webinars, seminars, oral presentations, workshops, individual and group meetings, launch events, and poster presentations.

2.5.3 What does setting goals involve?

Setting goals helps guide and focus the development of your dissemination strategy. Setting a goal for each strategy also enables you to evaluate its success and identify any barriers to achieving the goal. It may be useful to structure your dissemination strategies around the following SMART goals:

Specific—Make your goal(s) specific; think about exactly what you want to achieve

Measurable—Set a measurable target (metrics or other) against which you will evaluate the performance of your dissemination strategy

Attainable—Is your goal realistic to achieve?

Relevant—Make sure your goals are relevant to your research aims and objectives

Time-based—Give your goal a realistic deadline

You should review and refine your dissemination strategies based on performance relative to the set goals.

See "Application Exercise—Scenario" for example goals for passive and active dissemination strategies.

Download the GuiDiR framework for more information about each step and its activities: https://charmerstudy.org/download-guide-to-disseminating-research-guidir/

3 Discussion

GuiDiR complements existing knowledge translation models and frameworks by providing detailed guidance on how to plan and execute dissemination activities across the lifetime of a research project. GuiDiR is primarily intended to support researchers and practitioners in ensuring that learning from health services research reaches the right people at the right time ("Disseminate research | NIHR. Accessed April 20, 2023. https://www.nihr.ac.uk/partners-and-industry/charities/disseminate-research.htm," n.d.) and, in turn, influences policy and/or practice. It may also have utility for research funders as a standard for evaluating the dissemination plans included in research proposals. The benefits of GuiDiR are thus multifaceted, as prioritizing prioritizes dissemination as a distinct component of research projects that must be appropriately planned, resourced, and undertaken throughout the lifespan of a project. In doing so, GuiDiR can contribute toward closing the translational gap between evidence generation and policy/practice impact ("Paul Glasziou and Iain Chalmers: Is 85% of health research really 'wasted'?—The BMJ. Accessed April 20, 2023. https://blogs.bmj.com/bmj/2016/01/14/paul-glasziou-and-iain-chalmers-is-85-of-health-research-really-wasted/," n.d.).

4 Questions for further discussion

- Why is dissemination often underemphasized in knowledge translation frameworks, and what are the consequences of this oversight?
- How can researchers support inclusivity when identifying target audiences and dissemination partners?
- What role should research funders play in evaluating and supporting dissemination plans?

5 Application exercise/scenario

The application exercise includes two examples: one of passive dissemination and one of active dissemination.

5.1 Example 1: Passive dissemination

Let's return to our example of a **passive** dissemination strategy informed by a potential **enabler** (Fig. 19.3), as illustrated in Step 3.

The table below provides an example goal for this dissemination strategy (Fig. 19.4):

The article could include a link to a full report hosted on the research website. The charity newsletter metrics can

Barriers/enablers	Passive dissemination strategy
Patients trust information that is disseminated via a particular charity (enabler)	Article in monthly newsletter distributed by the charity

FIG. 19.3 Passive dissemination strategy example.

inform the research team about the number of people who received the newsletter, the number of people who opened it, and the number of people who clicked on the link. The website metrics can indicate how long people interacted with the report.

5.2 Example 2: Active dissemination

Now, let's return to our example of an **active** dissemination strategy informed by a potential **barrier**, as illustrated in Step 3 (Fig. 19.5).

The table below provides an example goal for this dissemination strategy (Fig. 19.6):

The webinar could involve multiple speakers beyond the research team, such as dissemination partners who enhance credibility. The webinar should include interactive components, such as polling and breakout groups, to help the research team assess whether the dissemination messages are understood.

SMART Goals	Description of goal
Specific	Disseminate new research evidence to patients diagnosed with a relevant health condition via charity newsletter.
Measurable	10,000 people diagnosed with a relevant health condition receive communication about the new research evidence.
Attainable	The charity newsletter has 20,000 contacts, thus a conservative 50% opening the article is attainable.
Relevant	A core objective of the research is to disseminate findings to the patient population that the research evidence will affect.
Time-based	Research team to work with dissemination partners to plan co-production of the article and full report before the target charity newsletter is distributed.

FIG. 19.4 Example goal for a passive dissemination strategy.

Barriers/enablers	Active dissemination strategy
Practitioners do not have sufficient capacity to engage with new sources of knowledge in work time (barrier)	Convene an interactive webinar outside of work time and incentivise attendance by awarding continuing professional development points

FIG. 19.5 Active dissemination strategy example.

SMART Goals	Description of goal
Specific	Disseminate new research evidence to practitioners specialising in the relevant clinical area to which the evidence relates.
Measurable	10% of the practitioner population in the UK attend the webinar 70% of all attendees engage with polling during webinar
Attainable	Communication with professional body of the practitioner population indicates typical uptake of 10-20% for webinars hosted out of work time
Relevant	A core objective of the research is to disseminate findings to the practitioner population that the research evidence will affect.
Time-based	Research team to host the webinar before approaching policy makers. This permits polling results to bolster arguments for a change in national guidance in response to the new research evidence.

FIG. 19.6 Example goal.

References

Government of Canada CI of HR. Knowledge mobilization—CIHR [Internet], 2005. Available from: https://cihr-irsc.gc.ca/e/29529.html.

Allen, J.D., Towne, S.D., Maxwell, A.E., DiMartino, L., Leyva, B., Bowen, D.J., Linnan, L., Weiner, B.J., 2017b. Measures of organizational characteristics associated with adoption and/or implementation of innovations: a systematic review. BMC Health Serv. Res. 1472-6963. 17 (1). doi:10.1186/s12913-017-2459-x.

Allen, J.D., Towne, S.J.D., Maxwell, A.E., Dimartino, L., Leyva, B., Bowen, D.J., Linnan, L., Weiner, B.J., 2017a. Meausures of organizational characteristics associated with adoption and/or implementation of innovations: a systematic review. BMC Health Serv. Res. 14726963. 17 (1). Available from: http://www.biomedcentral.com/bmchealthservres/. doi:10.1186/s12913-017-2459-x.

Baumann, A.A., Hooley, C., Kryzer, E., Morshed, A.B., Gutner, C.A., Malone, S., Walsh-Bailey, C., Pilar, M., Sandler, B., Tabak, R.G., Mazzucca, S., 2022. A scoping review of frameworks in empirical studies and a review of dissemination frameworks. Implement. Sci. 17485908. 17 (1). Available from: http://www.implementationscience.com/. doi:10.1186/s13012-022-01225-4.

Cowdell, F., Dyson, J., Sykes, M., Dam, R., Pendleton, R., 2022. How and how well have older people been engaged in healthcare intervention design, development or delivery using co-methodologies: a scoping review with narrative summary. Health Soc. Care Commun. 0966-0410. 30 (2), 776–798. doi:10.1111/hsc.13199.

Damschroder, L.J., Reardon, C.M., Widerquist, M.A.O., Lowery, J., 2022. The updated consolidated framework for implementation research based on user feedback. Implement. Sci. 17485908. 17 (1). Available from: https://implementationscience.biomedcentral.com. doi:10.1186/s13012-022-01245-0.

Davidoff, F., Dixon-Woods, M., Leviton, L., Michie, S., 2015a. Demystifying theory and its use in improvement. BMJ Qual. Saf. 20445415. 24 (3), 228–238. Available from: http://qualitysafety.bmj.com/content/24/3/228.full.pdf+html. doi:10.1136/bmjqs-2014-003627.

Davidoff, F., Dixon-Woods, M., Leviton, L., Michie, S., 2015b. Demystifying theory and its use in improvement. BMJ Qual. Saf. 2044-5415. 24 (3), 228–238. doi:10.1136/bmjqs-2014-003627.

Davies, P., Walker, A.E., Grimshaw, J.M., 2010. A systematic review of the use of theory in the design of guideline dissemination and implementation strategies and interpretation of the results of rigorous evaluations. Implement. Sci. 17485908. 5 (1). Available from: http://www.implementationscience.com/content/5/1/14. doi:10.1186/1748-5908-5-14.

Disseminate research | NIHR. Accessed April 20, 2023. https://www.nihr.ac.uk/partners-and-industry/charities/disseminate-research.htm.

Doran, T., Fullwood, C., Gravelle, H., Reeves, D., Kontopantelis, E., Hiroeh, U., Roland, M., 2006. Pay-for-performance programs in family practices in the United Kingdom. N. Engl. J. Med. 0028-4793. 355 (4), 375–384. doi:10.1056/NEJMsa055505.

Esmail, R., Hanson, H.M., Holroyd-Leduc, J., Brown, S., Strifler, L., Straus, S.E., Niven, D.J., Clement, F.M., 2020. A scoping review of full-spectrum knowledge translation theories, models, and frameworks. Implement. Sci. 17485908. 15 (1). Available from: http://www.implementationscience.com/. doi:10.1186/s13012-020-0964-5.

Glasziou, P., Chalmers, I., 2016. Is 85% of health research really "wasted. https://blogs.bmj.com/bmj/2016/01/14/paul-glasziou-and-iain-chalmers-is-85-of-health-research-really-wasted/. (Accessed 20 April 2023).

Glasziou, P., Chalmers, I., Is 85% of health research really "wasted"? The BMJ. Available from: https://blogs.bmj.com/bmj/2016/01/14/paul-glasziou-and-iain-chalmers-is-85-of-health-research-really-wasted/.

Government of Canada CI of HR. Knowledge mobilization—CIHR. October 27, 2005. Accessed April 20, 2023. https://cihr-irsc.gc.ca/e/29529.html.

Grindell, C., Coates, E., Croot, L., O'Cathain, A., 2022. The use of co-production, co-design and co-creation to mobilise knowledge in the management of health conditions: a systematic review. BMC Health Serv. Res. 1472-6963. 22 (1). doi:10.1186/s12913-022-08079-y.

Grol, R., Grimshaw, J., 2003. From best evidence to best practice: effective implementation of change in patients' care. Lancet. 01406736. 362 (9391), 1225–1230. doi:10.1016/s0140-6736(03)14546-1.

Jones, M.D., McGrogan, A., Raynor, D.K., Watson, M.C., Franklin, B.D., 2021. User-testing guidelines to improve the safety of intravenous medicines administration: a randomised in situ simulation study. BMJ Qual. Saf. 20445415. 30 (1), 17–26. Available from: http://qualitysafety.bmj.com/content/by/year. doi:10.1136/bmjqs-2020-010884.

Lorenc, T., Khouja, C., Harden, M., Fulbright, H., Thomas, J., 2024. Defensive healthcare practice: systematic review of qualitative evidence. BMJ Open. 2044-6055. 14 (7), e085673. doi:10.1136/bmjopen-2024-085673.

Nieuwland, A., O'Mara, J.R., Mackenbach, J.D., 2024. Exploring public health researchers' approaches, barriers, and needs regarding dissemination: a mixed-methods exploration. J. Clin. Transl. Sci. 2059-8661. 8 (1). doi:10.1017/cts.2024.527.

Nilsen, P., 2015. Making sense of implementation theories, models and frameworks. Implement. Sci. 17485908. 10 (1). Available from: http://www.implementationscience.com/. doi:10.1186/s13012-015-0242-0.

Oliver, K., Innvar, S., Lorenc, T., Woodman, J., Thomas, J., 2014. A systematic review of barriers to and facilitators of the use of evidence by policymakers. BMC Health Serv. Res. 1472-6963. 14 (1). doi:10.1186/1472-6963-14-2.

Paul Glasziou and Iain Chalmers: Is 85% of health research really "wasted"?—The BMJ. Accessed April 20, 2023. https://blogs.bmj.com/bmj/2016/01/14/paul-glasziou-and-iain-chalmers-is-85-of-health-research-really-wasted/.

Rabin, B.A., Brownson, R.C., Haire-Joshu, D., Kreuter, M.W., Weaver, N.L., 2008. A glossary for dissemination and implementation research in health. J. Public Health Manag. Pract. 10784659. 14 (2), 117–123. doi:10.1097/01.PHH.0000311888.06252.bb.

Raynor, D.K., Knapp, P., Silcock, J., Parkinson, B., Feeney, K., 2011. "User-testing" as a method for testing the fitness-for-purpose of written medicine information. Patient Educ. Couns. 18735134. 83 (3), 404–410. doi:10.1016/j.pec.2011.03.016.

Scott, S., Atkins, B., D'Costa, T., Rendle, C., Murphy, K., Taylor, D., Smith, C., Kellar, I., Briggs, A., Griffiths, A., Hornak, R., Spinewine, A., Thompson, W., Tsuyuki, R., Bhattacharya, D., 2024. Development of the Guide to Disseminating Research (GuiDiR): a consolidated framework. Res. Soc. Adm. Pharm. 15517411. 20 (11), 1047–1057. Available from: https://www.sciencedirect.com/science/journal/15517411. doi:10.1016/j.sapharm.2024.08.001.

Seaton, T.L., 2017. Dissemination and implementation sciences in pharmacy: a call to action for professional organizations. Res. Soc. Adm. Pharm. 15517411. 13 (5), 902–904. Available from: http://www.journals.elsevierhealth.com/periodicals/rsap. doi:10.1016/j.sapharm.2017.05.021.

Straus, S.E., Tetroe, J., Graham, I., 2009. Defining knowledge translation. CMAJ. 14882329. 181 (3–4), 165–168. Available from: http://www.cmaj.ca/cgi/reprint/181/3-4/165. doi:10.1503/cmaj.081229.

Strifler, L., Cardoso, R., McGowan, J., Cogo, E., Nincic, V., Khan, P.A., Scott, A., Ghassemi, M., MacDonald, H., Lai, Y., Treister, V., Tricco, A.C., Straus, S.E., 2018a. Scoping review identifies significant number of knowledge translation theories, models, and frameworks with limited use. J. Clin. Epidemiol. 18785921. 100, 92–102. Available from: www.elsevier.com/locate/jclinepi. doi:10.1016/j.jclinepi.2018.04.008.

Strifler, L., Cardoso, R., McGowan, J., Cogo, E., Nincic, V., Khan, P.A., Scott, A., Ghassemi, M., MacDonald, H., Lai, Y., Treister, V., Tricco, A.C., Straus, S.E., 2018b. Scoping review identifies significant number of knowledge translation theories, models, and frameworks with limited use. J. Clin. Epidemiol. 08954356. 100, 92–102. Available from: https://www.nihr.ac.uk/partners-and-industry/charities/disseminate-research.htm. doi:10.1016/j.jclinepi.2018.04.008.

CHAPTER

20

Using design thinking and journey mapping to inform person-centered service design

Logan Thomas Murry[a,b] *and Matthew Witry*[c]

[a]Accreditation Council for Pharmacy Education, Continuing Pharmacy Education and Continuing Professional Development, Chicago, IL, United States

[b]Pharmacy Practice and Science, The University of Iowa College of Pharmacy, Iowa City, IA, United States

[c]Department of Pharmacy Practice and Science, University of Iowa, Iowa City, IA, United States

CHAPTER OBJECTIVES

- Define design thinking, user experience, journey mapping, and patient personas
- Explain how user-centered tools and methodologies can be useful when improving or creating health services
- Describe the specific elements of the journey mapping process and the value of empathy-driven insights in understanding "touchpoints," including "pain points" and moments when patients experience positive emotions
- Outline the process of developing a journey map to describe a patient persona or experience
- Identify ways in which the insights gathered from journey mapping can be used and evaluated to enhance person-centricity in health services

1 Introduction

Designing effective healthcare interventions requires a nuanced understanding of patients' and healthcare providers' experiences across complex systems of care. Journey mapping is a human-centered design method that visualizes the sequence of steps, emotions, and touchpoints that an individual experiences as they navigate a service,

https://doi.org/10.1016/B978-0-443-44607-8.00020-0

make decisions, or use a tool or device. Journey mapping has emerged as a valuable tool for uncovering critical insights into the lived experiences of patients, caregivers, and healthcare providers (Davies et al., 2023). By capturing the dynamic interplay between people, processes, and environments, journey maps facilitate the identification of barriers, inefficiencies, and unmet needs that often remain hidden in traditional approaches to intervention design and evaluation, which have historically emphasized outcomes over processes (Bulto et al., 2024; Flood et al., 2021, 2022; Ly et al., 2021).

In the context of healthcare intervention design, journey mapping offers more than a descriptive framework; it serves as a strategic instrument for innovation driven by empathy for the user's lived experience. Using journey mapping to inform service design enables interprofessional, multidisciplinary teams to co-create solutions that are grounded in user experiences (UXs) and aligned with the goals of safety, equity, and effectiveness in Healthy People (2030). As health systems shift toward value-based care and person-centered models, the integration of journey mapping into design processes can be a useful approach for enhancing patient engagement, improving service delivery, and optimizing health outcomes and equity.

This chapter explores the conceptual foundations, practical applications, and methodological considerations of journey mapping within healthcare intervention design. Drawing from case studies and current literature, we examine how journey maps can be leveraged to inform intervention planning, foster collaboration, and support the development of responsive, sustainable healthcare solutions.

2 Defining concepts: Design thinking, user experience, journey mapping, and personas

To begin designing person-centered interventions through the journey mapping process, a foundational understanding of several interrelated concepts that guide human-centered design is required. Among these, *design thinking, UX, journey mapping*, and *personas* serve as core concepts that support the systematic exploration of individuals' interactions with healthcare systems, services, and technologies.

Design thinking is a human-centered, iterative approach to creative problem-solving that emphasizes empathy, collaboration, and experimentation. It can be defined as "a process that uses design-specific cognitive activities to acquire and apply knowledge of users' needs and creatively generate effective solutions" (Roberts et al., 2016). Originally rooted in engineering and computer science, design thinking now spans multiple disciplines and is increasingly applied in healthcare to improve service delivery and patient experiences (PXs). Central to design thinking is understanding users' needs, desires, and behaviors, which can be achieved through methods like journey mapping, prototyping, and formative evaluation (Flood et al., 2021, 2022; Trebble et al., 2010; Sanders and Stappers, 2014; Eldridge et al., 2016). Structured frameworks like the Stanford d.school's five-stage model (empathize, define, ideate, prototype, test) and the Design Council's Double Diamond (discover, define, develop, deliver) guide multidisciplinary teams through iterative problem-solving cycles (Roberts et al., 2016; Stickdorn et al., 2018). Despite persistent misconceptions that design is limited to esthetics or product development, evidence shows that design thinking enables experience-centric innovation across complex health systems (Zomerdijk and Voss, 2010; Valentine et al., 2017). Design thinking underpins person-centered service design and informs all elements of person-centered service design methodologies, from instrument design and data collection to implementation. Principles from design thinking offer a powerful framework for transforming healthcare through deeper user engagement and more meaningful solutions, with health services researchers and individuals involved in intervention design using the journey mapping process to embed empathy and creativity into service redesign.

UX refers to the totality of an individual's perceptions, emotions, and responses resulting from the use or anticipation of a product, service, or system (Berni et al., 2023). In healthcare, the concept of UX has been referred to as PX and encompasses not only the functionality of a service, clinical tool, or digital platform but also the interpersonal, environmental, and emotional factors that shape how care is delivered and received (Kessler et al., 2021). A 2021 study by Newton et al. (2021) identified six components of UX for eHealth interventions, which include satisfaction, acceptability, credibility, perceived impact, user-reported adherence, and usability. A positive UX often correlates with improved engagement, satisfaction, and adherence to interventions, while negative experiences may lead to frustration, avoidance, or distrust in the system. Importantly, UX in healthcare is multidimensional, involving patients, caregivers, clinicians, administrators, and other key groups,each with distinct and sometimes conflicting goals and pain points.

Journey mapping is a design method informed most commonly by qualitative data collection and augmented with quantitative data to visualize and analyze the sequence of events, interactions, and emotional states a user encounters while engaging with a service or navigating a process (Bulto et al., 2024; Murry et al., 2021a). Importantly, journey mapping can be used to collect and depict information within the UX with a product or service (Murry et al., 2021a). In healthcare, journey maps can capture an individual's longitudinal experience across care settings. For example, the steps taken from symptom onset to posttreatment recovery. Journey maps typically include stages (e.g., awareness, access, treatment), touchpoints (e.g., appointments, new services, digital care), and user sentiments (e.g., anxiety, relief, confusion) (Murry et al., 2021a). By externalizing the lived experience in a visual format, journey mapping helps multidisciplinary teams identify gaps, inefficiencies, and both positive and negative elements within care experiences that might otherwise remain invisible in conventional workflows or outcome metrics.

Personas are hypothetical profiles or archetypes representing composites of key user segments derived from qualitative and/or quantitative data (Dominello et al., 2025). In healthcare, personas may embody the goals, needs, behaviors, and contextual challenges of different patient groups or key partners,such as a working mother managing a chronic illness or a rural clinician navigating telehealth adoption. While not real individuals, personas are grounded in real-world data and are used to humanize the design process, ensuring that interventions are tailored to specific patient realities rather than generalized assumptions about the care process or experience. When paired with journey maps, personas enrich the design process by providing depth and context around the UX, enabling healthcare teams to envision how different patients may interact with the same intervention in unique and individualized ways.

Together, using principles from design thinking, UX data, journey mapping, and personas forms a toolkit of human-centered approaches and methodologies that can improve the relevance, acceptability, and impact of healthcare interventions. They facilitate a shift from designing *for* users to designing *with* users, helping to inform the development of innovative and enhanced services within the complex environments and experiences of our patients.

3 Foundational steps to journey mapping

Improving the UX in healthcare requires empathy for patients' unique circumstances, environments, and prior care experiences. While a variety of research methodologies can help collect UX data and information, journey mapping is uniquely designed to help researchers, designers, and care providers understand and empathize with the patient perspective. Several leading organizations in UX offer practical frameworks to guide this process and support insight generation, service design, and organizational alignment (Stevens, 2023; Figma., Figma., Figma, User journey mapping: What it is + how to do it, n.d.). The steps below outline a general approach to developing a patient journey, as illustrated in Fig. 20.1. Generally, the process is designed to understand and depict the PX by creating personas and visualizing the care continuum experienced by these personas from start to finish.

3.1 Step 1: Clarify the purpose and project goals

The first step in effective journey mapping is clarifying the purpose and objectives of the journey mapping process. As the UX Design Institute suggests, journey maps should be used not simply as visual aids but as tools to cultivate empathy, identify user pain points, and build cross-functional understanding (Stevens, 2023). To accomplish this, the importance of setting clear project goals, such as diagnosing inefficiencies in an existing process or exploring opportunities in a new service, cannot be overstated. To identify the purpose and goals of the project, it may be especially useful for researchers to evaluate existing primary literature and obtain preliminary data and insights from content experts, patients, and clinicians. Before setting out to improve a service, it is important to identify services that both need and could benefit from this process.

3.2 Step 2: Persona ideation and defining the scenario

With a clear understanding of the purpose and goals of the project, it is essential that we begin thinking about the patients and associated personas that we are interested in understanding. During persona ideation, the extent to which we can truly identify personas depends on the amount of information (i.e., data) we already have. In some instances, we may have robust data that describe a variety of patient demographic information (i.e., age, financial status, health literacy, etc.), which can be invaluable in developing accurate personas. In other instances, we may have a general appreciation or understanding of our patients, and more information will be required to triangulate personas (more on persona triangulation later in the chapter). Regardless of the extent to which we can be certain of our patient personas, it is essential that we keep them front-of-mind in the journey mapping process.

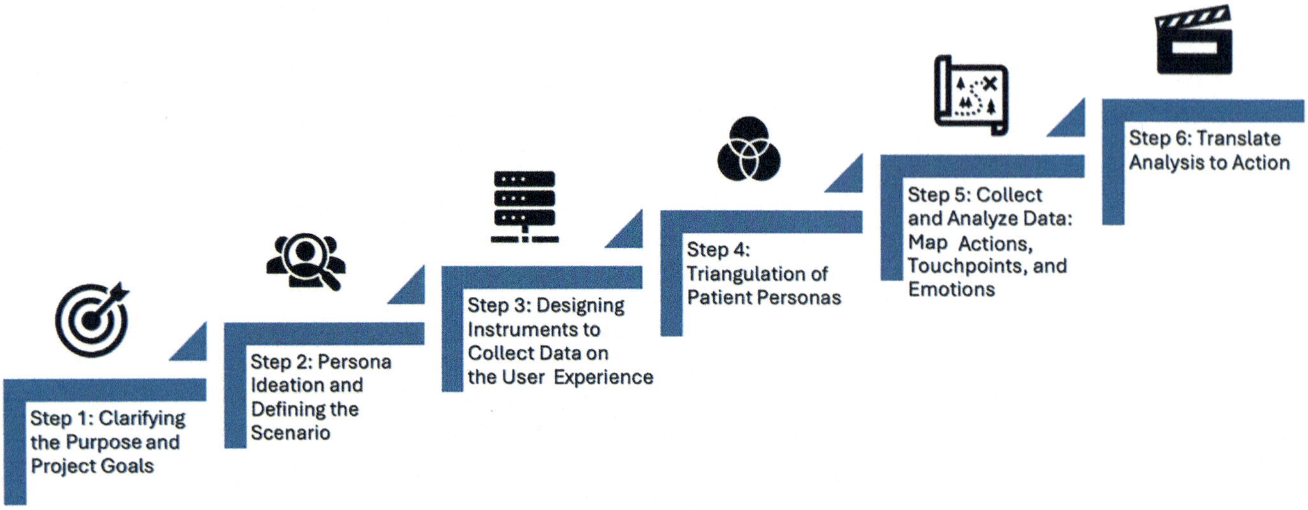

FIG. 20.1 Developing a patient journey. Outlined are the general steps for mapping the patient experience. While the steps may be completed in a specific order, it is important to note that this is an iterative process, with additional data and contexts introduced at various points throughout the journey-mapping process.

While identifying our patients and their associated personas, it is critical to consider the specific contexts and scenarios they will experience during their healthcare "journey," as patients will encounter different services and experience those services differently based on their own specific factors and circumstances. A journey map should reflect a specific experience, such as "refilling a prescription" or "accessing postdischarge care." Within this specific experience, there will be different journey stages that the individual will go through throughout the care process. The UX Design Institute recommends structuring these into sequential stages,for example: discover → decide → act → reflect (Stevens, 2023). When considering the patient journey, researchers and intervention designers are encouraged to define scenarios that reflect the full scope of the user's engagement, from the moment of need recognition to follow-up interactions. Selecting the right scope is key: it should be broad enough to capture context and cross-channel interactions but focused enough to allow for actionable insights.

3.3 Step 3: Designing instruments to collect qualitative and quantitative data on the UX

Once we have clarified the purpose and project goals, the specific scenario, and the PX we are interested in understanding, we can begin to think about the tools and instruments to use in order to collect the information required to accurately identify and describe both patient personas and the healthcare journeys they experience. For most journey mapping projects, a mixed-methods approach often provides the specific, nuanced information required to understand service experiences in great detail, with the volume of data that is often required to ensure consistent and reliable results. When creating journey maps using mixed methods, the process and the generated journey map contribute to the integration process, a pillar of mixed-methods research (Murry et al., 2023a). When designing instruments and tools to collect data that will inform journey maps, there are several points to consider, which are outlined below. In both instances below, specific questions and survey items should be informed by existing data, expectations, literature, and anything else that might provide preliminary insight into the PX. For example, if we know certain elements of the service are falling short, these could be a focus to further explore *why* and *what* specifically our patients experience. Throughout the instrument design process, it is essential to consider what we already know and what we need to know to improve our service offerings and care experiences.

3.3.1 *UX interviews*

UX interviews are a primary data source for creating a journey map that can help the team understand the process users go through, enabling them to identify potential areas for improvement through better design. Like other health services and qualitative research, choosing to conduct interviews depends on the specific question and the PX you are interested in understanding. More recently, the setting for data collection (virtual versus in-person) plays an increasingly important role in how data collection can and should occur (Carter et al., 2021). Interviews may be best suited for highly personal and nuanced care experiences, whereas other data collection approaches (e.g., focus groups) may help uncover more universally experienced pain points or highly positive elements of a service or healthcare interaction (Knott et al., 2022; Santhosh et al., 2021; Taherdoost, 2021). As mentioned previously, qualitative data collection should be approached with empathy and curiosity for understanding the PX. Data collection should be guided by the objectives and goals from Stage 1, using an interview guide with a flexible set of open-ended questions that encourage users to share their lived experiences, motivations, barriers, and emotions related to the target service or product.

As with qualitative research in general, rapport can be developed during the interview through open body language, active listening, and reassuring participants that there are no right or wrong answers, only valuable perspectives. During the interview, probes should be used liberally, with follow-up questions, encouragement to "tell me more about that," and allowance for silence to encourage reflection. Leading questions should be avoided,we want to understand their experience, not their agreement or disagreement with your assumptions. Interviewers should seek disconfirming evidence, as well as varying experiences and points of view, since these can highlight areas of divergence for potentially different individuals. Having two team members conduct the interview can be beneficial, as one investigator can focus on asking questions while the other concentrates on note-taking and thinking of alternative questions. Recording the interviews can provide a valuable record of the conversation.

These interviews should not only focus on the process but also interrogate the decision-making and emotions encountered along the way. Coding the data into the different stages of the process can help craft the journey map, as can creating codes for emotional reactions, high points, low points, decision points, and unmet needs. This process ensures that journey maps are more than process diagrams; they become empathetic narratives that bring the user's voice to the forefront of the design process. An example of what an interview guide might look like for a journey mapping project is included in Table 20.1 below. Keep in mind that the questions asked should be reflective of the specific service, technology, or care process you want to better understand.

These interview questions serve as a starting point for researchers who are beginning to think about the specific information that can and should be captured to inform the development of a patient journey map. While the examples provided above are predominantly designed for interviewing patients, we know that healthcare journeys often involve multiple perspectives, including those of caregivers, clinicians, and administrators. While potentially secondary to the PX and journey, these perspectives can play an important role in understanding the contextual and environmental factors that contribute to the current care experience and can inform intervention design. As such, researchers and service designers can consider the perspectives of other key groups and, where appropriate, collect supplemental information to capture these perspectives. Table 20.2 shows several additional prompts that may be relevant to key groups outside of patients.

3.3.2 *UX surveys*

In addition to qualitative data collected through interviews, quantitative data can play an important role in substantiating and triangulating findings. Creating a UX survey involves carefully designing questions that capture users' perceptions, behaviors, and pain points while ensuring the data collected is actionable. In the survey design process, it is critical to consider general best practices related to survey design, structure, and pretesting, as well as how the data collected will be supported by, inform, or further elaborate on qualitative findings to more holistically represent the journey of interest. Once we understand the survey purpose and how it intersects with our existing data, we can structure the survey with a balance of quantitative and qualitative questions. For example, Likert-type scale questions (e.g., "On a scale of 1–5, how easy was it to use this service?") provide measurable insights, while open-ended questions ("What frustrated you most about this process?") reveal deeper motivations and barriers. Generally, it can be helpful to develop specific questions for specific touchpoints or sequential stages within the journey. For example, if the sequential stages identified above were relevant—Discover → Decide → Act → Reflect in Stage 2—it would be important to align and categorize survey items within each sequential stage. This helps ensure you are measuring experience across all identified stages of the PX. When designing survey items, keep the language simple, unbiased, and user-centered to avoid leading responses. Finally, pilot test the survey with a small group of representative users to identify confusing wording or gaps in coverage before deploying it widely. In some instances, cognitive interviews and other instrument-evaluation methods can be helpful in understanding how respondents might interpret and respond to items, further contributing to and strengthening the inputs of the patient journey map (Meadows, 2021; Park and Kwon, 2021; Wolcott and Lobczowski, 2021). Table 20.3 shows example items for collecting information on PX, both generally and across specific stages. As was the case with the interview prompt examples, the items used should be reflective of the specific service, technology, or care process you want to better understand. It is important to note that these items are examples, and it is up to the researchers to develop optimal survey items, in addition to survey design and administration.

TABLE 20.1 Example of text, categories, and prompts for conducting an interview to inform the journey mapping process.

Topic	Prompts
1 Moderator introduction and expectations	
Moderator Introduction	**Welcome participants, introduce yourself, explain the purpose of the study, and describe the goal: to understand patient experiences with XXXX plan selection assistance.**
Interview Expectations	• The interview lasts approximately 1 hour • No right or wrong answers—participants are the experts • Passing on any question is allowed • Comments remain confidential • Recording is used for accuracy and is erased after transcription • Participants may ask questions or stop at any time
2. Setting the stage: Understanding context—warm-up questions to get participants to reflect on their healthcare experiences.	
• Walk me through the last time you needed care for this condition, from the moment you realized something was wrong to your most recent appointment. • What were your expectations before visiting your provider or clinic? • How do you usually decide where to seek care when you have a health concern? • When you think about your healthcare journey, what is the first word that comes to mind? • How do you typically feel when you start the process of seeking care? • What resources, people, or tools do you rely on when making healthcare decisions?	
3. Capturing key journey touchpoints—identify the major steps, transitions, and interactions in the patient's journey.	
• Describe the steps you went through, from scheduling your appointment to receiving care. • How did you first learn about your treatment options? Did anyone help you understand them? • What role, if any, does technology (e.g., patient portals, apps) play in your journey? • Tell me about your experience from beginning to end. What are the biggest steps along the way? • At which points did you feel the most supported, and when did you feel most on your own? • What's one point in the process where you wish things had been handled differently?	
4. Exploring emotional highs and lows—understand the emotional journey alongside functional steps.	
• Tell me about a moment during your care when you felt especially reassured or cared for. • Tell me about a time during this process when you felt frustrated, overwhelmed, or confused. What happened? • If you could describe your overall emotional journey during this process in three words, what would they be? • If we think about your healthcare journey as a rollercoaster, where are the biggest peaks and valleys? • How do emotions like anxiety, hope, or frustration influence your decision-making along the way? • What specific moments made you feel heard by your care team? What about moments when you did not feel heard?	
5. Identifying barriers and pain points—identify the biggest friction points and gaps in the patient experience.	
• Tell me about the moments when the process felt unnecessarily complicated. • What challenges did you face when trying to schedule care, understand instructions, or manage follow-ups? • Was there any information you needed but couldn't find, or that you wished had been explained differently? • What gets in the way of receiving the care you need when you need it? • If you could remove one major pain point from the process, what would it be?	
6. Looking ahead: hopes, needs, and ideal journeys—explore what patients want to improve and their vision for an ideal experience.	
• If you could redesign this healthcare experience from start to finish, what would you change first? • What tools, support, or communication would make the process easier? • What does an ideal healthcare experience or service look like for you? • Imagine a healthcare system designed specifically for your needs … what would it do differently? • What kinds of support would make you feel more confident at each step? • If a new service, app, or resource could make your experience smoother, what would it need to provide?	

TABLE 20.2 Additional prompts for other key groups.

Key group	Example prompt
Caregivers	"Tell me about a time when you had to coordinate care for a loved one. What worked, and what didn't?"
Clinicians	"From your perspective, where do patients seem most confused or overwhelmed during this process?"
Administrators	"Where do you see the most breakdowns between scheduling, care delivery, and follow-up?"

TABLE 20.3 Example survey items to inform a patient journey map.

1. Overall healthcare experience items—these questions capture **general experiences and impressions of the journey.**	
How satisfied are you with your overall healthcare experience?	Scale: 1 = Very Dissatisfied → 5 = Very Satisfied
How easy was it for you to navigate the healthcare process from start to finish?	Scale: 1 = Very Difficult → 5 = Very Easy
How confident do you feel about managing your healthcare needs?	Scale: 1 = Not Confident → 5 = Very Confident
What word or short phrase best describes your recent healthcare experience?	Open-Ended Response
2. Journey touchpoints and process mapping—helps identify which stages in the journey are smooth versus frustrating.	
Stage: Discover	
How challenging was it to obtain information about [service]?	Scale: 1 = Not Challenging at All → 5 = Very Challenging
What was most memorable about your experience learning about [service] for the first time?	Open-Ended Response
Stage: Decide	
When making the decision to use [service], how difficult did you find the decision?	Scale: 1 = Not Difficult at All → 5 = Very Difficult
What made the decision harder or easier?	Open-Ended Response
Stage: Act	
How do you feel about receiving [service]?	Scale: 1 = Very Unhappy → 5 = Very Happy
What were the best parts of choosing to receive [service]? What were the worst?	Open-Ended Response
Stage: Reflect	
How satisfied are you with your overall healthcare experience?	Scale: 1 = Very Dissatisfied → 5 = Very Satisfied
Which part of the process was the most challenging for you?	Scheduling appointments/Understanding instructions/Managing medications/Billing/insurance/Other:_______
How satisfied are you with the communication you received at each stage of your care?	Awareness/Scheduling/Provider Visit/Follow-Up/Billing (Scale: 1 = Very Dissatisfied → 5 = Very Satisfied)
Who helped you to understand or navigate this process?	Open-Ended Response
3. Emotional experience along the journey—UX surveys should capture emotional highs and lows, not just functional outcomes.	
At what point in your care did you feel the most stressed or overwhelmed?	Before appointment/During appointment/After results/Managing treatment/Not stressed
How often did you feel confident in the information you were given?	Scale: Never/Rarely/Sometimes/Often/Always
Describe one moment during your journey when you felt especially supported or reassured.	Open-Ended Response
4. Identifying barriers and pain points—pinpointing where breakdowns or friction occur in the experience.	
How easy was it to understand the instructions provided by your care team?	Scale: 1 = Very Difficult → 5 = Very Easy
Did you experience any delays in scheduling, receiving results, or accessing treatment?	Yes/No → If yes, please describe.
How satisfied are you with the tools or resources provided to manage your care?	Examples: portals, apps, printed instructions. Scale: 1 = Very Dissatisfied → 5 = Very Satisfied.
What's one thing that made the process harder than it needed to be?	Open-Ended Response

In the evolving healthcare landscape, patient portals, smartphone applications, and telehealth are playing an increasingly important role in both access to and delivery of care. When appropriate, it may be necessary to include assessment items that evaluate how these elements contribute to the care experience and whether they could or should be improved. Some basic assessment items related to digital tools that might contribute to the care experience are included in Table 20.4.

In addition to developing the patient journey, researchers or organizations might have specific questions related to service use, willingness-to-pay, or other engagement metrics that are aligned with organizational initiatives or evaluations of sustainability. These questions extend beyond current experiences and aim to explore potential future use and specific opportunities for improvement. More recently, the quantification of PX and the identification of optimal evaluation methods have been of increased focus, with patient-reported experience measures (PREMs) and

TABLE 20.4 Example survey items to inform a patient journey map for digital and technology experience.

Item—Since many healthcare journeys involve portals, apps, and telehealth, it's useful to evaluate UX there too	Scale/Response
Did you use any digital tools to manage your healthcare during this process?	Yes/No → If yes, select which:Patient portal/ Mobile app/ Telehealth platform/ Other:______
How easy was it to use these tools to access the information you needed?	Scale: 1 = Very Difficult → 5 = Very Easy
What features would improve your experience in using digital tools for your care?	Open-Ended Response

patient-reported outcome measures (PROMs) increasingly recommended (Benson, 2023; Kaneko et al., 2025; Murry and Desselle, 2023; Bull, 2021). In addition to PREMs and PROMs, there has been an increase in the use of the Net Promoter Score (NPS) to quantify PX and, importantly, identify the extent to which patients would or would not repeat service use or recommend the service to a friend. NPS consists of a two-part questionnaire. Firstly, respondents are presented with a rating question: "How likely is it that you would recommend our business/service to a friend or colleague?" This is a scaled item, and while NPS is most commonly a 10-point scale, it is up to the researchers to determine if a 5-point, 10-point, or some other scale is most appropriate. This is followed by an open-ended, free-text item, which enables respondents to provide the main reason for their score (Adams et al., 2022; Bonilla et al., 2025; Diliasari and Sulistiadi, 2024). While there is no universally recommended metric by which to evaluate PX, using items that are both actionable and aligned with person-centered care and organizational initiatives helps to enhance the usefulness of the data. Examples of survey items that align with service redesign and service use are included in Table 20.5.

Finally, demographic information plays a crucial role in developing patient personas when creating journey maps. This is especially true if we only have a general understanding of our patient population, with data collection informing more robust persona development. Demographic information provides essential context for understanding patient behaviors, preferences, and needs. For instance, collecting data like age, gender, and race/ethnicity helps identify patterns and disparities in healthcare experiences. Information about insurance type (e.g., private, Medicare, Medicaid, or uninsured) offers insights into access to care and financial constraints. Understanding the primary reason for seeking care, whether for routine checkups, urgent needs, or chronic condition management, further refines personas by highlighting differences in motivations and priorities. Moreover, distinguishing between first-time and repeat patient journeys reveals variations in expectations, familiarity with the healthcare process, and potential pain points. By incorporating these demographic and contextual details, patient personas become realistic, representative, and better aligned with the diverse experiences of the populations being served. Table 20.6 provides some examples of demographic and contextual questions that may be relevant and useful for persona development.

3.3.3 *Step 4: Collect and analyze data: Triangulation of patient personas*

Prior to launching larger data collection initiatives, we usually have a general idea of who our patients are and the personas they embody. In instances where we have insufficient data to make larger generalizations about patient personas, we can develop them throughout the data collection process. Often, in mixed methods, we may start to get an idea of who our patient groups are, and through an iterative process, we will develop this knowledge more completely as we gather additional data. Once key user types have been identified through data analysis, the archetypal user profiles can serve as powerful design tools. In pharmacy practice, for example, personas might include:

- "The tech-savvy caregiver"—managing complex medication regimens for an elderly parent using a mobile application.
- "The distrustful chronic pain patient"—wary of pharmacological treatment and skeptical of the healthcare system.
- "The busy professional"—who values convenience, reminders, and discreet interventions.

These personas should be used not only as references but also as *stand-ins* during ideation, prototyping, and evaluation phases. Furthermore, while a key contribution of personas is helping designers identify and build interventions around specific needs and users/patients, researchers should be cautious about stereotyping and overgeneralizing. In the persona design and development stage, it is critical to be judicious and create personas that effectively support the design process. Teams can ask: *How would this intervention meet the needs of Persona A? What barriers might Persona B face when accessing this service?*

TABLE 20.5 Example survey items for service redesign and service use.

Item—Helps inform service redesign and future improvements	Scale/Response
How likely are you to recommend this provider or facility to others? *(Net Promoter Score)*	Scale: 0 = Not at all likely → 10 = Extremely likely
What would make your healthcare journey smoother or less stressful?	Open-Ended Response
If you could change one thing about your experience, what would it be?	Open-Ended Response

TABLE 20.6 Example survey items for demographic and context information.

Items—These provide important context for interpreting survey results and developing personas.
Age, gender, race/ethnicity *(optional)*
Type of insurance (Private/Medicare/Medicaid/None)
Whether this is a first-time or repeat experience,

When developing patient personas, it is crucial that we rely on substantive and triangulated data. This involves collecting qualitative insights through interviews and focus groups (and other qualitative methods), quantitative metrics such as surveys and usage analytics, and anecdotal observations. Personas must be research-driven and triangulated, reducing one-size-fits-all assumptions and helping designers and clinicians anticipate diversity in health literacy, access, motivation, and social context. By grounding journey maps in authentic user stories, healthcare interventions can better address the experiences of patients in the real world.

3.3.4 *Step 5: Collect and analyze data: Map actions, touchpoints, and emotions*

The heart of journey mapping lies in documenting user actions, interactions, and touchpoints at each stage of the care or intervention experience. These include every component of the experience or service the user engages with: hospital or pharmacy, electronic healthcare system, outpatient or home health, and follow-up phone calls. Gathering data from each stage often requires mixed methods: user analytics, service logs, survey results, interviews, and field observations. The goal is to chart not just what users do, but where, when, and with whom they do it. This multitouchpoint awareness is essential for uncovering inconsistencies and service gaps that might otherwise go unnoticed.

In addition to interactions, emotions and internal responses are equally important. Effective journey maps visualize not just behaviors but also thoughts, emotions, and pain points. The UX Design Institute recommends integrating emotional tracking into each stage to highlight where users may feel confused, frustrated, relieved, or empowered. Designorate, a website committed to design thinking and healthcare design, run by Dr. Rafiq Elmansy, echoes this by suggesting the inclusion of effort metrics (such as delays, repeated steps, or uncertainty) as indicators of friction. Identifying "moments of truth," or emotionally charged experiences that significantly influence a user's overall impression, is particularly valuable for prioritizing improvements. To enhance usability and engagement, journey maps should be visualized in a way that is both detailed and digestible. The UX Design Institute encourages incorporating personas, stages, emotional arcs, and responsibility assignments. Visualization tools like Miro, Canva, or Lucidchart can be used to create dynamic and shareable maps that support collaboration across diverse teams.

3.3.5 *Step 6: Translate analysis to action*

Analyzing the completed journey map is where the process moves from insight to action. The UX Design Institute highlights how identifying pain points can lead to targeted improvements (Stevens, 2023). Other organizations focus on the use of additional tools and strategies, such as the Five Whys, Fishbone Diagrams, and mind maps, to help uncover root causes and ideate solutions. During this process, early iteration and stakeholder feedback are vital. Specifically, patient feedback plays an essential role in developing actionable results from journey maps to avoid designing and implementing assumption-driven interventions. The UX Design Institute also encourages using draft maps to align stakeholders and co-create change plans. Iterative mapping (through rounds of feedback, refinement, and validation) builds credibility and promotes organizational buy-in.

Insights from the journey map must ultimately be translated into action. Implementation plans should include assigned responsibilities, timelines, and outcome measures. Once changes are enacted, repeating the mapping process helps assess whether interventions are working as intended, or whether new gaps have emerged. Journey mapping, then, is not a static exercise but an ongoing method for learning and adaptation. It enables organizations to align strategy with lived experience, driving improvements that are not only effective but also empathetic and sustainable.

4 Case study: Journey mapping in healthcare research

To further illustrate the journey mapping process, we explore an example of journey mapping in healthcare research below. Within this examples, it is important for the reader to recognize both how the journey mapping process was conducted to address each of the steps as described above, and to consider areas or opportunities where these studies could use additional research methodology to maximize the impact of the journey mapping process.

4.1 Journey mapping the medicare Part D experience: A patient-centered evaluation of pharmacy consultation services

In the United States, older individuals are eligible for Medicare, an insurance benefit that includes multiple components to cover hospital stays, outpatient care, and prescription medications, albeit often with patient cost-sharing. The process of selecting a prescription medication benefit, a Medicare Part D plan, is a complex and often confusing task for older adults, involving dozens of plan options with varying costs and benefits. Community pharmacies have begun offering consultation services to support this decision-making process (Murry et al., 2023c, 2021b). However, despite positive experiences and potential cost savings, few patients use these services repeatedly or act on the advice provided. Traditional satisfaction surveys may fail to capture the full complexity of the PX (Murry et al., 2021b). In this study, we combined traditional data collection and research methods with principles from patient/person-centered service design. This example was a cross-sectional study conducted in a single rural, independently owned pharmacy in the Midwest United States. Thirty-six participants aged 65 + currently enrolled in Medicare Part D were surveyed (18 had used the pharmacy consultation service and 18 had not). We used an online journey mapping platform that created patient journeys using data collected from a 44-item survey, including 7 demographic items, 30 Likert-type items, and 7 open-ended questions.

4.1.1 Step 1: Clarify the purpose and project goals

Community pharmacies offering Medicare Part D consultations struggle with repeat service use and meaningful patient engagement. Patients often report confusion, a lack of trust, and an overload of plan details, which undermines the potential value of these services. The challenge lies in understanding the emotional and cognitive journey patients undergo during plan selection to refine services accordingly. The goal of the project was to journey map the experiences of patients who did and did not use a pharmacy-led Medicare Part D consultation service, with the goal of improving service design and delivery (Murry et al., 2021a).

4.1.2 Step 2: Persona ideation and defining the scenario

Prior to developing the patient journey maps, we conducted extensive research on Medicare Part D consultation services offered in the community pharmacy (Murry et al., 2021a, 2021b). This research supplemented our experiences as pharmacists working with older adults to select their Medicare Part D plans. Through interviews, survey responses, and interactions with patients, we were able to generate personas for individuals who had and had not used a Medicare Part D consultation service in the community pharmacy setting. In our study, these personas were labeled as "Beverly" and "Susan" for patients who did and did not use a service, respectively. From our collected data, it was evident that individuals who availed themselves of a Medicare Part D consultation service offered in the community pharmacy setting had a lower income than those who did not use the service but were otherwise comparable. Fig. 20.2 depicts the persona for "Beverly," our service user, and Fig. 20.3 depicts the persona for "Susan," our service nonuser.

In our example, the specific scenario of interest was selecting a Medicare Part D insurance plan. We examined individuals who both did and did not use a service to better understand the current intervention as it compared to the experience of selecting a plan without pharmacist and pharmacy support. In our study, we used software to facilitate the development of a journey map, which specified the following processes mapped to the Medicare Part D plan selection experience: discover → search → assess → decide → assist. This process effectively captures the experience of selecting a Medicare Part D plan from start to finish, where individuals: (1) discover the need or

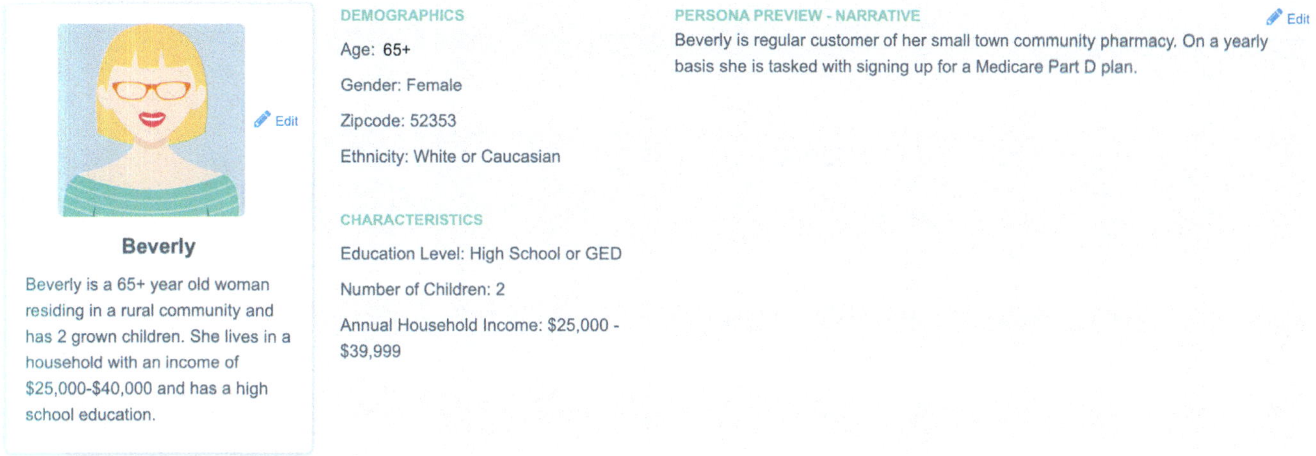

FIG. 20.2 "Beverly" persona for service user. A created persona for a Medicare Part D consultation service user. *From Journimap 3LC.*

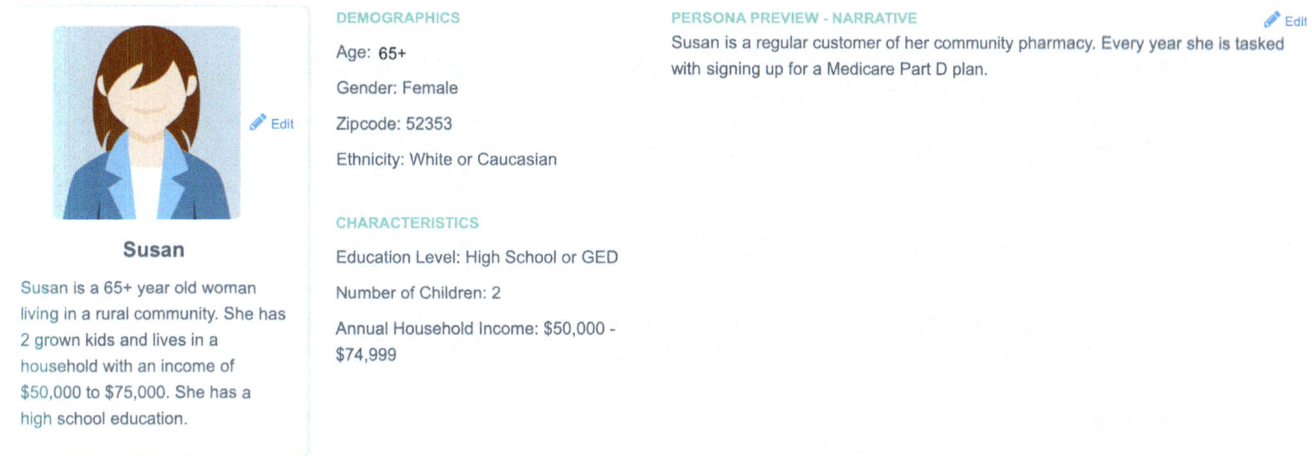

FIG. 20.3 "Susan" persona for service nonuser. A created persona for a Medicare Part D consultation service nonuser. *From Journimap 3LC.*

opportunity to select or change Medicare Part D plans during the open-enrollment period, (2) search for additional information and support to select a Medicare Part D plan, (3) compare different plans, (4) make a selection based on the support and information obtained, and (5) reflect on future sentiment about the process and how changes in the process could assist in improving the PX. Fig. 20.4 includes a blank journey map from the software used in this work, which shows both the different stages of the PX and the emotions and pain points experienced throughout the process.

4.1.3 Step 3: Designing instruments to collect qualitative and quantitative data on the UX

Within this study, we used an online journey mapping platform that created patient journeys using data collected from a 44-item survey, including 7 demographic items, 30 Likert-type items, and 7 open-ended questions. While this survey collected information to create personas and develop patient journeys, this work was informed by previous research focused on the Medicare Part D experience (Murry et al., 2020). For demographic items to further develop personas, we asked participants for their age, gender, zip code, education level, number of children, annual household income, and race/ethnicity. For the 30 Likert-type items and 7 open-ended response items, we mapped questions to each of the patient journey stages: discover, search, assess, decide, and assist. Examples of items for each stage are listed in Table 20.7.

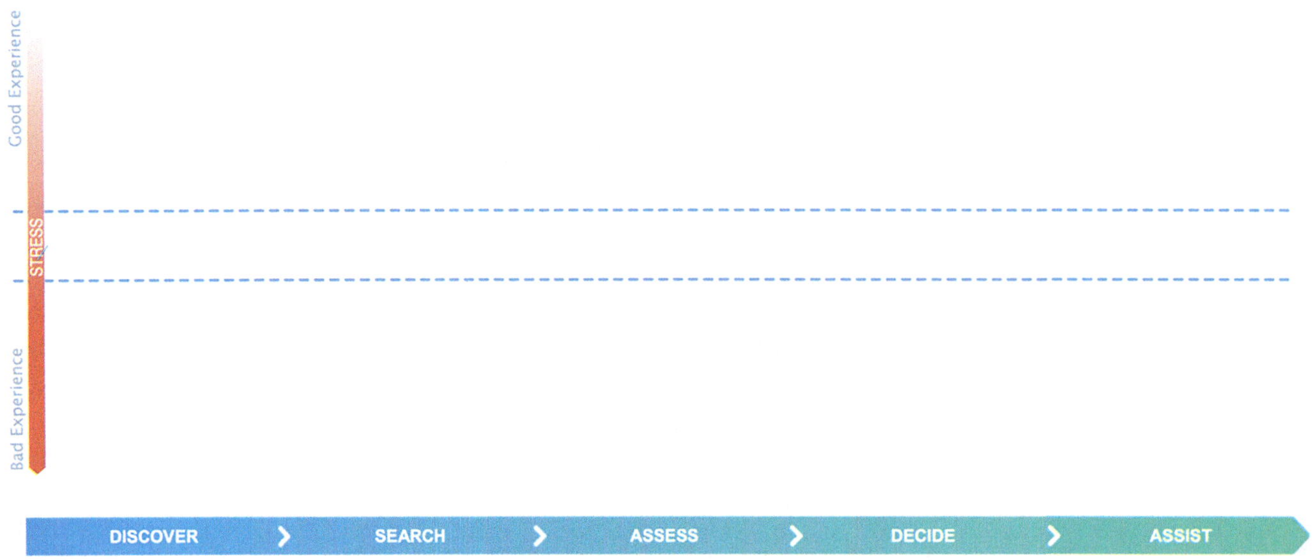

FIG. 20.4 A blank map prior to mapping the patient journey for selecting a Medicare Part D plan. *From Journimap L3C.*

TABLE 20.7 Survey Items for each stage of the patient journey.

Journey map stage	Example item
Discover	Gaining a good understanding of signing up for a Medicare Part D plan was easy. [5-point Likert-type item, 1 = Strongly Disagree → 5 = Strongly Agree]How did you first hear about signing up for a Medicare Part D plan? [Open-ended]
Search	I did not consult others when seeking to learn more about signing up for a Medicare Part D plan. [5-point Likert-type item, 1 = Strongly Disagree → 5 = Strongly Agree] Briefly describe what was the most enjoyable or least enjoyable about your process of finding information about signing up for a Medicare Part D plan. [Open-Ended]
Assess	Comparing Medicare Part D plans was frustrating and difficult. [5-point Likert-type item, 1 = Strongly Disagree → 5 = Strongly Agree] Briefly describe what it was like to compare Medicare Part D plans during the sign-up process. [Open-ended]
Decide	When it came time to sign up for a Medicare Part D plan, I found it difficult to decide. [5-point Likert-type item, 1 = Strongly Disagree → 5 = Strongly Agree] How would you describe what it was like deciding between Medicare Part D plans? Please share a few words that best describe the experience of making a decision. [Open-ended]
Assist	I wish that I had more and/or better information before signing up for a Medicare Part D plan. [5-point Likert-type item, 1 = Strongly Disagree → 5 = Strongly Agree]I I look forward to signing up for a Medicare Part D plan in the future. [5-point Likert-type item, 1 = Strongly Disagree → 5 = Strongly Agree] What I liked best about signing up for a Medicare Part D plan was: (please add your comments below) [Open-ended] What I liked least about signing up for a Medicare Part D plan was: (please add your comments below) [Open-ended]

From Journimap L3C.

4.1.4 Step 4: Collect and analyze data: Triangulation of patient personas

Once we collected our responses, we were able to triangulate our patient personas, ensuring that they reflect a comprehensive and accurate understanding of older adults' decision-making processes. Quantitative findings, such as demographics and insurance coverage, were integrated with qualitative insights, including patient frustrations, knowledge gaps, and emotional responses when comparing plans. By cross-referencing these multiple data sources, the researchers were able to identify consistent patterns, such as widespread confusion about plan costs and coverage, as well as key points where beneficiaries needed additional support. This rigorous triangulation strengthened the development of evidence-based patient personas, ensuring they accurately represented the diverse experiences, challenges, and priorities faced by Medicare beneficiaries selecting Part D plans.

In our study, individuals who used the Medicare Part D service were slightly older and generally had a lower income than those who did not use the Medicare Part D consultation service. One such individual was named

"Beverly," who could be described as a cost-conscious patient inherently needing additional support in Part D plan selection by using the pharmacy service. Alternatively, an individual who did not use the service, "Susan," was potentially less restricted by a fixed income during the Part D decision-making process. More on advanced persona development will be discussed later in the chapter.

4.1.5 Step 5: Collect and analyze data: Map actions, touchpoints, and emotions

Using quantitative and qualitative data from the survey, the PX with selecting a Medicare Part D plan was mapped for both personas (service users and nonusers). In both journey maps, several pain points and emotions were identified throughout the service experience. Empathy mapping revealed that pharmacy service users experienced more emotional highs and lows, with both positive and negative touchpoints, than nonusers. Despite receiving expert guidance, they reported greater frustration and uncertainty, whereas nonusers tended to trust their external advisors. Journey mapping showed that pharmacy service users encountered more touchpoints and greater emotional fluctuations throughout the selection process. However, both groups ended with low optimism about their final plan choice, suggesting ongoing decision fatigue or dissatisfaction. Quantitatively, pharmacy service users demonstrated significantly greater awareness of plan options and more opportunities to compare features ($P < .05$), yet they also struggled more with plan selection and required additional assistance late in the process. Qualitative themes underscored that patients found the decision-making process overwhelmingly complex regardless of service use, and that trust played a key role: nonusers relied on agents or family, while pharmacy service users were more skeptical, often perceiving pharmacy staff as "salespeople".

After data collection, responses can be used to map out PXs visually. We can map out different stages of the care experience, various touchpoints within the intervention or service, the emotions patients experience, and identify opportunities for service improvement. Patient journeys from our study are included in Fig. 20.5 and Fig. 20.6.

We compared the PX to the current service delivery. At the community pharmacy, these services were offered as one-on-one appointments where patients came in, discussed plans with a pharmacist using the Medicare website, and had the option of signing up for the plan at the community pharmacy. For the service user, this comparison and the option to make a choice immediately following the discussion of plans seemingly resulted in additional pain points compared to those who did not use the service. Despite these pain points, service users appeared to feel more supported throughout the process. Both groups ultimately left the Part D plan selection process feeling uncertain. From these patient journeys, several service improvements were identified and are discussed in the next section.

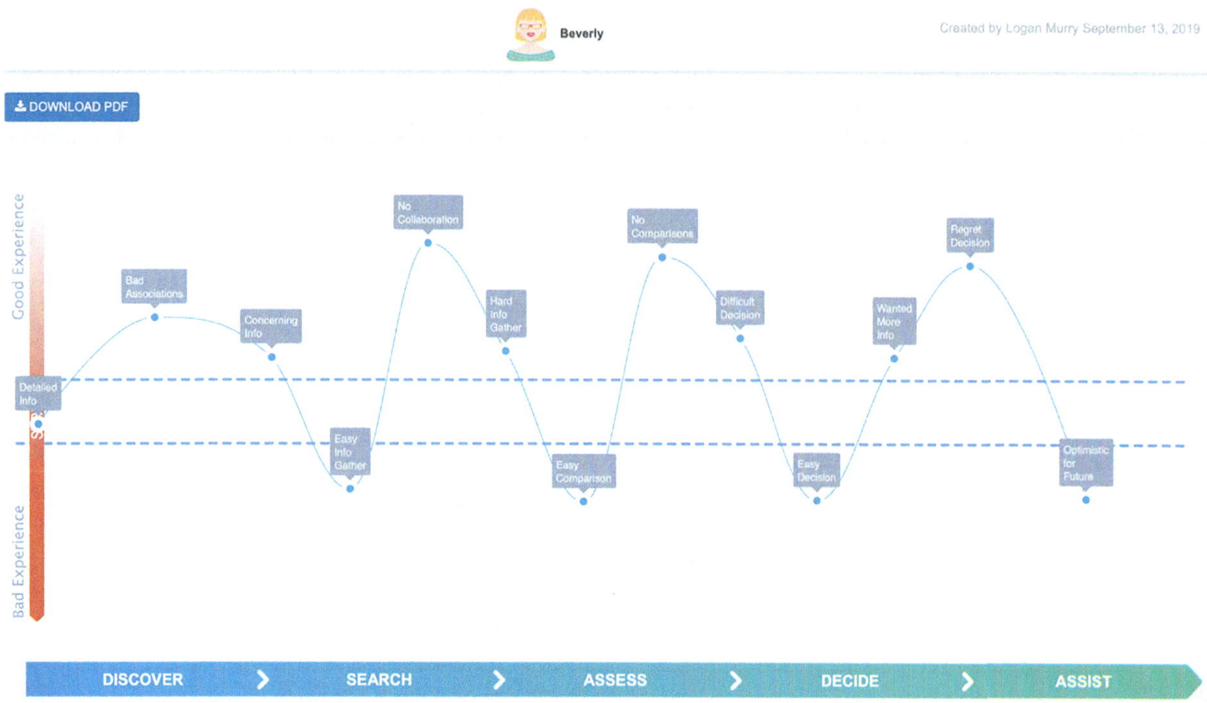

FIG. 20.5 "Beverly" patient experience and journey as service user. *From Journimap 3LC.*

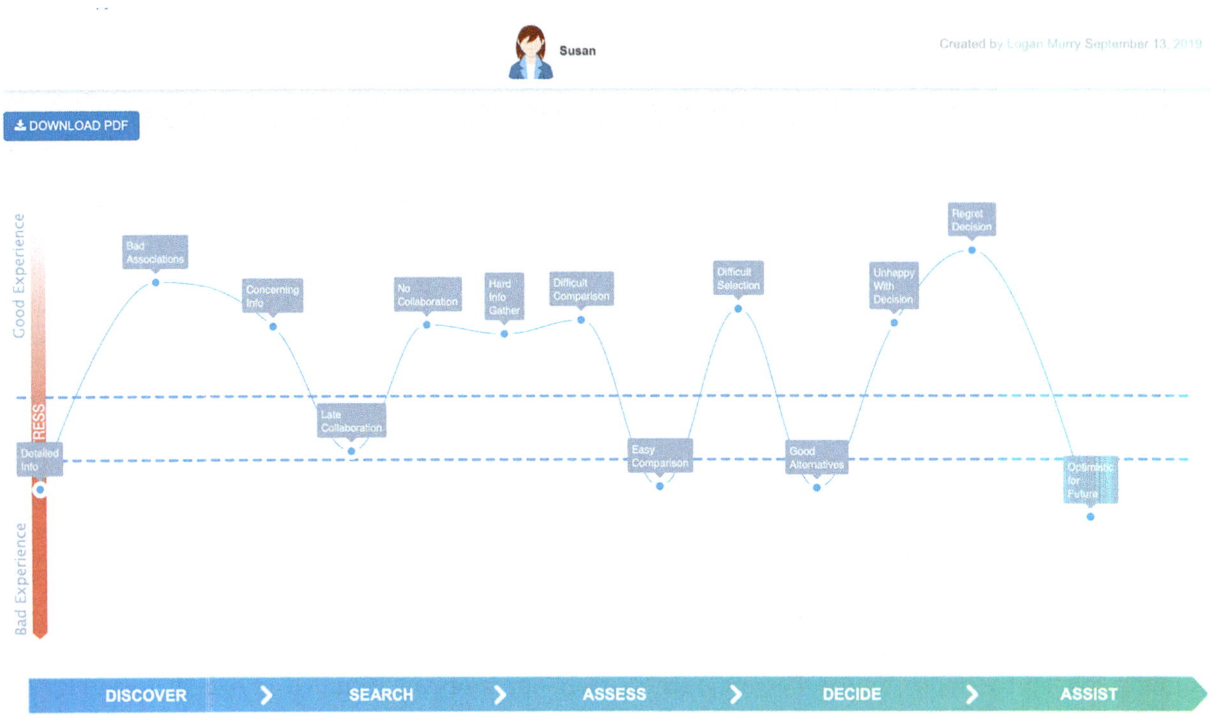

FIG. 20.6 "Susan's" patient expereince and journey as a service nonuser. *From Journimap 3LC.*

4.1.6 Step 6: Translate analysis to action

From these journey maps, several opportunities for process and service improvement were identified. From an intervention design perspective, the pharmacist-led Medicare Part D consultation service may unintentionally overload patients with complex plan data. Instead, information should be framed around patient-relevant benefits, not just costs or coverage specifics. Further, based on the patient journey from using the service, trust is more critical than information volume. Patients often default to trusted individuals or brands rather than analyzing detailed data. Finally, patients appeared to struggle with the complexity of insurance information being presented (i.e., insurance literacy). Consultation services should consider a patient's insurance literacy and cognitive capacity, especially for older adults with lower numeracy skills. From these findings, the research team recommended that the service be revised in several ways, including creating handouts of the information discussed, conducting a follow-up call to provide additional information or answer questions surrounding the Part D plan decision, and involving a trusted relative or other advocate in the information delivery and decision-making process. These findings were also used to inform additional studies to further improve the PX while identifying financially sustainable service offerings, which will be discussed later in this chapter (Murry et al., 2023c, 2023b).

5 Conclusions

While the pharmacy consultation service increased awareness of Medicare plan options, it may not consistently improve PX due to information overload and trust gaps. Journey mapping revealed emotional complexities and provided a richer understanding of decision-making challenges. To increase engagement and impact, pharmacies should redesign services to simplify plan information and focus on building trust rather than delivering excessive detail.

6 Additional ways to operationalize personas and patient preference

In addition to the journey mapping process, there are supportive and supplementary approaches to design or refine healthcare and pharmacy interventions that align with patient needs and preferences, as identified through the PX lens. Building upon PX research and personas has the potential to increase patient engagement and service use. Some of these strategies are described below.

6.1 Eliciting and synthesizing patient preferences

Operationalizing patient preferences begins with systematically capturing what matters most to patients. This may include their values, goals, communication preferences, logistical needs, and perceptions of risk, burden, or benefit associated with different treatment options or service models. In pharmacy settings, for instance, patients may express preferences regarding medication delivery (e.g., home versus in-pharmacy), frequency of follow-ups, language used in counseling, or the use of digital adherence tools.

Several methodologies can be used to gather and analyze patient preferences:

- Qualitative interviews and focus groups are conducted to uncover nuanced motivations and barriers
- Discrete choice experiments (DCEs) or conjoint analysis are used to quantify the trade-offs patients are willing to make
- Shared decision-making tools and PROMs are used to integrate preferences directly into care

By embedding these methods early in the design cycle, developers can ensure interventions reflect real-world patient priorities, increasing their relevance, usability, and acceptability. In the Medicare Part D service journey map process described above, these findings were used to inform a DCE study to identify attributes of a service that aligned with patient preferences (Murry et al., 2023b). This is just one example of how journey mapping and additional methodologies can build upon earlier findings to optimize person-centered services.

6.2 Designing with preference alignment in mind

Aligning interventions with patient journeys and preferences means offering flexibility, choice, and responsiveness. As identified in the example of journey mapping completed in Australia, no two patient journeys are completely identical, requiring as much specificity and adaptability within our interventions as possible (Shafei et al., 2024). In pharmacy settings, this might manifest as:

- Tiered intervention models (e.g., offering both digital and in-person medication therapy management options)
- Customizable communication strategies (e.g., SMS, apps, phone calls)
- Visual and language adaptations for diverse cultural and health literacy needs
- Incorporation of motivational interviewing techniques for populations with low readiness for behavior change

Integrating personas and preferences into logic models, user journeys, or implementation frameworks ensures they influence not just front-end design but also evaluation criteria and sustainability planning.

6.3 Continuous feedback and iteration

As described earlier, designing patient or person-centered interventions is not a one-time exercise but an ongoing process. Persona-based usability testing, preference-sensitive outcome tracking, and codesign sessions with target users should be built into continuous quality improvement cycles. This is particularly vital in rapidly evolving areas such as digital health, pharmacogenomics, or chronic disease management, where patient needs and technological possibilities frequently shift.

7 Conclusion

Journey mapping provides a flexible, patient-centered framework for understanding the complex and often fragmented experiences of patients, caregivers, and healthcare professionals. By focusing on how individuals think, feel, and navigate care systems, journey maps offer more than a descriptive account of tasks or processes; they help to identify actionable insights that reflect real-world care delivery and PX. When grounded in empathy, supported by qualitative and quantitative methodologies, combined with additional patient preference findings, and co-created with key parties, journey maps can drive the design of interventions that are not only effective but deeply resonant with those they intend to serve.

Unlike traditional process improvement tools that emphasize efficiency or throughput, journey mapping places particular emphasis on the way patients think and feel throughout the healthcare process. Journey mapping has the ability to identify hidden barriers and points of friction that profoundly influence engagement, satisfaction, and outcomes. Structured approaches, like those advanced by the UX Design Institute, operationalize this method through clearly defined objectives, research-informed personas, purposeful data collection, and iterative visualization. These practices ensure that intervention design remains responsive to lived experience rather than constrained by internal assumptions or rigid workflows.

In pharmacy and broader healthcare settings, journey mapping has been used both to enhance existing services and to guide service development. When informed by patient preferences, persona archetypes, and cross-disciplinary input, journey maps enable interventions to reflect the priorities and constraints of real-world patients across diverse populations and care contexts. Using additional methodologies, such as discrete choice experiments and other ways of quantifying patient preferences, can extend journey maps beyond static visualization into continuous improvement frameworks that support implementation, measurement, and iteration.

Importantly, journey maps should not be treated as fixed or exhaustive models. The value of journey maps lies in their ability to promote reflection, facilitate dialog, and align interdisciplinary teams around a shared understanding of UX. Journey maps offer a common language for navigating a complex care experience. As healthcare systems continue to prioritize value-based care, equity, and person-centered outcomes, the strategic application of journey mapping can play an essential role in the design of interventions rooted in the needs and experiences of patients.

8 Questions for further discussion

Identifying needs

- How can journey mapping help uncover needs or pain points that traditional needs assessments might overlook?
- In what ways might patient-reported experiences differ from clinicians' or administrators' assumptions about patient needs?

Methodological considerations

- What are the strengths and limitations of journey mapping compared to other qualitative research methods in healthcare intervention design?
- How might the scale and scope of a journey map (e.g., high-level versus detailed) influence the types of insights generated?

Patient and key party

- What strategies can ensure that the voices of marginalized or hard-to-reach patient populations are authentically represented in a journey map?
- How can involving patients in the mapping process improve the accuracy and relevance of the resulting interventions?

Application to intervention refinement

- How can insights from a journey map be translated into actionable design changes without losing the nuances of PXs?
- What role should journey mapping play in ongoing quality improvement cycles—should it be a one-time exercise or a repeated process?

Measuring impact

- How can the effectiveness of journey map–informed interventions be measured in terms of patient outcomes, satisfaction, and engagement?
- What metrics or qualitative indicators best capture the impact of changes inspired by journey mapping?

Future directions

- How might emerging technologies (e.g., digital ethnography, AI-assisted analysis) change the way journey maps are created and used?
- What opportunities exist for integrating journey mapping into broader human-centered design or implementation science frameworks in healthcare?

9 Application exercise/scenario

Consider a service or intervention that patients may struggle with, or that could be improved to make it more person-centered.

1. How could you apply journey mapping to improve the service?
2. What specific pain points or other touchpoints might be identified where improvements could occur?
3. How would you go about evaluating and quantifying the PX as a result of these changes?

Acknowledgment

This work was supported by a grant from the Iowa Pharmacy Association's Outcomes Innovative Pharmacy grant program.

References

Adams, C., Walpola, R., Schembri, A.M., Harrison, R., 2022. The ultimate question? evaluating the use of net promoter score in healthcare: a systematic review. Health Expect. 13697625. 25 (5), 2328–2339. Available from: http://onlinelibrary.wiley.com/journal/10.1111/(ISSN)1369-7625. doi:10.1111/hex.13577.

Benson, T., 2023. Why it is hard to use PROMs and PREMs in routine health and care. BMJ Open Qual. 2399-6641. 12 (4), e002516. doi:10.1136/bmjoq-2023-002516.

Berni, A., Borgianni, Y., Basso, D., Carbon, C.C., 2023. Fundamentals and issues of user experience in the process of designing consumer products. Des. Sci. 20534701. 9. Available from: https://www.cambridge.org/core/journals/design-science. doi:10.1017/dsj.2023.8.

Bonilla, P., Elizondo, V., Flanagan, J.P., 2025. Assessing patient satisfaction: the role of net promoter scores in healthcare. 125. https://scholarworks.utrgv.edu/somrs/2025/posters/125.

Bull, C., 2021. Patient satisfaction and patient experience are not interchangeable concepts. Int. J. Qual. Health Care. 1353-4505. 33 (1). doi:10.1093/intqhc/mzab023.

Bulto, L.N., Davies, E., Kelly, J., Hendriks, J.M., 2024. Patient journey mapping: emerging methods for understanding and improving patient experiences of health systems and services. Eur. J. Cardiovasc. Nurs. 18731953. 23 (4), 429–433. Available from: https://academic.oup.com/eurjcn. doi:10.1093/eurjcn/zvae012.

Carter, S.M., Shih, P., Williams, J., Degeling, C., Mooney-Somers, J., 2021. Conducting qualitative research online: challenges and solutions. Patient. 1178-1653. 14 (6), 711–718. doi:10.1007/s40271-021-00528-w.

Davies, E.L., Bulto, L.N., Walsh, A., Pollock, D., Langton, V.M., Laing, R.E., Graham, A., Arnold-Chamney, M., Kelly, J., 2023. Reporting and conducting patient journey mapping research in healthcare: a scoping review. J. Adv. Nurs. 13652648. 79 (1), 83–100. Available from: http://onlinelibrary.wiley.com/journal/10.1111/(ISSN)1365-2648. doi:10.1111/jan.15479.

Diliasari, K., Sulistiadi, W., 2024. Use of net promoter score (NPS) in hospital marketing strategy to increase patient satisfaction and loyalty. Int. J. Soc. Serv. Res. 2807-8691. 4 (03), 907–911. doi:10.46799/ijssr.v4i03.615.

Dominello, A., Cheek, C., Clay-Williams, R., 2025. The use of personas to involve consumers in healthcare co-design: a scoping review. BMC Health Serv. Res. 1472-6963. 25 (1). doi:10.1186/s12913-025-12786-7.

Eldridge, S.M., Lancaster, G.A., Campbell, M.J., Thabane, L., Hopewell, S., Coleman, C.L., Bond, C.M., Lazzeri, C., 2016. Defining feasibility and pilot studies in preparation for randomised controlled trials: development of a conceptual framework. PLOS ONE. 1932-6203. 11 (3), e0150205. doi:10.1371/journal.pone.0150205.

Figma. User journey mapping: what it is + how to do it https://www.figma.com/resource-library/user-journey-map/

Flood, M., Ennis, M., Ludlow, A., Sweeney, F.F., Holton, A., Morgan, S., Clarke, C., Carroll, P., Mellon, L., Boland, F., Mohamed, S., De Brún, A., Hanratty, M., Moriarty, F., 2021. Research methods from human-centered design: potential applications in pharmacy and health services research. Res. Soc. Adm. Pharm. 15517411. 17 (12), 2036–2043. Available from: http://www.journals.elsevierhealth.com/periodicals/rsap. doi:10.1016/j.sapharm.2021.06.015.

Flood, M., Gleeson, L.L., Flynn, S., Ludlow, A., Sweeney, F.F., Holton, A., Carroll, P., Mohamed, S., Moriarty, F., Morgan, S., Ennis, M., Clarke, C., Mellon, L., Boland, F., De Brún, A., Hanratty, M., Kelly, S., 2022. Using methods from human-centered design in health research: an introduction for pharmacy and health services researchers. In: Contemporary Research Methods in Pharmacy and Health Services. Elsevier, Ireland, pp. 103–113. Available from: https://www.sciencedirect.com/book/9780323918886. doi:10.1016/B978-0-323-91888-6.00011-9.

Healthy People 2030. U.S Department of Health and Human Services. Office of Disease Prevention and Health Promotion. https://odphp.health.gov/healthypeople.

Kaneko, C., Suzuki, S., Tanaka, I., Hiruma, H., Okada, H., 2025. Patient experience in community pharmacy services: a scoping review. J. Gen. Fam. Med. 2189–7948. doi:10.1002/jgf2.70040.

Kessler, M.M., Breuch, L.A.K., Stambler, D.M., Campeau, K.L., Riggins, O.J., Feedema, E., Doornink, S.I., Misono, S., 2021. User experience in health & medicine: building methods for patient experience design in multidisciplinary collaborations. J. Tech. Writ. Commun. 15413780. 51 (4), 380–406. Available from: http://jtw.sagepub.com/content/by/year. doi:10.1177/00472816211044498.

Knott, E., Rao, A.H., Summers, K., Teeger, C., 2022. Interviews in the social sciences. Nat. Rev. Methods Primers. 26628449. 2 (1). Available from: https://www.nature.com/nrmp/journal-information. doi:10.1038/s43586-022-00150-6.

Meadows, K., 2021. Cognitive interviewing methodologies. Clin. Nurs. Res. 1054-7738. 30 (4), 375–379. doi:10.1177/10547738211014099.

Murry, L., Gerleman, B., Deng, H., Urmie, J., 2020. Cost-savings and patient experience with a pharmacy-led medicare part D consultation service. Innov. Pharm. 2155-0417. 11 (2), 10. doi:10.24926/iip.v11i2.3191.

Murry, L.T., Al-Khatib, A., Witry, M.J., 2021a. Using journey mapping to understand the patient experience with selecting a medicare part D plan using a pharmacy consultation service. Explor. Res. Clin. Soc. Pharm. 26672766. 1, 100006. doi:10.1016/j.rcsop.2021.100006.

Murry, L.T., Desselle, S.P., 2023. Beyond satisfaction in person-centered pharmacy services. Explor. Res. Clin. Soc. Pharm. 26672766. 12 (100355). doi:10.1016/j.rcsop.2023.100355.

Murry, L.T., Fadare, O.O., Al-Khatib, A., Witry, M.J., 2023a. Integration in mixed-methods studies: existing practices, considerations and recommendations for pharmacy research. Int. J. Pharm. Pract. 20427174. 31 (4), 431–437. Available from: https://academic.oup.com/ijpp. doi:10.1093/ijpp/riad033.

Murry, L.T., Murry, R.C., Deng, H., Viyyuri, B., Gerleman, B.L., Urmie, J., 2021b. Community pharmacy medicare part D consultations: plan-switching decisions and chronic medication adherence. J. Pharm. Pract. 15311937. 34 (5), 727–733. Available from: https://journals.sagepub.com/home/jpp. doi:10.1177/0897190020903852.

Murry, L.T., Viyurri, B., Chapman, C.G., Witry, M.J., Kennelty, K.A., Nayakankuppam, D., Doucette, W.R., Urmie, J., 2023b. Patient preferences and willingness-to-pay for community pharmacy-led Medicare Part D consultation services: a discrete choice experiment. Res. Soc. Adm. Pharm. 15517411. 19 (5), 764–772. Available from: http://www.journals.elsevierhealth.com/periodicals/rsap. doi:10.1016/j.sapharm.2023.01.008.

Murry, L.T., Witry, M.J., Urmie, J.M., 2023c. A qualitative exploration of patient preferences for Medicare Part D consultation services offered in a community pharmacy setting. J. Am. Pharm. Assoc. 15443450. 63 (1), 97. Available from: http://www.japha.org/issues.aspx?journalid=63. doi:10.1016/j.japh.2022.08.020.

Newton, A.S., March, S., Gehring, N.D., Rowe, A.K., Radomski, A.D., 2021. Establishing a working definition of user experience for ehealth interventions of self-reported user experience measures with ehealth researchers and adolescents: scoping review. J. Med. Internet Res. 1438-8871. 23 (12), e25012. doi:10.2196/25012.

Park, E., Kwon, M., 2021. Testing the digital health literacy instrument for adolescents: cognitive interviews. J. Med. Internet Res. 1438-8871. 23 (3), e17856. doi:10.2196/17856.

Roberts, J.P., Fisher, T.R., Trowbridge, M.J., Bent, C., 2016. A design thinking framework for healthcare management and innovation. Healthcare. 22130772. 4 (1), 11–14. Available from: http://www.journals.elsevier.com/healthcare-the-journal-of-delivery-science-and-innovation. doi:10.1016/j.hjdsi.2015.12.002.

Sanders, E.B.N., Stappers, P.J., 2014. Probes, toolkits and prototypes: three approaches to making in codesigning. CoDesign. 17453755. 10 (1), 5–14. doi:10.1080/15710882.2014.888183.

Santhosh, L., Rojas, J.C., Lyons, P.G., 2021. Zooming into focus groups: strategies for qualitative research in the era of social distancing. ATS Scholar. 26907097. 2 (2), 176–184. Available from: https://www.atsjournals.org/doi/full/10.34197/ats-scholar.2020-0127PS. doi:10.34197/ats-scholar.2020-0127PS.

Shafei, I., Karnon, J., Crotty, M., 2024. Process mining and customer journey mapping in healthcare: enhancing patient-centred care in stroke rehabilitation. Digit. Health. 2055-2076. 10. doi:10.1177/20552076241249264.

Stephanie, L., Runacres, F., Poon, P., 2021. Journey mapping as a novel approach to healthcare: a qualitative mixed methods study in palliative care. BMC Health Serv. Res. 1472-6963. 21 (1). doi:10.1186/s12913-021-06934-y.

Stevens, E., 2023. How to design a customer journey map (A step-by-step guide). https://www.uxdesigninstitute.com/blog/design-a-customer-journey-map/

Stickdorn, M., Hormess, L., Schneider, J., 2018. This Is Service Design Doing: Applying Service Design Thinking in the Real World. O'Reilly Media, Inc.

Taherdoost, H., 2021. Data collection methods and tools for research; a step-by-step guide to choose data collection technique for academic and business research projects. Int. J. Acad. Res. Manag. 10 (1), 10–38.

Trebble, T.M., Hansi, N., Hydes, T., Smith, M.A., Baker, M., 2010. Process mapping the patient journey: an introduction. BMJ. 0959-8138. 341 (aug13 1), c4078. doi:10.1136/bmj.c4078.

Valentine, L., Kroll, T., Bruce, F., Lim, C., Mountain, R., 2017. Design thinking for social innovation in health care. Des. J. 1460-6925. 20 (6), 755–774. doi:10.1080/14606925.2017.1372926.

Wolcott, M.D., Lobczowski, N.G., 2021. Using cognitive interviews and think-aloud protocols to understand thought processes. Curr. Pharm. Teach. Learn. 18771300. 13 (2), 181–188. Available from: http://www.elsevier.com/wps/find/journaldescription.cws_home/718643/description#description. doi:10.1016/j.cptl.2020.09.005.

Zomerdijk, L.G., Voss, C.A., 2010. Service design for experience-centric services. J. Serv. Res. 15527379. 13 (1), 67–82. doi:10.1177/1094670509351960.

CHAPTER

21

Health information technology in pharmacy: A concept-mapping approach to evaluation

Ayomide Ogundipe, Tin Fei Sim, and Lynne Emmerton

Curtin School of Diagnostic and Therapeutic Sciences, Curtin University, Perth, WA, Australia

CHAPTER OBJECTIVES

- Explore the principles of concept mapping and describe its relevance to evaluating health information technologies in pharmacy practice
- Apply concept mapping methods to develop a structured evaluation framework for pharmacy-related health technologies
- Discuss the strengths, limitations, and best practices of concept mapping compared to other framework development methods

1 Introduction

1.1 Relevance of evaluating health information technologies in pharmacy practice

Health information communication technology (ICT) has accelerated globally, with the digitization of many aspects of the medication supply chain in recent years (Cheong et al., 2020). In contemporary pharmacy practice, ICT can be described as the platforms, software, computer networks, and communication devices available to pharmacists (Ogundipe et al., 2023a). Initiatives planned for the upcoming decade were implemented "almost overnight" following the emergence of the COVID-19 pandemic (Cheong et al., 2020). The Australian healthcare system has experienced a paradigm shift to real-time interconnectivity for practitioners and consumers alike (Connecting the dots: Digitally empowered pharmacists, 2019) through the introduction and widespread utilization of electronic prescribing and dispensing,[a] (Connecting the dots: Digitally empowered pharmacists, 2019) real-time prescription monitoring (Connecting the dots: Digitally empowered pharmacists, 2019), the *My Health Record*,[b] (Initiatives and Programs, 2022) telehealth (Initiatives and Programs, 2022), secure messaging (Initiatives and Programs, 2022) and the Clinician Vaccine Integrated Platform (2022).

[a] Australia's first prescription exchange service.
[b] Opt-in personally controlled electronic health records.

Contemporary Research Methods in Pharmacy and Health Services - Volume 2
https://doi.org/10.1016/B978-0-443-44607-8.00017-0

Despite the development of interoperable health ICT systems in developed countries, there is a lack of qualitative assessment of their benefits to current practice (Christopoulou et al., 2018; Bélanger et al., 2012; Fernald et al., 2017; Sockolow et al., 2016). Pharmacists may benefit from the interoperability of technology platforms for use within the pharmacy sector and to work collaboratively with other healthcare providers (Ogundipe et al., 2023b). Modeling pharmacist interactions with health ICT to undertake clinical decision-making and professional services can identify how ICT should evolve to meet the needs of pharmacists in existing and emerging roles (Ogundipe et al., 2023b). Identified barriers and facilitators for ICT adoption in pharmacy practice include pharmacist confidence and competence, workplace design and workflow, and internal and external regulatory requirements (Luetsch, 2017); these factors are likely relevant to the further adoption of health ICT.

Evaluation of health ICT may support the integration of new and existing technologies into contemporary pharmacy practice (Ogundipe et al., 2023a). Additionally, it can enhance the integration of new technologies into practice during the design and implementation of the technology. This allows researchers to examine predictors of success throughout the lifecycle of new or existing technology, future-proofing the rapidly evolving technology landscape (Ogundipe et al., 2023a, 2023b). Despite these advancements, no evaluation framework has been published or recommended for contemporary pharmacy practice (Ogundipe et al., 2023a).

1.2 Concept mapping as a methodological approach: Why concept mapping is useful

Concept mapping emerged over 30 years ago as a mixed-methods (qualitative and quantitative) approach to inquiry, enabling groups of people to conceptualize their thinking about a specific topic (McLinden, 2017). This methodology, with origins in the planning and evaluation of projects, has since been applied to a multitude of sectors, including not-for-profit, corporate, and government entities (McLinden, 2017). Contemporary healthcare is facing an array of challenges, including the assessment of quality of care and life, the planning and evaluation of services, and the effective utilization of new and evolving technologies (Trochim and Kane, 2005). To address these tasks, it is imperative that a variety of disciplines collaborate in a coordinated manner at all levels of the health system, including government and policy, health administrators, health professionals, and the public (Trochim and Kane, 2005). Concept mapping can be used to address these issues, as it generates ideas in an open brainstorming session that participants then rate independently. Like the Delphi technique, it combines collective data generation with subsequent independent rating rounds to refine and prioritize inputs, though concept mapping adds a visual structuring component that represents relationships among ideas.

Moreover, concept mapping is participatory in nature and, therefore, well-suited for research in which the engagement of a group of people is required to explore meaning and design solutions for complex issues (McLinden, 2017). Concept mapping has several key characteristics relevant to addressing problems in contemporary healthcare: it is intentionally designed to integrate input from multiple sources with varying expertise or interests; it creates a series of maps that visually demonstrate the composite thinking of a group; and the maps provide a framework that can immediately be leveraged to guide activities such as action planning, program development, and evaluation (Trochim and Kane, 2005).

2 Methodology overview

2.1 Principles of concept mapping

Structured conceptualization, colloquially known as concept mapping, refers to any process that can be described as a sequence of operationally-defined steps and yields a conceptual representation (Trochim, 1989). The term "concept mapping" refers to any methodology that is used to develop a picture or map of the ideas or concepts of an individual or group (Trochim and Kane, 2005). Concept mapping can be used by groups to create a conceptual framework to guide planning or evaluation (Trochim, 1989). There are several analogous approaches to concept mapping: "idea mapping", "mind maps", "causal mapping", or "cognitive mapping". These are distinctly different from concept mapping in that they were designed for use by individuals as a mechanism to enhance a person's creative thinking about a problem or improve the organization of thought (Trochim and Kane, 2005). In this chapter, the term "concept mapping" refers only to the structured group conceptualization, a mixed-methods participatory group idea mapping methodology that integrates processes such as brainstorming, unstructured sorting, and multivariate statistical methods of multidimensional scaling and hierarchical cluster analysis (Trochim and Kane, 2005).

2.2 Heuristic classification of concept maps

Nabitz et al. (2017) identified the following types of concept mapping approaches (Nabitz et al., 2017):

"Type A: Theory and model building—a concept map constructed to contribute to clarifying and improving a theory or model

Type B: Policy and management—a concept mapping approach used to structure questions and topics for policy making and organizational development

Type C: Planning and evaluation—a concept mapping approach to clarify goals for a project and specify evaluation criteria

Type D: Quality—a concept map developed to clarify, cluster, and prioritize quality criteria or quality improvement projects

Type E: Research—a concept mapping approach applied to design a classification system or operationalize dimensions of a complex concept."

2.3 Steps in concept mapping

Typically, concept mapping encompasses seven steps:

1. *Preparation* (Trochim, 1989)

Identify the purpose of the mapping, select participants, and develop a clear focus for conceptualization to ensure relevance and clarity.

2. *Generation of statements* (Trochim, 1989)

Collect a comprehensive set of ideas or statements, usually, though not necessarily, achieved through some form of brainstorming, either in person or online (Trochim and Kane, 2005).

3. *Structuring of statements* (Trochim, 1989) *(or organization phase)*

Concept mapping analysis encompasses the organization and representation phases. Participants sort and rate generated ideas for one or more variables of interest, e.g., relative importance and feasibility (Trochim and Kane, 2005). This step is decidedly judgmental and qualitative (Trochim and Kane, 2005). These sorts are converted into similarity matrices, which provide the basis for multivariate analyses such as multidimensional scaling and hierarchical cluster analysis (Trochim and Kane, 2005). The resulting maps show relationships among statements, and clusters are named and refined by participants. Ratings, if collected, can be overlaid to identify patterns and support planning or evaluation (Trochim and Kane, 2005).

4. *Representation of statements in the form of a concept map* (Trochim, 1989)

Data from sorting and rating are analyzed, usually but not always, through a sequence of multivariate statistical analyses to create visual maps that display the relationships among ideas in two dimensions for ease of interpretation (Trochim and Kane, 2005). Cross-links illustrate connections between domains in a concept map, helping to demonstrate how knowledge from one domain relates to another (Novak and Cañas, 2006).

5. *Interpretation of maps* (Trochim, 1989)

Participants review and discuss the resulting maps to identify themes, validate clusters, and ensure outputs align with project goals (Trochim and Kane, 2005).

6. *The utilization of maps* (Trochim, 1989)

The maps and findings are applied to support decision-making, communicate insights, or guide planning and evaluation efforts (Trochim and Kane, 2005).

7. *Continuous review*

Continuously review and update the concept map to reflect progress and adapt to environmental or circumstantial changes.

2.4 Validity and reliability

Traditional concepts of external and internal validity are difficult to operationalize in concept mapping and are often overlooked (Rosas and Kane, 2012). External representational validity—the extent to which a conceptualized model mirrors the reality it is designed to represent—and internal representational validity—the degree to which the conceptualized model reflects the judgments made by participants in organizing information to produce the model—have been proposed as approaches to determine validity (Rosas and Kane, 2012).

The consistency of participant input can be assessed using sorting and rating data by computing conventional item and rater reliability estimates (Rosas and Kane, 2012). However, this analysis was not conducted in the present study and, therefore, the reliability of the data could not be formally established. Traditionally, reliability assessments focus on the repeatability of test items or overall scores based on a known or assumed correct response (Rosas and Kane, 2012). However, concept mapping data differs in that there is no single correct answer; instead, sorting reliability focuses on evaluating the extent to which the structural arrangement of items, both individually and collectively, is consistent with expected or typical patterns (Rosas and Kane, 2012).

3 Case example: Development of an evaluation framework for health information communication technology in contemporary pharmacy practice using concept mapping

3.1 Context and objectives

This section describes an evaluation framework designed using a concept mapping approach for health ICT in contemporary pharmacy practice. The rationale for this model was informed by a systematic scoping review of evaluation frameworks for health ICT in health informatics literature, which confirmed the absence of literature exploring pharmacists' health ICT needs in contemporary pharmacy practice (Ogundipe et al., 2023a). Considering the unique practice environment of pharmacists, there is justification for the development of an evaluation framework specifically addressing the ICT needs of pharmacists and their practice environment. The approach was intentionally iterative, drawing on and adapting existing evaluation frameworks to provide a preliminary framework that could be refined and validated through future research.

3.2 Theoretical background

A systematic scoping review (Ogundipe et al., 2023a) informing the present work concluded that domains from the Technology Acceptance Model (TAM) (Venkatesh and Davis, 2000), Information System Success (DeLone and McLean, 2004) (ISS) model, and Human, Organization, Technology Fit (Yusof et al., 2008) (HOT-fit) model could be adapted to create an evaluation framework for health ICT in contemporary pharmacy practice, including pharmacist prescribing (Ogundipe et al., 2023a). While none of these evaluation frameworks had been applied to pharmacy, scope existed to broaden their application and tailor these frameworks to meet the requirements of pharmacy practice. The TAM, ISS, and HOT-fit collectively address user and organizational domains that may impact health ICT usability. However, these models are limited in their ability to describe the impact of health ICT on service provision and organizational outcomes in contemporary pharmacy practice. These component models, and their proposed contribution to a pharmacy-specific model, are summarized below (Table 21.1).

While several frameworks exist to evaluate user acceptance and system success—TAM, ISS, and HOT-fit—the focus of this chapter is on concept mapping rather than theoretical models. For this project, the qualitative data were derived from the research team, who generated, sorted, and rated statements related to the focus topic to form the basis for the concept maps and subsequent analysis.

3.3 Study design and concept mapping process

The proposed evaluation framework was developed following a critical appraisal of the TAM, ISS, and HOT-fit models, in addition to concept mapping (Jankowska, 2014) of the evaluation frameworks. Concept mapping was adopted as a means to "organize and represent knowledge in the form of a diagram which shows the relationships between concepts" (Jankowska, 2014). As the aim of the study was the development of a proposed framework rather than statistical generalization, an iterative, qualitative, consensus-based adaptation of concept mapping was used. No individual ratings, similarity matrices, or multivariate analyses were conducted. Participants were members of the research team.

3.3.1 *Step-by-step procedure*

1. Preparation—the mapping focus was defined, and the research team was convened as participants.
2. Generation of statements—candidate statements and key concepts were compiled by the research team, drawing on the TAM, ISS, and HOT-fit models, as well as other literature through discussion and document review (Table 21.1).
3. Structuring statements (sorting/grouping)—instead of collecting individual sorts and ratings, statements were iteratively grouped by the research team into thematically similar domains (Fig. 21.1).

TABLE 21.1 Summary of the TAM, ISS, and HOT-fit models.

Evaluation framework	Theoretical basis	Evaluation factors
Technology Acceptance Model (Venkatesh and Davis, 2000) (TAM)	Developed from the theory of reasoned action (TRA) (Ketikidis et al., 2012), the TRA proposes that users are rational decision-makers who *"consciously choose their course of action based on an analysis of potential costs and benefits attached to each of various behavior alternatives"* (Ketikidis et al., 2012).	• Perceived usefulness (Venkatesh and Davis, 2000) • Perceived ease of use (Venkatesh and Davis, 2000) • Behavioral intention (Venkatesh and Davis, 2000) • Use behavior (Venkatesh and Davis, 2000)
Technology Acceptance Model 2 (Venkatesh and Davis, 2000) (TAM2)	Incorporates additional theoretical constructs across social influence processes and cognitive instrumental processes (Venkatesh and Davis, 2000).	• Factors listed in TAM • Behavioral intention expanded to include voluntariness and experience (Venkatesh and Davis, 2000) • Perceived usefulness expanded to include subjective norm, which consists of image, job relevance, output quality, and result demonstrability (Venkatesh and Davis, 2000)
Technology Acceptance Model 3 (Venkatesh and Bala, 2008) (TAM3)	Incorporates determinants previously captured in TAM2, highlighting factors related to perceived ease of use and perceived usefulness (Venkatesh and Bala, 2008).	• Factors listed in the TAM and TAM2 • Perceived ease of use expanded to anchor and adjustment (Venkatesh and Bala, 2008) • Anchor further expanded to computer self-efficacy and perceptions of external control (Venkatesh and Bala, 2008) • Computer anxiety and computer playfuln ess (Venkatesh and Bala, 2008) • Adjustment further expanded to include perceived enjoyment and objective usability (Venkatesh and Bala, 2008)
Information Systems Success (DeLone and McLean, 2004) (ISS) model	Developed to provide a comprehensive evaluation of the performance of information systems in e-commerce (DeLone and McLean, 2004).	• System quality (DeLone and McLean, 2004) • Information quality (DeLone and McLean, 2004) • Service quality (DeLone and McLean, 2004) • Use (DeLone and McLean, 2004) • User satisfaction (DeLone and McLean, 2004) • Net Benefits (DeLone and McLean, 2004)
Human, Organization, and Technology Fit (Yusof et al., 2008) (HOT-fit) model	Developed from the Information System Success Model and the IT-Organization Fit Model (Yusof et al., 2008)	Human • System use (Yusof et al., 2008) • User satisfaction (Yusof et al., 2008) Organization • Structure (Yusof et al., 2008) • Environment (Yusof et al., 2008) Technology • System quality (Yusof et al., 2008) • Information quality (Yusof et al., 2008) • Service quality (Yusof et al., 2008) • Net benefits (Yusof et al., 2008)

From Ogundipe, A., Sim, T.F., Emmerton, L., 2023. Development of an evaluation framework for health information communication technology in contemporary pharmacy practice. Explor. Res. Clin. Soc. Pharm. 9, 100252. doi:10.1016/j.rcsop.2023.100252.

4. Representation—the evaluation frameworks were mapped manually according to their domains, and "cross-links" (Novak and Cañas, 2006) were used to demonstrate the relationships between domains.
5. Interpretation and consensus—differences in views were discussed until consensus was reached on the placement of domains and cross-links. Consensus was achieved qualitatively through discussion; no quantitative analysis was performed (Fig. 21.2).
6. Utilization—the final map served as the basis for the proposed evaluation framework.
7. Continuous review—the concept map was treated as a living resource, updated iteratively as the framework evolved. The research team considered the construct and face validity of the concept map, evaluating each domain and how they were interlinked, ensuring that the final concept map represented the initial intent of an evaluation framework for health ICT in contemporary pharmacy practice (Fig. 21.3).

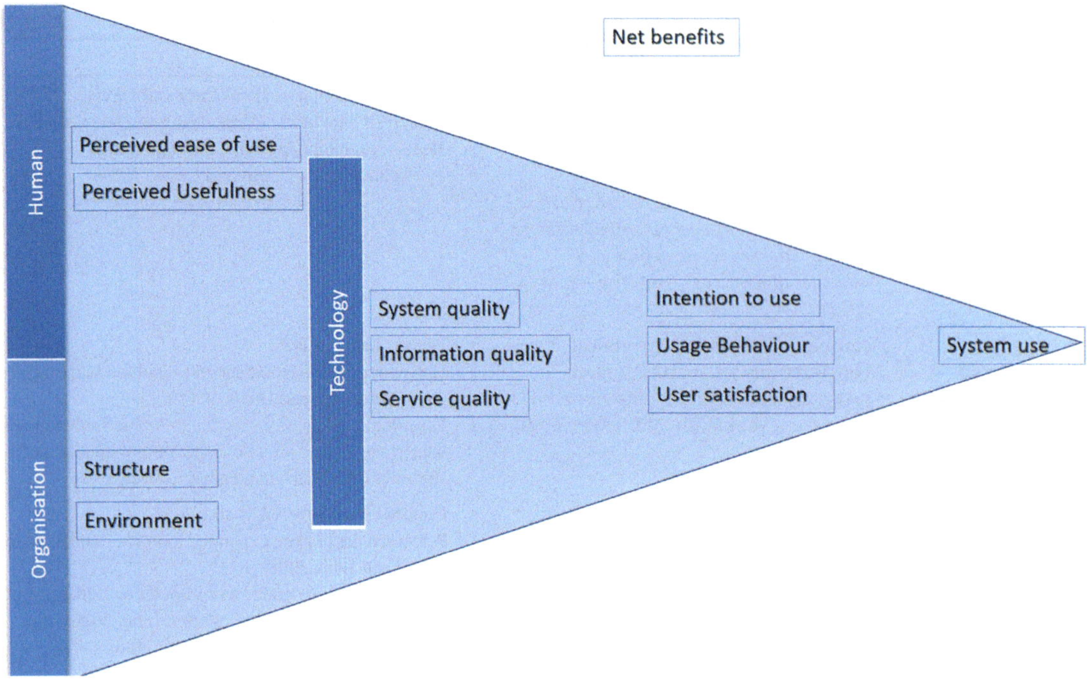

FIG. 21.1 Initial iteration of concept map.

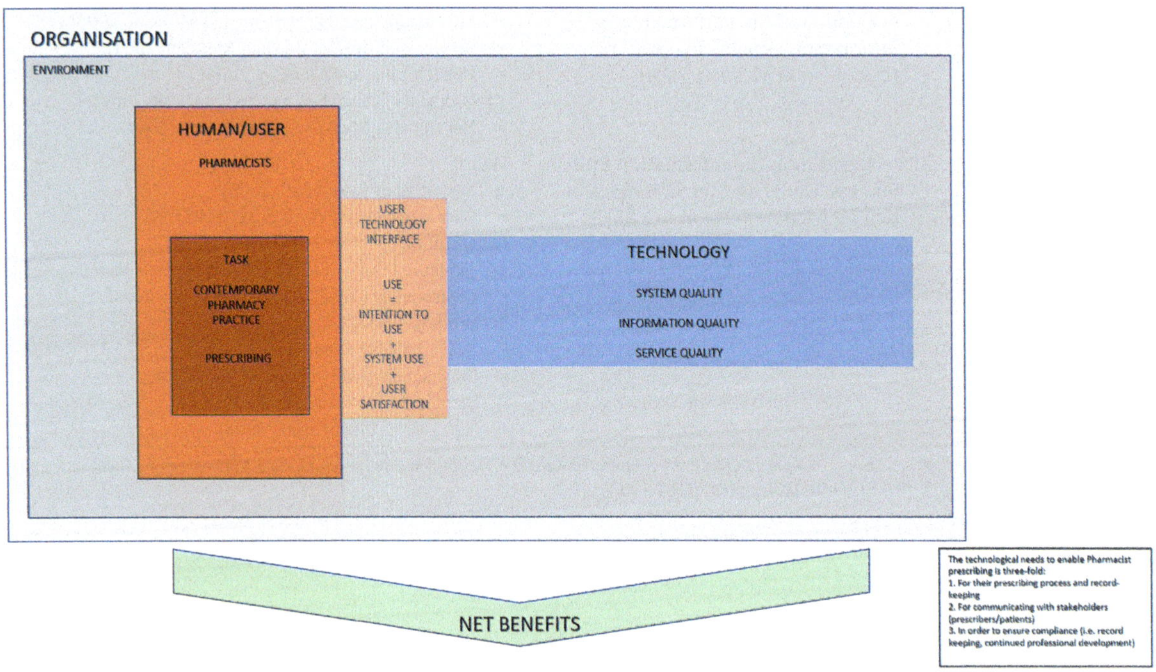

FIG. 21.2 Second iteration of the concept map.

3.4 Framework development

The design of an evaluation framework for health ICT in contemporary pharmacy practice must address the dynamic interactions of the environment, task, user, and tool (Shackel, 2009). The resulting model, named the Technology Evaluation Key (TEK) (Fig. 21.3), addresses this by illustrating how pharmacists' use of ICT is influenced by the overall healthcare system, the organization in which they practice, and the health ICT enabling their services or clinical decision-making.

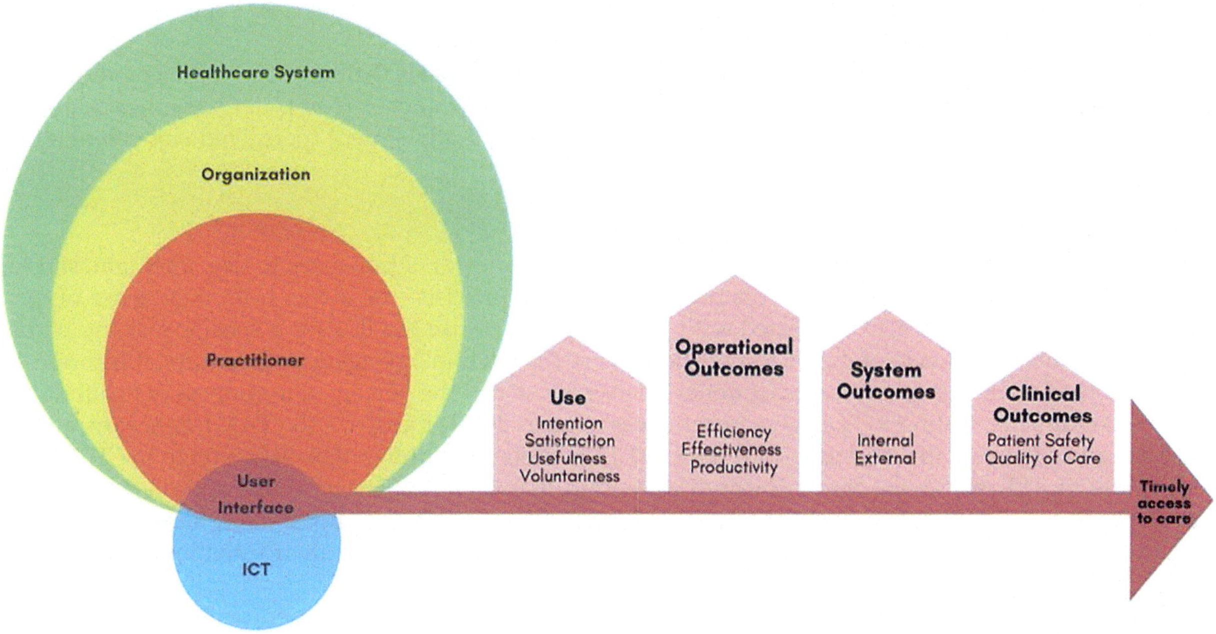

FIG. 21.3 Proposed technology evaluation key (TEK). *From Ogundipe, A., Sim, T.F., Emmerton, L., 2023. Development of an evaluation framework for health information communication technology in contemporary pharmacy practice. Explor. Res. Clin. Soc. Pharm. 9, 100252. doi:10.1016/j.rcsop.2023.100252.*

These describe the "system" in which the pharmacist uses a specific health ICT. The second feature of the TEK is the additional components drawn from the TAM, ISS, and HOT-fit models to describe the "outputs" of a positive user experience with the specific health ICT. Each component of the TEK is described below. It should be noted that this illustration does not imply the relative contribution of each construct or the strength of associations between constructs. Indeed, the measurement of each construct may identify how the visual representation could be simplified.

ICT encompasses system quality, information quality, and service quality from the ISS and HOT-fit models. The information, system quality, and additional support for pharmacists can create different service quality outcomes. Therefore, these factors influence how ICT operates in practice. It is anticipated that ICT evaluation may occur through the various domains of the TEK framework to identify factors that can improve ICT adoption and usability by practitioners.

The overarching healthcare ecosystem in which pharmacists operate allows pharmacists in Australia to access patient information through electronic health records, real-time prescription monitoring, the Clinician Vaccine Integrated Platform, and secure messaging (Shackel, 2009). While these specific systems may vary internationally, pharmacists in other countries often have access to analogous digital tools to support patient care, such as shared health records, immunization registries, and electronic communication platforms. Pharmacists should utilize this information in accordance with the corresponding legal and ethical frameworks governing data privacy and security. In the proposed TEK framework, the healthcare system domain was adapted from the environment, as previously seen in the HOT-fit evaluation framework. This domain may help capture the importance of integration and alignment of ICT used throughout the healthcare system to better support pharmacists. In addition, legislative updates, training for consumers and clinicians, as well as promotional advocacy or policy to encourage the adoption of updated or newly introduced ICT, may be part of the measures used to evaluate policy implementation of ICT in the healthcare system.

As previously stated, the evaluation of health ICT may consider the organization in which it is used and its goals in using health ICT in practice. This domain was adapted from the HOT-fit framework. In the TEK framework, the organization acknowledges different contexts in which pharmacists work within the healthcare system and, hence, the impact of organizational culture, access to technology, and services provided within the context of that organization. This domain was considered to encompass the subjective norm from the TAM2 model. Additionally, the organization's readiness to implement and adopt the ICT, its training and professional development of staff, as well as its organizational policies and procedures for ICT use in practice, may constitute part of the evaluation process.

Whilst numerous studies exist on health ICT usability (Ogundipe et al., 2023a; Yen and Bakken, 2012; Ammenwerth, Iller and Mahler, 2006; Shaw, 2002; Jacob et al., 2020; Garavand et al., 2016), none are available in the context of pharmacy practice (Ogundipe et al., 2023a). The lack of evaluation at the interface between pharmacists and technology results in an inability to measure the impact of health ICT on workflow, user experience, and outcomes for professional tasks and services in a fast-evolving practice landscape.

Practitioner in the TEK is an adaptation of the human domain in the HOT-fit model. At the convergence of the practitioner and their ICT is the user interface, which encompasses the anchor (computer self-efficacy, perceptions of external control, computer anxiety, and computer playfulness) and adjustment (perceived enjoyment and objective usability) domains from the TAM3 model.

3.4.1 *Use*

A combination of domains from the TAM, ISS, and HOT-fit frameworks translates to use, intention, satisfaction, usefulness, and voluntariness in the TEK. It is proposed that pharmacists' use stems from their sense of the ICT's relevance to their tasks. Use is also associated with their intention to use the ICT for a specific task, based on their experiences, and directly influences their voluntariness to use that technology again in the future. It is proposed that user satisfaction may negatively affect a practitioner's sense of use and the perceived usefulness of health ICT. There are semantic arguments relating to "perceived usefulness" versus "usefulness" (in the TAM); hence the adaptation.

User satisfaction, in both the ISS model and the HOT-fit model, is simplified to satisfaction in the TEK. The hierarchical nature of TEK places the user (practitioner) within the context of their organization and the healthcare system. Experience (TAM2), intention (TAM), and voluntariness (TAM2) encompass the pharmacists' experience with health ICT, training, or continued professional development and influence their intention and voluntariness to utilize the technology for the task at hand.

Importantly, the domains within TEK were derived from established frameworks and market research, providing a strong theoretical foundation that enhances the rigor and enduring relevance of the model, even in a rapidly evolving practice environment. While the content, scope, and depth within each domain may change as practice advances, the domains themselves are likely to remain relevant. As these domains evolve, it will be necessary to return to Step 7 (continuous review) to revisit and refine the concept map, ensuring that the framework reflects current priorities and maintains its usefulness.

It is proposed that the unification of the above factors leads to net benefits, as previously illustrated in the ISS and HOT-fit models but re-envisioned as an output of user experience with technology in practice. The practitioner's user experience may influence their overall use, encompassing intention, satisfaction, usefulness, and voluntariness. The follow-on effects of practitioner use are operational outcomes (efficiency, effectiveness, productivity), system outcomes (internal, external), and clinical outcomes (patient safety, quality of care). These domains each highlight areas for both potential benefit and hindrance of health ICT use in practice, encompassing system and patient-related outcomes.

3.4.2 *Operational outcomes, system outcomes, clinical outcomes, and timely access to care*

Operational outcomes, derived from service quality and net benefits (ISS and HOT-fit), represent the overall impact of the use of ICT in practice. System outcomes, derived from system quality in the ISS and HOT-fit models, represent the measurable outcomes of ICT use in practice. While both domains were adapted from existing models, they are bespoke to the TEK framework as they demonstrate that these are measurable outcomes. Furthermore, they signal an end outcome that can satisfy stakeholders, i.e., policymakers and developers, by evaluating health ICT as a priority in ensuring a range of outputs and patient safety. Operational, clinical, and system outcomes are intertwined and must be considered concurrently during implementation.

Operational and system outcomes potentially address the lack of measurable outcomes from existing evaluation frameworks in relation to ICT adoption. From an operational standpoint, organizations should consider the need to update and maintain hardware and software, implement changes to workflows and operational layouts, as well as establish formalized procedures and policies to ensure regular maintenance and updates of systems. As a follow-on effect of ICT use in practice, clinical outcomes and timely access to care are proposed as additional patient-centric outcomes to be further explored during validation and stakeholder consultation. It is anticipated that effective ICT use by practitioners may have a positive impact on clinical outcomes for patients, improving patient experience and, therefore, timely access to care.

4 Applying concept mapping in pharmacy practice

> One thing a person cannot do, no matter how rigorous their analysis or heroic their imagination, is to draw up a list of things that would never occur to him.
>
> ***—Thomas Schelling, Economist and Nobel Laureate.***

Where concept mapping could be advantageous is in presenting the collective wisdom of a crowd, namely by encompassing diverse viewpoints, ensuring the independence of each view from the influence of others, and serving as a mechanism for aggregating many individual viewpoints into a collective (McLinden, 2017).

Concept mapping could be a useful approach to increase community participation or involvement in research, especially in circumstances where practice is fast-evolving and the buy-in of personnel involved becomes critical (Windsor, 2013). Windsor (2013) utilized concept mapping to develop culturally tailored and community-based health interventions for priority populations by examining the social dynamics and consequences of alcohol and substance use with 75 individual participants in Newark, New Jersey (Windsor, 2013). This example demonstrates the utility of concept mapping as a methodology to meaningfully engage consumers in community-based participatory research, leveraging the collaborative approach of concept mapping with scientific inquiry to develop capacity-building strategies that meet consumer needs (Windsor, 2013). Rising et al. (2019) utilized concept mapping to identify factors that contribute to consumer emergency department use and, as such, were able to identify several factors, including uncertainty about consequences, primary care options, and psychological concerns (Rising et al., 2019). These example studies used concept mapping alongside observational study designs and codesign, with concept mapping providing structure and clarity to the concepts, while observational data and codesigned approaches enriched the findings and ensured practical relevance.

Concept mapping offers several benefits for pharmacy practice and research. It allows input from diverse stakeholders—such as policymakers, pharmacists, technicians, and other health professionals—bringing together different areas of expertise and perspectives (Scahill, 2015). Through structured brainstorming and, where relevant, multivariate analysis, the process can systematically support the capture and organization of concepts and ideas relevant to pharmacy (Scahill, 2015). The resulting maps and visuals provide clear, impactful representations that can enhance understanding during meetings and discussions (Scahill, 2015). Most importantly, concept mapping supports action and planning, helping pharmacy teams move initiatives forward effectively (Scahill, 2015).

4.1 Strengths and limitations of the method

While concept mapping has great utility in the conceptualization and planning of interventions, its utility in evaluation remains largely untapped (Trochim, 2017). This limitation is partly due to the reliance on specialized software to conduct analysis, which is only one step of the concept mapping methodology (Trochim, 2017). The more challenging step is the process of data collection, specifically sorting the data, as it requires participants to make subjective judgments about how ideas relate to each other, ensure consistency across different perspectives, and capture complex concepts in a structured way (Trochim, 2017). Although concept mapping is mixed-methods in approach, it can be time-intensive for both researchers and participants, so this should be communicated upfront. The quality of the focus statements is crucial, as these should be grounded in the literature and research questions, be clear, specific, and framed in positive or neutral language, with only one idea per statement (Scahill, 2015). Careful wording is especially important because statements are rated relative to one another (Scahill, 2015). Finally, successful facilitation requires the facilitator to apply group leadership skills and have training in the relevant software.

5 Conclusion

This chapter has described concept mapping as a research method, using a case example involving the design of an initial evaluation framework for health information and communication technologies in pharmacy practice. By combining evidence from a systematic scoping review with structured stakeholder input, the framework highlights the distinct needs of pharmacists and the environments in which they work. The iterative design reflects its status as a preliminary model, adapted from existing validated frameworks to provide a foundation for further testing and refinement. Concept mapping has proven valuable for integrating diverse perspectives, generating visual outputs, and guiding action, but attention to validity, participant engagement, and methodological rigor remains essential. Future work should look to apply concept mapping methodology in varied practice settings, incorporating the full process—including quantitative steps—to strengthen its evidence base. In doing so, pharmacy practice and research can more effectively assess and optimize the use of health ICT, as well as broader professional, organizational, and policy innovations that collectively support patient care, safety, and sustainable practice development.

6 Questions for further discussion

- How does concept mapping compare to other evaluation methods used in pharmacy practice research?
- What are the key challenges in adapting existing health ICT evaluation frameworks to pharmacy settings?
- How might online tools or digital platforms improve the efficiency and scalability of concept mapping?
- What factors influence the validity and reliability of concept-mapping outcomes in practice?

7 Application scenario

Scenario:
A community pharmacy is preparing to implement a new electronic medication management system to improve workflow, patient safety, and staff communication. The pharmacy management team wishes to evaluate the system's impact using a structured participatory approach.
Exercise:
1. Stakeholder identification

- List the key groups that should be invited to participate in the concept mapping exercise
- For each group, briefly describe the perspective or expertise they bring, and explain how their inclusion strengthens the validity of the findings

2. Focus statement development

- Draft 3–5 focus statements to guide brainstorming about the new system. Consider how existing literature can be used to inform or justify the focus statements

Ensure statements are:

- Clear and easy to understand
- Grounded in outcomes or experiences relevant to evaluation
- Positively or neutrally phrased

3. Process design

Outline how you would:

- Collect ideas from stakeholders (e.g., workshops, surveys)
- Organize and sort ideas into clusters or themes
- Develop rating criteria (e.g., importance, feasibility, impact)
- Summarize how these steps contribute to building a preliminary evaluation framework

4. Application, reflection, and reporting
Discuss how the resulting concept map could be used by the pharmacy team to:

- Inform implementation decisions
- Identify areas for system improvement
- Support ongoing evaluation and adaptation

Reflect on the methodological strengths and limitations of concept mapping in this setting.
If preparing to report the study in a scholarly outlet, consider the following:

- Describing the process in a step-by-step manner so readers can follow the method clearly
- Providing sufficient details for the work to be replicable
- Making explicit any assumptions, adaptations, or additional steps taken to establish validity and reliability is essential

References

Connecting the dots: digitally empowered pharmacists, 2019. Available from: https://www.psa.org.au/wp-content/uploads/2019/07/Connecting-the-dots-Digitally-Empowered-Pharmacists.pdf.
Ammenwerth, E., Iller, C., Mahler, C., 2006. IT-adoption and the interaction of task, technology and individuals: a fit framework and a case study. BMC Med. Inform. Decis. Mak. 1472-6947. 6 (1). doi:10.1186/1472-6947-6-3.

Bélanger, E., Bartlett, G., Dawes, M., Rodríguez, C., Hasson-Gidoni, I., 2012. Examining the evidence of the impact of health information technology in primary care: an argument for participatory research with health professionals and patients. Int. J. Med. Inform. 1386-5056. 81 (10), 654–661. doi:10.1016/j.ijmedinf.2012.07.008.

Cheong, M.W.L., Brock, T., Karwa, R., Pastakia, S.D., 2020. COVID-19 and clinical pharmacy worldwide—a wake up call and a call to action. JACCP. 2574-9870. 3 (5), 860–863. Available from: https://onlinelibrary.wiley.com/journal/25749870. doi:10.1002/jac5.1286.

Christopoulou, S., Kotsilieris, T., Anagnostopoulos, I., 2018. Assessment of health information technology interventions in evidence-based medicine: a systematic review by adopting a methodological evaluation framework. Healthcare. 2227-9032. 6 (3), 109. doi:10.3390/healthcare6030109.

Clinician vaccine integrated platform, 2022. Available from: https://www.digitalhealth.gov.au/healthcare-providers/cvip.

DeLone, W.H., McLean, E.R., 2004. Measuring e-commerce success: applying the DeLone and McLean information systems success model. Int. J. Electron. Commer. 1086-4415. 9 (1), 31–47. Available from: http://www.tandfonline.com/toc/mjec20/current. doi:10.1080/10864415.2004.11044317.

Fernald, D., Wearner, R., Dickinson, W.P., 2017. Supporting primary care practices in building capacity to use health information data. EGEMS. 2327-9214. 2 (3), 4. doi:10.13063/2327-9214.1094.

Garavand, A., Mohseni, M., Asadi, H., Etemadi, M., Moradi-Joo, M., Moosavi, A., 2016. Factors influencing the adoption of health information technologies: a systematic review. Electron. Physician. 2008-5842. 8 (8), 2713–2718. doi:10.19082/2713.

Initiatives and programs, 2022. Available from: https://www.digitalhealth.gov.au/healthcare-providers/initiatives-and-programs.

Jacob, C., Sanchez-Vazquez, A., Ivory, C., 2020. Understanding clinicians' adoption of mobile health tools: a qualitative review of the most used frameworks. JMIR mHealth uHealth. 2291-5222. 8 (7), e18072. doi:10.2196/18072.

Jankowska, M., 2014. Concept Mapping: A Tool of Multiple Purposes in Research. SAGE Publications, Ltd. doi:10.4135/978144627305013514688.

Ketikidis, P., Dimitrovski, T., Lazuras, L., Bath, P.A., 2012. Acceptance of health information technology in health professionals: an application of the revised technology acceptance model. Health Inform. J. 1460-4582. 18 (2), 124–134. doi:10.1177/1460458211435425.

Luetsch, K., 2017. Attitudes and attributes of pharmacists in relation to practice change—a scoping review and discussion. Res. Soc. Adm. Pharm. 1551-7411. 13 (3), 440. doi:10.1016/j.sapharm.2016.06.010.

McLinden, D., 2017. And then the internet happened: thoughts on the future of concept mapping. Eval. Program Plann. 0149-7189. 60, 293–300. doi:10.1016/j.evalprogplan.2016.10.009.

Nabitz, U., van Randeraad-van der Zee, C., Kok, I., van Bon-martens, M., Serverens, P., 2017. An overview of concept mapping in Dutch mental health care. Eval. Program Plann. 0149-7189. 60, 202–212. doi:10.1016/j.evalprogplan.2016.08.012.

Novak, J., Cañas, A., 2006. The theory underlying concept maps and how to construct them. Technical Report IHMC CmapTools. http://cmap.ihmc.us/Publications/ ResearchPapers/TheoryUnderlyingConceptMaps.pdf.

Ogundipe, A., Sim, T.F., Emmerton, L., 2023a. Health information communication technology evaluation frameworks for pharmacist prescribing: a systematic scoping review. Res. Soc. Adm. Pharm. 1551-7411. 19 (2), 218–234. Available from: http://www.journals.elsevierhealth.com/periodicals/rsap. doi:10.1016/j.sapharm.2022.09.010.

Ogundipe, A., Sim, T.F., Emmerton, L., 2023b. The case to improve technologies for pharmacists' prescribing. Int. J. Pharm. Pract. 0961-7671. 31 (1), 113–115. doi:10.1093/ijpp/riac075.

Rising, K.L., Doyle, S.K., Powell, R.E., Doty, A.M.B., LaNoue, M., Gerolamo, A.M., 2019. Use of group concept mapping to identify patient domains of uncertainty that contribute to emergency department use. J. Emerg. Nurs. 0099-1767. 45 (1), 46–53. doi:10.1016/j.jen.2018.05.015.

Rosas, S.R., Kane, M., 2012. Quality and rigor of the concept mapping methodology: a pooled study analysis. Eval. Program Plann. 0149-7189. 35 (2), 236–245. doi:10.1016/j.evalprogplan.2011.10.003.

Scahill, S.L., 2015. Concept mapping and pattern matching in pharmacy practice research. In: Pharmacy Practice Research Methods. Springer International Publishing, New Zealand, pp. 175–195. doi:10.1007/978-3-319-14672-0_10.

Shackel, B., 2009. Usability—context, framework, definition, design and evaluation. Interact. Comput. 0953-5438. 21 (5–6), 339–346. doi:10.1016/j.intcom.2009.04.007.

Shaw, N.T., 2002. 'CHEATS': a generic information communication technology (ICT) evaluation framework. Comput. Biol. Med. 0010-4825. 32 (3), 209–220. Available from: www.elsevier.com/locate/compbiomed. doi:10.1016/S0010-4825(02)00016-1.

Sockolow, P., Dowding, D., Randell, R., Favela, J., 2016. Using mixed methods in health information technology evaluation. In: Studies in Health Technology and Informatics, vol. 225. IOS Press, United States, pp. 83–87. 18798365. Available from: http://www.iospress.nl/bookserie/studies-in-health-technology-and-informatics/. doi:10.3233/978-1-61499-658-3-83.

Trochim, W., Kane, M., 2005. Concept mapping: an introduction to structured conceptualization in health care. Int. J. Qual. Health Care. 1464-3677. 17 (3), 187–191. doi:10.1093/intqhc/mzi038.

Trochim, W.M., 2017. Hindsight is 20/20: reflections on the evolution of concept mapping. Eval. Program Plann. 01497189. 60, 176–185. Available from: www.elsevier.com/inca/publications/store/5/9/3/. doi:10.1016/j.evalprogplan.2016.08.009.

Trochim, W.M.K., 1989. An introduction to concept mapping for planning and evaluation. Eval. Program Plann. 0149-7189. 12 (1), 1–16. doi:10.1016/0149-7189(89)90016-5.

Venkatesh, V., Bala, H., 2008. Technology acceptance model 3 and a research agenda on interventions. Decis. Sci. 0011-7315. 39 (2), 273–315. doi:10.1111/j.1540-5915.2008.00192.x.

Venkatesh, V., Davis, F.D., 2000. Theoretical extension of the technology acceptance model: four longitudinal field studies. Manag. Sci. 0025-1909. 46 (2), 186–204. doi:10.1287/mnsc.46.2.186.11926.

Windsor, L.C., 2013. Using concept mapping in community-based participatory research: a mixed methods approach. J. Mix. Methods Res. 1558-6901. 7 (3), 274–293. doi:10.1177/1558689813479175.

Yen, P.Y., Bakken, S., 2012. Review of health information technology usability study methodologies. J. Am. Med. Inform. Assoc. 1527-974X. 19 (3), 413–422. Available from: http://jamia.bmj.com/content/19/3/413.full.pdf+html. doi:10.1136/amiajnl-2010-000020.

Yusof, M.M., Kuljis, J., Papazafeiropoulou, A., Stergioulas, L.K., 2008. An evaluation framework for health information systems: human, organization and technology-fit factors (HOT-fit). Int. J. Med. Inform. 1386-5056. 77 (6), 386–398. doi:10.1016/j.ijmedinf.2007.08.011.

C H A P T E R

22

Methodological guidance on patient and public involvement and engagement in social pharmacy research

Lourdes Cantarero Arevalo[a], *Anna Birna Almarsdóttir*[a], *Lotte Stig Nørgaard*[a], *Suanne Kaae*[a], *Ramune Jacobsen*[a], *Caroline Buhl*[a], *Aimo Strömberg*[b], *and Katri Hämeen-Anttila*[b]

[a]Department of Pharmacy, Faculty of Health and Medical Sciences, University of Copenhagen, Copenhagen, Denmark

[b]School of Pharmacy, Faculty of Health Sciences, University of Eastern Finland, Kuopio, Finland

CHAPTER OBJECTIVES

- Explain what Patient and Public Involvement and Engagement (PPIE) means within social pharmacy
- Provide step-by-step methodological guidance to design and implement PPIE
- Highlight common challenges and practical solutions based on lessons learned
- Discuss the importance of PPIE in improving research quality and relevance
- Demonstrate how PPIE can be adapted in diverse and resource-constrained settings

1 Introduction

In recent years, there has been growing recognition of the importance of Patient and Public Involvement and Engagement (PPIE) in Social Pharmacy Research (Cantarero-Arevalo et al., 2024). PPIE moves beyond viewing patients and the community as mere subjects of study and instead embraces them as active contributors to the research process. In social pharmacy—a field that focuses on the complex interplay between medicines, users, pharmacists, and health systems—PPIE offers a powerful means to enhance the relevance, equity, and impact of research (Adesanoye and Guirguis, 2017; Fredriksson et al., 2025). Within the context of social pharmacy, PPIE refers to the meaningful involvement of patients, carers, and members of the public in shaping the research agenda, codesigning studies, interpreting findings, and ensuring that research outcomes resonate with the lived experiences of medicine users (Price et al., 2022; Carroll et al., 2023; Cantarero-Arevalo et al., 2024). This approach acknowledges the unique expertise patients and communities bring, especially in addressing issues such as medication adherence, access to care, acceptability of treatments, and the broader social and cultural dimensions of medication use.

Contemporary Research Methods in Pharmacy and Health Services - Volume 2
https://doi.org/10.1016/B978-0-443-44607-8.00018-2

PPIE in research is not only ethically compelling but also methodologically enriching (Cantarero-Arevalo and Nørgaard, 2025). PPIE is also enriching for researchers for a variety of reasons. A scoping review aimed at studying the experiences of academic researchers involved in PPIE suggested that PPIE enriches researchers by broadening their perspectives and helping them understand patients' and the public's real-world experiences. It improves research quality, ethical awareness, and communication skills by making studies more relevant, inclusive, and collaborative. In addition, PPIE provides personal fulfillment and professional development through seeing the impact of research and building networks for future opportunities (Pratte et al., 2023).

PPIE helps ensure that research questions are grounded in real-world concerns, that study designs are sensitive to patient realities, and that findings are more likely to inform policy and practice (Greenhalgh et al., 2019; Staniszewska et al., 2017). Particularly in social pharmacy, where the goal is often to improve how medicines are used and understood in everyday life, PPIE aligns naturally with the discipline's focus on societal impact.

This chapter provides practical and methodological guidance for implementing PPIE in social pharmacy research. Drawing on well-established frameworks such as Guidance for Reporting Involvement of Patients and the Public (GRIPP2) (Staniszewska et al., 2017), the Patient-Centered Outcomes Research Institute (PCORI) Engagement Rubric (PCORI, 2021), and the Patients Active in Research and Dialogs for an Improved Generation of Medicines (PARADIGM) tools for cocreation in medicines research, it offers step-by-step advice for researchers—especially those working in diverse and resource-constrained settings. Special attention is given to how methods and tools can be adapted to fit local contexts.

To illustrate the practical application of PPIE, the chapter includes examples from social pharmacy projects conducted in the Nordic countries, where collaborative research cultures, strong welfare systems, and increasing attention to citizens' voices provide a fertile ground for participatory approaches (Villarba et al., 2025; van Leersum et al., 2024). These examples reflect both the promise and the complexity of involving patients and the public meaningfully in the coproduction of knowledge.

By grounding the discussion in social pharmacy's core values—equity, responsiveness, and contextual sensitivity—this chapter aims to empower researchers to design and conduct participatory research with the potential to make momentous impacts on various stakeholders, which is inherently more inclusive and responsive to community needs.

2 Methods: How to implement patient and public involvement and engagement

Implementing PPIE in social pharmacy research requires careful methodological planning, guided by values of inclusivity, transparency, and respect for lived experiences and preferences. This section provides a step-by-step guide to designing, executing, and sustaining meaningful engagement with patients and the public across the research cycle. Drawing on existing frameworks and examples from recent research in Nordic countries, the section highlights key models, practical tools, and ethical considerations. It also provides a summary of practical tips to engage and involve patients and the public as research partners in social pharmacy research.

	Summary of practical tips proposed to engage and involve patients as research partners in social pharmacy research
1	Understand the nuances of legal, ethical, and cultural norms across different research contexts, including awareness of varying preunderstandings (Cavaller-Bellaubi et al., 2021; Ocloo and Matthews, 2016)
2	Create the right mindset and a safe culture through inclusive methods, icebreaking activities, and by avoiding pharmaceutical jargon (which may require extra time and patience) (Cavaller-Bellaubi et al., 2021; Ocloo and Matthews, 2016)
3	Conduct formative evaluations throughout the different stages by checking in regularly with patients (Cavaller-Bellaubi et al., 2021; Ocloo and Matthews, 2016; Vat et al., 2020; Manafo et al., 2018; Deane et al., 2019)
4	Recruit the relevant patients/caregivers. Ensure diversity in the sampling (age, geography, socioeconomic position, disease severity, attitudes toward medicines) (Cavaller-Bellaubi et al., 2021; Ocloo and Matthews, 2016)
5	Be aware of conflicting interests (consider carefully if "professional" patient advocates and individual patients are in the same room, and consider the role of industry) (Cavaller-Bellaubi et al., 2021; Ocloo and Matthews, 2016)
6	Understand, motivate, and create trust by defining, together with patients, incentives for engagement and participation (Pokhilenko et al., 2021)
7	Define a retention plan based on patients' interests and expertise, ensuring long-term engagement (Sheridan, et al., 2017)
8	Prepare yourself in an evidence-based manner regarding patient engagement (theories of engagement) (Pokhilenko et al., 2021)

	Summary of practical tips proposed to engage and involve patients as research partners in social pharmacy research
9	Clearly define and redefine the patient engagement plan (through regular renegotiation), including roles, duties, and expectations (Ocloo and Matthews, 2016)
10	Provide ongoing support, payment, encouragement, and recognition for patient contributions (Ocloo and Matthews, 2016; Manofo, 2018)
11	Remove tightly defined boundaries between professionals and patients to enable shared control and responsibility (flexible interaction) (Ocloo and Matthews, 2016)
12	Engage patients early in the process and enhance ownership (Deane et al., 2019; Manofo, 2018)
13	Listen to patients' priorities. Align with patients' potential research competencies and interests (Vat et al., 2020; Sacristán et al., 2016; Patalano et al., 2020; Ocloo and Matthews, 2016)
14	Assess internal expertise (eventually including other researchers and experts if internal expertise is unavailable) (Chudyk et al., 2018)
15	Establish an ethical, trust-based collaboration (power balance) and ensure transparency (18) (Cavaller-Bellaubi et al., 2021; Ocloo and Matthews, 2016)
16	Share scientific literature with patients in a layperson's manner (Chudyk et al., 2018) (7)
17	Contemplate theory when defining the research question and when deciding how to engage patients, such as by considering social theories on engagement (25)
18	Incorporate external expert validation of the research process when needed (Chudyk et al., 2018)
19	Secure comprehensive training in research methods for patients and the public, and support their growth as researchers if they wish (Deane et al., 2019; Manofo, 2018)
20	Ensure dedicated leadership, operational time, resources, and funding (Cavaller-Bellaubi et al., 2021)
21	Engage patient networks and networks of networks (Ocloo and Matthews, 2016)
22	Share conclusions with relevant networks and stakeholders, and ask for feedback (Ocloo and Matthews, 2016)
23	Create advocacy and dissemination plans, with patients and patients' networks serving as catalysts at this point (Ocloo and Matthews, 2016; Sheridan et al., 2017)
24	Conduct a summative evaluation of patient engagement (quality criteria: learning, changes, impact, action, support) (Cavaller-Bellaubi et al., 2021; Deane et al., 2019)

2.1 Key approaches and models of PPIE

Several conceptual models guide PPIE practices in health research, ranging from consultative approaches to full coproduction. These include consultation, where patients and the public are asked for feedback on specific issues (e.g., reviewing a questionnaire); collaboration, where patients and the public work with researchers throughout a project but do not have shared decision-making authority; and coproduction, where patients and the public are equal partners with shared power and responsibility across all research stages.

These models exist on a spectrum and can be adapted depending on the project's scope, aims, and resources (Greenhalgh et al., 2019; Price et al., 2022). Increasingly, scholars recognize that PPIE approaches are deeply entwined with implementation science, enhancing the design and conduct of implementation research by helping ensure interventions are acceptable, scalable, sustainable, and responsive to community and patient voices (e.g., Mathieson et al., 2025). The INVOLVE framework (National Institute for Health and Care Research (NIHR), UK) and the Canadian Institutes for Health Research (CIHR) Strategy for Patient-Oriented Research (SPOR) strategy (Canada) provide robust guidance for selecting and implementing suitable models for various contexts, and the chapter on implementation science offers further detail on how PPIE can be integrated into implementation frameworks to strengthen real-world uptake.

2.2 Step-by-step guide to implementing PPIE

2.2.1 Step 1: Planning and purpose definition

Begin by defining the purpose of involving patients or citizens. Is the aim to identify relevant research questions, improve study design, interpret findings, or enhance dissemination? This clarity helps shape recruitment, engagement methods, and roles (Adesanoye and Guirguis, 2017; Staniszewska et al., 2017).

Example: In autumn 2022, a patient expert joined the Pharmaceutical Policy Research Group at the University of Eastern Finland, with the collaboration documented over a year to explore and develop patient participation in social pharmacy research. An agreement outlined tasks, practicalities, and compensation. The patient expert contributed to shaping the group's research strategy, communicated it, participated in a research consortium on automatic substitution of biological medicines, helped develop a patient survey, and coorganized a workshop on patient involvement. Key strengths included the patient's role in ensuring patient-friendly communication, identifying relevant topics, leveraging networks, and fostering an open, trusting atmosphere. Challenges included limited organizational support and funding for broader patient participation. Lessons highlight the importance of building trust, providing patients with enough knowledge to engage meaningfully, and including patient participation in funding applications. Overall, the collaboration demonstrated how patient and researcher expertise complement each other, highlighting the need for further research on the impacts of patient involvement in social pharmacy.

2.2.2 *Step 2: Recruitment and representation*

Recruitment should aim for diversity across age, gender, health status, socioeconomic background, and ethnicity to avoid privileging dominant voices. Even when the research aim focuses on a specific population group, such as elderly refugees, we should strive to include diverse voices in terms of gender, socioeconomic background, or other relevant characteristics to ensure richness and representativeness in the insights collected. Use community networks, pharmacies, patient associations, and digital platforms to reach underrepresented groups.

Transparent communication about roles, expectations, compensation, and time commitments is essential (Carroll et al., 2023; PCORI, 2021). Coresearcher contracts or terms of reference can help formalize the partnership.

Example: In a Danish project exploring patient perspectives on new medication forms, patient representatives were engaged as partners from the design stage. Their involvement ensured that the study design was sensitive to patients' real-life experiences—both in terms of selecting appropriate patient groups for recruitment and in shaping specific elements, such as the interview guide. This collaboration helped ensure that the questions were relevant and communicated in a patient-friendly manner.

2.2.3 *Step 3: Training and support*

Both researchers and patient contributors benefit from training. Patients may need orientation on research processes, while researchers may need training in communication, facilitation, and partnership dynamics with patients. Tools from the European Patients' Academy (EUPATI) and PARADIGM offer practical training materials for building capacity in PPIE.

Example: In a Danish project involving young adults with chronic conditions, youth coresearchers were trained in basic qualitative methods before starting the research project, including recruitment techniques, interviewing skills, and thematic analysis. This step contributed significantly to validity and data richness.

2.2.4 *Step 4: Engagement activities*

Engagement methods should be tailored to participants' preferences and accessibility needs. Common approaches include workshops for idea generation and project planning, focus groups for refining intervention components, advisory panels to guide and evaluate project development, and community forums or digital platforms for broader public dialog.

Creative tools such as visual facilitation, storytelling, or journey mapping may enhance engagement for populations with low literacy or limited research experience (Villarba et al., 2025; van Leersum et al., 2024).

Example: In an Icelandic study on medication deprescribing among older adults, researchers codeveloped research questions with a community advisory board consisting of elderly patients and caregivers, ensuring alignment with the daily challenges of medicine use.

2.2.5 *Step 5: Reflexivity and evaluation*

Ongoing reflection on the process helps ensure quality and fairness in engagement. Use tools like the GRIPP2 reporting checklist (Staniszewska et al., 2017; Christiansen et al., 2023) to evaluate and document how PPIE influenced the research. Consider feedback from all parties on what worked, what did not, and what could improve future collaborations.

Example: In Denmark, the Social Pharmacy group at the University of Copenhagen led a research–practice project to develop a postcurriculum pharmacy communication training program promoting patient-centered counseling. Partners included pharmacy owners, universities, a public research institution, and a newly formed patient organization, which recruited patients, produced video interviews, and joined staff training. The blended learning program achieved positive outcomes, but the patient organization faced challenges such as unclear roles, limited participation in steering meetings, and frequent last-minute changes that increased workload and frustration—resulting in over 90% of their planned initiatives being altered or postponed. Lessons highlight the importance of early expectation alignment, clear communication, flexibility in research–practice collaborations, and buffer resources to support patient organizations effectively.

2.3 Tools and techniques

Several published resources can support the practical implementation of PPIE:
Published resources to support PPIE implementation

Tool/framework	Purpose	Source
GRIPP2 Checklists	Reporting and evaluating PPIE	(Staniszewska et al., 2017)
PCORI Engagement Rubric	Planning, executing, and sustaining engagement	(PCORI, 2021)
PARADIGM Toolbox	Patient engagement in medicines R&D	PARADIGM Initiative
EUPATI Training Modules	Educating patients and researchers for involvement	(EUPATI, 2022)
INVOLVE Guidance	Comprehensive PPIE practice guide	INVOLVE (UK NIHR)

2.4 Adapting to resource-constrained and culturally diverse settings

PPIE must be flexible enough to work in low-resource or culturally distinct settings. This may involve relying on existing community structures (e.g., pharmacies, local NGOs) for engagement, using informal meetings or radio discussions where formal literacy or access to technology is limited, and translating materials and consent processes into local languages or using oral consent.

In remote areas of Iceland, researchers used mobile clinics and trusted pharmacy staff to engage isolated older adults in research on polypharmacy. This context-sensitive approach enabled meaningful involvement despite geographic and logistical barriers.

3 Discussion: Lessons learned and methodological reflections

The implementation of PPIE in social pharmacy research has brought valuable methodological and ethical insights. While PPIE is widely promoted for improving research quality, equity, and legitimacy, its practice often reveals a complex mix of challenges, opportunities, and tensions. This section reflects on lessons learned from recent studies and collaborative experiences in the Nordic countries and internationally, highlighting key issues related to recruitment, expectations, power dynamics, sustainability, and methodological innovation.

3.1 Common challenges

3.1.1 Recruitment and representation

A recurring challenge in PPIE is the recruitment of diverse and representative patient and citizen partners. Research teams often rely on existing networks or convenience sampling, which can lead to the overrepresentation of individuals with prior engagement experience or high levels of education (Villarba et al., 2025; Carroll et al., 2023). Engaging marginalized, low-literacy, or digitally excluded populations requires deliberate outreach strategies, flexible meeting formats, and collaboration with trusted community intermediaries.

3.1.2 Sustaining involvement over time

Longitudinal engagement can be challenging to maintain, particularly when research timelines stretch over years. Patient or citizen contributors may face health setbacks, fatigue, or logistical constraints. Ensuring continuity may involve building capacity among multiple contributors and establishing mechanisms for rotating participation while maintaining institutional memory (Greenhalgh et al., 2019).

3.1.3 *Managing expectations*

Misalignment of expectations between researchers and patient partners can undermine trust. Patients may anticipate direct influence on decision-making, while researchers may limit their involvement to specific stages. Transparent communication, a trusting atmosphere, codeveloped terms of reference, and regular feedback loops are critical for managing expectations (PCORI, 2021; Price et al., 2022).

3.2 Dos and don'ts for effective engagement

Do:

- Plan engagement activities early and incorporate them throughout the project lifecycle
- Offer training and support for both researchers and patient partners
- Recognize contributions through authorship, acknowledgment, or compensation
- Be flexible and responsive to the needs and preferences of participants

Do not:

- Treat PPIE as a checkbox or token gesture
- Assume that one "patient voice" represents all experiences
- Overburden contributors with excessive tasks without appropriate support
- Underestimate the emotional labor involved in sharing lived experiences

These principles are echoed in the INVOLVE guidelines and the GRIPP2 reporting standards (Staniszewska et al., 2017; NIHR INVOLVE, 2019).

3.3 Benefits versus Drawbacks compared to traditional research approaches

PPIE has demonstrable benefits, including improved relevance of research questions, better recruitment strategies, enhanced outcome measures, and an increased likelihood of knowledge translation (Adesanoye and Guirguis, 2017; Staniszewska et al., 2017). Studies also report increased trust between researchers and communities.

However, drawbacks include increased time and resource demands, the potential for interpersonal conflict, and challenges in maintaining scientific rigor when lay perspectives diverge from academic norms. These tensions call for careful facilitation and methodological flexibility rather than rigid adherence to either traditional or participatory paradigms (Greenhalgh et al., 2019).

3.4 Power dynamics and trust

Power imbalances between researchers and patients are a central concern in PPIE. While coproduction aspires to equality, traditional hierarchies often persist in decision-making, authorship, and recognition. Building trust requires humility, reflexivity, and a willingness to share control over the research process (Price et al., 2022). In the Nordic context, where egalitarian values are culturally embedded, researchers may be well-positioned to challenge hierarchical norms—yet they must still actively dismantle subtle barriers to full participation and learn new ways of working and acknowledging patients' expertise. In cultures where hierarchical norms prevail, research involving patients and the public may require a longer and more in-depth inception phase to build the trust necessary for participants to feel comfortable and actively engage.

3.5 Scalability and sustainability

Sustainable PPIE requires long-term investment in relationships, structures, and institutional support. Embedding engagement in funding requirements, ethics review processes, and academic incentives can normalize participation as a standard rather than an exception. Initiatives such as patient panels at universities, pharmacy education programs including community partners, or permanent advisory groups contribute to sustainability.

However, scalability across projects and institutions must avoid standardization that undermines contextual relevance. The diversity of health systems, population needs, and research goals calls for adaptable engagement strategies that preserve local meaning and ownership (van Leersum et al., 2024).

3.6 Future directions and research gaps

Despite growing attention, several methodological gaps remain:

- Evaluation of impact: Few studies systematically assess how PPIE shapes research outcomes or patient experiences. Frameworks like GRIPP2 and the Impact Log from PCORI could be more widely applied.
- Engagement in digital settings: Postpandemic shifts to online methods offer both opportunities and barriers to inclusion. Research on hybrid and asynchronous engagement models is needed.
- Participatory methods in complex systems: As social pharmacy increasingly intersects with digital health, environmental sustainability, and artificial intelligence-driven interventions, new participatory methods are needed to engage citizens in these evolving contexts.

Strengthening the evidence base for PPIE in pharmacy requires interdisciplinary collaboration, funding support, and greater academic recognition of coproduced knowledge.

4 Questions for further discussion

The following discussion questions are designed to deepen understanding of the theoretical, practical, and ethical complexities of PPIE in social pharmacy research. Each question is intended to support reflection and encourage dialog among students, early-career researchers, and practitioners.

- How can PPIE improve the quality and relevance of social pharmacy research?
- What strategies can help engage hard-to-reach populations?
- How can power imbalances between researchers and citizens be minimized?
- What ethical considerations are unique to PPIE in this field?
- How might digital tools enhance or limit PPIE efforts?

5 Application exercise/scenario

Scenario title: Designing a Citizen Engagement Plan for Research on Deprescribing Anxiolytics among Young People

Context: The use of anxiolytics among young people (ages 16–25) is increasing across many high-income countries, including those in the Nordic region. Concerns have been raised about long-term dependency, limited non-pharmacological support, and inadequate deprescribing practices. A research team in social pharmacy aims to explore how young citizens can help design more relevant, accessible, and youth-friendly approaches to deprescribing interventions in community pharmacy or general practice settings.

Your task is to design a citizen engagement plan that outlines how you will involve young people—not as patients, but as citizens and cocreators of knowledge—throughout the project lifecycle. Pay special attention to digital engagement strategies suitable for this age group.

5.1 Mock citizen engagement plan

5.1.1 Identifying stakeholders

- **Primary stakeholders**: Young people (ages 16–25) with past or current experience of anxiolytic prescriptions (e.g., benzodiazepines or z-drugs).
- **Secondary stakeholders**: Youth advocacy groups, school counselors, student health services, mental health NGOs, and peer networks (e.g., online forums).
- **Professionals**: Pharmacists, general practitioners, youth mental health workers.
- **Community contributors**: Young digital creators, influencers, and artists engaged in mental health advocacy.

5.1.2 Engagement methods by research phase

New research shows that digital platforms can foster inclusion and expression among youth when designed collaboratively and with attention to privacy and digital literacy (Cantarero-Arevalo and Nørgaard, 2025; Reynolds and Sariola, 2018).

Engagement methods by research phase

Phase	Engagement activity	Method
Planning	Coidentify priority issues related to anxiolytic use and deprescribing	Online ideation workshops using Miro, Padlet, or Instagram polls
Design	Codevelop content for a youth-friendly digital deprescribing tool	Hackathon-style digital sprint with youth participants
Implementation	Pilot digital engagement strategies in pharmacy settings	Peer-led video storytelling shared on TikTok, YouTube, or a custom microsite
Evaluation	Joint reflection on the process and impact of engagement	Online journaling (via Discord or WhatsApp) and virtual debrief circles

5.1.3 *Anticipated challenges and solutions*

Anticipated challenges and solutions

Challenge	Solution
Stigma around mental health and medication use	Anonymous input options; partner with trusted youth-led organizations
Unequal digital access or burnout from online spaces	Offer hybrid formats and check-in to avoid overburdening contributors
Building trust with adult researchers	Use peer facilitators and decentralized platforms (e.g., private Discord servers)
Ethical concerns regarding minors or vulnerable youth	Involve ethics boards early; codevelop age-appropriate consent models

5.1.4 *Evaluation plan*

- Use GRIPP2 Short Form adapted for citizen-led initiatives
- Monitor engagement through built-in analytics on platforms (e.g., Instagram Insights, Discord participation logs)
- Conduct qualitative interviews or use feedback forms (text-based or voice notes) to assess experiences and satisfaction
- Cocreate a zine or digital comic summarizing what was learned and shared from the engagement, authored by youth collaborators

This approach values creative, nontraditional forms of reflection and dissemination, aligning with youth communication styles and preferences (Totzeck et al., 2024).

5.2 Guiding questions for learners

1. How can we ensure that young people feel safe and respected when sharing their perspectives on medication use?
2. What role can digital media and peer storytelling play in engaging youth around stigmatized topics like mental health and medication?
3. How do you manage ethical issues when working with citizens under 18 or young adults experiencing distress?
4. What does shared power look like in a youth–researcher partnership?
5. How can pharmacies become spaces for youth-informed deprescribing practices?

5.3 Model answer (summarized)

Involving young people as citizens, not just patients, is crucial for addressing the social, emotional, and cultural realities of anxiolytic use. We would start by recruiting a youth advisory group through schools, online forums, and youth mental health organizations. To break stigma and support creative expression, we would codesign a campaign using Instagram stories, meme challenges, and short YouTube videos where young people reflect on medication and mental health.

To minimize power imbalance, we would work with youth peer facilitators and use cocreated spaces like private Discord channels. All contributions would be optional and anonymized when requested. We would evaluate the engagement using both analytics (e.g., platform engagement) and participatory feedback methods like video diaries and digital art. Outputs would be shared back with communities in the form of a zine and an open-access digital toolkit for youth-friendly deprescribing conversations in pharmacies.

Through this process, we would ensure that youth feel heard, valued, and empowered to shape services that affect their wellbeing.

6 Conclusion

The integration of PPIE in social pharmacy research is no longer a peripheral or optional add-on—it is increasingly recognized as a foundational approach for producing ethically sound, socially relevant, and practically impactful research. This chapter has offered a comprehensive overview of how to conceptualize, design, and evaluate PPIE efforts, particularly within the context of community-based and health services research involving medicine users, carers, and citizens.

6.1 Recap of key methodological insights

- **Flexible models of engagement**—including consultation, collaboration, and coproduction—should be selected and adapted based on the research context, population, and available resources (Greenhalgh et al., 2019; PCORI, 2021).
- **Early planning and role clarity** are critical to ensuring meaningful engagement. Establishing shared goals, timelines, and expectations with contributors helps reduce misunderstandings and tokenism (Price et al., 2022; Staniszewska et al., 2017).
- **Diversity and inclusivity** must be actively pursued through tailored recruitment, culturally sensitive communication strategies, and accessible engagement methods—especially in underserved or hard-to-reach populations (Carroll et al., 2023; Reynolds and Sariola, 2018).
- **Digital platforms** offer valuable tools for reaching and engaging younger or geographically dispersed contributors but require careful attention to digital literacy, privacy, and fatigue (Cantarero-Arevalo and Nørgaard, 2025; Totzeck et al., 2024).
- **Evaluation of engagement**—using tools like the GRIPP2 checklist and participatory feedback mechanisms—supports transparency, learning, and accountability (Staniszewska et al., 2017).

6.2 The transformative potential of PPIE in social pharmacy

When implemented thoughtfully, PPIE has the power to reshape how social pharmacy research is conceptualized and conducted. It brings in new voices, centers lived experience, and strengthens the democratic legitimacy of health knowledge production. Whether through codesigned deprescribing interventions, youth-led digital campaigns, or advisory boards of older adults navigating polypharmacy, PPIE bridges the gap between scientific expertise and everyday realities.

More importantly, meaningful engagement challenges conventional power hierarchies in research. It fosters mutual respect, shared ownership, and a recognition that knowledge exists in many forms—not only in peer-reviewed articles but also in life stories, digital expressions, and collective action. In this way, PPIE not only improves methodological rigor but also contributes to social justice and health equity.

6.3 Encouragement for thoughtful and critical integration

For students, researchers, and practitioners in social pharmacy, the invitation is clear: integrate PPIE not as a trend or a requirement, but as a principled commitment to better, fairer, and more relevant research. Start small, but start early—partner with communities and not just individual patients. Be open to discomfort, to learning, and to relinquishing some control. Moreover, above all, remain critically reflective—on whose voices are being heard, whose are missing, and what changes when research becomes a shared endeavor.

The path to meaningful engagement is not linear or straightforward—but it is rich with possibility. In the words of Greenhalgh et al. (2019), "no one-size-fits-all framework exists." Instead, the most successful engagement emerges when we remain responsive to context, relationships, and the shifting landscape of participation itself.

Let this chapter serve as both a methodological guide and a call to action. The future of social pharmacy research depends not only on what we study but also on who is part of the journey.

Additional readings for consideration

Brett J, Staniszewska S, Mockford C, Herron-Marx S, Hughes J, Tysall C, et al. A systematic review of the impact of patient and public involvement on service users, researchers, and communities. *Patient*. 2014;7(4):387–95. doi:10.1007/s40271-014-0065-0.

Galmarini E, Marciano L, Schulz PJ. The effectiveness of visual-based interventions on health literacy in health care: a systematic review and meta-analysis. *BMC Health Serv Res*. 2024;24:718. doi: 10.1186/s12913-024-0718-x.

Green G, Johns T. Exploring the relationship (and power dynamic) between researchers and public partners working together in applied health research teams. *Front Sociol*. 2019;4:20. doi: 10.3389/fsoc. 2019.00020.

Greenhalgh T, Hinton L, Finlay T, Macfarlane A, Fahy N, Clyde B, et al. Frameworks for supporting patient and public involvement in research: systematic review and co-design pilot. *Health Expect*. 2019;22(4):785–801. doi: 10.1111/hex. 12,888.

Reynolds L, Sariola S. The ethics and politics of community engagement in global health research. *Crit Public Health*. 2018;28(3):257–68.

Myllylä M, Pantti M, Kivijärvi A. Participation paradox: asylum seekers' everyday participation in Finland. *Nord J Migr Res*. 2025;15(2):2, 1–18. doi: 10.33134/njmr.686.

Tembo D, Hickey G, Montenegro C, Chandler D, Nelson E, Porter K, et al. Effective engagement and involvement with community stakeholders in the co-production of global health research. *BMJ*. 2021;372:n178. doi: 10.1136/bmj.n178.

World Health Organisation. WHO Global Patient Engagement Framework: A Vision for Engaged and Empowered People-centred Health Systems. Geneva: World Health Organisation; 2023.

Case scenario references

Cantarero-Arevalo, L., **& Nørgaard,** L. **S.** (2025). Ethical integration of citizen science and youth participatory action research: Insights from the YouthChronic project. *Research Involvement and Engagement, 11*, 36. https://doi.org/10.1186/s40900-025-00699-y

Totzeck, C., van der Meer, A.S., Christiansen, H. et al. Systematic Review: Patient and Public Involvement of Children and Young People in Mental Health Research. *Clin Child Fam Psychol Rev***27**, 257–274 (2024). https://doi.org/10.1007/s10567-024-0047 Reynolds, L., **& Sariola, S.** (2018). The ethics and politics of community engagement in global health research. *Critical Public Health, 28*(3), 257–268. https://doi.org/10.1080/09581596.2018.1449598

AI disclosure

During the preparation of this work, the author(s) used Grammarly (paid version) because they are not native English speakers and needed support when writing in English. After using this tool/service, the authors reviewed and edited the content as needed and take full responsibility for the content of the publication.

Appendix: Additional guidelines that may aid readers

1. PARADIGM

- A European initiative providing practical tools and guidelines to involve patients meaningfully in medicines development and regulatory processes.
- Offers best practices, training materials, and frameworks to promote patient engagement at every stage of research.
- Official website & resources

2. GRIPP2
- A set of reporting checklists is designed to improve the quality, transparency, and consistency of patient and public involvement reporting in research publications
- Two versions: short and long forms for different study types
- Published in the BMJ, it is widely used internationally
- Paper: Staniszewska et al. (2017)
3. INVOLVE guidelines
- Developed by INVOLVE (UK National Institute for Health Research), these guidelines provide comprehensive support for involving patients and the public in health and social care research
- Includes practical advice on planning, recruiting, supporting, and evaluating involvement activities
- Website: https://www.invo.org.uk/
4. CIHR SPOR
- Canada's strategy promotes patient engagement in health research to improve outcomes
- Provides frameworks and tools for meaningful patient involvement at all stages of research
- Website: https://cihr-irsc.gc.ca/e/41204.html
5. EUPATI
- Focuses on educating patients and patient advocates about medicines research and development to enhance their participation as partners
- Offers training modules and guidance documents for patient engagement
- Website: https://www.eupati.eu/
6. PCORI Engagement Rubric
- A guide developed by PCORI (USA) for researchers and patients to foster effective engagement in patient-centered outcomes research
- Includes principles and practical strategies for collaboration
- Website: https://www.pcori.org/engagement/engagement-resources/pcori-engagement-rubric
7. WHO Patient Engagement Framework
- Provides a global perspective on patient engagement to improve healthcare quality and outcomes
- Highlights strategies, benefits, and challenges of meaningfully involving patients
- Document: WHO Patient Engagement

References

Adesanoye, D., Guirguis, L., 2017. Patient engagement in pharmacy practice research. Can. Pharm. J. 1715-1635. 150 (2), 94–97. doi:10.1177/1715163517690539.

Cantarero-Arevalo, L., Kaae, S., Jacobsen, R., Nielsen, A., Slyngborg, L., Smistrup, N., Kastrup, L.M., Hämeen-Anttila, K., Strömberg, A., Nørgaard, L.S., 2024. Empowering patients as co-researchers in social pharmacy: lessons learned and practical tips for meaningful partnership and impact. Res. Soc. Adm. Pharm. 1551-7411. 20 (3), 372–376. doi:10.1016/j.sapharm.2023.12.006.

Cantarero-Arevalo, L., Nørgaard, L.S., 2025. Ethical integration of citizen science and youth participatory action research: insights from the YouthChronic project. Res. Involv. Engagem. 2056-7529. 11 (1). Available from: https://researchinvolvement.biomedcentral.com/. doi:10.1186/s40900-025-00699-y.

Carroll, J.C., Jiang, C., Mook, H., McGivney, M.A.S., Coley, K.C., 2023. Patients' opinions on participation in patient-centered outcomes research in community pharmacies: a qualitative study. J. Am. Pharm. Assoc. 1544-3450. 63 (1), 182–187. Available from: http://www.japha.org/issues.aspx?journalid=63. doi:10.1016/j.japh.2022.09.001.

Cavaller-Bellaubi, M., Faulkner, S.D., Teixeira, B., Boudes, M., Molero, E., Brooke, N., McKeaveney, L., Southerton, J., Vicente, M.J., Bertelsen, N., García-Burgos, J., Pirard, V., Reid, K., Ferrer, E., 2021. Sustaining meaningful patient engagement across the lifecycle of medicines: a roadmap for action. Ther. Innov. Regul. Sci. 2168-4804. 55 (5), 936–953. Available from: https://www.springer.com/journal/43441. doi:10.1007/s43441-021-00282-z.

Christiansen, M.G., Pappot, H., Hamilton, C., Lund-Jacobsen, T., Kristensen, A.W., Nordentoft, S., Høeg, B.L., Bidstrup, P., Nielsen, I.H., Ulstrup, J., Trip, A.K., Jarden, M., Piil, K., 2023. Patient engagement in research scale (PEIRS-22): danish translation, applicability, and user experiences. Res. Involv. Engagem. 2056-7529. 9 (1). Available from: https://researchinvolvement.biomedcentral.com/. doi:10.1186/s40900-023-00526-2.

Chudyk, A.M., Waldman, C., Horrill, T., Demczuk, L., Shimmin, C., Stoddard, R., Hickes, S., Schultz, A.S.H., 2018. Models and frameworks of patient engagement in health services research: a scoping review protocol. Res. Involv. Engagem. 2056-7529. 4 (1). Available from: http://researchinvolvement.biomedcentral.com/. doi:10.1186/s40900-018-0111-5.

Deane, K., Delbecque, L., Gorbenko, O., Hamoir, A.M., Hoos, A., Nafria, B., Pakarinen, C., Sargeant, I., Richards, D.P., Skovlund, S.E., Brooke, N., 2019. Co-creation of patient engagement quality guidance for medicines development: an international multistakeholder initiative. BMJ Innov. 2055-642X. 5 (1), 43–55. Available from: http://innovations.bmj.com/. doi:10.1136/bmjinnov-2018-000317.

EUPATI, 2022. Training materials for patient involvement. Available from: https://www.eupati.eu.

Fredriksson, M., Sampaio, F., Moberg, L., 2025. The impact of patient and public involvement in healthcare services: a conceptual review spanning social sciences and health sciences. SSM Qual. Res. Health 2667-3215. 7. Available from: https://www.sciencedirect.com/science/journal/26673215. doi:10.1016/j.ssmqr.2024.100517.

Greenhalgh, T., Hinton, L., Finlay, T., Macfarlane, A., Fahy, N., Clyde, B., Chant, A., 2019. Frameworks for supporting patient and public involvement in research: systematic review and co-design pilot. Health Expect. 1369-6513. 22 (4), 785–801. doi:10.1111/hex.12888.

Manafo, E., Petermann, L., Mason-Lai, P., Vandall-Walker, V., 2018. Patient engagement in Canada: a scoping review of the 'how' and 'what' of patient engagement in health research. Health Res. Policy Syst. 1478-4505. 16 (1). doi:10.1186/s12961-018-0282-4.

Mathieson, A., Brunton, L., Wilson, P.M., 2025. The use of patient and public involvement and engagement in the design and conduct of implementation research: a scoping review. Implement. Sci. Commun. 2662-2211. 6 (1). Available from: https://www.springer.com/journal/43058. doi:10.1186/s43058-025-00725-w.

NIHR INVOLVE, 2019. Guidance on co-producing a research project. Available from: https://www.invo.org.uk.

Ocloo, J., Matthews, R., 2016. From tokenism to empowerment: progressing patient and public involvement in healthcare improvement. BMJ Qual. Saf. 2044-5415. 25 (8), 626–632. doi:10.1136/bmjqs-2015-004839.

Patalano, F., Gutzwiller, F.S., Shah, B., Kumari, C., Cook, N.S., 2020. Gathering structured patient insight to drive the PRO strategy in COPD: patient-centric drug development from theory to practice. Adv. Ther. 37 (1), 17–26.

PCORI, 2021. Engagement rubric. Patient-Centred Outcomes Research Institute. Available from: https://www.pcori.org/engagement/resources/engagement-rubric.

Pokhilenko, I., van Esch, T.E.M., Brabers, A.E.M., de Jong, J.D., 2021. Relationship between trust and patient involvement in medical decision-making: a cross-sectional study. PLoS ONE. 1932-6203. 16 (8). Available from: https://journals.plos.org/plosone/article/file?id=10.1371/journal.pone.0256698&type=printable. doi:10.1371/journal.pone.0256698.

Pratte, M.-M., Audette-Chapdelaine, S., Auger, A.-M., Wilhelmy, C., Brodeur, M., 2023. Researchers' experiences with patient engagement in health research: a scoping review and thematic synthesis. Res. Involv. Engagem. 2056-7529. 9 (1). doi:10.1186/s40900-023-00431-8.

Price, A., Clarke, M., Staniszewska, S., Chu, L., Tembo, D., Kirkpatrick, M., Nelken, Y., 2022. Patient and public involvement in research: a journey to co-production. Patient Educ. Couns. 0738-3991. 105 (4), 1041–1047. doi:10.1016/j.pec.2021.07.021.

Reynolds, L., Sariola, S., 2018. The ethics and politics of community engagement in global health research. Crit. Public Health. 28 (3), 257–68.

Sacristán, J.A., Aguarón, A., Avendaño-Solá, C., Garrido, P., Carrión, J., Gutiérrez, A., Kroes, R., Flores, A., 2016. Patient involvement in clinical research: why, when, and how. Patient Prefer. Adherence 10, 631–640. doi:10.2147/PPA.S104259.

Sheridan, S., Schrandt, S., Forsythe, L., Hilliard, T.S., Paez, K.A., 2017. The PCORI engagement rubric: promising practices for partnering in research. Ann. Fam. Med. 1544-1717. 15 (2), 165–170. Available from: http://www.annfammed.org/content/15/2/165.full.pdf. doi:10.1370/afm.2042.

Staniszewska, S., Brett, J., Simera, I., Seers, K., Mockford, C., Goodlad, S., Altman, D.G., Moher, D., Barber, R., Denegri, S., Entwistle, A., Littlejohns, P., Morris, C., Suleman, R., Thomas, V., Tysall, C., 2017. GRIPP2 reporting checklists: tools to improve reporting of patient and public involvement in research. BMJ. 0959-8138. 358, j3453. doi:10.1136/bmj.j3453.

Totzeck, C., van der Meer, A.S., Christiansen, H., et al., 2024. Systematic review: patient and public involvement of children and young people in mental health research. Clin. Child Fam. Psychol. Rev. 27, 257–274. doi:10.1007/s10567-024-0047.

van Leersum, C.M., Jaschinski, C., Bults, M., van der Zwart, J., 2024. Citizen involvement in research on technological innovations for health, care or well-being: a scoping review. Health Res. Policy Syst. 1478-4505. 22 (1). Available from: https://health-policy-systems.biomedcentral.com/. doi:10.1186/s12961-024-01152-4.

Vat, L.E., Finlay, T., Schuitmaker-Warnaar, T.J., Fahy, N., Robinson, P., Boudes, M., Diaz, A., Ferrer, E., Hivert, V., Purman, G., Kürzinger, M.L., Kroes, R.A., Hey, C., Broerse, J.E.W., 2020. Evaluating the "return on patient engagement initiatives" in medicines research and development: a literature review. Health Expect. 1369-7625. 23 (1), 5–18. Available from: http://onlinelibrary.wiley.com/journal/10.1111/(ISSN)1369-7625. doi:10.1111/hex.12951.

Villarba, J., Monnin, C., Turcotte, D., Maruf, A.A., Gunderson, J., Kedy, J., Mosel, J.A., Slaney, T., Chudyk, A.M., 2025. Protocol for a scoping review of patient engagement in pharmacy practice research. BMJ Open. 2044-6055. 15 (3). Available from: http://bmjopen.bmj.com/content/early/by/section. doi:10.1136/bmjopen-2024-089930.

CHAPTER

23

Enhancing the clinical pharmacy service of a large teaching hospital: Development of a new clinical prioritization tool

Rebecca Clarke[a], *Maeve Colleran*[a], *Gail Melanophy*[a], *and Margaret Bermingham*[b]

[a]Pharmacy Department, St James's Hospital, Dublin, Ireland

[b]School of Pharmacy, University College Cork, Cork, Ireland

CHAPTER OBJECTIVES

- To outline the current literature on clinical prioritization tools for use by pharmacists in general adult hospital settings.
- To describe the methodology for the selection of prioritization criteria, as well as the development and assessment of a clinical prioritization tool in a hospital pharmacy department.
- To appraise this methodology in the context of the current literature
- To challenge the reader to consider how to apply their learning from this chapter in their own clinical setting

1 Introduction

Drug-related problems can cause negative health outcomes and preventable harm for patients. Such problems encompass a lack of treatment efficacy or safety issues, including adverse drug events, and may arise from medication errors, nonadherence, or issues at transitions of care (Schindler et al., 2021). A recent study estimated that 1.8% of hospital inpatients had an admission related to an adverse drug reaction, and 6.6% of hospital inpatients experienced an adverse drug reaction at any time during their hospitalization (van Staa et al., 2024). A second recent study estimated that among people with an acute hospital admission, the adverse drug reaction rate was 18.4%, and that this equated to a health system cost of £2.21 billion (Osanlou et al., 2022). The adoption of clinical pharmacy

Contemporary Research Methods in Pharmacy and Health Services - Volume 2
https://doi.org/10.1016/B978-0-443-44607-8.00022-4

services in hospitals has been shown to have a positive impact on drug-related problems through the optimization of medicines use (Lombardi et al., 2018; Spinewine et al., 2006).

Hospital-based clinical pharmacists operate in patient-facing roles; they may be ward-based or team-based, and they conduct clinical reviews of patients' medications while working closely with other healthcare disciplines to ensure the safe and cost-effective use of medicines (Pharmaceutical Society of Ireland, 2016). In an ideal setting, clinical pharmacists could review patients daily, given the potential for drug-related problems, such as those arising from missed doses of medicines, a lack of pharmaceutical support for medical or nursing staff, and reduced medicines reconciliation services (Lord Carter of Coles, 2016). The number and complexity of patients being admitted to hospitals are on the rise without a corresponding increase in the number of clinical pharmacists employed (Lord Carter of Coles, 2016). As a result, some patients may not receive a full clinical pharmacy review or be reviewed as regularly as needed during their inpatient stay (Lord Carter of Coles, 2016). This is a known risk factor for medication errors (Lord Carter of Coles, 2016).

Patient prioritization may function to distinguish between those who are high-risk and most in need of a clinical pharmacy review and those whose needs are less, serving to optimize pharmacists' workload and alleviate time and resource pressures for pharmacy teams (Lewis, 2017). The goal of clinical pharmacy prioritization tools is to identify such high-risk patients and target finite pharmacy resources to those patients who will benefit the most (Lewis, 2017).

Several prioritization tools have been developed for use in a general adult inpatient setting (Alshakrah et al., 2021; Falconer et al., 2014; Geeson et al., 2019; Hickson et al., 2017; Martinbiancho et al., 2011; Roten et al., 2010; Kaufmann et al., 2018). There is some heterogeneity in the reported tools, with differences in terms of the health system in which they were developed, study design, outcome measures, prioritization criteria used, and validation methods reported (Table 23.1).

Clinical prioritization tools described in the literature use many different approaches to the development of the final tool. These tools assess an individual's risk of adverse drug events, drug-related problems, medication errors, or overall level of complexity based on a variety of disease-, medication, and patient-related factors to prioritize the delivery of pharmaceutical care (Table 23.2). The various criteria used for patient prioritization, also referred to as "flags" (Falconer et al., 2014), "risk factors" (Geeson et al., 2019; Hickson et al., 2017; Martinbiancho et al., 2011; Kaufmann et al., 2018), "components" (Alshakrah et al., 2021), or "queries" (Roten et al., 2010) among the different studies, can be grouped into three main categories: disease-related, medication-related, and patient-related criteria.

Common criteria used to determine patient priority are high-risk medicines (Alshakrah et al., 2021; Falconer et al., 2014; Geeson et al., 2019; Hickson et al., 2017; Martinbiancho et al., 2011; Roten et al., 2010; Kaufmann et al., 2018), polypharmacy (Alshakrah et al., 2021; Falconer et al., 2014; Geeson et al., 2019; Martinbiancho et al., 2011; Roten et al., 2010; Kaufmann et al., 2018), the presence of specific medical conditions (Alshakrah et al., 2021; Falconer et al., 2014; Geeson et al., 2019; Hickson et al., 2017; Martinbiancho et al., 2011; Kaufmann et al., 2018), renal or hepatic impairment (Alshakrah et al., 2021; Falconer et al., 2014; Geeson et al., 2019; Martinbiancho et al., 2011; Roten et al., 2010; Kaufmann et al., 2018), patient age (Alshakrah et al., 2021; Falconer et al., 2014; Geeson et al., 2019; Martinbiancho et al., 2011; Roten et al., 2010), laboratory results (Alshakrah et al., 2021; Falconer et al., 2014; Geeson et al., 2019; Roten et al., 2010), and medicines requiring therapeutic drug monitoring (Alshakrah et al., 2021; Falconer et al., 2014; Geeson et al., 2019; Hickson et al., 2017).

The presence of high-risk medicines is often used to support patient prioritization. The medicines most frequently represented in the tools reported here are anticoagulants (Alshakrah et al., 2021; Falconer et al., 2014; Hickson et al., 2017; Martinbiancho et al., 2011; Roten et al., 2010; Kaufmann et al., 2018), antiepileptics (Alshakrah et al., 2021; Falconer et al., 2014; Geeson et al., 2019; Hickson et al., 2017; Martinbiancho et al., 2011; Kaufmann et al., 2018), antimicrobials such as aminoglycosides, glycopeptides, antiretrovirals, and antifungals (Alshakrah et al., 2021; Geeson et al., 2019; Hickson et al., 2017; Martinbiancho et al., 2011; Roten et al., 2010), antidiabetic medicines including insulin (Alshakrah et al., 2021; Falconer et al., 2014; Hickson et al., 2017; Martinbiancho et al., 2011; Kaufmann et al., 2018), opioids (Alshakrah et al., 2021; Falconer et al., 2014; Hickson et al., 2017; Martinbiancho et al., 2011), and narrow therapeutic index medicines (Alshakrah et al., 2021; Hickson et al., 2017; Roten et al., 2010; Kaufmann et al., 2018). The Adult Complexity Tool for Pharmaceutical Care (ACTPC-2) contains the greatest number of prioritization criteria (n = 20) and was described by its authors as potentially the most comprehensive tool available when it was published in 2021 (Alshakrah et al., 2021).

Outside the tools described in detail above, other clinical prioritization tools have been reported that have a specialist clinical focus. The Adverse Inpatient Medication Event (AIME) is a risk prediction model for prioritization of hospitalized patients at risk of medication harm (Falconer et al., 2021). It is an important example of a clinical model that is continually reassessed to ensure it meets the needs of pharmacists and patients. The AIME tool was developed using clinical variables extracted from a hospital database (Falconer et al., 2021). That tool was later modified by the same research team to include frailty as a prioritization element and was developed into the modified AIME-Frail tool (Falconer et al., 2024). The inclusion of frailty in the tool was found to improve its predictive performance and differentiate it from the other tools described (Falconer et al., 2024).

TABLE 23.1 Characteristics of selected studies that describe the development of a clinical prioritization tool.

Reference	Design, setting & duration	Aim	Participants	Prioritization tool & type	Tool development	Perceived or actual tool outcome(s)	Tool validity	Tool limitations
Alshakrah et al., 2021, UK	Delphi method Online/phone Duration not reported	To obtain expert consensus on the design of a pharmacy screening tool	Delphi One: N = 33 (pharmacists, academics, physicians) Delphi Two: N = 40 (chief pharmacists, clinical pharmacists)	The Adult Complexity Tool for Pharmaceutical Care (ACTPC). Ranks patient acuity into three levels: red, amber, or green. Paper-based algorithm	Consensus methodology (pharmacists, academics, physicians)	May facilitate more patient-centered care, identify patients at greatest risk of drug-related problems, save pharmacy resources, and promote greater clinical involvement of pharmacy technicians	Not yet validated	Not validated in clinical settings
(Falconer et al., 2014), New Zealand	Eight-month prospective observational study in a New Zealand hospital	To develop a software-based tool to prioritize patients for initiatives to prevent adverse drug events	Adult inpatients (N = not reported)	The Assessment of Risk Tool (ART). Calculates risk scores to classify patients as low, medium, or high risk of adverse drug events. Electronic and fully automated for real-time ADE risk assessment	Literature review and consensus methodology (expert opinion – pharmacists)	Improved provision of medicines reconciliation and clinical review for high-risk patients, successfully targeted high-risk patients for discharge pharmacy services, and achieved a 1-hour daily time saving for pharmacists	Internal	Requires fully electronic patient medical records; no external validation.
(Geeson et al., 2019), UK	Prospective cohort study involving medical wards in two hospitals Two-month duration in each hospital	To develop a prognostic model to identify patients at high-risk of preventable, moderate-to-severe drug-related problems, and to assess its validity, feasibility, efficiency savings, and any potential risks	Adult inpatients (N = 1503)	The Medicines Optimization Assessment Tool (MOAT). Regression equation with 13 predictors that can be used to calculate the predicted risk of drug-related problems. Electronic pharmacists enter patient data on a Microsoft Excel® form	Multivariate logistic regression	Showed fair predictive performance and value in guiding decision-making; may positively impact pharmacist workload due to time savings from deprioritizing low-risk patients	Internal	No external validation is included and does not account for less commonly reported prioritization criteria, such as difficulty swallowing
(Hickson et al., 2017), UK	Quasiexperimental service evaluation in a 900-bed English teaching hospital; duration not reported	To design a pharmacy screening tool to help prioritize patient reviews and to assess pharmacist adherence to the tool	Random selection of adult inpatients (N = 35)	The Pharmaceutical Assessment Screening Tool (PAST). Ranks patient acuity into three levels, electronically recorded	Literature review and consensus methodology (expert opinion—pharmacists)	May identify those at greatest risk of developing adverse drug events and facilitate pharmacist prioritization	Not validated	Found to contain unused sections, not applicable to specialist areas, and not validated

Continued

TABLE 23.1 Characteristics of selected studies that describe the development of a clinical prioritization tool—cont'd

Reference	Design, setting & duration	Aim	Participants	Prioritization tool & type	Tool development	Perceived or actual tool outcome(s)	Tool validity	Tool limitations
(Kaufmann et al., 2018), Switzerland	Prospective validation study conducted within orthopedic geriatric, and internal medicine wards in two mid-sized hospitals (300–400 beds). Duration not reported	To develop and validate a self-assessment screening tool for completion by patients to help identify those at risk of drug-related problems	Adult inpatients N = 195: n = 164 in the initial study DART V1.0; and n = 31 in DART V2.0	Drug- Associated Risk Tool (DART). Questionnaire screening tool for use by patients to identify those at risk of drug-related problems. Paper-based	Literature review and consensus methodology (nominal group technique and Delphi study—pharmacists, physicians, and others). The 27 risk factors providing the basis for the DART were identified in an earlier study	Supports pharmacists in identifying patients who will benefit most from a pharmacy review, saves time and resources, and allows for patient involvement, which may reveal more drug-related problems	Internal and external	Reliant on patient involvement and the patient having a good understanding of the disease and medicines
(Martinbiancho et al., 2011), Brazil	Three-month prospective observational study in a 784-bed complex tertiary hospital	To build a tool to classify patients according to drug therapy risk and to optimize the use of pharmacy resources	Paediatric and adult inpatients (N = 1442)	Risk Score: Ssummation of risk scores to classify patients as high, moderate, or low risk. Paper-based	Literature review, univariate then multivariate analysis	May help to direct pharmacy resources, reduce adverse drug events, facilitate more rigorous patient monitoring, and improve patient care	Internal	Inclusion of intravenous medicines as a risk factor could result in a falsely high-risk score. The use of the score was limited in nonhigh-risk areas, and there was no external validation.
(Roten et al., 2010), Switzerland	A 3-month prospective observational comparative study was conducted in the general medical and geriatric wards of a multisite hospital	To develop and validate a screening tool for clinical pharmacists, comprising electronic queries, designed to identify inpatients at risk of drug-related problems	Adult inpatients (N = 501)	Electronic queries. A screening tool consisting of six risk factors to help identify at-risk patients. Electronic screening of medical records.	Literature review and consensus methodology (expert opinion - pharmacists)	Helps to detect inpatients at risk of drug-related problems and assists clinical pharmacists in prioritizing medication reviews, thus optimizing their workload	Internal	Does not define a list of high-risk medicines and that may affect reproducibility. The tool may not identify all at-risk patients due to missing criteria in the electronic queries, such as disease information, No external validation.

TABLE 23.2 A summary of (i) disease-related, (ii) medication-related, and (iii) patient-related prioritization criteria included in selected clinical prioritization tools. Abbreviations: CCU, cardiac care unit; HDU, high dependency unit; ICU, intensive care unit.

	Alshakrah et al. (2021)	Falconer et al. (2014)	Geeson et al. (2019)	Hickson et al. (2017)	Kaufmann et al. (2018)	Martinbiancho et al. (2011)	Roten et al. (2010)
Disease-related criteria							
Specific conditions	•	•	•	•	•	•	
Disease status (stable vs. unstable)	•			•			
Number of comorbidities			•		•		
Renal or hepatic impairment	•	•	•		•	•	•
Organ transplant	•			•			
Palliative care	•						
Pain	•						
National Early Warning Score	•						
Swallowing difficulty, nil by mouth, enteral tube, total parenteral nutrition	•					•	
Immunosuppression						•	
Laboratory results	•	•	•				•
Recent hospital admission	•	•					
High-risk transfer (ICU, HDU, CCU)		•	•				
High-risk speciality		•					
Home intravenous medicine			•				
Medication-related criteria							
Takes medicines not prescribed					•		
Polypharmacy	•	•	•		•	•	•
High-risk medicines	•	•	•	•	•	•	•
Drug interactions	•						•
Admission with a drug-related problem	•						
Restricted antibiotics	•						
Intravenous antibiotics		•					•
Other intravenous medicines						•	•
Medicines requiring therapeutic drug monitoring	•	•	•	•			
High-cost medicines				•			
Time since last pharmacy review		•					
Patient-related criteria							
Age	•	•	•			•	•
Extremes of weight	•						
Medication allergy or history of adverse drug events	•		•		•		
Pregnant or breastfeeding	•						
Not registered with a general practitioner or primary care provider.		•					
Nonadherence		•					•
Language barrier		•			•		
Poor understanding					•		
Medicines management difficulties					•		

Clinical prioritization tools that focus on specific patient cohorts and ambulatory care settings have also been described. Doherty et al. described a data-driven approach to delivering specialist clinical pharmacist care to outpatients with diabetes or heart failure in a tertiary hospital (Doherty et al., 2024). This study used validated prioritization criteria based on 4000 cases, supplemented by clinical data, with the aim of identifying people at risk of clinical deterioration while awaiting an outpatient appointment (Doherty et al., 2024). People were reviewed based on an algorithm that assigned risk to each patient (Doherty et al., 2024). The application of the tool created a pragmatic clinic waiting list, where patients who were identified as having emerging risks could be prioritized and an appointment arranged (Doherty et al., 2024). At the time of writing, a tool developed or implemented using an artificial intelligence or machine learning approach has not been published; however, the work of Doherty and colleagues suggests that such an approach is feasible (Doherty et al., 2024)

A number of potential benefits associated with clinical prioritization tools have been reported, including improvements in patient safety and greater efficiency for pharmacy teams (Alshakrah et al., 2021; Falconer et al., 2014; Geeson et al., 2019; Hickson et al., 2017; Martinbiancho et al., 2011; Roten et al., 2010; Kaufmann et al., 2018). Clinical prioritization tools may enhance safety by detecting patients at risk of drug-related problems or medication errors (Alshakrah et al., 2021; Falconer et al., 2014; Geeson et al., 2019; Hickson et al., 2017; Roten et al., 2010; Kaufmann et al., 2018) and by ensuring that complex patients are reviewed by a suitably experienced pharmacist at appropriate time intervals (Alshakrah et al., 2021; Hickson et al., 2017; Martinbiancho et al., 2011). These tools may also optimize workflow through ease of use (Falconer et al., 2014), de-prioritization of low-risk patients (Geeson et al., 2019), and the allocation of low-risk patients to suitably trained pharmacy technicians (Alshakrah et al., 2021). They may also play a role in training and supporting new or junior members of staff (Alshakrah et al., 2021). By these means, time and resource savings are possible for pharmacy departments. Indeed, Falconer et al. demonstrated a mean time saving of one hour per day of pharmacists' time as a result of using their fully automated clinical prioritization tool (Falconer et al., 2014).

Given the potential benefits of clinical prioritization tools, the development and implementation of such a tool are of interest to pharmacists working in clinical settings. This chapter will explore the methodology associated with the development of a clinical prioritization tool for use in a hospital pharmacy department and use a case study to demonstrate one approach to developing and implementing such a tool.

2 Methods

This methods section is informed by the development and testing of a clinical prioritization tool conducted by Clarke and colleagues in a large academic hospital, with reference to the broader literature on clinical prioritization tools (Clarke et al., 2023).

2.1 Study design

In the development of a clinical prioritization tool, Clarke et al. (2023) designed a study comprising two parts. Part 1 consisted of an anonymous cross-sectional survey of clinical pharmacists in one hospital, designed to evaluate existing methods used by those pharmacists for clinical prioritization. The results of this survey led to the development of a new clinical prioritization tool. Part 2 involved a preintervention and postintervention study that was conducted to assess the impact of the newly developed clinical prioritization tool on pharmacist activity and to evaluate pharmacist satisfaction with the tool.

2.2 Identifying clinical prioritization criteria

Criteria to be included in a clinical prioritization tool may be identified through a literature review, engagement with pharmacists in the setting where the tool will be used, adaptation of an existing clinical prioritization tool, or a combination of these approaches. Clarke et al. (2023) surveyed clinical pharmacists in their setting using a questionnaire based on a previously published instrument (Falconer et al., 2019) that was adapted to account for the needs of the clinical research setting. Expert peer review was conducted by the study team, all of whom were pharmacists, and a draft survey was piloted among 10% of clinical pharmacists in the study hospital to ensure face and content validity. The final questionnaire consisted of fifteen quantitative questions related to clinical prioritization criteria, two qualitative questions to gather opinions and ideas regarding clinical prioritization, and three demographic questions. The survey was completed exclusively by pharmacists. The results of this survey were then used to support the development of a clinical prioritization tool, which included an algorithm and an upgraded electronic health record (EHR) in the study setting. In the development of clinical prioritization tools, other researchers have incorporated a literature search to identify key prioritization criteria as part of tool development (Falconer et al., 2014; Hickson et al., 2017; Martinbiancho et al., 2011; Roten et al., 2010; Kaufmann et al., 2015).

2.3 Development of a clinical prioritization

The prioritization tool developed by Clarke et al. consisted of an algorithm designed to guide pharmacists in assessing and assigning patient priority levels (Clarke et al., 2023). The tool was designed with reference to the pharmacist survey and ACTPC-2 (Alshakrah et al., 2021). The ACTPC-2 was chosen as it was considered the most comprehensive and relevant tool for the study setting, though it was too detailed for the needs of the study hospital to be implemented in its entirety. Survey results and peer reviews from experienced and managerial-level pharmacists, as well as medication safety pharmacists in the study setting, led to the modification and refinement of the tool to produce the final version.

Criteria included in the tool should be predefined. The presence of polypharmacy is a key criterion included in many clinical prioritization tools; however, the term is defined differently across various tools, with Kaufmann et al. (2018) using a >5 medicines cut-off and Alshakrah et al. (2021) using a level of ≥15 medicines. Age is another common criterion included in clinical prioritization tools and is defined differently in different tools, with some using a definition of older age as ≥65 years (Falconer et al., 2014; Martinbiancho et al., 2011) and others using a definition of ≥80 years (Roten et al., 2010). Polypharmacy and older age were defined by Clarke et al. (2023) based on the results of the study survey. Other criteria frequently included in clinical prioritization tools and requiring definition include renal impairment, hepatic impairment, and a list of high-risk medicines.

When the final list of prioritization criteria is agreed upon, the method of patient prioritization should be decided. Alshakrah et al. prioritized patients using an algorithm, color-coding them into red, amber, or green categories (Alshakrah et al., 2021) whereas Hickson et al. assigned a patient acuity level of 1, 2, or 3 to signify high, moderate, or low risk, respectively (Hickson et al., 2017). Clarke et al. also employed a three-level approach, where high-risk medicines, drug-drug or drug-disease interactions with adverse effects, abnormal laboratory results relating to medication, certain disease states, and specific patient factors were classified as Level 1 or high priority (see Fig. 23.1) (Clarke et al., 2023). Some studies use a cumulative score or regression calculation to assign a risk category of high, moderate, or low (Falconer et al., 2014; Geeson et al., 2019; Martinbiancho et al., 2011) while others identify a defined

Priority Level	Prioritisation Criteria	Action
1 Highly complex patient or acute / unstable condition	• Patient in an unstable condition and has a chronic disease (e.g. Parkinson's, epilepsy, HIV, tuberculosis, porphyria) • Unstable acute condition (e.g. non-ST-elevation myocardial infarction, ST-elevation myocardial infarction, acute decompensated heart failure, thyroid crisis) • Acute serious infection (e.g. meningitis, sepsis, endocarditis) • Unstable renal/hepatic impairment • Pregnant or breastfeeding • Organ transplant • Polypharmacy (≥ 10 meds) ***with*** complex regimens (e.g. drug-drug / drug disease interaction) • Drug-drug or drug disease interaction(s) ***with*** toxic or sub-therapeutic effect • High risk medicines • Medicines requiring therapeutic drug monitoring with toxic/sub-therapeutic effect • Admission due to adverse drug reaction or medication error • Abnormal labs affecting medication • New intensive care unit step-down	Priority for review Review every 24 – 48 hours (Monday – Friday)
2 Moderately complex patient	• Stable and/or chronic disease (e.g. chronic kidney disease, chronic lung disease, Parkinson's disease, epilepsy, ischaemic heart disease, chronic heart failure, HIV) • Age ≥ 65 years (excluding MedEI wards) • Bodyweight very low (< 50 kg) or high (> 100 kg) • History of severe medication allergy • Recent admission (within one month) • Swallow issues, medicines by enteral feeding tube, *nil per os* • Polypharmacy (≥ 10 meds) without complex regimen (e.g. drug-drug or drug-disease interaction) • Newly prescribed/restricted antimicrobial • Palliative care patient • Drug-drug or drug-disease interaction ***without*** toxic or sub-therapeutic effect • Medicines requiring therapeutic drug monitoring ***without*** toxic or sub-therapeutic effect • Abnormal laboratory results ***not*** relating to or affecting medication(s)	Review after Level 1 patients Review every 48 – 72 hours (Monday – Friday)
3 Stable, non-acute patient	• No Level 1 or Level 2 criteria met	Review after Level 2 patients if time permits Review 1 – 2 times weekly (Monday – Friday)

FIG. 23.1 Clinical prioritization tool developed based on a survey of clinical pharmacists. *Modified from Clarke, R., Colleran, M., Melanophy, G., Bermingham, M., 2023. Enhancing the clinical pharmacy service of a large teaching hospital: development of a new clinical prioritisation tool. Explor. Res. Clin. Soc. Pharm. 26672766. 12, 100335. https://doi.org/10.1016/j.rcsop.2023.100335*

number of key risk factors for drug-related problems, which may be used to highlight high-risk patients for pharmacy review (Kaufmann et al., 2018; Roten et al., 2010).

2.4 Electronic versus paper-based clinical prioritization tools

Several studies have reported using paper-based clinical prioritization tools (Alshakrah et al., 2021; Kaufmann et al., 2018; Martinbiancho et al., 2011); however, the majority of reported tools are electronic or are integrated into an EHR. The choice of paper-based versus electronic clinical prioritization tools is influenced by the study setting and the resources available to the study team. Designing a tool that will seamlessly integrate into an existing EHR, having access to personnel with the skills to integrate the tool, and ensuring that the prioritization data for each patient can be accessed through the existing EHR will facilitate that integration.

2.5 Implementation and testing of the clinical prioritization tool

Prior to the initial testing of the clinical prioritization tool, a pilot should be undertaken to ensure that it is relevant and efficient to use in practice. Once piloting is complete, a study to assess the effectiveness of the tool can be undertaken. Clarke et al. (2023) conducted a preintervention and postintervention study to test the prioritization tool. Each phase consisted of 5 days of data collection over a 2-week period. Purposive sampling was used to identify ten pharmacists to take part in the preintervention and postintervention study. Five senior pharmacists and five basic-grade pharmacists working in different clinical specialties were invited to take part. This was to ensure that testing of the tool was conducted in a diverse and representative sample of the wider clinical pharmacy department.

Data collection forms were designed through peer review to capture desired information on pharmacists' clinical workflow during the intervention study. The preintervention data collection form captured information including (1) time spent on clinical prioritization on that day, (2) each pharmacist's level of satisfaction with clinical prioritization activities, and (3) the reasons why they chose to prioritize a patient using an alphabetized list of options provided. This list was modeled on the criteria within the final prioritization tool. A comments box was offered for pharmacists to note any other information of relevance on each day of the intervention study. Quantitative data collected included the number of medicines reconciliations and clinical reviews completed, the order in which patients were reviewed, and the time spent on clinical prioritization each day. Pharmacists recorded a priority level of 1, 2, or 3 for each patient reviewed. In this case, Level 1 was the highest priority level, Level 2 was moderate priority, and Level 3 was low priority. The post-intervention data collection form included all information captured by the preintervention form. In addition, on the post-intervention form, pharmacists were asked if the tool helped their clinical prioritization decisions.

Several studies have tested the agreement between the clinical prioritization tool and pharmacist judgment (Hickson et al., 2017; Martinbiancho et al., 2011; Roten et al., 2010). Roten et al. (2010) developed and validated a screening tool consisting of electronic queries within an EHR to identify and generate a list of patients deemed to be at risk of drug-related problems and requiring pharmacist review. Hickson et al. (2017) categorized patients according to a patient acuity level, the results of which were then recorded electronically to facilitate prioritization of patients at the highest risk of an adverse drug event. Like Roten et al., the aim was to quantify the agreement between the pharmacist-documented patient acuity level and the expected patient acuity level, as determined by the tool (Hickson et al., 2017; Roten et al., 2010).

2.6 Assessing the validity of the tool

Some studies have assessed the internal validation of their tools by evaluating sensitivity and specificity or by employing statistical methods such as bootstrap sampling, as demonstrated in the reporting of the Medicines Optimization Assessment Tool (Geeson et al., 2019; Kaufmann et al., 2018; Martinbiancho et al., 2011; Roten et al., 2010). In some cases, the internal validity of the tool was assessed in a separate study from the initial tool development study—for example, the Assessment of Risk Tool (Falconer et al., 2017)—or was externally validated, such as the Drug Associated Risk Tool (Stämpfli et al., 2018).

Roten et al. developed and validated a tool consisting of electronic queries within an EHR to identify and generate a list of patients deemed to be at risk of drug-related problems and requiring pharmacist review (Roten et al., 2010). Hickson et al. (2017) categorized patients according to a patient acuity level, the result of which was then recorded electronically to facilitate prioritization of patients at the highest risk of an adverse drug event. Like Roten et al., the aim was to quantify agreement between the pharmacist-documented patient acuity level and the expected patient acuity level determined by the tool (Hickson et al., 2017; Roten et al., 2010).

2.7 Data analysis

Statistical analysis may be required to support the assessment of the clinical prioritization tool. Consideration should be given to the need for statistical expertise among the study team prior to the initiation of the study.

3 Case study

This case study describes the development and testing of a clinical prioritization tool designed for use in the Pharmacy department of a large academic hospital. The process involved four steps:

- A survey of clinical pharmacists was conducted to identify their current approaches to clinical prioritization and the key patient factors they currently use to prioritize in their work.
- Development of a clinical prioritization tool, based on the results of a survey of clinical pharmacists. This tool was then integrated into the Electronic Patient Medication Administration Record (EMPAR).
- A preintervention and postintervention assessment of the impact of the tool on pharmacist prioritization activities and outcomes was conducted.
- An assessment of pharmacists' satisfaction with the tool.

3.1 Survey of clinical pharmacists

Survey respondents identified medicines reconciliation tasks, high-risk medicines, unverified medicines not yet reviewed by a pharmacist, pharmacist notes, and the prescription of antimicrobials as the most important features of the pharmacy care organizer. Methadone, insulin, systemic anticancer therapy, medication for Parkinson's disease, and clozapine were considered the highest-risk medications, and pharmacists also considered antiepileptic drugs, anticoagulants, and antimicrobials to be high-risk medication classes in their practice. Pharmacists identified acute and chronic kidney disease, infection, neurological disorders, and unstable illness as key disease states requiring clinical prioritization, while pregnancy and breastfeeding, drug misuse, poor historian, suspected nonadherence, and recent hospitalization were identified as key social factors. Table 23.3.

3.2 Development of clinical prioritization tool

A clinical prioritization tool was designed based on the outcomes of the survey. The clinical prioritization tool categorized patients into three levels: Level 1, highly complex or unstable patient; Level 2, moderately complex patient; and Level 3, stable or nonacute patient (Fig. 23.1). Each level is defined by prioritization criteria and specifies the ideal frequency of pharmacist review. The footnote emphasizes that a patient's priority level may change, duties such as patient education or medicines information queries must also be completed daily, and that the tool does not replace clinical judgment. The pharmacy care organizer was upgraded to incorporate the new tool in a *Clinical Pharmacy Review* column, which displays a patient's assigned priority level. Two new tasks were added to the pharmacy care organizer: (1) a *Clinical Pharmacy Review* task through which a pharmacist can view the clinical prioritization tool and assign the patient priority level, and (2) the *Critical Care Step-down* task that highlights patients transferred from the Intensive Care Unit to a general ward.

3.3 Preintervention and postintervention study

Preintervention, over a 5-day period, pharmacists reviewed 531 patients and conducted 168 medicine reconciliations. Post-intervention, over a 5-day period, pharmacists reviewed 516 patients and conducted 159 medicine reconciliations (Fig. 23.2). There was a statistically significant increase in the number of Level 1 patients reviewed preintervention compared to postintervention (220 patients versus 238 patients, $P < .05$).

Post-intervention, basic-grade pharmacists reviewed 222 patients. Their assigned priority levels matched those of the researcher (a pharmacist) in 188 (84.7%) cases (substantial $\kappa = 0.652$, $P < .001$). Senior pharmacists reviewed 319 patients, and their assigned priority levels matched those of the researcher in 212 (66.5%) cases (moderate $\kappa = 0.427$, $P < .001$). The sensitivity of the tool for each priority level was also determined using the pharmacist-assigned levels as the reference standard.

Among basic-grade pharmacists, the greatest number of disagreements between the clinical prioritization tool and pharmacist-assigned priority levels involved patients aged ≥ 65 years ($n = 19$, 35.8% of cases), while for senior pharmacists, the greatest disagreement occurred in patients with serious acute infections ($n = 57$, 50.4%).

TABLE 23.3 Top clinical prioritization criteria and subcriteria identified by pharmacists participating in the study.

Criteria	Subcriteria	Positive response (%)
Top five features of the Pharmacy Care Organizer that help you prioritize patients	Medicines reconciliation task	89
	High risk medicines	78
	Unverified medicines	78
	Pharmacist notes	70
	Antimicrobials	59
Top five high-risk medications or classes of medications	Methadone	89
	Insulin	86
	Systemic anticancer therapy	81
	Carbidopa/levodopa (± entacapone), co-beneldopa	81
	Clozapine	76
Top five medications or medication classes you consider high-risk	Parkinson's disease medications	89
	Insulin	73
	Antiepileptics	70
	Anticoagulants	68
	Antimicrobials	68
	Systemic anticancer therapy	68
What number of unverified medicines would you consider high-risk?	> 5 unverified medicines	32
Do you prioritize patients when you identify a drug-drug or drug-disease interaction with a suspected toxic or subtherapeutic effect?	Yes, prioritize	95
Do you prioritize patients when you identify a drug-drug or drug-disease interaction, even if there is no suspected toxic or subtherapeutic effect?	No, do not prioritize	60
What degree of polypharmacy do you consider a high priority?	> 10 medicines	46
What number of comorbidities would you consider a high priority?	No, do not prioritize	57
Top five conditions that you consider a high priority	Acute kidney injury	81
	Infection	57
	Chronic kidney disease (eGFR < 30 mL/min)	43
	Neurological disorders	43
	Any unstable disease	43
Do you prioritize your patient for review if they have abnormal lab results related to or affecting their medication?	Yes, prioritize	97
Do you prioritize your patient for review if they have abnormal lab results not related to or affecting medication?	Yes, prioritize	51
Do you prioritize a patient for review if they have transferred to your ward from the Intensive Care Unit or High Dependency Unit?	Yes, prioritize	97
At what age threshold would you prioritize an older adult?	≥ 65 years old	41
Top five patient-related or social risk factors that you consider high-priority	Pregnancy and/or breastfeeding	92
	Drug misuser	84
	Poor historian/confused	81
	Suspected nonadherence	65
	Recent hospitalization (readmission within 30 days of discharge)	51

Reproduced with permission from Clarke, R., Colleran, M., Melanophy, G., Bermingham, M., 2023. Enhancing the clinical pharmacy service of a large teaching hospital: development of a new clinical prioritisation tool. Explor. Res. Clin. Soc. Pharm. 26672766. 12, 100335. https://doi.org/10.1016/j.rcsop.2023.100335

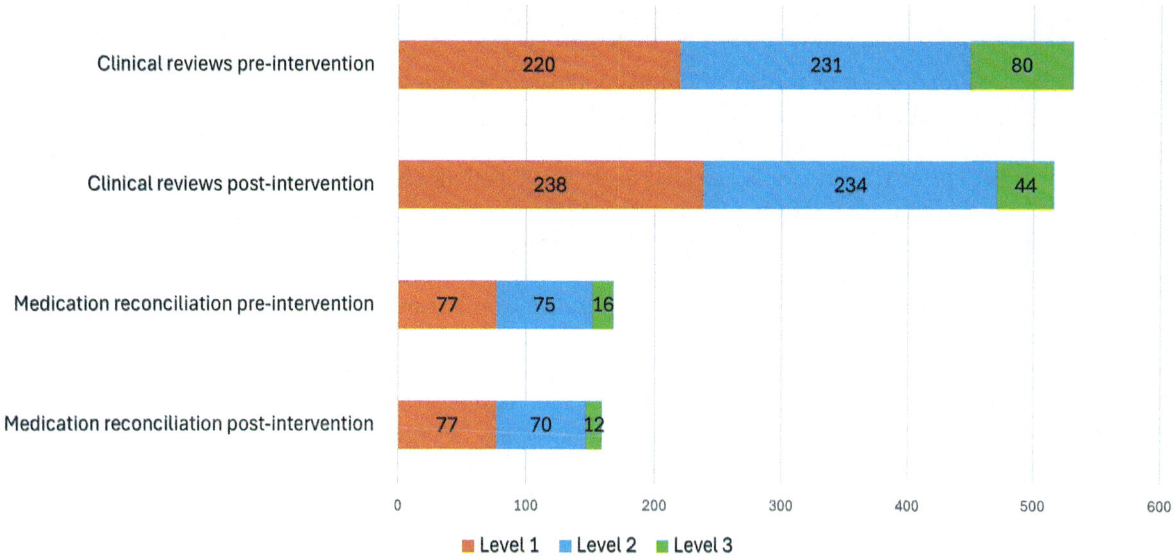

FIG. 23.2 Comparison of the number of medicine reconciliations and clinical reviews conducted by pharmacists preintervention and postimplementation of the clinical prioritization tool. *Modified from Clarke, R., Colleran, M., Melanophy, G., Bermingham, M., 2023. Enhancing the clinical pharmacy service of a large teaching hospital: development of a new clinical prioritisation tool. Explor. Res. Clin. Soc. Pharm. 26672766. 12, 100335. https://doi.org/10.1016/j.rcsop.2023.100335*

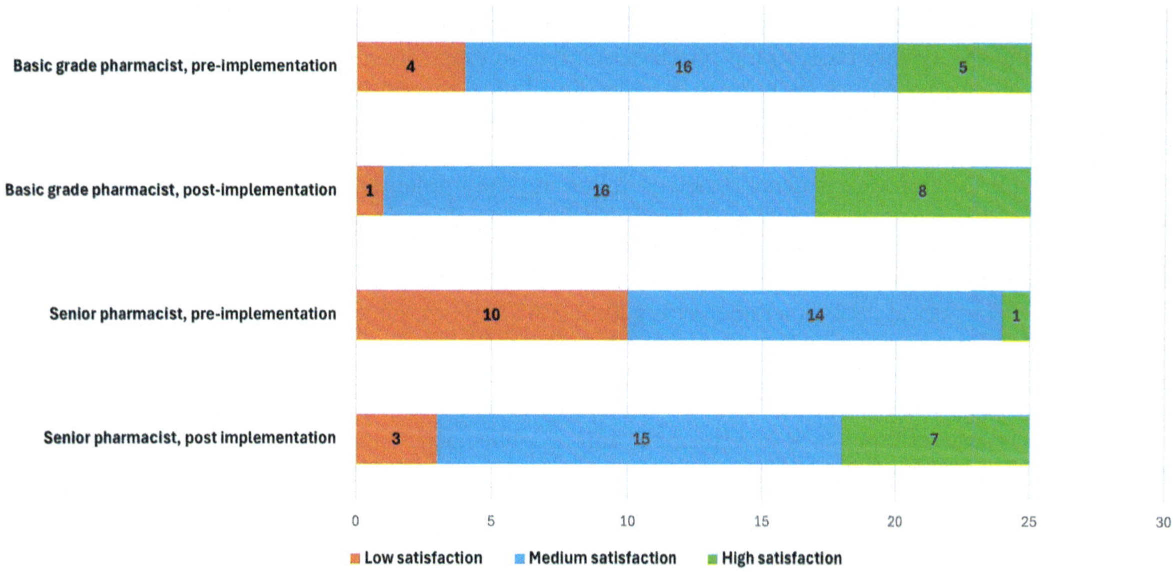

FIG. 23.3 Pharmacist satisfaction with their clinical prioritization activity during the preintervention and postimplementation study period. *Modified from Clarke, R., Colleran, M., Melanophy, G., Bermingham, M., 2023. Enhancing the clinical pharmacy service of a large teaching hospital: development of a new clinical prioritisation tool. Explor. Res. Clin. Soc. Pharm. 26672766. 12, 100335. https://doi.org/10.1016/j.rcsop.2023.100335*

The mean time spent on clinical prioritization each day was similar between basic grade and senior pharmacists, and there was no significant difference in the time spent preintervention or postintervention. Basic grade pharmacists spent 12.8 ± 1.3 minutes preintervention and 12.6 ± 1.5 minutes postintervention ($P = .85$), while senior pharmacists spent 15.4 ± 3.4 minutes preintervention and 12.4 ± 2.0 minutes postintervention ($P = .14$). Post-intervention, a mean time saving of 6.5 minutes per pharmacist per week was observed ($P = .63$).

3.4 Assessment of pharmacist satisfaction with the tool

Pharmacists recorded how satisfied they were with their clinical prioritization each day preintervention and postintervention (Fig. 23.3). Postintervention, the number of high levels of satisfaction recorded increased from 6 to 15, while the number of low ratings decreased from 14 to 4.

4 Discussion

Common criteria included in clinical prioritization tools, such as age ≥65 years and high-risk medicines, mirror known risk factors associated with medication-related harm and pharmaceutical interventions, as reported in a 2016 systematic review (Suggett and Marriott, 2016). Similar criteria were reported as the top-rated criteria identified in several reports of clinical prioritization tools (Alshakrah et al., 2021; Falconer et al., 2014; Geeson et al., 2019; Hickson et al., 2017; Martinbiancho et al., 2011; Roten et al., 2010; Kaufmann et al., 2018; Clarke et al., 2023) as well as those selected by a majority of respondents to a survey by Falconer et al. (2019). Specific target levels for clinical parameters were not included in some tools (Clarke et al., 2023) in order to maintain simplicity and to allow for individual clinical judgment. It is recommended that clinical prioritization tools should be concise in order to be practical and easy to use (da Costa et al., 2018).

Some tools described in the literature are paper-based or not automated (Alshakrah et al., 2021; Martinbiancho et al., 2011; Kaufmann et al., 2018) although the majority have been electronic to a greater or lesser extent (Falconer et al., 2014; Geeson et al., 2019; Hickson et al., 2017; Roten et al., 2010; Clarke et al., 2023). As the use of digital health records expands, ensuring that a clinical prioritization tool can be incorporated into an EHR is paramount. However, among the feedback received from pharmacists who took part in the study by Clarke et al. was the suggestion that pharmacists may prioritize patients based on criteria outside of the electronic clinical prioritization tool, such as referrals from other healthcare staff (Clarke et al., 2023). This feedback reinforces the concept that prioritization is multifactorial and that prioritization tools should support rather than replace clinical expertise (Falconer et al., 2019; Abuzour et al., 2021; Saxby et al., 2017). Furthermore, it is essential that healthcare systems investigate the role of artificial intelligence and machine learning in the identification of clinical prioritization criteria, the development of clinical prioritization tools, and the implementation of these tools.

In the evaluation of the clinical prioritization tool described by Clarke et al., there was a significant increase in high-priority patients clinically reviewed post-intervention compared to preintervention, with a greater increase in high-priority patients reviewed among basic grade pharmacists than among senior pharmacists (Clarke et al., 2023). One explanation is that senior pharmacists are more experienced in clinical prioritization and have established methods for prioritizing compared to basic grade pharmacists. These results suggest a more targeted delivery of pharmaceutical care through the use of a clinical prioritization tool, aligning with the findings of Falconer et al. (2014) who cited an increase in the number of high-risk patients reviewed following the implementation of the Assessment of Risk Tool. Furthermore, Geeson et al. have proposed that a reduction in low-priority patients being reviewed may lead to potential time and resource savings arising from the deprioritization of these low-risk patients (Geeson et al., 2019).

There was stronger agreement with the clinical prioritization tool developed by Clarke et al. compared with another instrument, the Pharmaceutical Assessment Screening Tool (PAST) (Hickson et al., 2017; Saxby et al., 2017). Hickson et al. (2017) calculated fair agreement when comparing patient-acuity levels assigned by the researchers applying the PAST versus those assigned by pharmacists (Hickson et al., 2017). Saxby et al. (2017) reported slight agreement between respondent pharmacists and the expected acuity levels based on the PAST. Both Hickson et al. (2017) and Saxby et al. (2017) concluded that a lack of agreement among pharmacists with the PAST warranted further review of the tool's prioritization criteria. Stronger agreement was reported by Clarke et al. (2023), and this may reflect the larger sample size and greater number of criteria (n = 25) in Clarke's tool compared to the PAST (n = 17), as well as the fact that these criteria are more clearly defined than those in the PAST (Clarke et al., 2023; Hickson et al., 2017).

Deviation between a clinical prioritization tool and the level of priority assigned by a pharmacist has been reported. Clarke et al. (2023) suggested that differing priority levels assigned for older-age patients may have arisen for reasons not documented by the pharmacist, such as unstable renal function, and this could have influenced the level assigned in this patient group. Other studies have explained deviations between prioritization tools and pharmacist agreement as being due to differences in pharmacists' perceptions of pharmaceutical complexity, their level of experience, and instances where a higher level was assigned than recommended by the tool to serve another purpose, such as a reminder to prioritize particular tasks (Hickson et al., 2017; Saxby et al., 2017). Ongoing review and modification of a clinical prioritization tool will ensure that it remains relevant and is applied consistently.

Roten et al. (2010) and Geeson et al. (2019) demonstrated tool sensitivity of 85.1% and 66%–90%, respectively, for the detection of drug-related problems. Sensitivity was prioritized over specificity by Clarke et al., who determined that the benefits of the tool in correctly categorizing patients outweighed the potential negative effects of including false positives (Clarke et al., 2023). Indeed, there are several examples in the literature where sensitivity may be prioritized over specificity when the goal is to identify patients with specific characteristics in a population (Chubak et al., 2012). Gaining consensus from all pharmacists on the clinical prioritization tool and its content is recommended and may enhance its sensitivity. Roten et al. (2010) concluded that refinement of the clinical prioritization criteria within their tool could yield a higher degree of sensitivity. Increasing the number of observations may also improve the reliability of sensitivity results.

The Assessment of Risk Tool reported one hour saved daily, or an 80% time saving relative to the time taken before tool implementation (Falconer et al., 2014), whereas Clarke et al. (2023) reported a time saving of just 6.5 minutes per pharmacist per week. The Assessment of Risk Tool is electronic, fully automated, and assigns priority levels without the need for pharmacist review, which may account for the differences reported. Additionally, the clinical prioritization tool assessed by Clarke was newly introduced to pharmacists for a five-day post-intervention study (Clarke et al., 2023). Pharmacists using the Assessment of Risk Tool familiarized themselves with the tool over an eight-month study period (Falconer et al., 2014). Therefore, time efficiencies may improve over time.

There are limitations and outstanding questions in the development and research of clinical prioritization tools. The tools reported in the literature have used an observational approach to assessing the tool's impact (Alshakrah et al., 2021; Clarke et al., 2023; Falconer et al., 2014; Geeson et al., 2019; Hickson et al., 2017; Martinbiancho et al., 2011; Roten et al., 2010; Kaufmann et al., 2018). Randomized controlled trials are the gold standard approach to assessing the clinical impact of any healthcare intervention and deliver robust methodology alongside definitive results. Therefore, assessing clinical prioritization tools in this way will provide a stronger evidence base for their use in clinical practice and potentially increase uptake of this formal approach to managing pharmacist clinical workload while optimizing patient care. The Assessment of Risk Tool demonstrated a quantifiable reduction in medication errors; however, the clinical benefits of many other tools have not yet been verified (Falconer et al., 2014). Therefore, assessment of the impact of clinical prioritization tools on patient outcomes, such as drug-related problems, adverse drug events, and length of hospital stay, remains outstanding. Alongside the assessment of patient outcomes and pharmacist workload, health economic evaluation must also be conducted on clinical prioritization tools to identify if, through impact on clinical outcomes, there is an economic benefit to the healthcare system. Again, it is necessary that robust clinical data are available in order to build reliable models for such research.

Assessing external validation is an essential step in developing a tool that can be used in a multisite study or clinically across several sites. Kaufmann et al. (2018) described a process of external validation for their Drug-Associated Risk Tool. However, the majority of tools published thus far lack external validation (Alshakrah et al., 2021; Falconer et al., 2014; Geeson et al., 2019; Hickson et al., 2017; Martinbiancho et al., 2011; Roten et al., 2010). Most tools, but not all, do include internal validation (Falconer et al., 2014; Geeson et al., 2019; Martinbiancho et al., 2011; Roten et al., 2010; Kaufmann et al., 2018). Aligned with this, most studies of clinical prioritization tools have been conducted in single sites, with only Geeson et al. (2019) and Kaufmann et al. (2015) applying their tool in two sites, and Roten et al. (2010) reporting data from a multisite hospital. Larger-scale studies and studies using a single clinical prioritization tool across multiple sites will help to identify if a clinical prioritization tool is standardizable across a health system or if a tool should be developed for individual hospitals.

In conclusion, clinical prioritization tools demonstrate several benefits to patient care and the delivery of clinical pharmacy services. They aim to optimize patient safety, pharmacist workload, and time management, as well as improve the allocation of hospital pharmacy resources through more targeted clinical reviews. Pharmacists who wish to implement a prioritization tool may be assured that the methodologies described here to develop and evaluate clinical prioritization tools have achieved these aims and can be adapted or further developed to better suit other contexts. It is essential that any clinical prioritization tool is current and meets the ongoing needs of patients and the health system in which it is used. This necessitates an ongoing review of the literature and stakeholder engagement to identify changes in the clinical landscape and emerging high-risk situations. Furthermore, qualitative and quantitative methods should be employed to obtain feedback from pharmacists who use the tool to continuously improve it and to identify any emerging issues.

5 Questions for further discussion

- What conditions in the changing landscape of healthcare might render the proposed tool even more useful or perhaps less useful in the years to come?

If you were designing a clinical prioritization tool, what key features would you include in your tool?
If you were evaluating a clinical prioritization tool, what outcome measures would you include in your evaluation?

- What are some things you might do upon developing a potentially successful or effective tool that was not greeted with favor among your clinical pharmacy staff?

6 Application exercise/scenario

Suppose you are a manager at a local hospital working on your PhD in health outcomes research at a nearby college or school of pharmacy. Hospital-level administrators have grappled with indecision about the pharmacy department's budget and staffing and have asked the department to provide ways to demonstrate its value. At the same time, you know that pharmacy services have been underutilized and that various outcomes, such as those associated with discharge planning and medication optimization, have been underwhelming. You decide to develop a clinical prioritization tool.

- How would you adapt an existing clinical prioritization tool to meet the needs of your scenario and setting?

You would like input from the pharmacists in the department regarding the design of the clinical prioritization tool. Describe how you would elicit their opinions and translate those into additional items for the tool.

- Once the clinical prioritization tool is developed, describe a process by which you would test it and how you would present these results to hospital administrators.

References

Abuzour, A.S., Hoad-Reddick, G., Shahid, M., Steinke, D.T., Tully, M.P., Williams, S.D., Lewis, P.J., 2021. Patient prioritisation for hospital pharmacy services: current approaches in the UK. Eur. J. Hosp. Pharm. 2047-9956. 28 (e1), e102. doi:10.1136/ejhpharm-2020-002365.

Alshakrah, M.A., Steinke, D.T., Tully, M.P., Abuzour, A.S., Williams, S.D., Lewis, P.J., 2021. Development of the adult complexity tool for pharmaceutical care (ACTPC) in hospital: a modified Delphi study. Res. Soc. Adm. Pharm. 15517411. 17 (11), 1907–1922. Available from: http://www.journals.elsevierhealth.com/periodicals/rsap. doi:10.1016/j.sapharm.2021.02.009.

Chubak, J., Pocobelli, G., Weiss, N.S., 2012. Tradeoffs between accuracy measures for electronic health care data algorithms. J. Clin. Epidemiol. 18785921. 65 (3), 343. Available from: https://www.elsevier.com/locate/jclinepi. doi:10.1016/j.jclinepi.2011.09.002.

Clarke, R., Colleran, M., Melanophy, G., Bermingham, M., 2023. Enhancing the clinical pharmacy service of a large teaching hospital: development of a new clinical prioritisation tool. Explor. Res. Clin. Soc. Pharm. 26672766. 12, 100335. doi:10.1016/j.rcsop.2023.100335.

da Costa, F.A., van Mil, J.W.F., Alvarez-Risco, A., 2018. The Pharmacist Guide to Implementing Pharmaceutical Care. Springer Science+Business Media, Portugal, pp. 1–506. Available from https://link.springer.com/book/10.1007/978-3-319-92576-9. doi:10.1007/978-3-319-92576-9.

Doherty, C., Campbell, G., French, O., Smith, A., Hodgkinson, A., Rajasingam, D., Webb, J., Karalliedde, J., 2024. A pharmacist-led, digital health informatics-based, insight-led care approach to aid clinical prioritization of people with diabetes and heart failure. Can. Pharm. J. (Ott. 1715-1635. 157 (6), 286–289. doi:10.1177/17151635241277547.

Falconer, N., Scott, I.A., Abdel-Hafez, A., Cottrell, N., Long, D., Morris, C., Snoswell, C., Aziz, E., Jie Lam, J.Y., Barras, M., 2024. The adverse inpatient medication event and frailty (AIME-frail) risk prediction model. Res. Soc. Adm. Pharm. 15517411. 20 (8), 796–803. Available from: https://www.sciencedirect.com/science/journal/15517411. doi:10.1016/j.sapharm.2024.05.003.

Falconer, N., Nand, S., Liow, D., Jackson, A., Seddon, M., 2014. Development of an electronic patient prioritization tool for clinical pharmacist interventions. Am. J. Health Syst. Pharm. 1079-2082. 71 (4), 311–320. doi:10.2146/ajhp130247.

Falconer, N., Liow, D., Zeng, I., Parsotam, N., Seddon, M., Nand, S., 2017. Validation of the assessment of risk tool: patient prioritisation technology for clinical pharmacist interventions. Eur. J. Hosp. Pharm. 2047-9956. 24 (6), 320–326. doi:10.1136/ejhpharm-2016-001165.

Falconer, N., Barras, M., Cottrell, N., 2019. How hospital pharmacists prioritise patients at high-risk for medication harm. Res. Soc. Adm. Pharm. 15517411. 15 (10), 1266–1273. doi:10.1016/j.sapharm.2018.11.003.

Falconer, N., Barras, M., Abdel-Hafez, A., Radburn, S., Cottrell, N., 2021. Development and validation of the adverse inpatient medication event model (AIME). Br. J. Clin. Pharmacol. 0306-5251. 87 (3), 1512–1524. doi:10.1111/bcp.14560.

Geeson, C., Wei, L., Franklin, B.D., 2019. Development and performance evaluation of the medicines optimisation assessment tool (MOAT): a prognostic model to target hospital pharmacists' input to prevent medication-related problems. BMJ Qual. Saf. 2044-5415. 28 (8), 645–656. doi:10.1136/bmjqs-2018-008335.

Hickson, R.P., Steinke, D.T., Skitterall, C., Williams, S.D., 2017. Evaluation of a pharmaceutical assessment screening tool to measure patient acuity and prioritise pharmaceutical care in a UK hospital. Eur. J. Hosp. Pharm. 20479964. 24 (2), 74–79. Available from: http://ejhp.bmj.com/content/by/year/2015. doi:10.1136/ejhpharm-2015-000829.

Kaufmann, C.P., Stämpfli, D., Mory, N., Hersberger, K.E., Lampert, M.L., 2018. Drug-Associated Risk Tool: development and validation of a self-assessment questionnaire to screen for hospitalised patients at risk for drug-related problems. BMJ Open. 2044-6055. 8 (3), e016610. doi:10.1136/bmjopen-2017-016610.

Kaufmann, C.P., Stämpfli, D., Hersberger, K.E., Lampert, M.L., 2015. Determination of risk factors for drug-related problems: a multidisciplinary triangulation process. BMJ Open. 20446055. 5 (3), 1–7. Available from: http://bmjopen.bmj.com/content/5/3/e006376full.pdf+html. doi:10.1136/bmjopen-2014-006376.

Lewis, P., 2017. Right patient, right time, right pharmacist: the time for clinical prioritisation tools? Eur. J. Hosp. Pharm. 2047-9956. 24 (6), 314. doi:10.1136/ejhpharm-2017-001395.

Lombardi, N., Wei, L., Ghaleb, M., Pasut, E., Leschiutta, S., Rossi, P., Troncon, M.G., 2018. Evaluation of the implementation of a clinical pharmacy service on an acute internal medicine ward in Italy. BMC Health Serv. Res. 1472-6963. 18 (1). doi:10.1186/s12913-018-2988-y.

Lord Carter of Coles, 2016. Operational Productivity and Performance in English NHS Acute Hospitals: Unwarranted Variations – An Independent Report for the Department of Health by Lord Carter of Coles. Department of Health London, United Kingdom. https://assets.publishing.service.gov.uk/government/uploads/system/uploads/attachment_data/file/499229/Operational_productivity_A.pdf.

Martinbiancho, J.K., Zuckermann, J., Mahmud, S.D.P., Dos Santos, L., Jacoby, T., da Silva, D., Vinhas, M., 2011. Development of risk score to hospitalized patients for clinical pharmacy rationalization in a high complexity hospital. Lat. Am. J. Pharm. 03262383. 30 (7), 1342–1347. Available from http://www.latamjpharm.org/trabajos/30/7/LAJOP_30_7_1_14_46565XP09J.pdf.

Osanlou, R., Walker, L., Hughes, D.A., Burnside, G., Pirmohamed, M., 2022. Adverse drug reactions, multimorbidity and polypharmacy: a prospective analysis of 1 month of medical admissions. BMJ Open. 2044-6055. 12 (7), e055551. doi:10.1136/bmjopen-2021-055551.

Pharmaceutical Society of Ireland. 2016. Future Pharmacy Practice in Ireland: Meeting Patients' Needs. https://www.psi.ie/information-and-resources/future-pharmacy-practice-ireland-meeting-patients-needs-report

Roten, I., Marty, S., Beney, J., 2010. Electronic screening of medical records to detect inpatients at risk of drug-related problems. Pharm. World Sci. 0928-1231. 32 (1), 103–107. doi:10.1007/s11096-009-9352-6.

Saxby, K.J.E., Murdoch, R., McGuinness, J., Steinke, D.T., Williams, S.D., 2017. Pharmacists' attitudes towards a pharmaceutical assessment screening tool to help prioritise pharmaceutical care in a UK hospital. Eur. J. Hosp. Pharm. 20479964. 24 (6), 315–319. Available from: http://ejhp.bmj.com/content/by/year/2015. doi:10.1136/ejhpharm-2016-001074.

Schindler, E., Richling, I., Rose, O., 2021. Pharmaceutical Care Network Europe (PCNE) drug-related problem classification version 9.00: german translation and validation. Int. J. Clin. Pharm. 2210-7703. 43 (3), 726–730. doi:10.1007/s11096-020-01150-w.

Spinewine, A., Dhillon, S., Mallet, L., Tulkens, P.M., Wilmotte, L., Swine, C., 2006. Implementation of ward-based clinical pharmacy services in Belgium-description of the impact on a geriatric unit. Ann. Pharmacother. 10600280. 40 (4), 720–728. doi:10.1345/aph.1G515.

Stämpfli, D., Boeni, F., Gerber, A., Bättig, V.A.D., Weidmann, R., Hersberger, K.E., Lampert, M.L., 2018. Assessing the ability of the drug-associated risk tool (DART) questionnaire to stratify hospitalised older patients according to their risk of drug-related problems: a cross-sectional validation study. BMJ Open. 2044-6055. 8 (6), e021284. doi:10.1136/bmjopen-2017-021284.

Suggett, E., Marriott, J., 2016. Risk factors associated with the requirement for pharmaceutical intervention in the hospital setting: a systematic review of the literature. Drugs Real World Outcomes. 2199-1154. 3 (3), 241–263. doi:10.1007/s40801-016-0083-4.

van Staa, T.P., Pirmohamed, M., Sharma, A., Ashcroft, D.M., Buchan, I., 2024. Adverse drug reactions and hospital admissions: large case-control study of patients aged 65–100 years using linked English primary care and hospital data. Pharmacoepidemiol. Drug Saf. 10991557. 33 (1). Available from: http://onlinelibrary.wiley.com/journal/10.1002/(ISSN)1099-1557. doi:10.1002/pds.5681.

CHAPTER

24

How can a behavioural economics lens contribute to deprescribing? Nudging taking fewer medicines

Nagham J. Ailabouni
The University of Queensland, Brisbane, QLD, Australia

CHAPTER OBJECTIVES

- To provide a broad overview of implementation science and behavioral economics
- To understand gaps in leveraging implementation science and behavioral economics in deprescribing research and practice
- To understand the value of using behavioral strategies to change behavior
- To outline avenues for the application of behavioral economics that can benefit the field of deprescribing
- To provide insights into the pros and cons of using behavioral economics in the field of deprescribing
- To discuss emerging future directions related to behavioral economics in deprescribing

1 Introduction

Changing the behavior of clinicians, prescribers, consumers, and organizations is key to addressing various global health challenges (Johnson and May, 2015; Grimshaw et al., 2012). However, changing and sustaining health behavior remains one of the most challenging goals to achieve (Chisholm et al., 2012). Think about the last time you made a commitment to change your behavior. Perhaps this involved setting a New Year's resolution or goal list, modifying your diet or lifestyle, or changing another long-standing habit. Despite your best intentions to make a positive change to improve your health or mindset, implementing the new desired behavior in your everyday life would have required making intensive, intentional, long-term changes. This includes breaking habits, introducing new resources, making different choices, and sometimes changing the structure of your life, including where you live or work. This may have discouraged you from committing to the new desired goal.

Contemporary Research Methods in Pharmacy and Health Services - Volume 2
https://doi.org/10.1016/B978-0-443-44607-8.00026-1

Similarly, changing behavior of key stakeholders to optimize medicine use can be challenging to implement in practice (Ailabouni et al., 2016a, 2024b; Ailabouni et al., 2022). Despite increased awareness related to medicine-related harm as a global health challenge, and research initiatives or programs to address this challenge worldwide, inappropriate medicine use remains highly prevalent (World Health Organization, n.d.). Potentially inappropriate medicines are medicines that may cause more harm than potential benefit (Zullo et al., 2018; Ailabouni et al., 2019). Deprescribing, the process of reducing or stopping potentially inappropriate medicines, is a component of optimizing medicine use (Scott et al., 2015). Optimizing medicine use may also involve prescribing medicines of therapeutic benefit that are not currently being taken by the patient (Ailabouni et al., 2021, 2019; Ailabouni et al., 2019).

Despite evidence that deprescribing is both feasible and safe, implementing deprescribing recommendations in practice remains challenging (Ailabouni et al., 2025b, 2022b). This has been partially explained by the underutilization of implementation science concepts in the field of deprescribing, which could limit sustained changes in behavior to improve medicine use (Ailabouni et al., 2022b; Baumgartner et al., 2020).

Implementation science emerged to close the gap between research and practice, or, in other words, to change the behavior of key stakeholders such as clinicians, consumers, healthcare institutions, and governmental bodies (Bauer et al., 2015). Implementation science has achieved landmark milestones in exploring and uncovering contextual determinants (barriers and facilitators) of interventions, conceptual implementation science frameworks, theories, and models, and testing the comparative effectiveness of implementation strategies (Chambers and Emmons, 2024). Despite this, the scalability and maintenance of implementation strategies outside of research environments, particularly those associated with high costs in certain contexts, have been limited in practice.

Successful deprescribing heavily depends on intentionally implementing strategies, often involving multiple components, within a multidisciplinary team, all whilst gaining buy-in from the consumer who is willing to take fewer medicines (Scott et al., 2015). Therefore, leveraging implementation science concepts may also improve the uptake of deprescribing recommendations in practice. A 2022 commentary highlighted that the deprescribing research field may benefit from leveraging implementation science to advance three main avenues (Ailabouni et al., 2022b). These include:

1. Define, differentiate, and apply the concepts of *"evidence-based intervention"* and *"implementation strategy"* in the field of deprescribing
2. Understand the importance of context and describe the contextual determinants at play by using implementation science determinant frameworks
3. Specify and evaluate deprescribing implementation outcomes according to existing typologies

Only considering the above avenues to intentionally design effective implementation strategies, however, may only be scratching the surface of improving the translation of deprescribing in practice (Hodson et al., 2024). In this chapter, a fourth additional avenue is proposed, which relates to applying behavioral economics in the field of deprescribing.

Behavioral economics is a field that could address this gap and enhance the implementation of deprescribing (Thaler and Sunstein, 2008). First developed in the mid-20th century, behavioral economics combines insights from psychology and economics to understand how people make decisions and why they behave the way they do in real-world settings (Heukelom, 2014). Behavioral economics has captured the attention of governments and policymakers, who have incorporated behavioral economic insights into various policy designs. Specific concepts of behavioral economics (Thaler and Sunstein, 2008) have been applied to support vaccine promotion and screening for medical conditions (Lucas et al., 2023), such as prostate cancer, by, for example, changing default options so people are automatically screened. In addition, these concepts have been applied to change prescribing or deprescribing behavior (Kullgren et al., 2024) by screening for potentially inappropriate medicine use, for example. Nevertheless, behavioral economic concepts and strategies remain underutilized in the field of deprescribing, offering opportunities for deprescribing research and translation into practice.

Behavioral economics could provide latitude to strengthen the translational impact of deprescribing research and improve deprescribing implementation in practice (Hodson et al., 2024). Given that deprescribing could be strengthened by applying implementation science concepts (Ailabouni et al., 2022b), and implementation science could leverage behavioral economics to increase its translation and impact, the potential value of leveraging behavioral economics could be extended to the field of deprescribing. This is because understanding how people behave and make choices can be pivotal in designing effective strategies that increase the uptake and translation of deprescribing (Kao and Velupillai, 2015).

To date, there is a paucity of literature regarding the use of behavioral economics in the field of deprescribing, in both research and practice contexts. Some research programs have specifically explored using behavioral economics to discourage the use and/or initiation of opioids after sharing with clinicians the number of their patients' deaths (Doctor et al., 2018). In addition, behavioral economics has been used to explore discontinuing low-value care among older people. However, a gap exists related to leveraging behavioral economics concepts and using their full potential in the field of deprescribing.

This book chapter explores leveraging the science of behavioral economics in the field of deprescribing. It explains behavioral economic concepts and suggests behavioral theory strategies that may enhance deprescribing research, facilitate the implementation of deprescribing recommendations in practice, and trigger reforms in health policies to drive and sustain deprescribing efforts.

2 Methods

2.1 Terminology

In implementation science, an interplay exists between three key independent variables, which include the *evidence-based clinical intervention*, the *implementation strategy*, and the *context* (Kemp et al., 2019). It has been recognized that, currently, in the field of deprescribing, studies do not define these three independent variables and that these terms have been variably applied in the deprescribing field (Ailabouni et al., 2022b) with some studies referring to *implementation strategies* (e.g., medicine reviews) as the *intervention*. This makes it challenging to synthesize findings across deprescribing studies.

This chapter will discuss implementation strategies dervied from behavioral economics. Therefore, understanding the definitions of certain terms related to implementation science concepts, such as *intervention* and *implementation strategy*, is important. To increase clarity, a general example (exercising) is used to describe the definition of these terms. These terms are also described in the context of the deprescribing process (Fig. 24.1), which includes(Curran, 2020):

- The *evidence-based clinical intervention* refers to the specific practice, program, or action that is intended to produce a desired health or service outcome (Curran, 2020). For example, exercise or the act of deprescribing itself—that is, stopping or reducing unnecessary or potentially harmful medicines to improve patient outcomes.
- *Effectiveness research* evaluates the outcomes of interventions in real-world settings (e.g., a drop in fat percentage; a reduction in the average number of medications) (Curran, 2020).

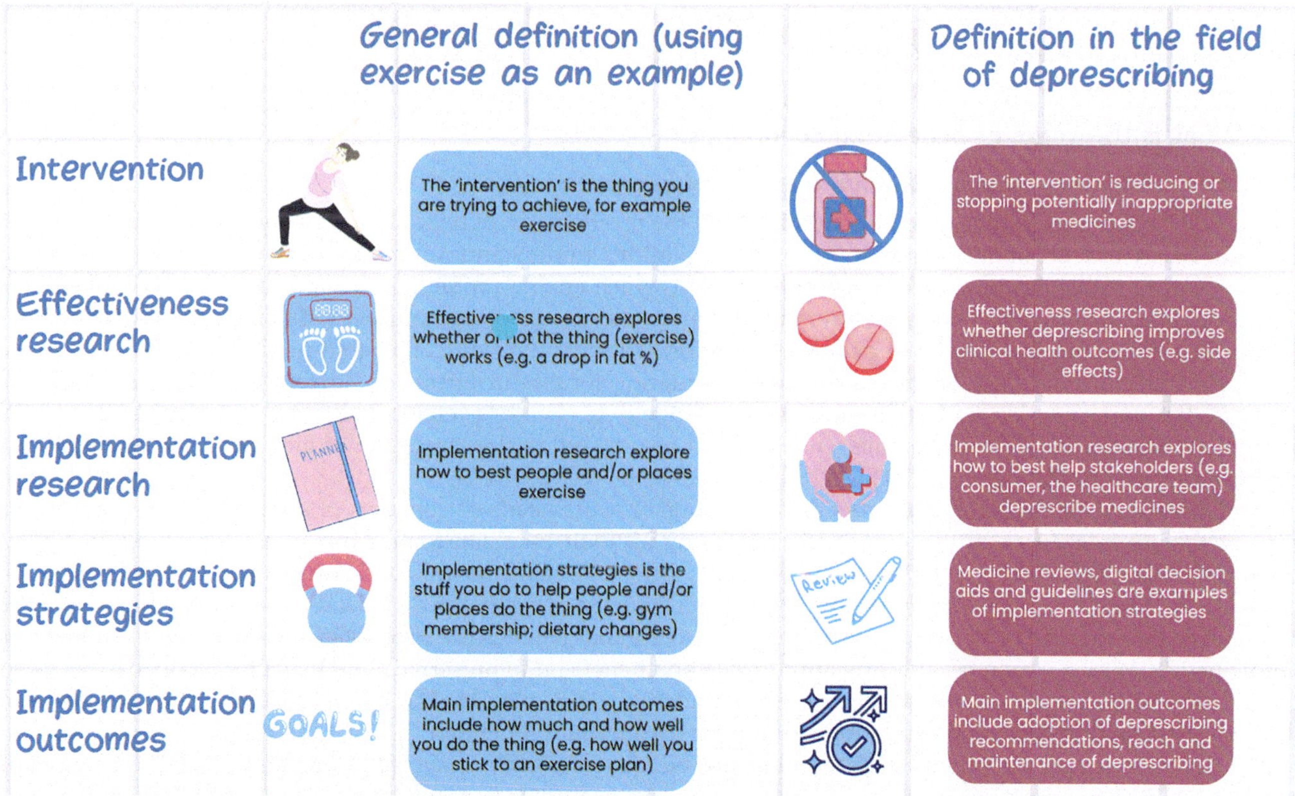

FIG. 24.1 Implementation science concepts: an example in the field of exercise.

- *Implementation research* is the scientific study of methods to promote the uptake of research findings into routine healthcare in clinical, organizational or policy settings (Curran, 2020).
- The *implementation strategy* is defined as a specific approach or combination of approaches that aids in translating or achieving a specific evidence-based intervention in a real-world setting. Examples of these strategies include using patient empowerment brochures, pharmacist-led medicine reviews, or roundtable multidisciplinary discussions to support the process of shared decision-making about medicines. Implementation strategies may specifically incorporate health behavioral theories to utilize behavioral economic concepts (Curran, 2020).
- *Implementation outcomes* are the effects of deliberate and purposive actions to implement new treatments, practices, and services (e.g., fidelity: how well a person sticks to an exercise plan; how closely a deprescribing plan is followed). These are distinct from clinical treatment or service system outcomes (Proctor et al., 2011).

2.2 Behavioral economics strategies to implement change

Choice architecture is a term used by behavioral economists to describe the ecosystem that influences a person's ability to make decisions (Thaler and Sunstein, 2008). It includes the way choices are presented or structured, which can influence the decisions that people make without taking away their freedom to choose (Johnson et al., 2012).

Behavioral economics changes the architecture of a person's choices. By acknowledging the role of the environment, social factors, and cognitive factors that may influence behaviors, strategies that leverage behavioral economic concepts may change choice architecture. Examples of such behavioral strategies include *nudging*, which involves subtly designing processes so that making the desired choice becomes more natural (Thaler and Sunstein, 2008). For example, setting an automatic medicine review reminder in the electronic medical record may prompt clinicians to review and rationalize medicine use.

De-sludging is another example, which involves removing unnecessary frictions or barriers that may otherwise provide roadblocks and prevent people from making better choices (Hodson, 2023). An example of this could be streamlining the process of deprescribing in the clinical workflow by integrating automatic discontinuation dates for medicines and using fewer paper forms to reduce the cognitive load on clinicians. *Social-norm feedback* can also be a valuable strategy that deliberately drives the uptake of medicine reviews and/or deprescribing in practice (Ivers et al., 2012). This has been applied to improve antibiotic prescribing (Zeng et al., 2023). Other examples include utilizing *opt-out designs*, incentives, and *choice bundling*, where less desirable behaviors are followed by desirable behaviors (i.e., rewards) to encourage follow-through (Ashe and Wilson, 2020).

2.3 What is the value of behavioral economics?

2.3.1 *Understanding human behavior, biases, and heuristics*

The key to changing behavior is to first understand the mechanisms of behavior and why people behave the way they do. Behavioral economics can help individuals gain this understanding in a more practical and realistic way. Biases, or predictable thinking patterns, and heuristics, which enable problem-solving or decision-making, impact the way we make decisions and, therefore, can influence various aspects of our everyday lives (Kahneman, 2011). *Present bias*, for example, means that people often prioritize short-term outcomes that provide immediate pleasure or satisfaction over delayed gratification when considering long-term effects or outcomes. Choosing a quick-fix extreme diet versus making a long-term lifestyle change (e.g., steady exercise, balanced nutrition, gradual habit formation) may provide the immediate reward of fast results, but in the long-term, it may not be as sustainable as the latter approach (Kahneman, 2011).

Similarly, some clinicians may address the immediate or acute needs or concerns of their patients by prescribing new medicines instead of, at the same time, reviewing all their medicines and rationalizing their use to achieve potential longer-term health benefits (Ailabouni et al., 2016a). Reasons for this occurring in practice include patient expectations to receive a prescription when they visit a clinician and pay for a medical consultation, time and other resource constraints, and the lack of existing infrastructure that enables the process of reviewing and rationalizing medicine use. Whilst it may be clinically appropriate and beneficial to prescribe a medicine for a patient, this inherent *present bias* and clinical inertia (Steinman and Landefeld, 2018) may lead to the overuse of certain medicines or the continuation of medicine prescriptions for longer than initially intended.

This behavior of prescribing medicine(s) may also be related to *commission bias* (Song et al., 2024), where people may be inclined to act rather than refrain from acting. An example of this is ordering additional diagnostic tests just "to be safe," even if they are not clinically indicated, or performing a medical invasive or surgical procedure even when a more conservative, noninvasive approach may have worked. The antonym of *commission bias* is *omission bias* (Baron and Ritov, 2004). This occurs when people avoid acting because of potential fear, discomfort, or the perception that the possible downsides are more immediate than the potential long-term benefits, thereby maintaining the status-quo (Ritov and Baron, 1992). For example, it has been reported that a barrier to deprescribing potentially inappropriate medicines is clinicians' experience of "fear of consequences" (Scott et al., 2014). A clinician may be reluctant to deprescribe a patient's aspirin, even if it is no longer likely to benefit them or if their life expectancy is limited. This reluctance arises from the fear that the patient may potentially experience a cardiovascular event (e.g., stroke or myocardial infarction) after the discontinuation of the medicine (e.g., aspirin) (Ailabouni et al., 2016b).

The concept of the *availability heuristic* is another way in which behavioral economics explains human behavior. *The availability heuristic*, or a "cognitive shortcut", occurs when people judge the likelihood of an event based on how easily they can think of examples that come to mind (Folkes, 1988). For example, a person may be easily influenced by famous people, influencers, or celebrities who have achieved significant weight loss by following a particular diet, taking certain medicines, drinking a special beverage, or exercising in a specific way. This may lead them to overestimate the effectiveness of these strategies for weight loss, even if the actual reliability of these strategies is lacking. Similarly, after watching a widely publicized news story about some people experiencing serious side effects from a medicine or a vaccine (e.g., the COVID-19 vaccine), a person may start to believe that all vaccines are very dangerous. This is because these narratives evoke vivid, emotional, and memorable feelings that could lead to an overestimation of the risk associated with the vaccine, resulting in vaccine avoidance altogether, even though the overall potential benefit outweighs the comparatively small risk of side effects (Luz et al., 2020).

In the field of deprescribing, the *availability heuristic* could provide an explanation for why clinicians and patients may be more amenable to deprescribing a medicine used for preventive purposes (e.g., a statin for lowering blood cholesterol) versus another medicine used for symptomatic relief (e.g., a sleeping tablet such as a benzodiazepine for insomnia) (Ailabouni et al., 2016b). This is because the potential drawbacks of deprescribing the sleeping tablet seem more tangible (i.e., having a bad night's sleep) in comparison to experiencing the benefits of taking a preventive medicine, which seem more invisible or abstract (i.e., you don't immediately feel healthier after taking your statin). *The framing heuristic* explains the tendency of people to be influenced when making decisions by the way information or choices are presented, for example, by explaining gains versus losses or the order in which choices are presented (Gong et al., 2013). This has been identified as a cognitive bias that impacts health decision-making.

Anchoring bias is the tendency to rely on initial information provided or previous decisions made in the past when making judgments in the present (Ly et al., 2023). For example, a person may feel attached to medicines that were initially prescribed by their clinician (e.g., a blood pressure tablet), even though new evidence has emerged showing that using this medicine for high blood pressure is not as effective as other medicines. In this scenario, the person is persistently holding on to the original prescription decision, which is the "anchor".

Anchoring bias is also experienced by clinicians who have just started treating a new person who may have had a long-standing relationship with a previous clinician who initiated most of their medicines many years ago (Hooper et al., 2016). The new clinician may be biased by the fact that another clinician started these medicines and by the perception that if their patient is still taking them, they must still be providing benefit (Coffin, n.d.). This is despite the fact that the person's goals of care may change over time as they age, and, hence, their medicine needs may no longer align with achieving their current goals of care. In this sense, inherited prescribing, which is the "anchor," brings significant *anchoring bias* and may be an impediment to reviewing and deprescribing medicines that may no longer be needed or helpful. Cumulatively, these biases and heuristics may seriously impact the quality and consistency of health decision-making, in turn affecting choices made and behavior behavior in the long-term (Featherston et al., 2020).

2.3.2 Designing and choosing implementation strategies to address biases and heuristics

Table 24.1 summarizes biases and heuristics that may play a role in the success of implementing deprescribing. It also offers specific implementation strategies, grounded in behavioral economics and theory, that may address inherent biases while overcoming known challenges in the context of a) designing and conducting deprescribing research and b) implementing deprescribing recommendations in practice.

2.4 Aiding collaborative decision-making

To date, incorporating heuristics, biases, and other aspects of how people make decisions has not been systematically integrated within the field of implementation science (Hodson et al., 2024). This extends to the field of

TABLE 24.1 Behavioral strategies that align with existing biases and heuristics.

		Evidence-based strategies to implement	
Bias or heuristic	**Example**	**Deprescribing research**	**Deprescribing in practice**
Present bias	Prescribing new medicines to address the acute needs of a person versus reviewing medicines and making decisions that affect long-term health outcomes	• Incorporate short-term incentives (e.g., increased remuneration) or feedback systems to sustain motivation (Olsen et al., 2025) • Design studies that examine long-term benefits or outcomes that may persist beyond the end of the study (Ailabouni et al., 2019)	• Utilize regular medicine-review services, such as pharmacist-led medicine reviews, periodic goal-setting, and annual comprehensive reviews, to sustain engagement that may continually assess the ongoing need for medicines, thereby mitigating present bias (Ailabouni et al., 2019) • Communicate potential health benefits or practical short-term gains from deprescribing (e.g., fewer side effects, lower risk of cognitive decline, reduction in the cost of medicines, etc.) (Ailabouni et al., 2025a)
Commission bias	Providing a medical prescription or continuing a medication beyond the recommended length of time "just in case"	• Explore using default discontinue functions on prescribing software to override clinical inertia (Ailabouni et al., 2016a). Overriding this default may require the clinician to enter an explanation of why they are choosing to prescribe the medicine beyond the recommended length of time	• Normalize not prescribing medicines or deprescribing medicines to be considered a clinical action rather than an inaction • Replace the action of prescribing with another. For example, offer a follow-up with the patient to check in with them rather than providing a prescriptions
Omission bias	Fear of consequences when deprescribing medications	• Explore the impact of education about inaction (i.e., maintaining the status-quo) as an active choice through the use of decision-aids or campaigns (Olsen et al., 2025) • Examine the impact of engaging local deprescribing champions who can mentor and encourage other clinicians to deprescribe (Ailabouni et al., 2016a)	• Share success stories with other clinicians about deprescribing decisions that did not result in harm to the patient and improved patient outcomes • Raise awareness about the potential negative consequences of continuing medications that may outweigh the possible consequences of deprescribing
Availability heuristic	Stories (e.g., on the news or via social media) related to unpleasant withdrawal effects or the return of the underlying disease after deprescribing medicines may discourage others from accepting deprescribing recommendations	• Explore the effectiveness of strategies (e.g., using videos from the patients' perspective after deprescribing medicines) that could strengthen the perception of positive deprescribing experiences and potential benefits (Ailabouni et al., 2022a)	• Use individualized tapering plans that outline a detailed process of deprescribing, along with the expected withdrawal effects, the risk of the underlying disease returning, and strategies to address unexpected outcomes (e.g., withdrawal effects) • Share positive patient experiences to demonstrate that safe deprescribing is feasible, and balance potential misinformation about deprescribing.
Framing heuristic	Patients or clinicians may feel influenced by their friends, relatives, peers, or colleagues to make deprescribing decisions depending on the information (e.g., positive or negative feedback, gains versus losses) they are presented with	• Explore the use of decision-aids or patient-centered information brochures that accurately present evidence-based gains versus losses of continuing medicines that may be harmful (Ailabouni et al., 2025a; Ailabouni et al., 2024a)	• Support and raise awareness among clinicians to discuss the benefits and harms, or gains versus losses, of continuing certain medicines versus deprescribing medicines in a shared decision-making process (Olsen et al., 2025)
Anchoring bias	• Patients may feel attached to medicines that were initiated a long time ago by another clinician who is different from their current clinician • Clinicians may feel pressured to continue prescribing medicines that they did not initiate, even if they are unsure about the clinical need for the medicines	• Explore the extent to which inherited prescribing could have potential negative consequences (Ailabouni et al., 2016a) • Gain an understanding of how initial prescribing decisions may shape later clinical judgments (Ailabouni et al., 2021)	• Utilize systems that require you to prescribe medicines one by one after a certain period has passed, instead of copying an existing medicine list or chart. This approach would compel the prescriber to reconsider the indication and re-evaluate the continued need for the medicine • Present patients with the most up-to-date evidence about the potential benefits or harms of using medicines

deprescribing, where early work has mainly focused on exploring the barriers and facilitators of deprescribing in practice. The next generation of studies explored, to some extent, unpacking these barriers using social-cognitive theories, mostly through models or frameworks such as the Theoretical Domains Framework (Atkins et al., 2017), the Capability, Opportunity, Motivation, Behavior model (Michie et al., Michie et al., n.d.) or the Consolidated Framework for Implementation Research (Damschroder et al., 2022). However, gaining knowledge by exploring and categorizing contextual determinants (barriers and facilitators) using these frameworks only scratches the surface of unpacking the drivers of the problem (Ailabouni et al., 2022b). The knowledge derived from applying such frameworks falls short and does not extend beyond the assumption that behavior change will mindfully occur after uncovering these factors (Hodson et al., 2024). This makes driving real behavior change challenging (see Chapter 26).

Behavioral economics could, therefore, provide a potential future direction to address these gaps. Specifically, behavioral economics could aid shared decision-making in the field of deprescribing (Hodson et al., 2024; Anderson et al., 2015). Shared decision-making should be a core component of clinicians making deprescribing decisions alongside the patient (Fariman et al., 2025). By accounting for how people behave rather than how we hope they behave, we can influence decision-making and, relatedly, change behavior in practice. Behavioral economics can support shared or collaborative decision-making to increase the uptake of deprescribing by:

1. **Enhancing patient engagement in the deprescribing process:** Behavioral economics demonstrates that patients value the choices they make and often value adequate self-advocacy (Ailabouni et al., 2024b), autonomy, and a sense of control when making these choices (Courtney et al., 2014). Asking patients about their goals, health priorities, and their preferences is essential to gaining buy-in and making a joint decision to deprescribe medicines (Ailabouni et al., 2022; Fariman et al., 2025).
2. **Counteracting existing biases by sharing perspectives:** Understanding and recognizing existing biases or patterns of decision-making may help tailor strategies that align with how the person behaves or thinks to enable success (Kahneman, 2011). This may include, for example, a person's attachment to their medicines (Weir et al., 2019), the perception that deprescribing medicines is burdensome and/or a hassle (Doherty et al., 2020), and/or their belief that their health will deteriorate after deprescribing the medicine (Ailabouni et al., 2019). A consultation that involves open communication between the prescriber and the patient can provide various viewpoints and challenge automatic assumptions, biases, or habitual behaviors that may no longer be of benefit. Raising awareness about current evidence-based medicine related to the use of certain medicines and the potential long-term benefits of deprescribing may address common misconceptions. This may shift decisions that clinicians and patients make, driving the uptake of deprescribing medicines in practice.
3. **Improving communication and framing:** Changing the framing of a decision by describing the potential gains, as opposed to the possible losses, can improve a person's willingness to accept a deprescribing recommendation from a clinician (e.g. pharmacist, medical doctor; Gong et al., 2013). Rebranding deprescribing as a process that will result in positive gains, such as better health and fewer side effects, as opposed to a process that will result in losses (e.g., withdrawal effects), may improve communication about potential medicine changes (Jones et al., 2024). This, in turn, may improve the acceptability and uptake of deprescribing recommendations in practice (Ailabouni et al., 2019).

2.5 Informing the field of deprescribing through a behavioral economic lens

Table 24.2 outlines how a behavioral economic lens can inform the field of deprescribing in three main avenues including, implementing deprescribing in practice, conducting deprescribing research, and changing health policies to promote deprescribing.

3 Examples of behavioral economics nudging in deprescribing

3.1 Definition of nudging

The theory of nudging is an example of a behavioral implementation strategy (Thaler and Sunstein, 2009). Nudging involves providing subtle cognitive cues that alter a person's choice architecture (Thaler and Sunstein, 2009). This may impact their decision-making and encourage them to make a different choice. We may not notice them, but nudges are all around us and influence thousands of micro-decisions we make in our everyday lives. Examples of nudges include placing vegetables and fruit at eye-level in cafés and fridges to encourage healthy eating habits or using brightly colored water bottles to help remind you to stay hydrated.

TABLE 24.2 Applying a behavioral economic lens to deprescribing practice, research, and policy.

	What does a behavioral economics lens offer?
Implementing deprescribing in practice	• Removes decision barriers and reorganizes choice architecture that influences decision-making (e.g., environment, social factors) which may limit the uptake of deprescribing in practice • Reconfigures inherent biases and heuristics that may demotivate clinicians or patients from implementing deprescribing recommendations in practice
Progressing deprescribing research	• Enhances the design of implementation strategies that can be tested for clinical effectiveness in deprescribing intervention studies • Explicitly explores and reports biases and heuristics from the perspectives of clinicians and patients that influence shared decision-making in deprescribing
Changing health policies to promote deprescribing	• By implementing automatic *default reminders* for medicine reviews at specific time points, behavioral economics can systematically increase the uptake of deprescribing recommendations by encouraging medication reviews that may result in deprescribing medicines that are no longer needed • By utilizing *opt-out* strategies, policies supporting medicine reviews and deprescribing can reach more patients, particularly older people who take multiple medications • By encouraging feedback and benchmark reporting on reviewing and deprescribing medicines, policies can motivate clinicians to deprescribe. Certain heuristics (e.g., framing) and strategies (e.g., social norm feedback) may encourage clinicians to align their behavior with what they believe others are doing, for example, after receiving messages that outline the deprescribing patterns of their peers

When designed cleverly, nudges are usually inexpensive to implement and are generally low-touch, requiring little to no effort to introduce into an existing organization or system. Nudges appeal to System 1 thinking, which refers to our automatic, unconscious, and emotional responses to stimuli, such as choosing the first thing you spot on the menu, even if it may not be the healthiest option (Thaler and Sunstein, 2009). Utilizing the power of effective and efficient nudging is potentially a cost-effective and sustainable approach to influencing a person's choices and ultimately changing their behavior long-term (Nudge Theory, n.d.).

In deprescribing research, nudging has been explored to a limited extent with mixed results. For example, Chua et al. conducted a broad overview of systematic reviews related to deprescribing interventional studies in older people and found that most studies did not isolate behavior strategies (e.g. choice architecture; nudging; Chua et al., 2024).

3.2 A nudging, codesigned conversation-starter tool to empower people to start conversations about their medicines

The World Health Organization's dementia global action plan outlines that it is a priority to provide consumers with person-centered resources to support them (World Health Organization [WHO], n.d.). Such resources can empower consumers to engage in a shared decision-making process with their clinician. To date, there is a limited number of co-designed (Anderson et al., 2016), user-friendly, patient-directed resources that have been evaluated and tested with patients, primarily older people and people living with dementia, to ensure they are acceptable and feasible to use in practice (Chan et al., 2023).

To address this gap, the PReparing people living with dementia and their caregivers to Initiate conversations about their MEdicines tool (PRIME) was co-designed with six consumers (people with dementia or caregivers) and five healthcare professionals who formed a stakeholder steering group (Ailabouni et al., 2024b). The PRIME tool is a low-touch, conversation-starter nudging tool that aims to empower people living with memory problems, including dementia or mild cognitive impairment, and their caregivers. People using the PRIME tool in clinical practice may feel more encouraged to have a conversation about their medicines. Such conversations may result in a collaborative decision with their healthcare professional to continue, reduce, or stop taking one or more of their medicines (Grant et al., 2025; Linsky et al., 2022).

The PRIME tool's usability and readability have been tested with 35 consumers (Ailabouni et al., 2025a). These consumers reported that the tool is valuable for broaching a conversation about their medicines with their healthcare professional. The PRIME tool's implementation has also been pilot-tested in practice and has been viewed by patients and clinicians as acceptable and feasible to use for starting a conversation about medicines in a clinical consultation (Ailabouni et al., 2025a).

3.3 Real-world example using the PRIME tool: Nudging toward fewer medicines in clinical practice

Given the nudging design of the PRIME tool, a hypothetical patient case is included in this chapter to explore how the tool can be used as a strategy to encourage people to take fewer medications in practice.

3.3.1 Background

Mrs. Lin is an 83-year-old woman of Chinese descent who lives alone. She has a limited ability to speak and understand English. She has limited caregiver or family support to help her with everyday needs. Her primary language is Traditional Chinese, and she relies on her daughter, Emma, for assistance with medical appointments and decision-making. Mrs. Lin was diagnosed with mild cognitive impairment six months ago after her family expressed concerns about confusion and a decline in her ability to make decisions. Up until now, Mrs. Lin has been managing her own daily medication regimen. Most of her medications are packed in a medicine blister pack (a dosage administration aid) as listed in Table 24.3.

3.3.2 Other (not packaged in a medicine blister pack)

Mrs. Lin also reports taking the following traditional Chinese medicines:

1. Gān Cǎo (Licorice root)
2. Língzhī (Reishi mushroom or Ganoderma)

3.3.3 Medical history

- Hypertension
- Peripheral edema—swelling in legs and ankles
- Stroke 8 years ago—residual weakness on her left side, which affects her balance and increases her risk of falling
- Mild cognitive impairment
- Osteoporosis
- Generalised anxiety disorder
- Insomnia

3.3.4 Concerns

1. **Cognitive function and decision-making:** Mrs. Lin's mild cognitive impairment has resulted in forgetfulness, confusion, and difficulty managing her medicines. Her daughter, Emma, has noticed that she sometimes forgets to take her medicines. Mrs. Lin told Emma that she occasionally has a difficult time understanding instructions from her healthcare team. Emma has also reported that she is unsure about Mrs. Lin's ability to engage in effective decision-making with the healthcare professional team regarding her health and medicines. Often, Emma reports that she has needed to attend medical appointments to translate for Mrs. Lin and assist with making health decisions. However, Emma is not always available due to her own work and family responsibilities. Emma reports that she sometimes feels overwhelmed by the decision-making burden and the responsibility of caring for Mrs. Lin.
2. **Family support:** Mrs. Lin's family is supportive; however, they have limited involvement in her healthcare. Her son lives in a neighboring city. Emma, her daughter, often assists with her medical appointments, but she is not always available, and it is difficult for Emma to remind Mrs. Lin to take her medicines several times during the day.

TABLE 24.3 Medicine list as per the medicine blister pack.

Medicine	Dose and frequency	Indication	Duration
Atorvastatin	40 mg mane and nocte	Initiated after stroke	8 years
Amlodipine	5 mg mane	Hypertension	12 years
Aspirin	100 mg mane	Initiated after stroke	8 years
Temazepam	20 mg nocte	Trouble sleeping	1 year
Alendronate	70 mg weekly	Low bone mineral density	6 years
Furosemide	20 mg at noon	Oedema	2 years

3. **Medicine "pill" burden:** Mrs. Lin takes more than five medicines (polypharmacy) and has a complex medication regimen. This, along with Mrs. Lin's limited English proficiency and cognitive function, has raised concerns for her family. Polypharmacy is associated with the use of one or more potentially inappropriate medicines and other harms such as falls, especially in older adults.
4. **Falls risk:** Mrs. Lin has a high risk of falling. She is prescribed some fall-risk-increasing drugs (e.g., temazepam). She reports feeling unstable on her feet, which is associated with weakness that developed on the left side of her body following a poststroke.

3.3.5 Implementation strategy

Mrs. Lin may benefit from a multicomponent strategy (Fig. 24.2) consisting of:

1. **Nudging using the PRIME tool:** Given Mrs. Lin's and her family's current concerns, she may benefit from reflecting on her health priorities and revising her current medication list. To assist Mrs. Lin in achieving this, a pharmacist could provide the PRIME tool (in Chinese) at the time of delivering her medication blister pack to her and Emma. Mrs. Lin and Emma would read and fill out the PRIME tool at their own pace. They could choose to use the hard copy tri-fold brochure, a PDF of the brochure, or complete the PRIME tool online as an interactive tool (accessible via www.kindmeds.org).
2. **A comprehensive medicine review:** A healthcare professional, such as a pharmacist, could meet with Mrs. Lin and Emma to conduct a comprehensive medicine review upon referral from her General Practitioner (GP). The aim of the review is to understand Mrs. Lin's current health priorities and review her medicines with the aim of rationalizing her medicine list and improving her health outcomes. The pharmacist would use Mrs. Lin and Emma's PRIME tool responses, in addition to their clinical notes and the interview with them, to make clinical recommendations to improve her medicines. This may involve suggesting deprescribing recommendations to the GP. These deprescribing recommendations would help align Mrs. Lin's medicine list with her current goals of care.

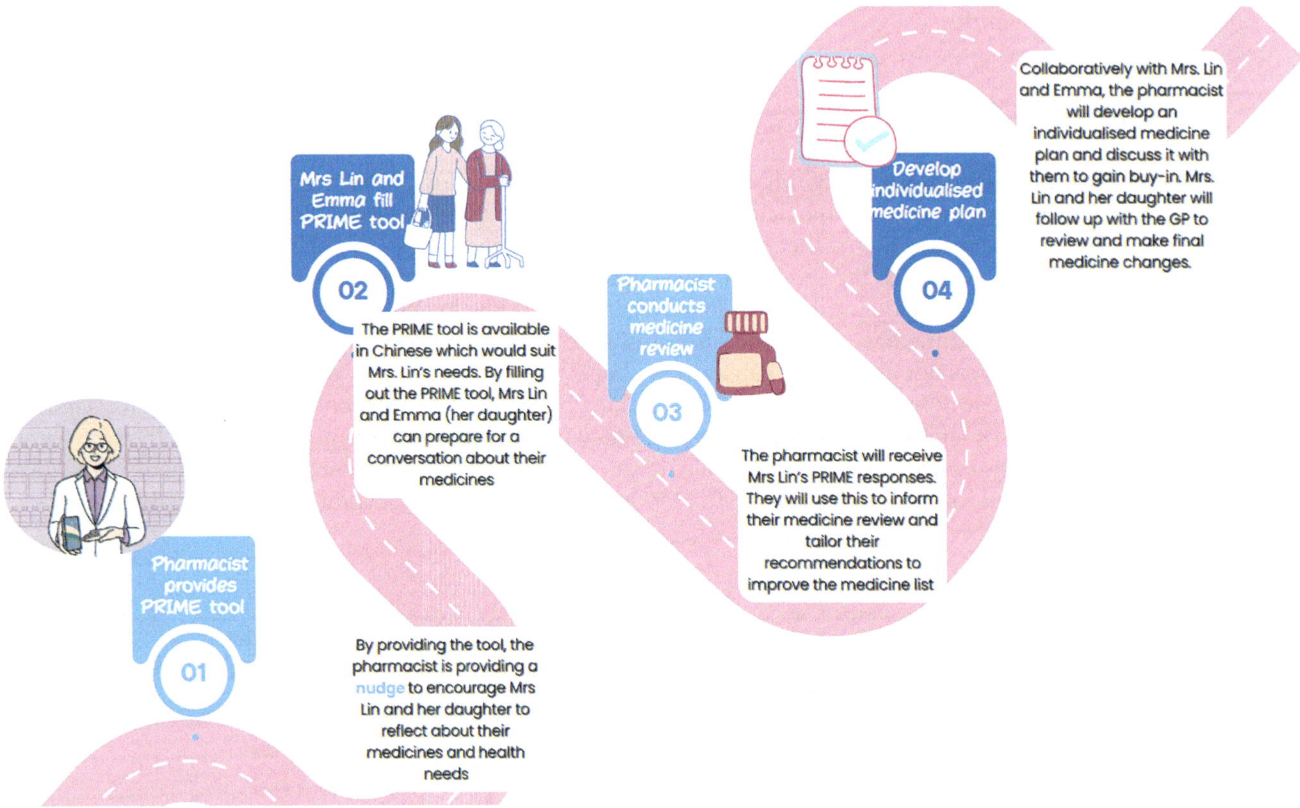

FIG. 24.2 **Roadmap illustrating the use of the PRIME tool in practice.** Using the PRIME tool in practice to start conversations about medicines.

3. **Follow-up and GP medical appointment:** To review the recommendations suggested by the pharmacist, Mrs. Lin and Emma would schedule a medical appointment with their GP. Their GP would receive a copy of the PRIME responses and the pharmacist's clinical report and individualized plan that was produced after the medicine review. The GP would have all the information they need to have an in-depth shared decision-making conversation with Mrs. Lin and Emma regarding the medicine list. They would review and finalize changes to their medicines and counsel them appropriately with the individualized medicine plan that has been developed for Mrs. Lin. Mrs. Lin and Emma would also have the chance to ask the GP any questions they have and raise any concerns they may have about the medicine list.

3.4 An example of nudging in research

Nudging can be applied to design effective strategies for use in research studies. Various studies have employed this strategy to improve health outcomes for patients. This example illustrates how nudging can be used to encourage patients and healthcare professionals to engage in shared decision-making conversations about medications.

3.4.1 *Background*

In a research environment or context (e.g., interventional study; model of care), the PRIME tool could be used as an implementation strategy to optimize medicine use in an interventional study (Ailabouni et al., 2024b, 2025a). The PRIME tool could be used on its own or in combination with other strategies to "nudge" the patient and the clinician to consider deprescribing medicines.

3.4.2 *Behavioural economic frameworks*

Messenger, **I**ncentives, **N**orms, **D**efaults, **S**alience, **P**riming, **A**ffect, **C**ommitments, and **E**go (MINDSPACE) is an example of a behavioral economic framework that focuses on nine different strategies or "cues" (Dolan et al., 2012). The MINDSPACE framework lists simple-to-implement nudges, such as *incentives, norms, and defaults,* that researchers and clinician-researchers may choose to implement to boost behavior change. The MINDSPACE framework incorporates heuristics and biases to design effective implementation strategies in a research context. Designing an implementation strategy using the MINDSPACE framework could later be leveraged to achieve large-scale behavior change.

3.4.3 *Application of the MINDSPACE framework using the PRIME tool*

Table 24.4 describes the application of the MINDSPACE framework in a research study that uses the PRIME conversation-starter tool to improve medicine use for people living with dementia and their caregivers. This example illustrates how this framework could assist researchers and clinician-researchers in scaling a nudging strategy to encourage optimization of medicines. It also lists the potential MINDSPACE strategies or "cues" to consider for successfully causing behavior change and explains the definitions of the strategies while providing examples of how these strategies could be utilized to design research implementation strategies. Implementing these strategies would cumulatively encourage meaningful conversations about medicines in a shared decision-making process with a clinician (e.g., medical doctor, pharmacist). In the future, generating this evidence base and knowledge could potentially be translated into improving the appropriateness of medicines used by people living with dementia. This could reduce their risk of experiencing medicine-related harm and improve their overall health and well-being.

3.5 Summary of nudging in deprescribing research

Examples of nudges in the Novel Uses of adaptive Designs to Guide provider Engagement in Electronic Health Records (NUDGE-EHR) study (Lauffenburger et al., 2021) included presenting information about medicine risks to make the information more impactful *(Behavioral principle: Salience)* or changing a pre-set course a prescriber might have normally chosen by automatically including deprescribing instructions when prescribing *(Behavioral principle: Default bias)* (Thaler and Sunstein, 2009). In this study, most behavioral design factors did not significantly increase deprescribing versus control. However, nudges based on the behavioral principle of *precommitment* significantly increased deprescribing versus control. This specifically involved prompting prescribers prior to the medical appointment to have a conversation about medicines and their potential harms with their patients using a patient-directed resource. The priming and preparation for the conversation showed a positive signal (Lauffenburger et al., 2021).

TABLE 24.4 Application of MINDSPACE framework using the PRIME tool.

MINDSPACE[a] framework strategy or cue	Relationship to our behaviour	How can the PRIME* tool aid the implementation of the strategy or cue?	Applications or considerations for a research study design
Messenger	We are heavily influenced by who communicates information to us (e.g., medical information provided to us by a clinician, such as our doctor or pharmacist)	A clinician, such as a medical doctor (e.g., GP* or geriatrician) or a pharmacist, who provides or recommends the PRIME tool to a patient may encourage the patient to use it. This is especially true if the patient has a long-standing relationship and established rapport with the healthcare professional.	Consider designing the study to include clinician-researchers or clinicians as interventionists who have an existing rapport with patients and can provide the PRIME tool to them as a resource. This will encourage the uptake of the tool.
Incentives	Our responses to incentives (taking or stopping medicines) are shaped by predictable mental shortcuts that relate to our beliefs about gaining (e.g., better health) or losing (e.g., side effects)	The PRIME tool provides information to patients in its "background" section about potential medicine harms and common side effects (e.g., drowsiness, confusion) that may be associated with using certain medicine classes. It also provides patients the opportunity to reflect on their health priorities and consider the benefits they may be receiving from their medicines. By presenting balanced information and the "trade-off" between the benefits and harms of medicines, an individual may feel more incentivized to have a conversation about taking fewer medicines.	Prior to conducting the study, provide training to the interventionists that offers a broad overview of optimizing medicine use, deprescribing, and the background information included in the PRIME tool. This will enable them to have a conversation with participants in the study and present the "gains" versus "losses" of continuing or deprescribing their medicines.
Norms	We are strongly influenced by what others do (e.g., our caregiver's or family's beliefs about medicines)	The PRIME tool can be used by the person with dementia separately, the caregiver separately, or by the person with dementia and their caregiver together. The tool's information and contents may allow both parties to reflect on what matters most to them and may influence and change their beliefs about their medicines. It may also aid the caregiver and the person with dementia in having a conversation about a potentially challenging topic using a structured and productive approach.	Design the research study in a way that provides an opportunity for the caregivers to be involved in the study as research participants, paired as dyads with the person they are caring for.
Defaults	Removes barriers, and we "go with the flow" of pre-set options (e.g., signing up for electronic health record systems that store our health information and aid clinicians in reviewing medicines and medical records)	Previous research testing the tool found that the tool would be most effective if it were embedded or integrated into the everyday clinical care flow so that it becomes a 'default' (Ailabouni et al., 2025a). For example, incorporating the tool as a prerequisite form as part of the comprehensive annual check or plan would remove barriers and improve the flow of patients filling out the form prior to their medical appointment with their doctor.	Tailor the study design to utilize existing systems and processes within the specific healthcare setting. If it is possible to add the tool to existing pre-medical appointment paperwork, this could remove barriers and improve communication.
Salience	Our attention is drawn to what is novel and seems relevant to us (e.g., being influenced by online or television advertising about medicines)	Previous research found that the PRIME tool, according to people's lived experiences, is relevant to individuals living with dementia and their caregivers who are managing multiple medicines. They also commented on the novelty of the tool and noted that the content, color and format of the tool are both attractive and effective in making it more noticeable to them.	Include specific information in the participant information sheet about the novelty and purpose of the tool.
Priming	Our actions are often influenced by subconscious cues (e.g., remembering to take medicine that is on your bedside table)	The PRIME tool has been reported to be potentially most useful if it is made available in medical centers waiting rooms or pharmacies while patients are waiting for their medicines to be prepared. These are examples of subconscious cues that could boost uptake of the tool.	Consider choice architecture in your research study design, whereby the tool is placed in a noticeable, easy-to-grab location and is made available in settings where the patient may already be considering reviewing their medicines (e.g., medical center, pharmacy).

MINDSPACE[a] framework strategy or cue	Relationship to our behaviour	How can the PRIME* tool aid the implementation of the strategy or cue?	Applications or considerations for a research study design
Affect	Our emotional associations, cultural beliefs, and values can powerfully shape our actions (e.g., some cultures have stronger feelings of attachment to medicines than others)	The PRIME tool has been adapted and tailored to suit the needs of certain groups of people who identify as culturally and linguistically diverse (e.g., Chinese or Italian people). By adapting the tool to include culturally appropriate information, it connects with individuals who may have diverse beliefs that impact their medicine-taking habits and values.	Ensure that the tools or resources you provide to participants are available in various forms, including different languages, and are adapted specifically to meet their culturally diverse needs.
Commitments	We seek to be consistent with our public promises and reciprocate acts (e.g., we are more likely to commit to a medication regimen or plan after discussing it with a clinician)	The PRIME tool incorporates a "self-reflection" section, which enables the patient and/or their caregiver to reflect on and document their health priorities and beliefs about their medicines. This can be a powerful resource that the patient can also use as a "commitment" to follow up with their healthcare professional and ask questions.	Incorporate follow-ups (e.g., a week, 3 months, or 6 months postmedical appointment) to ensure continuity of care. Reflect on commitments or statements made by patients in the self-reflection section of the PRIME tool to remind the patient and assess what changes the patient is willing to make to improve the use of medicines.
Ego	We act in ways that make us feel better about ourselves (e.g., taking medicine to provide symptomatic short-term relief, even if the potential long-term effects may be harmful)	The PRIME tool provides information to patients in its "background" section related to the potential harms of medicines and the possibility that, over the long-term, certain medicines may no longer align with their current goals of care. This information, along with education provided by a clinician, could shift the narrative and encourage patients to consider the long-term effects of their medicines, making them more willing to stop one or more of their medicines.	Include support and training in using the tool for the interventionists to enable them to have in-depth conversations about the benefits and harms of medicines. Specifically, highlight to participants the potential long-term effects of certain medicines that may be harmful.

[a]*MINDSPACE (Messenger, Incentives, Norms, Defaults, Salience, Priming, Affect, Commitments, and Ego) Framework.*

Nudges that were found to be less effective included pop-up EHR alerts that were presented to prescribers in high volumes. One study incorporated pop-up alerts to prompt deprescribing of anticholinergic medicines and found that 85% of alerts to providers and 95% of alerts to medical assistants went unread (Campbell et al., 2021). The multicomponent strategy in this study did not reduce the use of high-risk anticholinergic medicines among older people. Another study utilizing this approach to deprescribe glycemic medicines, as aligned with the Choosing Wisely guidelines, found that of the 67,412 alerts that had been sent, approximately 1.15% were actioned by prescribers, often accompanied by negative or disagreeing comments (Viswanadham et al., 2025).

In summary, the effectiveness of nudges in health services research and deprescribing specifically is variable (Nagtegaal et al., 2019). Nudges that relied on a multitude of prompts and simple reminders were not accepted by prescribers and were not effective at changing behavior (Viswanadham et al., 2025). This is likely due to prompt fatigue and the nudges not being specifically individualized to their patient or the clinical situation, which often led to them being ignored or unread (Gani et al., 2025).

To date, nudges that have been found to be most promising and effective have incorporated empowering prescribers and patients to have a conversation about medicines and their benefits and harms prior to the medical appointment. It is likely that multiple symbiotic bundles of nudges are required to make a real change and not just one stand-alone nudge (Lauffenburger et al., 2021). In addition, choosing, designing, and embedding such nudges that are mindful and match the specific clinical context, such as the examples included in adaptive trial designs (e.g., NUDGE-EHR), may have a higher likelihood of success. More high-quality studies, including pragmatic, randomized controlled trials (RCTs), are needed to test nudge designs to improve patient-level health outcomes. Using mixed methods in studies will also enable capturing why prescribers and/or patients may have responded or not responded to specific nudges.

3.5.1 Pros and cons of nudging deprescribing

Before considering using nudging to deprescribe medicines, it is important to consider its possible pros and cons (Ewert, 2020; Tannenbaum, 2022). These include:

Pros

1. Nudges are low-cost strategies that may be relatively easy to implement in comparison to large-scale education campaigns to raise awareness about deprescribing.
2. Nudges maintain patients' autonomy.Providing nudges or cues to patients to consider deprescribing may be less coercive than a deprescribing decision, which might feel forced. The nudge encourages deprescribing but doesn't force the prescriber or the patient to implement it.
3. Nudges may address the behavioral barrier of clinical inertia, where the medication may have been prescribed a long time ago, and continuing it might seem easier *(status-quo bias).*
4. Nudges may be easily scalable and maintained: By embedding nudges in the clinical workflow and adapting them to the specific context, they can be applied to various clinical scenarios and tailored to different healthcare settings with relative ease.

Cons

1. Nudges have had variable efficacy, with some nudges (e.g., pop-up alerts on EHRs) being less effective than others (e.g., priming a conversation about health or medicines prior to a medical appointment).
2. Nudges may undermine a patient's autonomy. Even though nudges are less coercive, they may be viewed by some as manipulative. Changing the choice architecture without transparently discussing it with patients may undermine the trust patients have in their prescriber and/or the healthcare system.
3. Nudges, specifically alerts, have not been found to be acceptable to most prescribers due to overwhelming prompt fatigue and the fact that the alerts may not be applicable to their specific patients.
4. Nudges are not a substitute for shared decision-making between a patient and a prescriber. Nudging does not replace the role of the prescriber in following up after deprescribing has been implemented to ensure the medicine has been stopped or withdrawn safely.

4 Discussion

Deprescribing efforts being lost in translation in practice and lacking scalability have been recognized as important challenges (Baumgartner et al., 2020). This chapter provides an overview of leveraging behavioral economics and implementation science concepts to design and conduct deprescribing research or to increase the translation of deprescribing into practice.

Using behavioral economics and related behavioral strategies could offer low-touch approaches to create sustainable translation of deprescribing during interventional studies and beyond in clinical practice (Hodson, 2023; Hodson et al., 2024). By utilizing patients' and other stakeholders' subconscious ways of decision-making and thinking, behavioral economic principles can transform research studies, policies, and clinical practice strategies to mitigate existing barriers that may limit deprescribing. This, in turn, may encourage the view among stakeholders (e.g., doctors, pharmacists) that deprescribing is a natural component of the prescribing continuum and an integral part of providing quality care to patients.

To date, various deprescribing interventional studies have aimed to improve the appropriateness of prescribing by implementing strategies that aid shared decision-making in practice. Whilst some of these studies, primarily RCTs or cluster-RCTs, have achieved relatively high discontinuation rates of potentially inappropriate medicines (e.g., proton pump inhibitors, nonsteroidal antiinflammatory medicines), their long-term sustainability and scalability often diminish after the trial period ends (Ailabouni, Mangin and Nishtala, 2019; Martin et al., 2018). The rate of re-prescribing medicines that had initially been discontinued usually increases after the conclusion of an interventional study (Thompson et al., 2019). This is because it requires significant effort to intentionally review and make changes to medicines, especially at points of transition from one healthcare setting to another (e.g., upon hospital discharge) (Freeman et al., 2021).

In addition, awareness about applying implementation science concepts, specifically strategies to improve the uptake of deprescribing recommendations, is growing. However, to date, most implementation strategies used in deprescribing interventional studies have primarily included education initiatives, training of healthcare staff (e.g., medical doctors, pharmacists), and medicine reviews implemented by a healthcare professional (Ailabouni et al., 2019; Chua et al., 2024). Whilst successful in the short term, these strategies may be difficult to scale and maintain using a cost-effective approach. Evidence suggests that utilizing behavioral economics could drive sustainable and cost-effective implementation of deprescribing.

Exploring behavioral economic theories could also contribute to the existing large and growing knowledge base related to people's attitudes toward deprescribing and their willingness to take fewer medicines (Weir et al., 2019). Behavioral economic theories may provide deeper insights and explain patients' deprescribing intentions and the reasons behind their beliefs related to their medicines and health. This may strengthen clinicians' understanding of patients' overall attitudes and willingness to deprescribe these medicines (Conner and Norman, 2025) offering insights into how to potentially modify them. Specifically, distinct information related to biases that drive patient choices to deprescribe medicines could be explored and articulated. This could help clinicians in real-world practice settings gain buy-in from their patients to deprescribe their medicines, thereby improving deprescribing uptake in practice. In addition, researchers may use this knowledge to design and implement strategies that specifically address those biases. In turn, this may encourage improved implementation of deprescribing in research contexts.

4.1 Future directions

Unanswered questions regarding the acceptability, feasibility, and clinical effectiveness of behavioral strategies to encourage deprescribing remain. The application of behavioral science concepts in the field of deprescribing and optimizing medicine use more generally has been conservative to date (Chua et al., 2024). Future studies could focus on designing and testing the acceptability and feasibility of specific behavioral strategies. In addition, information related to the effectiveness of these strategies in effectiveness-implementation study designs could inform which of these strategies are likely to result in changes in decision-making patterns and improved translation of deprescribing into practice (Curran et al., 2012). For example, it may be worthwhile to develop and evaluate decision support tools, with a user-centered design, to explicitly address behavioral barriers (e.g., clinical inertia, status quo bias).

Emerging future directions may also include personalizing people's "choice architecture" for deprescribing decisions by using behavioral economic theories in combination with machine-learning and/or artificial intelligence (AI). Predictive AI-powered tools, using big data sets, could provide accurate signals for which patients would benefit and be amenable to deprescribing long-term antidepressants (Ranwala and Andrade, 2025). Strategies focused on pre-commitment of clinicians and patients, using, for example, priming and prompting conversations about medicines prior to medical appointments, have shown the most promise to date (Lauffenburger et al., 2021). Commitment from patients could be improved by using commitment devices such as structured deprescribing plans, reminders, and follow-ups, which could encourage sustainable deprescribing of potentially harmful medicines, improving people's health and wellbeing (Ailabouni et al., 2024b; Lamprell et al., 2021). This, however, needs to be balanced against respecting the patient's autonomy, as questions related to the ethical considerations of behavioral strategies remain. In particular, communication and transparency related to strategies (e.g., nudging) that subtly influence patient choices ought to be explored further.

5 Conclusion

Behavioral economics, and specifically behavioral strategies such as nudging, offer powerful tools that could accelerate the translation of deprescribing. However, evidence related to the use and effectiveness of behavioral strategies in high-quality deprescribing research studies is limited. Leveraging behavioral economic concepts and implementation science concepts in future deprescribing research and practice may uncover unexplored new avenues to improve the uptake of deprescribing and the use of medicines, as well as the health and well-being of patients, using pragmatic, sustainable approaches.

6 Questions for further discussion

- How are the mechanisms of behavioral economic strategies (e.g., nudging) examined and evaluated in interventional deprescribing studies?
- What considerations and/or scaffolds are needed to strengthen the implementation of nudges (e.g., electronic health record prompts) for deprescribing in practice?

- How would you describe the human behavior heuristics and biases evident in deprescribing qualitative literature (e.g., barriers and enablers of deprescribing)?
- What ethical considerations are important when modifying people's choice architecture to encourage use of fewer potentially inappropriate medicines?
- What behavioral economic strategies are considered culturally appropriate for culturally and linguistically diverse populations?
- How could artificial intelligence and/or machine learning personalize behavioral economic strategies (e.g., choice architecture) for targeted implementation?
- What would a high-quality, effectiveness-implementation hybrid study evaluating a behavioral economics deprescribing strategy involve?

7 Application exercise/scenario

Scenario:

A primary healthcare clinic has conducted an audit which revealed the prevalent and potentially inappropriate use of antidepressants among older people. The clinic's management team would like to reduce the potentially inappropriate long-term use of antidepressants, particularly those with anticholinergic and/or sedative properties, among older people.

The audit found that most people have been taking antidepressants for longer than potentially needed, or that use continues in people whose goals of care have significantly changed since the initial prescriptions. However, clinicians (e.g., primary healthcare physicians, nurse practitioners) report reluctance to raise deprescribing during medical appointments, citing time constraints and concerns about complex tapering schedules and symptom recurrence.

The clinic's leadership aims to design, implement, and evaluate an effectiveness-implementation hybrid study using behavioral economic strategies. The goal is to encourage antidepressant deprescribing through more person-centered conversations about stopping or reducing use, thereby translating the theory and evidence from this chapter into a practical, actionable plan.

Exercise:

1. **Identify relevant biases and heuristics**
   - Drawing on Table 24.1, identify at least two biases or heuristics (e.g., present bias, omission bias, availability heuristic, anchoring bias) contributing to the challenges of appropriately prescribing antidepressants, from both clinician and patient perspectives.
   - For each bias identified, briefly explain the mechanism by which it might be reinforcing continued antidepressant prescribing.
2. **Choose and/or design at least two behavioral strategies**
   - Propose at least two behavioral strategies (e.g., nudging, de-sludging, social-norm feedback, choice bundling) that could prompt deprescribing conversations and explain the rationale for each using concepts from this chapter.
   - Consider how a conversation-starter tool, like the PRIME tool, could be leveraged within this context.
3. **Apply the MINDSPACE framework to design an effectiveness-implementation hybrid study to deprescribe antidepressants**
   - Select three MINDSPACE cues (e.g., Messenger, Defaults, Salience) and describe how each could be applied to design the effectiveness-implementation hybrid study at the clinic.
4. **Anticipate limitations**
   - Referring to Section 3.5.1, identify at least two risks or limitations of your proposed interventional study (e.g., prompt fatigue, transparency about change in choice architecture).
   - Propose mitigation strategies for these risks.

5. Reflection and evaluation

- Describe how you would evaluate your interventional study and specify both effectiveness outcomes (e.g., number of antidepressant prescriptions) and implementation outcomes (e.g., fidelity, reach) and how you would measure them.
- Reflect on how the future directions discussed in Section 4.1 would apply to this scenario.

References

Ailabouni, N.J., Hanjani, L.S., Weir, K.R., Reeve, E., Abdulla, A., Bohill, R., Brandt, N., 2025a. Empowerment to have a conversation with healthcare professionals: co-designing the PRIME (PReparing people living with dementia and carers to Initiate conversations about their MEdicines) tool. J. Alzheimers Dis. 1387-2877. doi:10.1177/13872877251406907.

Ailabouni, N.J., Marcum, Z.A., Schmader, K.E., Gray, S.L., 2019. Medication use quality and safety in older adults: 2018 update. J. Am. Geriatr. Soc. 15325415. 67 (12), 2458–2462. Available from: http://onlinelibrary.wiley.com/journal/10.1111/(ISSN)1532-5415. doi:10.1111/jgs.16243.

Ailabouni, N.J., Marcum, Z.A., Schmader, K.E., Gray, S.L., 2021. Medication use quality and safety in older adults: 2019 update. J. Am. Geriatr. Soc. 15325415. 69 (2), 336–341. Available from: http://onlinelibrary.wiley.com/journal/10.1111/(ISSN)1532-5415. doi:10.1111/jgs.17018.

Ailabouni, N.J., Nishtala, P.S., Mangin, D., Tordoff, J.M., 2016b. General practitioners' insight into deprescribing for the multimorbid older individual: a qualitative study. N. Z. Int. J. CliN. Pract. 17421241. 70 (3), 261–276. Available from: http://onlinelibrary.wiley.com/journal/10.1111/(ISSN)1742-1241. doi:10.1111/ijcp.12780.

Ailabouni, N.J., Nishtala, P.S., Mangin, D., Tordoff, J.M., Cox, D., 2016a. Challenges and enablers of deprescribing: a general practitioner perspective. PLOS ONE. 1932-6203. 11 (4), e0151066. doi:10.1371/journal.pone.0151066.

Ailabouni, N.J., Reeve, E., Helfrich, C.D., Hilmer, S.N., Wagenaar, B.H., 2022b. Leveraging implementation science to increase the translation of deprescribing evidence into practice. Res. Soc. Adm. Pharm. 15517411. 18 (3), 2550–2555. Available from: http://www.journals.elsevierhealth.com/periodicals/rsap. https://www.sciencedirect.com/science/article/pii/S1551741121001844. doi:10.1016/j.sapharm.2021.05.018.

Ailabouni, N.J., Terrill, B., Freeman, C.R., 2025b. The Power of the Consumer Voice in Knowledge Translation of Deprescribing. Springer Science and Business Media LLC, pp. 131–157. doi:10.1007/978-3-031-77314-3_5.

Ailabouni, N.J., Thompson, W., Hilmer, S.N., Quirke, L., McNeece, J., Bourke, A., Furst, C., Reeve, E., 2024a. Co-designing a consult patient decision aid for continuation versus deprescribing cholinesterase inhibitors in people living with dementia. Adis, Australia Drug. Aging. 11791969. 41 (10), 821–831. Available from: https://www.springer.com/journal/40266. doi:10.1007/s40266-024-01146-5.

Ailabouni, N.J., Weir, K.R., Brandt, N., Hanjani, L.S., Green, A., Thompson, W., Freeman, C.R., Mangin, D., Bohill, R., Furst, C., Reeve, E., 2024b. Partnering with a stakeholder steering group to co-design the PRIME deprescribing conversation tool: reflections and recommendations. Basic Clin. Pharmacol. Toxicol. 17427843. 134 (1), 121–125. Available from: http://onlinelibrary.wiley.com/journal/10.1111/(ISSN)1742-7843. doi:10.1111/bcpt.13938.

Ailabouni, N.J., Weir, K.R., Reeve, E., Turner, J.T., Norton, J.W., Gray, S.L., 2022a. Barriers and enablers of older adults initiating a deprescribing conversation. Patient Educ. Couns. 18735134. 105 (3), 615–624. Available from: https://www.elsevier.com/locate/pateducou. doi:10.1016/j.pec.2021.06.021.

Ailabouni, N., Mangin, D., Nishtala, P.S., 2019. DEFEAT-polypharmacy: deprescribing anticholinergic and sedative medicines feasibility trial in residential aged care facilities. Int. J. Clin. Pharm. 22107711. 41 (1), 167–178. Available from: http://springerlink.metapress.com/content/2210-7703/. doi:10.1007/s11096-019-00784-9.

Anderson, K., Foster, M.M., Freeman, C.R., Scott, I.A., 2016. A multifaceted intervention to reduce inappropriate polypharmacy in primary care: research co-creation opportunities in a pilot study. Med. J. Aust. 13265377. 204 (7), S41. Available from: https://www.mja.com.au/system/files/issues/204_07/10.5694mja16.00125.pdf. doi:10.5694/mja16.00125.

Anderson, K., Freeman, C., Rowett, D., Burrows, J., Scott, I., Rigby, D., 2015. Polypharmacy, deprescribing and shared decision-making in primary care: the role of the accredited pharmacist. J. Pharm. Pract. Res. 1445-937X. 45 (4), 446–449. doi:10.1002/jppr.1164.

Ashe, M.L., Wilson, S.J., 2020. A brief review of choice bundling: a strategy to reduce delay discounting and bolster self-control. Addict. Behav. Rep. 23528532. 11, 100262. doi:10.1016/j.abrep.2020.100262.

Atkins, L., Francis, J., Islam, R., O'Connor, D., Patey, A., Ivers, N., Foy, R., Duncan, E.M., Colquhoun, H., Grimshaw, J.M., Lawton, R., Michie, S., 2017. A guide to using the theoretical domains framework of behaviour change to investigate implementation problems. Implement. Sci. 1748-5908. 12 (1). doi:10.1186/s13012-017-0605-9.

Baron, J., Ritov, I., 2004. Omission bias, individual differences, and normality. Organ. Behav. Hum. Decis. Process. 07495978. 94 (2), 74–85. doi:10.1016/j.obhdp.2004.03.003.

Bauer, M.S., Damschroder, L., Hagedorn, H., Smith, J., Kilbourne, A.M., 2015. An introduction to implementation science for the non-specialist. BMC Psychol. 20507283. 3 (1). Available from: http://bmcpsychology.biomedcentral.com/. doi:10.1186/S40359-015-0089-9.

Baumgartner, A.D., Clark, C.M., LaValley, S.A., Monte, S.V., Wahler, R.G., Singh, R., 2020. Interventions to deprescribe potentially inappropriate medications in the elderly: lost in translation? J. Clin. Pharm. Ther. 13652710. 45 (3), 453–461. Available from: http://onlinelibrary.wiley.com/journal/10.1111/(ISSN)1365-2710. doi:10.1111/jcpt.13103.

Campbell, N.L., Holden, R.J., Tang, Q., Boustani, M.A., Teal, E., Hillstrom, J., Tu, W., Clark, D.O., Callahan, C.M., 2021. Multicomponent behavioral intervention to reduce exposure to anticholinergics in primary care older adults. J. Am. Geriatr. Soc. 15325415. 69 (6), 1490–1499. Available from: http://onlinelibrary.wiley.com/journal/10.1111/(ISSN)1532-5415. doi:10.1111/jgs.17121.

Chambers, D.A., Emmons, K.M., 2024. Navigating the field of implementation science towards maturity: challenges and opportunities. Implement. Sci. 17485908. 19 (1). Available from: https://implementationscience.biomedcentral.com. doi:10.1186/s13012-024-01352-0.

Chan, B., Isenor, J.E., Kennie-Kaulbach, N., 2023. Categorization of deprescribing communication tools: a scoping review. Basic Clin. Pharmacol. Toxicol. 17427843. 133 (6), 640–652. Available from: http://onlinelibrary.wiley.com/journal/10.1111/(ISSN)1742-7843. doi:10.1111/bcpt.13886.

Chisholm, A., Hart, J., Lam, V., Peters, S., 2012. Current challenges of behavior change talk for medical professionals and trainees. Patient Educ. Couns. 18735134. 87 (3), 389–394. doi:10.1016/j.pec.2011.12.001.

Chua, S., Todd, A., Reeve, E., Smith, S.M., Fox, J., Elsisi, Z., Hughes, S., Husband, A., Langford, A., Merriman, N., Harris, J.R., Devine, B., Gray, S.L., Arab-Zozani, M., 2024. Deprescribing interventions in older adults: an overview of systematic reviews. PLOS ONE. 1932-6203. 19 (6), e0305215. doi:10.1371/journal.pone.0305215.

Coffin, P.O., Barreveld, A.M., 2022. Inherited patients on opioids for chronic pain–considerations for primary care. N. Engl. J. Med. 386 (7), 611.

Conner, M., Norman, P., Attitudes, 2025. Intentions, and behavior change. Annu. Rev. Psychol. 0066-4308. doi:10.1146/annurev-psych-013125-042110.

Courtney, M.R., Spivey, C., Daniel, K.M., 2014. Helping patients make better decisions: how to apply behavioral economics in clinical practice. Patient Prefer. Adherence. 1177889X. 8, 1503–1512. Available from: http://www.dovepress.com/getfile.php?fileID=22221. doi:10.2147/PPA.S71224.

Curran, G.M., 2020. Implementation science made too simple: a teaching tool. Implement. Sci. Commun. 26622211. 1 (1). Available from: https://www.springer.com/journal/43058. doi:10.1186/s43058-020-00001-z.

Curran, G.M., Bauer, M., Mittman, B., Pyne, J.M., Stetler, C., 2012. Effectiveness-implementation hybrid designs: combining elements of clinical effectiveness and implementation research to enhance public health impact. Med. Care. 15371948. 50 (3), 217–226. doi:10.1097/MLR.0b013e3182408812.

Damschroder, L.J., Reardon, C.M., Widerquist, M.A.O., Lowery, J., 2022. The updated consolidated framework for implementation research based on user feedback. Implement. Sci. 17485908. 17 (1). Available from: https://implementationscience.biomedcentral.com. doi:10.1186/s13012-022-01245-0.

Doctor, J.N., Nguyen, A., Lev, R., Lucas, J., Knight, T., Zhao, H., Menchine, M., 2018. Opioid prescribing decreases after learning of a patient's fatal overdose. Science. 10959203. 361 (6402), 588–590. Available from: http://science.sciencemag.org/content/361/6402/588/tab-pdf. doi:10.1126/science.aat4595.

Doherty, A.J., Boland, P., Reed, J., Clegg, A.J., Stephani, A.M., Williams, N.H., Shaw, B., Hedgecoe, L., Hill, R., Walker, L., 2020. Barriers and facilitators to deprescribing in primary care: a systematic review. BJGP Open. 23983795. 4 (3). Available from: https://bjgpopen.org/content/bjgpoa/4/3/bjgpopen20X101096.full.pdf. doi:10.3399/bjgpopen20X101096.

Dolan, P., Hallsworth, M., Halpern, D., King, D., Metcalfe, R., Vlaev, I., 2012. Influencing behaviour: the mindspace way. J. Econ. Psychol. 01674870. 33 (1), 264–277. doi:10.1016/j.joep.2011.10.009.

Ewert, B., 2020. Moving beyond the obsession with nudging individual behaviour: towards a broader understanding of behavioural public policy. Public Policy Adm. 0952-0767. 35 (3), 337–360. doi:10.1177/0952076719889090.

Fariman, S., Arabshomali, A., Goordeen, D., Niznik, J.D., Hemati, H., Lafata, J.E., 2025. Shared decision making interventions for deprescribing in older adults with polypharmacy: a scoping review. J. Am. Geriatr. Soc. 0002-8614. 73 (12), 3884–3894. doi:10.1111/jgs.70059.

Featherston, R., Downie, L.E., Vogel, A.P., Galvin, K.L., Kumar, S., 2020. Decision making biases in the allied health professions: a systematic scoping review. PLOS ONE. 1932-6203. 15 (10), e0240716. doi:10.1371/journal.pone.0240716.

Folkes, V.S., 1988. The availability heuristic and perceived risk. J. Consum. Res. 0093-5301. 15 (1), 13. doi:10.1086/209141.

Freeman, C.R., Scott, I.A., Hemming, K., Connelly, L.B., Kirkpatrick, C.M., Coombes, I., Whitty, J., Martin, J., Cottrell, N., Sturman, N., Russell, G.M., Williams, I., Nicholson, C., Kirsa, S., Foot, H., 2021. Reducing medical admissions and presentations into hospital through optimising medicines (REMAIN HOME): a stepped wedge, cluster randomised controlled trial. Med. J. Aust. 13265377. 214 (5), 212–217. Available from: https://www.mja.com.au. doi:10.5694/mja2.50942.

Gani, I., Litchfield, I., Shukla, D., Delanerolle, G., Cockburn, N., Pathmanathan, A., 2025. Understanding "Alert Fatigue" in primary care: qualitative systematic review of general practitioners attitudes and experiences of clinical alerts, prompts, and reminders. J. Med. Internet Res. 1438-8871. 27, e62763. doi:10.2196/62763.

Gong, J., Zhang, Y., Yang, Z., Huang, Y., Feng, J., Zhang, W., 2013. The framing effect in medical decision-making: a review of the literature. Psychol. Health Med. 1354-8506. 18 (6), 645–653. doi:10.1080/13548506.2013.766352.

Grant, R.W., Peterson, I., McCloskey, J.M., Lipska, K.J., Nugent, J., Karter, A.J., Gilliam, L.K., 2025. Diabetes deprescribing in older adults a randomized clinical trial. JAMA Intern. Med. 21686114. Available from: http://archinte.jamanetwork.com/issues.aspx. doi:10.1001/jamainternmed.2025.2015.

Grimshaw, J.M., Eccles, M.P., Lavis, J.N., Hill, S.J., Squires, J.E., 2012. Knowledge translation of research findings. Implement. Sci. 17485908. 7 (1). Available from: http://www.implementationscience.com/content/7/1/50. doi:10.1186/1748-5908-7-50Canada.

Heukelom, F., 2014. Behavioral Economics: A History. Cambridge University Press. doi:10.1017/CBO9781139600224.

Hodson, N., 2023. De-sludging healthcare systems. doi:10.1136/bmj.p2916.

Hodson, N., Powell, B.J., Nilsen, P., Beidas, R.S., 2024. How can a behavioral economics lens contribute to implementation science? Implement. Sci. 17485908. 19 (1). Available from: https://implementationscience.biomedcentral.com. doi:10.1186/s13012-024-01362-y.

Hooper, L.M., Tomek, S., Roter, D., Carson, K.A., Mugoya, G., Cooper, L.A., 2016. Depression, patient characteristics, and attachment style: correlates and mediators of medication treatment adherence in a racially diverse primary care sample. Prim. Health Care Res. Dev. 14771128. 17 (2), 184–197. Available from: http://journals.cambridge.org/action/displayJournal?jid=PHC. doi:10.1017/S1463423615000365.

Ivers, N., Jamtvedt, G., Flottorp, S., Young, J.M., Odgaard-Jensen, J., French, S.D., O'Brien, M.A., Johansen, M., Grimshaw, J., Oxman, A.D., 2012. Audit and feedback: effects on professional practice and healthcare outcomes. Cochrane Database Syst. Rev. 14651858. 2012 (7). doi:10.1002/14651858.cd000259.pub3.

Johnson, E.J., Shu, S.B., Dellaert, B.G.C., Fox, C., Goldstein, D.G., Häubl, G., Larrick, R.P., Payne, J.W., Peters, E., Schkade, D., Wansink, B., Weber, E.U., 2012. Beyond nudges: tools of a choice architecture. Mark. Lett. 09230645. 23 (2), 487–504. doi:10.1007/s11002-012-9186-1.

Johnson, M.J., May, C.R., 2015. Promoting professional behaviour change in healthcare: what interventions work, and why? A theory-led overview of systematic reviews. BMJ Open. 20446055. 5 (9). Available from: http://bmjopen.bmj.com/content/5/9/e008592full.pdf+html. doi:10.1136/bmjopen-2015-008592.

Jones, K.F., Stolzmann, K., Wormwood, J., Pendergast, J., Miller, C.J., Still, M., Bokhour, B.G., Hanlon, J., Simon, S.R., Rosen, A.K., Linsky, A.M., 2024. Patient-directed education to promote deprescribing: a nonrandomized clinical trial. JAMA Intern. Med. 21686114. 184 (11), 1339–1346. Available from: http://archinte.jamanetwork.com/issues.aspx. doi:10.1001/jamainternmed.2024.4739.

Kahneman, D., New York, NY: Farrar, Straus and Giroux, 2011. Thinking, Fast and Slow 2011. Allen Lane and Penguin Books, New York.

Kao, Y.F., Velupillai, K.V., 2015. Behavioural economics: classical and modern. Eur. J. Hist. Econ. Thought. 14695936. 22 (2), 236–271. Available from: https://www.tandf.co.uk/journals/titles/09672567.asp. doi:10.1080/09672567.2013.792366.

Kemp, C.G., Wagenaar, B.H., Haroz, E.E., 2019. Expanding Hybrid Studies for Implementation Research: intervention, Implementation Strategy, and Context. Front. Public Health. 22962565. 7. Available from: http://journal.frontiersin.org/journal/public-health/section/public-health-education-and-promotion#archive. doi:10.3389/fpubh.2019.00325.

Kullgren, J.T., Kim, H.M., Slowey, M., Colbert, J., Soyster, B., Winston, S.A., Ryan, K., Forman, J.H., Riba, M., Krupka, E., Kerr, E.A., 2024. Using behavioral economics to reduce low-value care among older adults a cluster randomized clinical trial. JAMA Intern. Med. 21686114. 184 (3), 281–290. Available from: http://archinte.jamanetwork.com/issues.aspx. doi:10.1001/jamainternmed.2023.7703.

Lamprell, K., Tran, Y., Arnolda, G., Braithwaite, J., 2021. Nudging clinicians: a systematic scoping review of the literature. J. Eval. Clin. Pract. 13652753. 27 (1), 175–192. Available from: http://onlinelibrary.wiley.com/journal/10.1111/(ISSN)1365-2753. doi:10.1111/jep.13401.

Lauffenburger, J.C., Isaac, T., Trippa, L., Keller, P., Robertson, T., Glynn, R.J., Sequist, T.D., Kim, D.H., Fontanet, C.P., Castonguay, E.W.B., Haff, N., Barlev, R.A., Mahesri, M., Gopalakrishnan, C., Choudhry, N.K., 2021. Rationale and design of the novel uses of adaptive designs to guide provider engagement in electronic health records (NUDGE-EHR) pragmatic adaptive randomized trial: a trial protocol. Implement. Sci. 17485908. 16 (1). Available from: http://www.implementationscience.com/. doi:10.1186/s13012-020-01078-9.

Linsky, A.M., Kressin, N.R., Stolzmann, K., Pendergast, J., Rosen, A.K., Bokhour, B.G., Simon, S.R., 2022. Direct-to-consumer strategies to promote deprescribing in primary care: a pilot study. BMC Prim. Care. 27314553. 23 (1). Available from: https://bmcfampract.biomedcentral.com/. doi:10.1186/s12875-022-01655-5.

Lucas, T., Rogers, C.R., Aspiras, O., Manning, M., Dawadi, A., Thompson, H.S., 2023. Message framing for men? gender moderated effects of culturally targeted message framing on colorectal cancer screening receptivity among African Americans. Psychol. Men Masc. 15249220. 24 (2), 103–112. Available from: https://www.apa.org/journals/men.html. doi:10.1037/men0000418.

Luz, P.M., Nadanovsky, P., Leask, J., 2020. How heuristics and cognitive biases affect vaccination decisions. Cadernos de Saúde Pública. 1678-4464. 36 (suppl 2). doi:10.1590/0102-311x00136620.

Ly, D.P., Shekelle, P.G., Song, Z., 2023. Evidence for anchoring bias during physician decision-making. JAMA Intern. Med. 21686114. 183 (8), 818–823. Available from: http://archinte.jamanetwork.com/issues.aspx. doi:10.1001/jamainternmed.2023.2366.

Martin, P., Tamblyn, R., Benedetti, A., Ahmed, S., Tannenbaum, C., 2018. Effect of a pharmacist-led educational intervention on inappropriate medication prescriptions in older adults: the D-PRESCRIBE randomized clinical trial. JAMA. 15383598. 320 (18), 1889–1898. Available from: http://jama.jamanetwork.com/journal.aspx. doi:10.1001/jama.2018.16131.

Michie, S., Atkins, L., West, R., 2014. The Behaviour Change Wheel. A Guide to Designing Interventions, Vol. 1. Guide to Designing Interventions, pp. 1003–1010.

Nagtegaal, R., Tummers, L., Noordegraaf, M., Bekkers, V., 2019. Nudging healthcare professionals towards evidence-based medicine: a systematic scoping review. J. Behav. Public Adm. 2576-6465. 2 (2). doi:10.30636/jbpa.22.71.

Nudge Theory. https://thedecisionlab.com/reference-guide/psychology/nudge-theory. (Accessed 5 November 2025).

Olsen, W.M., St Pierre, K., Thompson, W., Weir, K.R., Freeman, C.R., Bohill, R., Farrell, B., Langford, A.V., O'Donnell, L.K., Reeve, E., Liau, S.J., McEvoy, A.M., Shrestha, S., Tesfaye, W., Breen, J., Etherton-Beer, C., Yik, J., Turner, J., Ailabouni, N.J., 2025. Shaping future deprescribing priorities: outcomes of a World Café stakeholder workshop. Expert Rev. Clin. Pharmacol. 17512441. Available from: https://www.tandfonline.com/loi/ierj20. doi:10.1080/17512433.2025.2609659.

Proctor, E., Silmere, H., Raghavan, R., Hovmand, P., Aarons, G., Bunger, A., Griffey, R., Hensley, M., 2011. Outcomes for implementation research: conceptual distinctions, measurement challenges, and research agenda. Adm. Policy Ment. Health. 0894-587X. 38 (2), 65–76. doi:10.1007/s10488-010-0319-7.

Ranwala, R.A.D.L.M.K., Andrade, A.Q., 2025. Predicting Antidepressant Deprescription with Machine Learning Using Administrative Data, Vol. 329. IOS Press. doi:10.3233/shti250959.

Ritov, I., Baron, J., 1992. Status-quo and omission biases. J. Risk Uncertain. 15730476. 5 (1), 49–61. doi:10.1007/BF00208786.

Scott, I.A., Anderson, K., Freeman, C.R., Stowasser, D.A., 2014. First do no harm: a real need to deprescribe in older patients. Med. J. Aust. 13265377. 201 (7), 390–392. Available from: https://www.mja.com.au/system/files/issues/201_07/sco00146.pdf. doi:10.5694/mja14.00146.

Scott, I.A., Hilmer, S.N., Reeve, E., Potter, K., Couteur, D.L., Rigby, D., Gnjidic, D., Del Mar, C.B., Roughead, E.E., Page, A., Jansen, J., Martin, J.H., 2015. Reducing inappropriate polypharmacy: the process of deprescribing. JAMA Intern. Med. 21686114. 175 (5), 827–834. Available from: http://archinte.jamanetwork.com/article.aspx?articleid=2204035. doi:10.1001/jamainternmed.2015.0324.

Song, F., Shou, Y., Olney, J., Yeung, F.S.H., 2024. Moral judgments under uncertainty: risk, ambiguity and commission bias. Curr. Psychol. 19364733. 43 (11), 9793–9804. Available from: https://www.springer.com/journal/12144. doi:10.1007/s12144-023-05050-w.

Steinman, M.A., Landefeld, C.S., 2018. Overcoming inertia to improve medication use and deprescribing. JAMA. 15383598. 320 (18), 1867–1869. Available from: http://jama.jamanetwork.com/journal.aspx. doi:10.1001/jama.2018.16473.

Tannenbaum, D., 2022.Are nudges sinister psychological tricks? Or are they useless? Actually they are neither. The Conversation. Retrieved November 5, 2025, https://theconversation.com/are-nudges-sinister-psychological-tricks-or-are-they-useless-actually-they-are-neither-192496.

Thaler, R.C., Sunstein, C.R., 2008. Nudge: Improving Decisions about Health, Wealth, and Happiness. New Haven: Yale University Press.

Thaler, R.H., Sunstein, C.R., 2009. Nudge: Improving Decisions about Health, Wealth, and Happiness. Penguin Books.

Thompson, W., Reeve, E., Moriarty, F., Maclure, M., Turner, J., Steinman, M.A., Conklin, J., Dolovich, L., McCarthy, L., Farrell, B., 2019. Deprescribing: future directions for research. Res. Soc. Adm. Pharm. 15517411. 15 (6), 801–805. doi:10.1016/j.sapharm.2018.08.013.

Viswanadham, R.V.N., Belli, H.M., Martinez, T.R., Wong, C., Blecker, S., Troxel, A.B., Mann, D.M., 2025. When nudges don't budge: a mixed methods study of why EHR-based deprescribing nudges failed to change provider behavior. Res. Sq. Available from https://www.researchsquare.com/browse. doi:10.21203/rs.3.rs-7466262/v1.

Weir, K.R., Bonner, C., McCaffery, K., Naganathan, V., Carter, S.M., Rigby, D., Trevena, L., McLachlan, A., Jansen, J., 2019. Pharmacists and patients sharing decisions about medicines: development and feasibility of a conversation guide. Res. Soc. Adm. Pharm. 15517411. 15 (6), 682–690. Available from: http://www.journals.elsevierhealth.com/periodicals/rsap. doi:10.1016/j.sapharm.2018.08.009.

World Health Organisation (WHO). n.d. Global action plan on the public health response to dementia 2017–2025 https://www.who.int/publications/i/item/9789241513487. (Accessed 13 September 2025).

World Health Organisation. n.d. Medication without harm. https://www.who.int/initiatives/medication-without-harm. (Accessed 26 November 2025).

Zeng, Y., Shi, L., Liu, C., Li, W., Li, J., Yang, S., Yang, X., Huang, Q., Yang, L., 2023. Effects of social norm feedback on antibiotic prescribing and its characteristics in behaviour change techniques: a mixed-methods systematic review. Lancet Infect. Dis. 14733099. 23 (5), e175. doi:10.1016/s1473-3099(22)00720-4.

Zullo, A.R., Gray, S.L., Holmes, H.M., Marcum, Z.A., 2018. Screening for medication appropriateness in older adults. Clin. Geriatr. Med. 18798853. 34 (1), 39–54. Available from: http://www.elsevier.com/inca/publications/store/6/2/3/3/6/4/index.htt. doi:10.1016/j.cger.2017.09.003.

CHAPTER

25

Concept mapping: An integrated, mixed methods approach for collaboratively building consensus

Jenny Leigh Newlon[a] *and Kimberly Illingworth*[b]

[a]Birth Control Pharmacist, Oak Park, CA, United States

[b]Faculty Affairs and Pharmacy Practice, Purdue University, West Lafayette, IN, United States

CHAPTER OBJECTIVES

After reading this chapter, the reader should be able to:

- Develop a study protocol using concept mapping methodology
- Compare the pros and cons of using concept mapping
- Identify topics that are appropriate for study using concept mapping

1 Introduction

While the outcome of most research leads to a call for more research, concept mapping takes a more proactive and tangible approach. Concept mapping starts with a problem that needs to be not only understood but also solved. The findings of concept mapping serve as a roadmap for those who wish to translate research findings into real-world impact and solve the problem (Green et al., 2012).

Both qualitative and quantitative methods have strengths and weaknesses, but mixed methods address the inherent weaknesses by drawing on and combining the strengths of both (Creswell and Plano Clark, 2018; Aarons et al., 2012). Blending the two methodologies meaningfully can be challenging, but four main approaches are typically used: convergent parallel design, explanatory sequential design, exploratory sequential design, and embedded design (Creswell and Plano Clark, 2018).

Convergent parallel design involves qualitative and quantitative data collection taking place separately and possibly simultaneously, with the results being brought together to interpret the findings (Creswell and Plano Clark, 2018). Explanatory sequential design starts with a quantitative component and then uses qualitative methods to explain the quantitative results in greater depth (Creswell and Plano Clark, 2018). Exploratory sequential design begins with qualitative data collection to identify phenomena and then uses quantitative methods to quantify the phenomena (Creswell and Plano Clark, 2018). Concept mapping does not use any of these mixed methods designs; instead, it is an embedded, integrated mixed methodology that aims to build consensus among various stakeholders (Kane and Trochim, 2007). The qualitative and quantitative portions of concept mapping are interwoven and interdependent, requiring active participant engagement in data collection and analysis. This active engagement is what

Contemporary Research Methods in Pharmacy and Health Services - Volume 2
https://doi.org/10.1016/B978-0-443-44607-8.00028-5

makes concept mapping a participatory approach. Participants go beyond being the subjects of the research and become actively involved in analyzing the data as well, as is discussed in Section 2.5.

Concept mapping can rapidly guide alignment on a topic, as well as prioritize the most actionable ideas. Therefore, it is a useful methodology when studying topics in which you hope to see rapid change, such as public health, advocacy, or even pharmacy practice. Several studies that may be relevant to the field of pharmacy have sought to:

- Increase the implementation of evidence-based HPV vaccination strategies (Tsui et al., 2024)
- Advance health equity in preventive intervention research (Boyd et al., 2023)
- Reduce barriers to pharmacist-prescribed contraceptive services (Newlon et al., 2024)
- Optimize the scope of practice for pharmacists, nurse practitioners, and physician assistants (Newlon et al., 2023)
- Improve access to affordable medications (Yaphe et al., 2019)
- Eliminate chronic disease disparities (Soule et al., 2024)

In the next section, we will discuss how to conduct a concept-mapping study

2 Methods

2.1 Research question and goal

The first stage of concept mapping is to determine the goal of the study. While most research methodologies strive to remain unbiased and observe whatever outcome may naturally occur, concept mapping uses research to effect change. Therefore, a goal must be chosen. Some recent examples include identifying best practices for scope determination and regulation of various healthcare providers (Newlon et al., 2023), prioritizing resources needed to increase the implementation of pharmacist-prescribed contraception services (Newlon et al., 2024), and improving family engagement in youth residential treatment for mental health (Herbell et al., 2025).

2.2 Participant identification and recruitment

After the research question (or goal) has been determined, the next step is to choose the participants. When considering who can help achieve the research goal, take into account all relevant groups. For example, if the goal of your research is to prioritize resources needed to increase the implementation of pharmacist-prescribed contraception services, then you must consider who has an impact on implementation. For this project, you would likely wish to include not only pharmacists who would provide the service but also pharmacy management, who make the ultimate decision whether to implement the service, pharmacy technicians, who are also involved in service provision, and patients, who receive the service. Although patients are not directly involved in implementation, the service cannot be implemented without them. In other words, a pharmacy cannot truly implement pharmacist-prescribed contraception services if no patients use the service due to unaddressed barriers, such as a lack of awareness of the service. However, it would not be necessary to include participants who have no direct impact on service implementation, such as physicians or academics.

Next you must determine the appropriate number of participants to recruit. For the first phase of data collection, brainstorming (discussed below), the data collection is qualitative and, therefore, no hard sample size numbers can be calculated. It is only necessary to include enough participants to represent all relevant stakeholder groups. For the second phase of data collection, sorting and rating (discussed below), the target sample size will be influenced by the intended analyses. To create a go-zone map, as few as 10 participants have been recommended (Kane and Trochim, 2007). However, if you wish to conduct subgroup analyses, such as "Does this subgroup rate this idea as statistically significantly more important than this other subgroup?", then a sample size calculation prior to recruitment is advisable.

Prior to recruitment, you must decide whether concept mapping will be conducted in-person, virtually, or in a hybrid format. Concept mapping studies have been conducted since before the internet became readily available to the public (Kane and Trochim, 2007), but in recent years, technological advancements have made virtual concept mapping possible. Virtual focus groups reduce barriers to participation and may allow for greater access to study participation for individuals from a wider geographic area, which can strengthen research findings (Eiguren et al., 2021; Keen et al., 2021).

2.3 Prompt development

Once a goal is determined, the concept mapping prompt should be developed. The purpose of the prompt is to guide participants in the brainstorming portion of the study. The prompt must be specific enough to keep participants on track, but it must also not be leading. The prompt must be open-ended to allow participants to contribute any ideas that may achieve the end goal of the project, no matter how unorthodox.

Pretesting the prompt prior to the brainstorming phase of concept mapping is recommended. Similarly to developing a new survey instrument (Ruel et al., 2016), it is important to test the prompt with an audience that closely resembles your target sample. Ask your volunteers how they would respond to the prompt or share what they think the prompt is asking. Revise the prompt as needed.

2.4 Data collection 1: Focus group brainstorming

The first phase of data collection for concept mapping consists of brainstorming focus groups. A facilitator will begin the session and play an important role in gently redirecting the conversation when it strays from the prompt and encouraging the momentum of the discussion. The facilitator is also responsible for setting the ground rules for the brainstorming session. Although participants are encouraged to build on one another's ideas, they should not use the brainstorming session to argue the merit of the ideas. Participants will have a chance to provide input on their perceptions of each idea's importance and feasibility during the second phase of data collection: sorting and rating.

The facilitator, or a second study team member, should record all participant-provided responses to the prompt ("ideas" or "statements"). These ideas should be displayed to all participants in real time. For in-person sessions, this can be achieved by writing the ideas on a board, and for virtual sessions, this can be achieved by sharing a screen where the ideas are being documented.

The purpose of sharing the ideas with the participants is two-fold: (1) it ensures that the participants' ideas are being captured accurately, and (2) participants can more easily build on and revise other participants' ideas. This collaborative approach to developing ideas aids with consensus-building that may be missing from other consensus-building techniques, such as the Delphi method (Linstone and Turoff, 1976) which allows for ideas to be submitted by participants separately.

The session may be concluded when saturation has been reached. In other words, the session is finished when participants have no new ideas to share. If the end of the scheduled session occurs before participants run out of ideas, another session may need to be scheduled. After the session, the researchers will compile the ideas ("statements") and prepare them for sorting and rating.

2.5 Data collection 2: Sorting and rating

Concept mapping is a participatory research method. One of the elements that makes it participatory is the sorting portion of concept mapping. By asking individual participants to sort the ideas ("statements") into groups based on similarity, participants play an active role in the qualitative analysis of the data collected during the brainstorming session. The results of the sorting provide insight into the participants' perceptions of the ideas generated, while also streamlining the overwhelming number of raw ideas into a more manageable number of themes.

In addition to sorting the ideas, participants are also asked to rate each idea twice. Participants are asked how important each idea is to achieving the goal referenced in the prompt during the brainstorming session and how feasible it is to follow through on each idea. For example, a participant may think that an idea is extremely important, but it may be nearly impossible to carry out. These ratings will be used to plot all of the ideas into the four quadrants of the go-zone map and identify the most actionable ideas that are most likely to successfully achieve the goal set forth by the prompt.

Although importance and feasibility are two common rating scales used in concept mapping (Herbell et al., 2025; Kane and Trochim, 2007; Newlon et al., 2023, 2024), different combinations of rating scales can be used. For example,

Yampolskaya et al. (2004) asked participants to rate statements in terms of importance and effectiveness, and Aarons et al. (2009) used rating scales for importance and changeability. In a larger departure from the gold standard, Laustsen et al. (2021) used the prompt, "Involvement of professionals in research on aging and health can lead to … ?" and asked participants to rate ideas in terms of (1) the extent to which ideas strengthen *practice* when conducting research, and (2) the extent to which ideas can strengthen *research*. Ultimately, the rating scales chosen for a given research study should reflect the goal of the study.

2.6 Analysis: Multidimensional scaling, hierarchical cluster analysis, and go-zone maps

After all of the sorting and rating data has been collected, it is time for analysis.

For sorting data, multidimensional scaling (MDS) can combine all participants' idea groupings into a single two-dimensional plot. To prepare the data, a similarity matrix must be created (Table 25.1). This similarity matrix can be created using software specific to concept mapping, or it can be done manually. To create the similarity matrix, the number of participants who grouped each pair of statements must be summed. For example, in Table 25.1, five participants were asked to sort five statements. One participant sorted statement #1 and statement #2 into the same group (column 1, row 2). Two participants sorted statement #1 and statement #3 into the same group (column 1, row 3).

After the similarity matrix has been created, MDS can be used to graphically represent the sorting data in a two-dimensional plot (Kruskal and Wish, 1978). Each point within the plot represents a statement or idea. Statements that are closer together are considered more similar, and statements that are further apart are considered less similar. The stress value of the MDS plot should be calculated to assess the overall fit of the data to a two-dimensional plot, with lower stress values indicating a better fit (Kruskal and Wish, 1978). If the stress value does not indicate a good fit, it means that a two-dimensional plot is not the best way to represent the sorting data. More practically, this means there is little agreement between participants on how to best group the statements, and it may be necessary to conduct additional brainstorming sessions.

If the stress value indicates a good fit, then hierarchical cluster analysis can be conducted to guide cluster identification. Hierarchical cluster analysis (Anderberg, 1973; Everitt, 1980) uses the X-Y coordinates generated by the MDS to create a tree structure or hierarchy of all possible cluster solutions. To determine the appropriate number of clusters, the researcher must review the statements in each cluster and decide which groupings make the most sense.

The rating data will be used to construct go-zone maps. The "go-zone" refers to the upper-right quadrant of the graph (or "map") where all of the statements/ideas that participants rated as the most important and feasible are located. These statements are the most actionable—they are the ideas that should be prioritized to make the biggest impact toward achieving the goal of your research. To construct the go-zone map, average scores must be calculated for each statement for both rating scales. Each rating scale will serve as an axis for the go-zone map. For example, if you asked participants to rate statements in terms of importance and feasibility using a four-point scale, then the average importance rating could serve as the x-axis coordinate, and the average feasibility rating could be the y-axis coordinate for the statement. It is inconsequential which rating scale (importance or feasibility) is assigned to which axis. An example go-zone map with fictitious data may be found in Fig. 25.1.

The map will be divided into quadrants by calculating the average of all importance ratings for all statements and the average of all feasibility ratings for all statements. These averages will correspond to straight lines, or

TABLE 25.1 Example similarity matrix.

		Statements				
		#1	#2	#3	#4	#5
Statements	#1	5				
	#2	1	5			
	#3	2	0	5		
	#4	0	1	3	5	
	#5	0	1	4	1	5

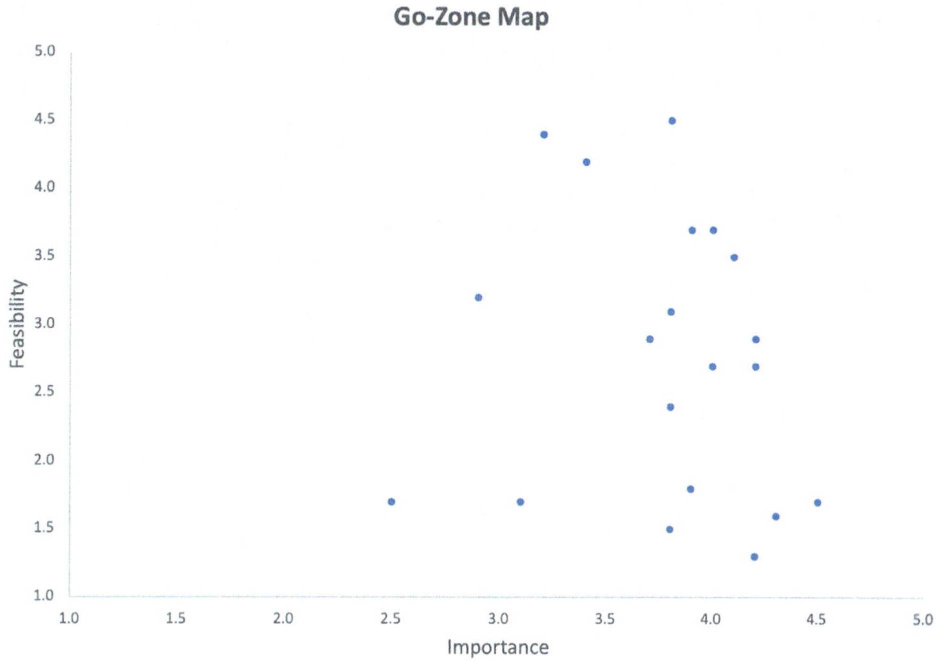

FIG. 25.1 Example go-zone map. For this example, the average feasibility rating was 2.6, and the average importance rating was 3.8 out of 4.

boundaries, for the go-zone map. Therefore, anything found in the go-zone, or upper-right quadrant, will be the items rated above average in terms of both importance and feasibility. The go-zone in Fig. 25.1 is highlighted.

Go-zone maps can be created for all items or for items from different clusters separately. Once again, the analysis and interpretation of the data depend on what makes sense for the goal of your research.

3 Discussion

3.1 Strengths and weaknesses of concept mapping

Concept mapping has many strengths and potential applications in pharmacy policy and health services research. The strengths of concept mapping include the use of integrated mixed-methods research, the encouragement of a collaborative, participatory approach, the ability to support consensus building, and the creation of actionable insights.

Integrated mixed methods refers to the interconnected use of both qualitative and quantitative data (Caracelli and Greene, 1993). Concept mapping contains several elements that make it an integrated mixed methods design. Concept mapping uses quantitative data from the sorting process to assess qualitative themes among the statements or ideas. Additionally, quantitative data (i.e., the rating data) is collected with regard to the qualitative data (i.e., statements) captured in the brainstorming sessions to inform go-zone map creation. This integration of both qualitative and quantitative data draws on the benefits of both methodologies and provides a richer, holistic view of the study topic than either could provide alone.

Concept mapping is well-suited for consensus building due to its collaborative, participatory approach. The brainstorming session provides an opportunity for various stakeholders to come together and bounce ideas off each other, which can facilitate consensus-building. One potential downside to concept mapping is that it is not ideal for heterogeneous focus groups if the different stakeholder groups do not feel safe sharing their thoughts with each other. For example, bringing pharmacists and their employers into the same focus group to discuss medication errors may not be successful if pharmacists fear being disciplined or terminated for sharing their true thoughts and experiences. Stakeholders play a crucial role in data analysis as well by sorting statements and ideas into groups to drive the identification of major themes. However, the most crucial part of participatory research comes at the conclusion of concept mapping: using and disseminating findings to enact positive changes (Vaughn and Jacquez, 2020).

3.2 Virtual versus in-person

Another important decision when designing a concept mapping study is whether to conduct it virtually or in-person. For the brainstorming focus groups, virtual participation can offer many benefits: it is less expensive (Roberts et al., 2021), does not require travel (Marley et al., 2023), and may take less effort to coordinate. Allowing virtual participation in focus groups helps to recruit more diverse participants in terms of race, education, and health status (Rupert et al., 2017). In addition, virtual participation may be the best choice for studies that are exploring more controversial or stigmatized topics because virtual participation can provide anonymity and increase candidness (Marley et al., 2023; Woodyatt et al., 2016). Regardless of the modality used, both virtual and in-person focus groups can result in equally rich, quality data (Richard et al., 2021).

3.3 Tools

Video conferencing software, such as Zoom (2025) or Webex (2025), can make virtual focus groups easier to host. Online survey tools, such as Qualtrics (Qualtrics, 2025), can be used for sorting and rating data collection. However, data collation for sorting data can be cumbersome if done with a tool that is not specifically designed for creating the similarity matrix. Several software tools exist that support sorting data collection and automatic similarity matrix compilation, including GroupWisdom (Groupwisdom, 2025), Simple Card Sort (Simple Card Sort, 2025), and Optimal Sort (Optimal Sort, 2025). These tools can streamline the research process and shorten the time from research planning to evidence-based implementation.

3.4 Next steps

The most important part of concept mapping comes at the very end: putting results into action. Concept mapping facilitates consensus building and prioritization of ideas, but the real impact of concept mapping comes from taking action on the results. Theoretically, if concept mapping has been done well, your team will have identified several steps that are likely to be impactful (i.e., important) and successful (i.e., feasible).

4 Questions for further discussion

- What might you consider when determining whether concept mapping is the best design for your research?
- How can concept mapping be used in social and administrative pharmacy research?
- What challenges might you face when using concept mapping as a research design?

5 Application exercise/scenario

For this application exercise, let's assume that you are interested in the working conditions of community pharmacies in the United States.

5.1 Research question and goal

Most research studies may approach this topic by attempting to better understand the barriers and facilitators to improving pharmacy working conditions. However, for concept mapping, you should think about the goal that you want your research to achieve. In this case, you might decide that your goal is to improve community pharmacy working conditions. **What other goals might you want to achieve?**

5.2 Participant identification and recruitment

To determine who your stakeholders are, you need to identify who is involved in pharmacy working conditions. Pharmacy executives and pharmacy owners choose company policies that may impact working conditions, board of pharmacy members can regulate some aspects of pharmacy practice within their state, legislators can write and pass bills regulating pharmacy practice, and pharmacists are directly affected by pharmacy working conditions;

therefore, all should be considered stakeholders. **Are there any other stakeholders whom you feel may be relevant to this study?**

5.3 Prompt development

It is important to create a clear and concise prompt. One possible prompt could be, "How do we improve community pharmacy working conditions?" A more targeted prompt might be, "How do we reduce burnout among community pharmacists?" **Which prompt would you choose, and why?**

5.4 Data collection 1: Focus group brainstorming

For the brainstorming session, it may be necessary to consider providing anonymity for participants. Pharmacists impacted by poor working conditions may not feel comfortable sharing candid responses while sharing a space with pharmacy executives, owners, and board of pharmacy members out of fear of retaliation (Clabaugh et al., 2021). Additionally, pharmacy executives and pharmacy owners may be unwilling to share how working conditions can potentially impact patient safety in front of legislators. If anonymity is not feasible, it may be worthwhile to consider separate focus groups to ensure participants are able to share their ideas freely (Newlon et al., 2023). **How might you provide participants with anonymity while participating in the brainstorming focus group?**

5.5 Data collection 2: Sorting and rating

After the focus groups are complete, sorting and rating can take place. For the rating portion, you will likely want to ask participants to rate each statement or idea in terms of importance and feasibility in order to prioritize actionable items. **What other rating scales might you consider for this study?**

5.6 Analysis

If the sample size allows, subgroup analyses of ratings between different stakeholder groups could provide useful insights. By comparing ratings between the different stakeholders, it may be possible to assess the level of agreement between stakeholder groups. For a topic as polarizing as pharmacy working conditions, you may find that consensus has not been achieved and additional focus groups may be necessary. However, if you feel a reasonable level of agreement has been reached, then you will be able to identify the prioritized list of actions that can be taken to improve pharmacy working conditions, with reasonable assurance that the actions will be successful and will not be met with resistance from stakeholders. **How would you determine whether a "reasonable level of agreement" has been reached?**

References

Groupwisdom, 2025. https://groupwisdom.com/groupconceptmapping.

Simple Card Sort, 2025.

Aarons, G.A., Fettes, D.L., Sommerfeld, D.H., Palinkas, L.A., 2012. Mixed methods for implementation research: application to evidence-based practice implementation and staff turnover in community-based organizations providing child welfare services. Child Maltreat. 15526119. 17 (1), 67–79. doi:10.1177/1077559511426908.

Aarons, G.A., Wells, R.S., Zagursky, K., Fettes, D.L., Palinkas, L.A., 2009. Implementing evidence-based practice in community mental health agencies: a multiple stakeholder analysis. Am. J. Public Health. 15410048. 99 (11), 2087–2095. Available from: http://www.ajph.org/cgi/reprint/99/11/2087. doi:10.2105/AJPH.2009.161711.

Anderberg, M.R., 1973. Cluster Analysis for Applications, Academic Press.

Boyd, R.C., Castro, F.G., Finigan-Carr, N., Okamoto, S.K., Barlow, A., Kim, B.K.E., Lambert, S., Lloyd, J., Zhang, X., Barksdale, C.L., Crowley, D.M., Maldonado-Molina, M., Obasi, E.M., Kenney, A., 2023. Strategic directions in preventive intervention research to advance health equity. Prev. Sci. 15736695. 24 (4), 577–596. Available from: https://www.springer.com/journal/11121. doi:10.1007/s11121-022-01462-5.

Caracelli, V.J., Greene, J.C., 1993. Data analysis strategies for mixed-method evaluation designs. Educ. Eval. Policy Anal. 0162-3737. 15 (2), 195–207. doi:10.3102/01623737015002195.

Clabaugh, M., Newlon, J.L., Plake, K.S.I., 2021. Perceptions of working conditions and safety concerns in community pharmacy. J. Am. Pharm. Assoc. 15443450. 61 (6), 761–771. Available from: http://www.japha.org/issues.aspx?journalid=63. doi:10.1016/j.japh.2021.06.011.

Creswell, J.W., Plano Clark, V.L., 2018. Designing and Conducting Mixed Methods Research, third ed. SAGE Publications, Inc.

Eiguren, A., Idoiaga, N., Berasategi, N., Picaza, M., 2021. Exploring the social and emotional representations used by the elderly to deal with the COVID-19 pandemic. Front. Psychol. 1664-1078. 11. doi:10.3389/fpsyg.2020.586560.

Everitt, B., 1980. Cluster analysis. Qual. Quant. 0033-5177. 14 (1), 75–100. doi:10.1007/bf00154794.

Green, A.E., Fettes, D.L., Aarons, G.A., 2012. A concept mapping approach to guide and understand dissemination and implementation. J. Behav. Health Serv. Res. 10943412. 39 (4), 362–373. doi:10.1007/s11414-012-9291-1.

Herbell, K., Albright, N., Berger, S., Stanek, C., Helsabeck, N.P., 2025. Identifying family engagement priorities in youth residential treatment settings: a group concept mapping study. Child. Youth Serv. Rev. 01907409. 168, 108037. doi:10.1016/j.childyouth.2024.108037.

Kane, M., Trochim, W., 2007. Concept Mapping for Planning and Evaluation. SAGE Publications, Inc. doi:10.4135/9781412983730.

Keen, S., Lomeli-Rodriguez, M., Williams, A.C.D.C., 2021. Exploring how people with chronic pain understand their pain: a qualitative study. Scand. J. Pain. 1877-8860. 21 (4), 743–753. doi:10.1515/sjpain-2021-0060.

Kruskal, J., Wish, M., 1978. Multidimensional Scaling. SAGE Publications, Inc. doi:10.4135/9781412985130.

Laustsen, C.E., Petersson, P., Westergren, A., Haak, M., 2021. Involvement of professionals in research: knowledge integration, development of practice, and challenges: a group concept mapping study. Health Res. Policy Syst. 1478-4505. 19 (1). doi:10.1186/s12961-021-00763-5.

Linstone, H.A., Turoff, M., 1976. The Delphi method: techniques and applications. Technometrics. 00401706. 18 (3), 363. doi:10.2307/1268751.

Marley, G., Tan, R.K.J., Wang, T., Li, C., Byrne, M.E., Wu, D., Wang, C., Tang, W., Ramaswamy, R., Luo, D., Sylvia, S.S., Tucker, J.D., 2023. Online focus group discussions to engage stigmatized populations in qualitative health research: lessons learned. Int. J. Qual. Methods. 16094069. 22. Available from: https://journals.sagepub.com/home/IJQ. doi:10.1177/16094069231204767.

Newlon, J.L., Campi, J.A., Rafie, S., Meredith, A.H., 2024. Determining user implementation needs for pharmacist-prescribed contraception using concept mapping: a participatory, multiple stakeholder approach. Explor. Res. Clin. Soc. Pharm. 26672766. 16. Available from: https://www.sciencedirect.com/science/journal/26672766. doi:10.1016/j.rcsop.2024.100525.

Newlon, J.L., Murphy, E.M., Ahmed, R., Illingworth, K.S., 2023. Determining and regulating scope of practice for health care professionals: a participatory, multiple stakeholder approach. Res. Soc. Adm. Pharm. 15517411. 19 (3), 457–467. Available from: http://www.journals.elsevierhealth.com/periodicals/rsap. doi:10.1016/j.sapharm.2022.11.005.

Optimal Sort, 2025 https://www.optimalworkshop.com/.

Qualtrics, 2025. https://www.qualtrics.com/.

Richard, B., Sivo, S.A., Orlowski, M., Ford, R.C., Murphy, J., Boote, D.N., Witta, E.L., 2021. Qualitative research via focus groups: will going online affect the diversity of your findings? Cornell Hosp. Q. 19389663. 62 (1), 32–45. Available from: https://journals.sagepub.com/home/CQX. doi:10.1177/1938965520967769.

Roberts, J.K., Pavlakis, A.E., Richards, M.P., 2021. It's more complicated than it seems: virtual qualitative research in the COVID-19 era. Int. J. Qual. Methods. 16094069. 20. Available from: http://ijq.sagepub.com/content/by/year. doi:10.1177/16094069211002959.

Ruel, E., Wagner, W.E., Gillespie, B.J., 2016. The Practice of Survey Research: Theory and Applications. SAGE Publications, Inc. doi:10.4135/9781483391700.

Rupert, D.J., Poehlman, J.A., Hayes, J.J., Ray, S.E., Moultrie, R.R., 2017. Virtual versus in-person focus groups: comparison of costs, recruitment, and participant logistics. J. Med. Internet Res. 14388871. 19 (3). Available from: http://www.jmir.org/article/viewFile/jmir_v19i3e80/2. doi:10.2196/jmir.6980.

Soule, E.K., Jones, D.M., Lovelady, N., Thomas, L., Du, R., Prewitt, T.E., Taylor, E., Baker, S., Guy, M.C., Cornell, C.E., Fagan, P., 2024. Using concept mapping to identify community partners' and researchers' perceptions of social justice: a path toward eliminating chronic disease disparities. Health Equity. 24731242. 8 (1), 426–436. Available from: home.liebertpub.com/publications/health-equity/641/. doi:10.1089/heq.2023.0230.

Tsui, J., Shin, M., Sloan, K., Mackie, T.I., Garcia, S., Fehrenbacher, A.E., Crabtree, B.F., Palinkas, L.A., 2024. Use of concept mapping to inform a participatory engagement approach for implementation of evidence-based HPV vaccination strategies in safety-net clinics. Implement. Sci. Commun. 26622211. 5 (1). Available from: https://www.springer.com/journal/43058. doi:10.1186/s43058-024-00607-7.

Vaughn, L.M., Jacquez, F., 2020. Participatory research methods: choice points in the research process. J. Particip. Res. Methods 1, 1–14.

Webex, 2025. https://www.webex.com/.

Woodyatt, C.R., Finneran, C.A., Stephenson, R., 2016. In-person versus online focus group discussions: a comparative analysis of data quality. Qual. Health Res. 15527557. 26 (6), 741–749. Available from: www.sageltd.co.uk/journals/details/j0331.html. doi:10.1177/1049732316631510.

Yampolskaya, S., Nesman, T.M., Hernandez, M., Koch, D., 2004. Using concept mapping to develop a logic model and articulate a program theory: a case example. Am. J. Eval. 25 (2), 191–207. doi:10.1016/j.ameval.2004.03.003.

Yaphe, H., Adekoya, I., Steiner, L., Maraj, D., O'campo, P., Persaud, N., 2019. Exploring the experiences of people in Ontario, Canada who have trouble affording medicines: a qualitative concept mapping study. BMJ Open. 20446055. 9 (12). Available from: http://bmjopen.bmj.com/content/early/by/section. doi:10.1136/bmjopen-2019-033933.

Zoom, 2025. https://www.zoom.com/.

SECTION IV

Technology advancing pharmacy research

CHAPTER

26

Modularity encoding: A network-based approach for representing healthcare coding systems in machine learning models

Mohsen Askar[a] *and Kristian Svendsen*[b]

[a]Department of Drug statistics, Norwegian Institute of Public Health, Oslo, Norway
[b]Department of Pharmacy, Faculty of Health Sciences, UiT-The Arctic University of Norway, Tromsø, Norway

CHAPTER OBJECTIVES

In this chapter, readers are introduced to modularity encoding (ME), a network-based approach for representing healthcare coding systems (HCSs) in machine learning (ML) models. ME reduces model dimensionality while enhancing interpretability, offering an alternative to conventional encoding strategies. By the end of this chapter, readers should be able to:

- Recognize the limitations of conventional encoding methods for HCSs (e.g., binary encoding, hierarchy-based grouping, etc.)
- Learn how to construct patient-level cooccurrence networks using healthcare data
- Apply Network Analysis modularity (community detection) to identify meaningful clinical HCS code groupings (modules) within the dataset population
- Compare the performance of ML models using ME to other commonly used encoding approaches
- Discuss how ME can enhance model interpretations with a real-world example
- Discuss the applications of ME in different HCSs, as well as the advantages and limitations of the approach

Contemporary Research Methods in Pharmacy and Health Services - Volume 2
https://doi.org/10.1016/B978-0-443-44607-8.00033-9

1 Introduction

1.1 Background

The integration of artificial intelligence (AI), ML, automation, and big data analytics is transforming modern healthcare and pharmacy research (Khan et al., 2023). AI is increasingly being adopted across different domains such as drug discovery, clinical outcome prediction, and clinical decision support, enabling researchers to gain insights from complex datasets (Chalasani et al., 2023; Varnosfaderani and Forouzanfar, 2024; Raghupathi and Raghupathi, 2014).

One primary component of these healthcare datasets is HCSs. HCSs are standardized taxonomies used to classify diagnoses, medications, procedures, and hospital services. Common examples of these systems include the International Classification of Diseases (ICD) (International Classification of Diseases (ICD), 2023), Anatomical Therapeutic Chemical classification (ATC) (Organization WH, 2023), diagnosis-related groups (DRG) (Fetter et al., 1980), Current Procedural Terminology (CPT) (Hirsch et al., 2015), and the Healthcare Common Procedure Coding System (HCPCS) (Medicine USNL of UMLS Metathesaurus, 2023). These systems enable consistent documentation, data analysis, research, and related uses.

These systems can be hierarchical, for example, ICD and ATC codes, where broader categories are at the top and categories become more specific toward the bottom, or nonhierarchical, where the system does not follow a hierarchical structure, such as the CPT. One common feature of these systems is that they are high-dimensional, meaning that they often contain thousands of codes. In real-world datasets, thousands of these distinct codes may be present, posing a significant challenge for modeling.

1.2 What is the challenge, and what are the current approaches?

For most ML algorithms, converting categorical values to numerical ones is necessary so that algorithms are able to process this information, a process called *encoding* (Dahouda and Joe, 2021). The required prediction model should usually balance reliable performance, an efficient training process, and the ability to interpret the model output as transparently as possible. The methods used for encoding can heavily influence these factors, leading to either enhancing or worsening the prediction model.

While these mentioned HCSs offer valuable clinical information when they are used as input features in ML models, encoding them using conventional methods usually poses a challenge and is considered one of the limitations in preprocessing data for prediction models (Wang et al., 2018). For example, encoding these HCSs with traditional methods, such as binary encoding-representing each single code as a separate variable and assigning a value of 0 or 1 according to the presence or absence of the code for each patient in the dataset-, produces a binary vector whose length corresponds to the total number of codes. This results in a dramatic increase in model dimensionality, memory requirements, and computational power, introduces high model sparsity, and ultimately limits model performance (Johnson and Khoshgoftaar, 2022; Jiang et al., 2019). In the ML field, this is called the "curse of dimensionality" (Keogh and Mueen, 2017) and often leads to a worsening of the algorithm's discrimination performance.

A variety of encoding methods have been suggested and illustrated in the literature. These methods can be categorized into, *first*, direct encoding approaches such as binary, one-hot encoding, and hash encoding (Pargent et al., 2022). These approaches are simple to apply but are usually high-dimensional. *Second*, supervised encoding based on a target variable, such as target encoding, which depends on the predictive relationship between codes and the outcome (Pargent et al., 2022). These methods are efficient but risk information leakage from the outcome variable to the model, which is one of the common model training mistakes (Kaufman et al., 2011). *Third*, semantic representation learning, such as Word2Vec (Johnson and Khoshgoftaar, 2022) and entity embedding (Guo and Berkhahn, 2016). *Fourth*, automated feature synthesis, such as Deep Feature Synthesis, which generates higher levels of features from raw data using relational structures and aggregation (Kanter and Veeramachaneni, 2015). These methods are powerful but make the model outputs less interpretable. And *fifth*, similarity-based encoding, which encodes categories by their similarity and the distances between them rather than treating them as independent (Cerda and Varoquaux, 2022).

Many approaches have been trialed to simplify these HCSs. Some studies have used the total count of codes (e.g., diagnoses or medications) as a single numerical indicator (Kulkarni et al., 2016), calculated relevant indexes such as the Charlson Comorbidity Index (Hegselmann et al., 2022), or grouped the codes to a higher hierarchical level if the HCS is hierarchical (Yu and Xie, 2020; Pakbin et al., 2018). While grouping to broader levels can preserve the hierarchical structure of classification systems such as ICD-10, it has been shown that models using the most detailed codes often perform worse than those using higher-level groupings (Deschepper et al., 2019). In addition, this strategy is not applicable to coding systems that are nonhierarchical. Moreover, although such approaches effectively reduce the dimensionality of the data, they result in the loss of a significant amount of information contained at the complete code level, which may be essential for developing reliable model interpretation (Shameer et al., 2017).

Another commonly used strategy is to group, or aggregate, the levels of HCSs according to predefined, more clinically relevant schemes (Fenn et al., 2021; Zhao et al., 2021; Panicacci et al., 2018; Moran et al., 2009). While this approach is more convenient, it is limited by the hierarchical design of the schemes themselves and by the need for continuous upgrades of these schemes to suit different versions of the HCSs. The impact of such grouping methods on model performance was examined and demonstrated that the choice of grouping strategy significantly influences predictive accuracy, with some methods yielding better results than others. Notably, there is no evidence-based framework for how to handle HCSs in ML models (Kansal et al., 2021).

1.3 Suggested method

In this chapter, we introduce ME, a new method to represent HCSs in ML models. The method is meant to be applicable to all HCSs, both hierarchical and nonhierarchical. ME can reduce model dimensions, model training time, and required computational power. It can increase clinical relevance and enhance the interpretation of model outputs.

To illustrate its utility, we applied ME to two widely used coding systems: ICD and DRG. A series of experiments were conducted to evaluate the method from multiple perspectives: benchmarking it against binary encoding, evaluating its performance under different resolution thresholds, and comparing it with other common encoding schemes. Finally, we provide a publicly available Python package to support future research and practical implementation of ME. This tool makes it straightforward for researchers and practitioners to apply the method to diverse healthcare datasets.

2 Methods

2.1 Data source description

We utilized the Medical Information Mart for Intensive Care (MIMIC-III) dataset, which comprises 58,976 intensive care unit (ICU) encounters from 46,467 unique patients at Beth Israel Deaconess Medical Center between 2001 and 2012. MIMIC-III dataset is a publicly available dataset and its full description is provided elsewhere (Johnson et al., 2016). We excluded patients younger than 18 years, elective and newborn admissions, patients who died during hospitalization, and admissions with missing or invalid ICD codes. The final cohort comprised 29,247 patients and 37,762 admissions. The prediction models input variables included demographic, administrative, and clinical variables, such as patient and admission identifiers, admission and discharge locations, insurance type, marital status, length of stay, emergency department utilization, age group, gender, and ICD-9 diagnosis codes. The outcome was defined as ICU readmission within 90 days of the previous admission. A detailed description of variable engineering, exclusions, model features, and exploratory data analysis (EDA) are attached in supplementary material I, II to our article (Askar et al., 2024). To ensure methodological rigor, we followed the *International Journal of Medical Informatics* checklist (Cabitza and Campagner, 2021) for reporting medical AI studies. The checklist is attached to the mentioned article, supplementary material III (Askar et al., 2024).

2.2 Modularity encoding steps

ME is carried out in three main steps: network construction, modularity detection, and mapping codes to module identifiers.

2.3 Network construction

A network consists of two main components: *nodes,* which represent the entities of interest, and *edges,* which are the connections between these nodes and represent a type of relationship between them (Prell, 2012). In our case, we created a network in which the HCS codes are the nodes, and the edges between them represent the number of patients who combined both HCS codes in our dataset.

For our study, we constructed a multimorbidity network using patient identifiers and ICD-9 codes, where nodes correspond to individual ICD-9 diagnosis codes and edges represent the number of patients sharing pairs of diagnoses. The method for generating such networks has been described in detail in previous work (Askar et al., 2021). The resulting network comprised 6840 nodes (ICD-9 codes) and 952,676 edges. The same method has been applied to create a network for DRG codes. The DRG network comprised 1661 nodes and 41,274 edges.

In practice, these networks would represent the multimorbidity patterns in the patient population in the case of ICD and DRG codes. For example, if we were creating a network for ATC codes, the network would represent the comedication patterns in the population in this case.

2.4 Modularity detection

Network modularity, or community detection, is a useful feature of network structure that identifies groups of nodes that are more strongly connected to each other than to the rest of the network (Ji et al., 2015). There are several community detection techniques to identify such modules, including density-based, centrality-based, partition-based, and hierarchical clustering approaches (Zhang and Long Jason, 2013; Newman, 2006). After constructing the networks, we identified modules (communities) in the network, which represented the patterns of multimorbidity that tend to cooccur in the population.

In our experiments, we used the Louvain algorithm for community detection (Blondel et al., 2008). The Louvain method is a popular community detection algorithm due to its simplicity, speed, and effectiveness in detecting network modules (Hu et al., 2016). One of the important parameters of the Louvain method is the modularity resolution, which controls the number and size of the generated modules (Hu et al., 2016; Fortunato and Barthélemy, 2007). Applying higher resolution thresholds results in fewer but larger modules, while lower resolution thresholds result in several smaller ones. After running the community detection algorithm, all codes are grouped under the corresponding detected module IDs.

2.5 Mapping codes to detected module IDs

After detecting the modules, we assigned each HCS code to its corresponding module ID. Ultimately, we will have one variable for the HCS codes, in which each code is now encoded with the module ID it belongs to. We then binary encoded this variable in ML models. This resulted in substantially fewer binary variables in the final model. Table 26.1 represents the number of modules and features (dimensions) in the created datasets after these steps. The workflow of the ME approach is illustrated in Fig. 26.1.

TABLE 26.1 The number of detected modules and total model features (dimensions) in the datasets created after binary encoding.

Dataset	Description	No. of detected modules	No. of all features after binary encoding
Original dataset ICD	All ICD codes were dummy-encoded into separate binary variables.	–	4403
Resolution = 1 (R1)	ICD codes are grouped into 8 modules, detected at a resolution threshold of 1.	8 modules	56
Resolution = 0.8 (R08)	ICD codes are grouped into 16 modules, detected at a resolution threshold of 0.8.	16 modules	63
Resolution = 0.6 (R06)	ICD codes are grouped into 32 modules, detected at a resolution threshold of 0.6.	32 modules	95
Resolution = 0.5 (R05)	ICD codes are grouped into 47 modules, detected at a resolution threshold of 0.5.	47 modules	80
Resolution = 0.1 (R01)	ICD codes are grouped into 314 modules, detected at a resolution threshold of 0.1.	314 modules	362
Resolution = 0.01 (R001)	ICD codes are grouped into 1078 modules detected at a resolution threshold of 0.01.	1078 modules	1123
Clinical Classification Software (CCS)	ICD codes are grouped into 285 categories of single-level clinical classification software.	285 groups	322
Highest ICD hierarchy (ICD_Highest)	The ICD codes are grouped at the highest level of the hierarchy.	18 groups	66
Original dataset DRG	The raw form of the dataset: all DRG codes were dummy-encoded into separate binary variables.	–	1482
Resolution = 1 (R1 DRG)	The DRG codes are grouped into 24 modules by resolution threshold 1.	24 modules	64

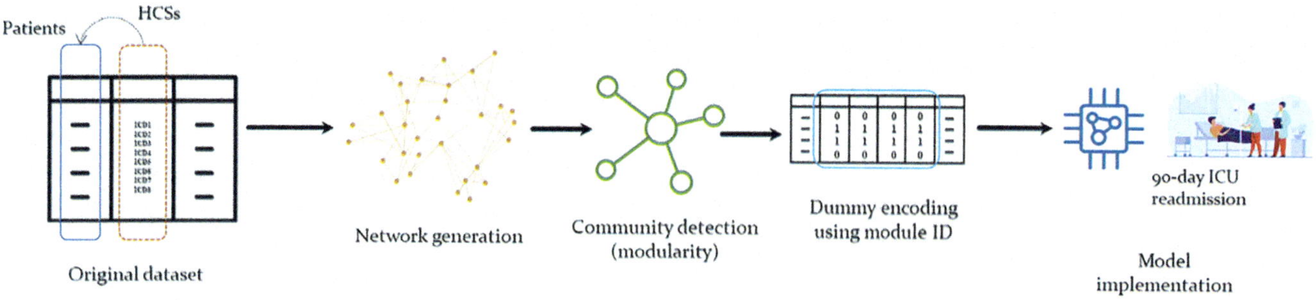

FIG. 26.1 ME steps. The steps for conducting modularity encoding are as follows: (1) A network is generated where the nodes represent the HCS codes, and the edges represent the cooccurrences of these codes within the patient population. (2) Community detection is used to identify modules of HCS codes that are strongly connected to each other. (3) Each code is then assigned to the module ID to which it belongs in the network. (4) The HCS variable is binary encoded, reducing the number of generated dimensions to correspond to the total number of detected modules in the network. (5) These binary variables are subsequently used as input variables in the ML prediction models.

2.6 Machine learning models

We followed standard ML modeling steps. Categorical variables were binary-encoded, while numerical variables were standardized. Standardization was performed separately on the training set and then applied to the testing set to prevent information leakage. The datasets were then randomly split into training and testing sets in a 70%–30% ratio. Three ML algorithms belonging to different algorithm families were implemented, namely a linear algorithm: logistic regression (LR); support vector machine (SVM) with a nonlinear kernel Radial Basis Function (RBF); and a tree-based algorithm: gradient boosting machine (GBM) to retrospectively predict 90-day ICU readmissions.

The output variable was imbalanced, meaning that the number of patients readmitted within 90 days from a previous admission was less than the number of patients who were not readmitted. To address this class imbalance (He and Garcia, 2009) and its potential impact on model performance, we applied random undersampling (Tanha et al., 2020). We randomly paired each instance of the minority class (ICU readmissions) with an instance from the majority class (nonreadmissions), resulting in balanced class distributions and enabling fair performance comparisons across models.

Model performance was evaluated using five evaluation metrics: accuracy, precision, recall, F1-score, and Area Under the Receiver Operating Characteristic (ROC) Curve (AUC). To estimate variability, 95% confidence intervals were computed via 1000 nonparametric bootstrap replicates on the test set. The code used in the study is publicly available here: https://anonymous.4open.science/r/modularity_encod_article-1FCC/.

2.7 Software

Data preprocessing and network generation were conducted using Stata 17, community detection and network visualization were performed with Gephi 0.10, and ML model implementation was done in Python 3.6.12 using scikit-learn 0.24.2.

2.8 Different comparisons with other methods

To test the utility of ME, we conducted four experiments: three on ICD codes and one on DRG codes. The *first experiment* compared model performance between traditional binary encoding, where each code is encoded in a separate binary variable (Original dataset), and ME at the highest resolution (R1 dataset). The *second experiment* evaluated models trained on ICD codes grouped into modules derived from different modularity resolution thresholds to assess whether specific thresholds yield better performance than others. The *third experiment* compared ME at the highest resolution with two alternative grouping strategies: aggregation to the highest ICD hierarchy and the Clinical Classification Software (CCS) scheme (Clinical Classifications Software, 2023). The *fourth experiment* replicated the second experiment using DRG codes instead of ICD codes. In a separate publication, we extended our experiments to demonstrate that ME provides meaningful clinical interpretations of models.

2.8.1 Experiment 1: Binary encoding versus ME on ICD and DRG codes

The experiment demonstrated better results for models trained using ME than binary encoding of the ICD codes in the original dataset in terms of most metrics for the three algorithms; see Table 26.2.

TABLE 26.2 A comparison of different performance metrics comparing the original dataset's binary encoding to modularity encoding.

Algorithm	Dataset	Accuracy (95% CI)	Precision (95% CI)	Recall (95% CI)	F1-score (95% CI)	AUC (95% CI)
LR	Original ICD	0.727 (0.723–0.731)	0.764 (0.759–0.77)	**0.656** (0.649–0.662)	**0.71** (0.701–0.711)	0.804 (0.800–0.808)
	R1	**0.736** (0.727–0.746)	**0.782** (0.769–0.795)	0.654 (0.640–0.668)	**0.71** (0.701–0.723)	**0.813** (0.805–0.823)
SVM	Original ICD	0.73 (0.726–0.735)	**0.787** (0.781–0.793)	0.632 (0.626–0.639)	0.7 (0.696–0.707)	0.822 (0.816–0.824)
	R1	**0.778** (0.769–0.787)	0.765 (0.753–0.777)	**0.802** (0.790–0.815)	**0.78** (0.774–0.793)	**0.837** (0.828–0.845)
GBM	Original ICD	0.779 (0.775–0.783)	0.751 (0.746–0.757)	0.835 (0.831–0.840)	**0.79** (0.787–0.795)	**0.837** (0.834–0.842)
	R1	**0.78** (0.772–0.789)	**0.752** (0.740–0.764)	**0.836** (0.826–0.847)	**0.79** (0.783–0.8)	0.836 (0.828–0.845)

Notes: Bold font indicates the best performance in the comparison metric.

TABLE 26.3 A comparison of different performance metrics for models where ICD codes are encoded using different modularity resolutions.

	Accuracy (95% CI)	Precision (95% CI)	Recall (95% CI)	F1-score (95% CI)	AUC (95% CI)
Logistic regression					
R1	**0.736** (0.727–0.746)	**0.782** (0.769–0.795)	0.654 (0.640–0.668)	0.71 (0.701–0.723)	**0.813** (0.805–0.823)
R08	0.734(0.728–0.741)	0.773(0.763–0.783)	0.663(0.653–0.673)	0.71(0.706–0.722)	0.81(0.804–0.817)
R06	0.73 (0.724–0.736)	0.772 (0.763–0.781)	0.651 (0.642–0.661)	0.71 (0.699–0.714)	0.812 (0.807–0.817)
R05	0.733 (0.728–0.739)	0.777 (0.770–0.785)	0.653 (0.645–0.662)	0.71 (0.704–0.717)	0.811 (0.806–0.817)
R01	0.724 (0.720–0.730)	0.762 (0.756–0.770)	0.652 (0.645–0.659)	0.7 (0.697–0.709)	0.803 (0.799–0.808)
R001	0.728 (0.724–0.733)	0.763 (0.757–0.770)	**0.661** (0.656–0.668)	0.71 (0.704–0.714)	0.804 (0.801–0.809)
Nonlinear support vector machine					
R1	0.778 (0.769–0.787)	0.765 (0.753–0.777)	0.802 (0.790–0.815)	0.78 (0.774–0.793)	0.837 (0.828–0.845)
R08	**0.786** (0.780–0.793)	0.767 (0.758–0.776)	**0.822** (0.814–0.830)	**0.79** (0.787–0.800)	0.841 (0.835–0.847)
R06	**0.786** (0.781–0.792)	0.775 (0.768–0.783)	0.806 (0.799–0.814)	**0.79** (0.784–0.796)	**0.847** (0.840–0.851)
R05	0.782 (0.777–0.788)	**0.779** (0.772–0.787)	0.788 (0.781–0.796)	0.78 (0.778–0.789)	0.845 (0.841–0.850)
R01	0.752 (0.748–0.757)	0.769 (0.763–0.776)	0.72 (0.714–0.727)	0.74 (0.739–0.750)	0.83 (0.825–0.834)
R001	0.741 (0.737–0.746)	**0.779** (0.773–0.786)	0.674 (0.668–0.681)	0.72 (0.718–0.728)	0.828 (0.820–0.828)
Gradient boosting machine					
R1	**0.78** (0.772–0.789)	**0.752** (0.740–0.764)	0.836 (0.826–0.847)	**0.79** (0.826–0.847)	**0.836** (0.828–0.845)
R08	**0.78** (0.774–0.786)	0.751 (0.743–0.760)	0.836 (0.829–0.844)	**0.79** (0.785–0.798)	0.831 (0.825–0.837)
R06	0.779 (0.774–0.785)	0.747 (0.740–0.755)	**0.843** (0.836–0.850)	**0.79** (0.786–0.798)	0.835 (0.830–0.841)
R05	**0.78** (0.775–0.786)	**0.752** (0.746–0.761)	0.834 (0.827–0.842)	**0.79** (0.786–0.797)	0.836 (0.831–0.841)
R01	0.771 (0.766–0.776)	0.741 (0.735–0.747)	0.833 (0.828–0.839)	0.78 (0.780–0.789)	0.83 (0.826–0.834)
R001	**0.78** (0.776–0.785)	0.752 (0.746–0.758)	0.836 (0.830–0.841)	**0.79** (0.788–0.796)	**0.836** (0.832–0.840)

Notes: Bold font indicates the best performance in the comparison metric.

The great reduction in dimensionality achieved using ME also led to a significant decrease in model training time, particularly for the SVM, which is typically computationally intensive. The training time was reduced from 83 minutes on the original ICD dataset to less than 30 seconds on the R1 dataset.

2.8.2 *Experiment 2: Different modularity resolution thresholds*

The findings suggested that higher resolution thresholds, which produce fewer modules, generally yield better performance compared to lower thresholds. However, for the SVM algorithm, recall, F1-score, and accuracy declined greatly as the number of modules increased, raising questions about the stability of SVM performance in this experiment (see Table 26.3 and Fig. 26.2). Based on these observations, we selected the R1 resolution for use in the third experiment.

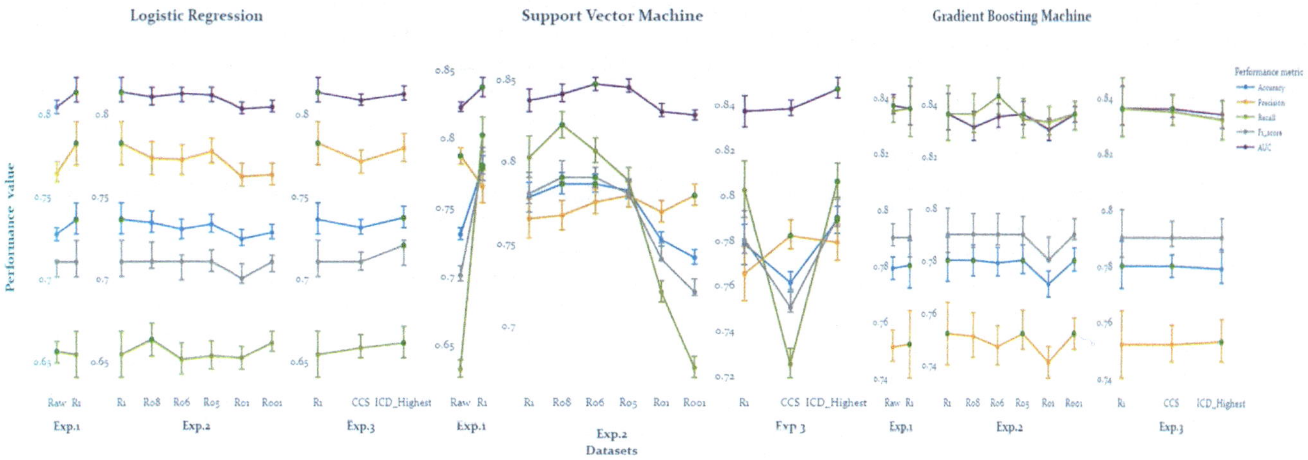

FIG. 26.2 A summary of the results from Experiments I, II, and III. This figure represents the outcomes of the first three ICD code experiments. LR, SVM, and GBM were used in all experiments. For all models, accuracy, precision, recall, F1-score, and AUC metrics with 95% confidence intervals were used to evaluate the models' performances. Green markers indicate the highest value of the evaluation metric in the respective comparison. Experiment 1 (binary vs modularity encoding), shown to the left of each subfigure, generally demonstrates better results for modularity grouping compared to dummy encoding of the raw ICD codes. In experiment 2 (different resolution threshold encoding), the performance results across different resolutions are close. The LR and GBM models suggest that R1 is the best resolution threshold, while the SVM model suggests that R08 is the best. In experiment 3 (comparison of modularity, highest hierarchy, and CCS encoding), grouping ICD codes to the highest level of the system hierarchy yielded the best results overall, followed by modularity grouping and CCS.

TABLE 26.4 A comparison of different performance metrics for various grouping strategy models.

	Accuracy (95% CI)	Precision (95% CI)	Recall (95% CI)	F1-score (95% CI)	AUC (95% CI)
Logistic regression					
R1	0.736 (0.727–0.746)	**0.782** (0.769–0.795)	0.654 (0.640–0.668)	0.71 (0.701–0.723)	**0.813** (0.805–0.823)
CCS	0.731 (0.727–0.736)	0.771 (0.764–0.778)	0.658 (0.652–0.666)	0.71 (0.705–0.716)	0.808 (0.804–0.813)
ICD Highest	**0.737** (0.731–0.744)	0.779 (0.771–0.788)	**0.661** (0.652–0.671)	**0.72** (0.708–0.723)	0.812 (0.807–0.819)
Nonlinear support vector machine					
R1	0.778 (0.769–0.787)	0.765 (0.753–0.777)	0.802 (0.790–0.815)	0.78 (0.774–0.793)	0.837 (0.828–0.845)
CCS	0.761 (0.757–0.766)	**0.782** (0.776–0.789)	0.725 (0.719–0.732)	0.75 (0.748–0.758)	0.838 (0.833–0.841)
ICD Highest	**0.789** (0.783–0.795)	0.779 (0.771–0.787)	**0.806** (0.799–0.814)	**0.79** (0.786–0.798)	**0.847** (0.841–0.853)
Gradient boosting machine					
R1	**0.78** (0.772–0.789)	0.752 (0.740–0.764)	**0.836** (0.826–0.847)	**0.79** (0.826–0.847)	**0.836** (0.828–0.845)
CCS	**0.78** (0.776–0.784)	0.752 (0.746–0.759)	0.835 (0.830–0.841)	**0.79** (0.787–0.796)	**0.836** (0.833–0.841)
ICD Highest	0.779 (0.774–0.786)	**0.753** (0.746–0.761)	0.832 (0.825–0.839)	**0.79** (0.785–0.797)	0.834 (0.828–0.839)

Notes: Bold font indicates the best performance in the comparison metric.

2.8.3 *Experiment 3: ME versus other grouping approaches*

Overall, the three grouping methods produced comparable performance; however, some differences were observed. Models trained on the R1 dataset and those grouped at the highest level of the ICD hierarchy generally outperformed models trained on the CCS scheme. Between these two, the ICD Highest models tended to perform slightly better than R1 in terms of accuracy, recall, and F1-score (LR, SVM), while R1 achieved the best results for AUC (LR, GBM), precision (LR), and recall (GBM). Both the ICD Highest and R1 consistently outperformed CCS across most metrics and algorithms. Notably, the SVM models trained with CCS grouping showed declines in accuracy, F1-score, and recall (Table 26.4 and Fig. 26.2). Fig. 26.2 summarizes the results from these three experiments.

2.8.4 *Experiment 4: Binary encoding vs ME on DRG codes*

Consistent with the ICD results, models trained on modularity-grouped DRG codes outperformed those using binary-encoded DRG codes in the original dataset, showing improvements across nearly all metrics and algorithms (see Table 26.5).

TABLE 26.5 The performance of predictions from models trained on the original binary-encoded DRG codes dataset compared to the modularity-encoded DRG codes dataset.

	Accuracy (95% CI)	Precision (95% CI)	Recall (95% CI)	F1-score (95% CI)	AUC (95% CI)
Logistic regression					
Original DRG	0.68 (0.675–0.688)	0.694 (0.684–0.705)	**0.644** (0.635–0.654)	0.67 (0.661–0.677)	0.749 (0.742–0.756)
R1_M24	**0.701** (0.691–0.712)	**0.734** (0.719–0.750)	0.629 (0.615–0.645)	**0.68** (0.665–0.691)	**0.771** (0.761–0.782)
Nonlinear support vector machine					
Original DRG	0.682 (0.676–0.689)	0.688 (0.679–0.698)	0.667 (0.658–0.676)	0.68 (0.670–0.685)	0.756 (0.751–0.762)
R1_M24	**0.721** (0.711–0.731)	**0.72** (0.707–0.734)	**0.723** (0.709–0.738)	**0.72** (0.710–0.733)	**0.794** (0.785–0.805)
Gradient boosting machine					
Original DRG	0.715 (0.709–0.722)	0.688 (0.680–0.698)	0.786 (0.778–0.794)	0.73 (0.727–0.741)	0.787 (0.781–0.794)
R1_M24	**0.73** (0.720–0.741)	**0.701** (0.689–0.716)	**0.8** (0.788–0.814)	**0.75** (0.737–0.759)	**0.798** (0.788–0.809)

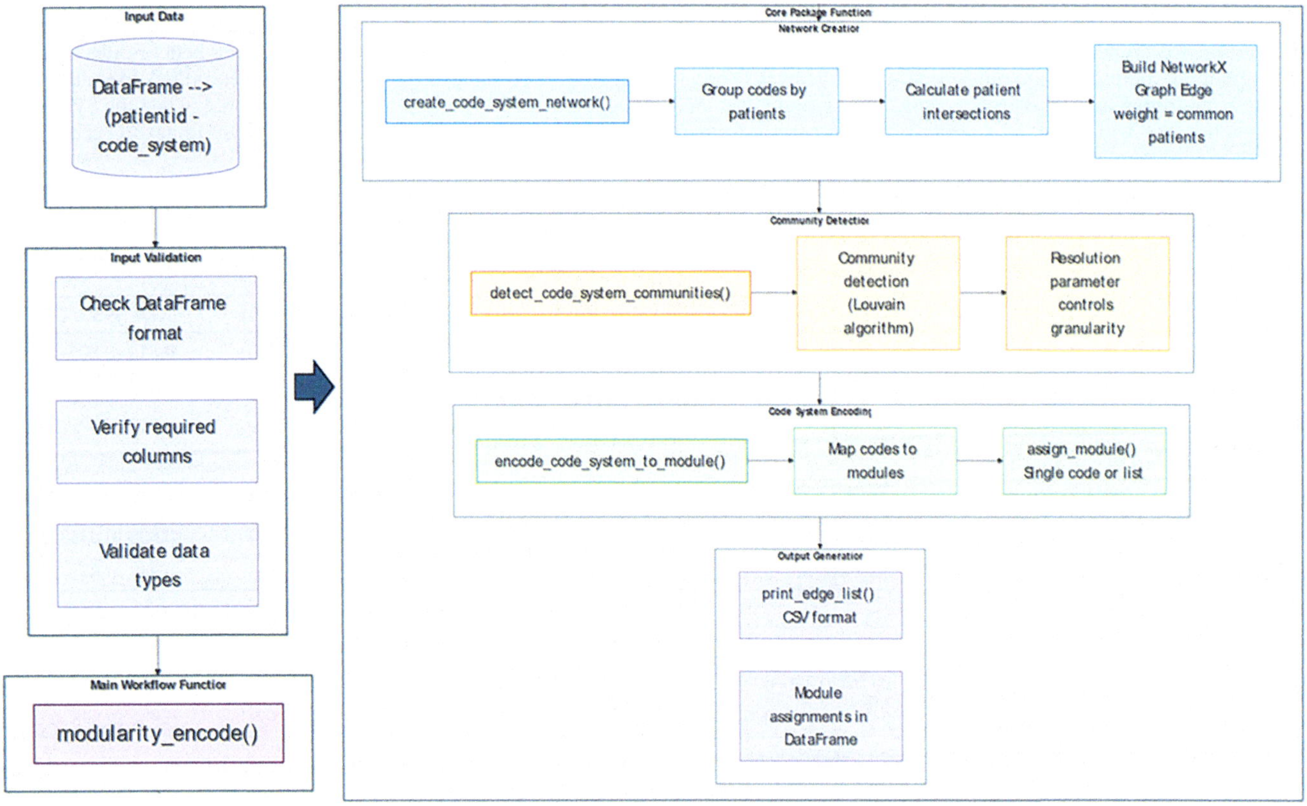

FIG. 26.3 ME Python package function structure. **The** Modularity Encoding package includes a structured set of functions. ME can be performed using a single function, "modularity_encode()". The package also contains detailed functions for users who need to track every step of the procedure. A detailed description of the package's functionality is available on its webpage on PyPI.

2.9 ME python package

To facilitate the use of this approach for future research, we developed a Python package called "*ME*", which is publicly available for download on the Python Package Index (PyPI) and can be installed using "pip install modularity-encoding". The package allows users to implement the full workflow through a single function, `*modularity_encode()*`. Fig. 26.3 presents the structure of the package functions. Comprehensive documentation, including a user guide and demonstration examples, is publicly available here: https://pypi.org/project/modularity-encoding/ and in supplementary material 4 of our article (Askar et al., 2024).

3 Discussion

ME is a data-driven method that utilizes Network Analysis (NA) community detection to detect clusters of HCS codes based on how often they cooccur together in the dataset population. These clusters form meaningful clinical patterns based on the type of HCS, such as multimorbidity or comedication. All approaches to encoding HCSs involve a trade-off between good model performance and potential information loss. Choosing the right encoding method is, therefore, critical for achieving reliable performance, as suboptimal techniques may fail to capture important patient characteristics and ultimately weaken predictive accuracy (Wang et al., 2018).

Unlike data-driven approaches that rely on the outcome variable, the relation between the target variable and HCS codes, and can cause overfitting, such as target encoding, ME is a data-driven approach that derives its grouping apart from the outcome variable. It extracts the patterns of occurrences of HCS codes in the dataset, providing a more interpretable representation of the information and making it less prone to overfitting.

3.1 Key findings from experiments

The experiments demonstrated the value of ME as an approach for handling high-dimensional HCSs. Across all three ML algorithms tested, ME improved or maintained predictive performance compared to the original dataset binary encoding. This improvement was achieved while greatly reducing the input model features (low model dimensionality), consequently decreasing the computational burden. For example, the number of features in the original ICD dataset exceeded 4000, whereas grouping the same codes through ME reduced this to only 56 features without compromising predictive accuracy.

When compared with other grouping strategies, such as single-level CCS or grouping to the highest ICD hierarchy, ME achieved comparable or slightly superior performance in most cases. Although the ICD hierarchy-based grouping performed marginally better in certain metrics, ME retained other key advantages, such as being data-driven, independent of static classification schemes, and therefore more flexible and adaptive to the studied dataset. The results also confirmed the practical benefits of ME in reducing training time, such as with SVM, where training time decreased from more than an hour to under a minute. Such efficiency is especially needed in the case of large-scale healthcare datasets, where computational costs and resource constraints can otherwise limit the feasibility of applying advanced ML models.

Overall, the experiments highlight three main findings: (a) ME yields *prediction performance* that is superior or at least comparable to other established grouping methods, (b) ME is more efficient and offers substantial reductions in feature dimensionality and training time, and (c) ME is not constrained by predefined hierarchies, making it applicable across both hierarchical and nonhierarchical HCSs. These findings establish ME as a promising alternative to existing encoding strategies in healthcare prediction modeling, with both methodological and practical advantages.

3.2 Universality of ME for hierarchical and nonhierarchical HCS systems

Many HCSs are designed with a hierarchical structure, such as the ICD or the ATC classification, where codes are organized from broad categories down to specific subgroups. Traditional grouping methods, such as collapsing codes to the highest hierarchy or using predefined classification schemes like CCS, take advantage of this structure but are inherently limited to hierarchical systems. Moreover, schemes like CCS must be regularly updated to stay aligned with new versions of ICD, requiring ongoing maintenance and manual curation.

Other HCSs, as mentioned before, such as CPT or the HCPCS, don't follow a hierarchical structure. For these systems, existing grouping strategies are less effective, as there is no built-in taxonomy to guide aggregation.

ME overcomes this limitation by relying on data-driven clustering rather than predefined taxonomies. Since ME groups the codes based on their observed cooccurrence patterns in the study population, it can be applied equally well to hierarchical and nonhierarchical systems. Moreover, ME may confirm or refine the clinical groupings that hierarchies suggest in hierarchical systems, while in nonhierarchical systems, it can reveal new, clinically meaningful clusters that would otherwise remain hidden.

This universality makes ME a flexible and widely applicable tool for reducing dimensionality in healthcare datasets. Regardless of the coding framework used, ME adapts to the underlying data structure and provides compact, interpretable representations that support both predictive modeling and clinical insights.

3.3 Clinical relevance and model interpretations

One of the general challenges facing ML prediction models in healthcare is what is called a "black box" problem (Hassija et al., 2024), where models may achieve high predictive accuracy but offer little insight into the interpretation behind these predictions. This lack of transparency limits the clinical adoption of ML models, as clinicians need to understand not only what the model predicts but also why. ME provides a way to bridge this gap. By grouping codes into modules that reflect actual cooccurrence patterns in the population, ME yields predictors that have direct clinical meaning. Each module represents a cluster of diagnoses or treatments that are commonly observed together, which can often be interpreted as a multimorbidity or comedication pattern. This allows clinicians to connect model outputs to recognizable clinical phenomena rather than abstract statistical constructs. The difference in interpretation between ME and approaches that use grouping to a higher level of hierarchy as a grouping method is that these methods implicitly assume that similarity within the same HCS hierarchy improves model predictions and makes sensible clinical interpretations, which may not be true in practice.

Many studies have investigated clinical patterns of diseases using the Network Analysis approach, revealing meaningful clinical patterns in each module (Guo et al., 2019; Chen and Xu, 2014; Zhou et al., 2022; Mu et al., 2020; Jones et al., 2023). In a complementary study, we applied the same network-based community detection approach to chronic conditions in the Norwegian elderly population (Askar et al., 2025). This analysis revealed eight distinct multimorbidity patterns that could be clinically interpreted and validated. The results are publicly available at https://for-articles.github.io/Multimorbidity_0.8_Resolution/. This exploration illustrates how ME, in addition to its performance and technical advantages, can also be used to uncover clinically relevant groupings and enhance the interpretability of predictive models. Beyond improving computational efficiency and predictive accuracy, ME has the potential to make ML outputs more actionable in healthcare settings. For example, one major pattern linked diabetes with cardiovascular and kidney diseases (cardiorenal syndrome), reflecting the well-known clinical trajectory where metabolic dysfunction increases the risk of cardiovascular complications and renal impairment. Such findings not only confirm established medical knowledge but also highlight the ability of ME to recover meaningful structures directly from registry data. By producing modules that align with real-world patterns of disease and treatment, ME strengthens both the interpretability and the trustworthiness of ML models for clinical decision-making. Fig. 26.4 summarizes the advantages and disadvantages of ME compared to other commonly used approaches.

Aspect	Binary encoding	Clinical Grouping (e.g., CCS)	Highest hierarchy	Modularity Encoding
Training time	-	+	+	+
Dimension reduction	-	+	+	+
Prediction performance	-	+	+	+
Clinical relevancy	-	+	-	+
Enhance interpretation	-	+	-	+
Universality for code systems	+	-	+	+
Suitability for hierarchical/non-hierarchical systems	-	-	-	+
Need updating	+	-	+	+
Introducing additional clinical info.	-	+	-	+
Easy implementation	+	-	+	-

(+) advantage, (−) disadvantage

FIG. 26.4 ME vs other approaches pros and cons. A comparison summary of the advantages and disadvantages of commonly used HCS encoding approaches.

3.4 Limitations and future directions

While ME provides several advantages compared to conventional grouping strategies, it also comes with important limitations that should be considered when applying it in practice. These limitations are linked both to the underlying modularity detection algorithms, such as the Louvain method, and to the way the resulting groupings depend on the data from which they are derived.

As mentioned before, the modules produced by ME are inherently data-driven. They reflect cooccurrence patterns present in the study population, which means that results may vary between different populations, healthcare settings, or time periods. For example, a module capturing diabetes, cardiovascular disease, and kidney disease may emerge in one population but appear differently in a younger or healthier population. This dependence on local data structure enhances flexibility but also limits generalizability.

ME relies on the method of modularity detection used and will consequently inherit its limitations. For example, in this study, we used the Louvain method for modularity detection. Despite the fact that the method is efficient and widely used, it comes with known limitations such as stochasticity, as it involves random initializations, which can lead to slightly different partitions of the network across runs and can limit reproducibility. Adapting the resolution parameter is crucial in this method, as different resolution thresholds will produce different numbers of modules and will also limit the reproducibility of results. Other algorithms can be used for community detection, such as the Leiden algorithm, which was developed as a modification of the Louvain method (Traag et al., 2019). Another limitation of the Louvain method is that it is a hard partitioning method, meaning it does not allow one node to appear in more than one module. This could be unrealistic in practical scenarios, as one disease can be linked to more than one morbidity pattern (Holden et al., 2011).

Although ME improves interpretability compared to other approaches, the clinical meaning of some modules may still be ambiguous without the use of expertise and domain knowledge to interpret the modules correctly. Not all clusters neatly align with established clinical categories, and some may appear as statistical associations rather than well-established disease or treatment patterns. This requires careful validation and, ideally, input from clinical experts before drawing conclusions from ME-derived modules.

One important future direction is testing alternative community detection methods beyond the Louvain method to overcome its limitations. It is also important to test algorithms that allow nodes to appear in more than one module to enhance the clinical interpretation of the modules (Ding et al., 2016).

Since ME is data-driven, there is also a need for cross-population validation. Comparing results across healthcare systems, time periods, and demographic groups could clarify which modules are universal and which are specific to a given context. Finally, benchmarking ME against other dimensionality reduction techniques, such as autoencoders or embeddings, could highlight its advantages and limitations.

4 Questions for further discussion

- What are the potential pitfalls of data-driven grouping, and what value does integrating clinical oversight add to the trained ML model?
- What trade-offs should you consider when applying different grouping approaches? Reflect on how you should proceed with your choice. Consider aspects such as predictive performance, interpretability, reproducibility, and generalizability.
- In what scenarios do you think ME would be less appropriate than more traditional encoding approaches?

5 Application exercises/scenarios

5.1 Scenario A: Applying ME to medication data

Using the same pipeline presented in this chapter, apply ME to the medication data available in the MIMIC dataset. Instead of using ICD-9 diagnosis codes, construct a cooccurrence network based on prescribed medications. Run community detection to identify modules of commonly coprescribed drugs.

- How many modules do you find, and what comedication patterns do they represent?
- Compare the predictive performance of models trained on the original medication codes versus models trained on ME modules.

5.2 Scenario B: Comparing Louvain and Leiden algorithms

The Leiden algorithm is a community detection algorithm developed as a modification of the Louvain method. Run both the Louvain and Leiden community detection algorithms on the same dataset (ICD-9 or medications).

- Explore how much the modules differ between the two algorithms
- Train identical ML models using the two sets of modules. Report differences in training time, predictive performance, and interpretability
- Reflect: do the algorithmic differences produce modules that are clinically distinct, or are they largely overlapping? Does one algorithm yield more coherent or clinically meaningful clusters?

AI Disclosure

During the preparation of this work, the author(s) used ChatGPT to edit text, reformulate sentences, and improve word choice. After using this tool/service, the author(s) reviewed and edited the content as needed and take full responsibility for the content of the publication.

References

Askar, M., Cañadas, R.N., Svendsen, K., 2021. An introduction to network analysis for studies of medication use. Res. Soc. Adm. Pharm. 15517411. 17 (12), 2054–2061. doi:10.1016/j.sapharm.2021.06.021.

Askar, M., Garcia, B.H., Svendsen, K., 2025. Exploring multimorbidity patterns in older hospitalized Norwegian patients using network analysis modularity. Int. J. Med. Inform. 13865056. 201, 105954. doi:10.1016/j.ijmedinf.2025.105954.

Askar, M., Småbrekke, L., Holsbø, E., Bongo, L.A., Svendsen, K., 2024. Using network analysis modularity to group health code systems and decrease dimensionality in machine learning models. Explor. Res. Clin. Soc. Pharm. 26672766. 14, 100463. doi:10.1016/j.rcsop.2024.100463.

Blondel, V.D., Guillaume, J.-L., Lambiotte, R., Lefebvre, E., 2008. Fast unfolding of communities in large networks. J. Stat. Mech. Theory Exp. 1742-5468. 2008 (10), 10008. doi:10.1088/1742-5468/2008/10/p10008.

Cabitza, F., Campagner, A., 2021. The need to separate the wheat from the chaff in medical informatics. Int. J. Med. Inform. 13865056. 153, 104510. doi:10.1016/j.ijmedinf.2021.104510.

Cerda, P., Varoquaux, G., 2022. Encoding high-cardinality string categorical variables. IEEE Trans. Knowl. Data Eng. 1041-4347. 34 (3), 1164–1176. doi:10.1109/tkde.2020.2992529.

Chalasani, S.H., Syed, J., Ramesh, M., Patil, V., Kumar, T.M.P., 2023. Artificial intelligence in the field of pharmacy practice: a literature review. Explor. Res. Clin. Soc. Pharm. 26672766. 12, 100346. doi:10.1016/j.rcsop.2023.100346.

Chen, Y., Xu, R., 2014. Network Analysis of Human Disease Comorbidity Patterns Based on Large-Scale Data Mining, Vol. 8492. Springer Science and Business Media LLC, pp. 243–254. doi:10.1007/978-3-319-08171-7_22.

Clinical Classifications Software, 2023. Clinical Classifications Software (CCS) for ICD-9-CM, pp. 8–9. https://hcup-us.ahrq.gov/toolssoftware/ccs/ccs.jsp.

Dahouda, M.K., Joe, I., 2021. A deep-learned embedding technique for categorical features encoding. IEEE Access. 21693536. 9, 114381–114391. Available from: http://ieeexplore.ieee.org/xpl/RecentIssue.jsp?punumber=6287639. doi:10.1109/ACCESS.2021.3104357.

Deschepper, M., Eeckloo, K., Vogelaers, D., Waegeman, W., 2019. A hospital wide predictive model for unplanned readmission using hierarchical ICD data. Comput. Methods Programs Biomed. 01692607. 173, 177–183. doi:10.1016/j.cmpb.2019.02.007.

Ding, Z., Zhang, X., Sun, D., Luo, B., 2016. Overlapping community detection based on network decomposition. Sci. Rep. 2045-2322. 6 (1). doi:10.1038/srep24115.

Fenn, A., Davis, C., Buckland, D.M., Kapadia, N., Nichols, M., Gao, M., Knechtle, W., Balu, S., Sendak, M., Theiling, B.J., 2021. Development and validation of machine learning models to predict admission from emergency department to inpatient and intensive care units. Ann. Emerg. Med. 01960644. 78 (2), 290–302. doi:10.1016/j.annemergmed.2021.02.029.

Fetter, R.B., Shin, Y., Freeman, J.L., Averill, R.F., Thompson, J.D., 1980. Case mix definition by diagnosis-related groups. Med. Care. 00257079. 18 (2), 1–53.

Fortunato, S., Barthélemy, M., 2007. Resolution limit in community detection. Proc. Natl. Acad. Sci. U. S. A. 0027-8424. 104 (1), 36–41. doi:10.1073/pnas.0605965104.

Guo, C., Berkhahn, F., 2016. Entity Embeddings of Categorical Variables. Available from: http://arxiv.org/abs/1604.06737.

Guo, M., Yanan, Y., Wen, T., Zhang, X., Liu, B., Zhang, J., Zhang, R., Zhang, Y., Zhou, X., 2019. Analysis of disease comorbidity patterns in a large-scale China population. BMC Med. Genomics. 1755-8794. 12 (S12). doi:10.1186/s12920-019-0629-x.

Hassija, V., Chamola, V., Mahapatra, A., Singal, A., Goel, D., Huang, K., Scardapane, S., Spinelli, I., Mahmud, M., Hussain, A., 2024. Interpreting black-box models: a review on explainable artificial intelligence. Cogn. Comput. 1866-9956. 16 (1), 45–74. doi:10.1007/s12559-023-10179-8.

He, H., Garcia, E.A., 2009. Learning from imbalanced data. IEEE Trans. Knowl. Data Eng. 1041-4347. 21 (9), 1263–1284. doi:10.1109/tkde.2008.239.

Hegselmann, S., Ertmer, C., Volkert, T., Gottschalk, A., Dugas, M., Varghese, J., 2022. Development and validation of an interpretable 3 day intensive care unit readmission prediction model using explainable boosting machines. Front. Med. 2296-858X. 9. doi:10.3389/fmed.2022.960296.

Hirsch, J.A., Leslie-Mazwi, T.M., Nicola, G.N., Barr, R.M., Bello, J.A., Donovan, W.D., Raymond, T., Alson, M.D., Manchikanti, L., 2015. Current procedural terminology; a primer. J. Neurointerv. Surg. 1759-8478. 7 (4), 309–312. doi:10.1136/neurintsurg-2014-011156.

Holden, L., Scuffham, P.A., Hilton, M.F., Muspratt, A., Ng, S.K., Whiteford, H.A., 2011. Patterns of multimorbidity in working Australians. Popul. Health Metr. 14787954. 9. Available from: http://www.pophealthmetrics.com/content/9/1/15. doi:10.1186/1478-7954-9-15Australia.

Hu, B., Li, W., Huo, X., Liang, Y., Gao, M., Pei, P., 2016. Improving Louvain algorithm for community detection. In: Proceedings of the 2016 International Conference on Artificial Intelligence and Engineering Applications. doi:10.2991/aiea-16.2016.20.

International Classification of Diseases (ICD), 2023. https://www.who.int/standards/classifications/classification-of-diseases, p. 9.

Ji, X., Machiraju, R., Ritter, A., Yen, P.Y., 2015. Examining the distribution, modularity, and community structure in article networks for systematic reviews. Annu. Symp. Proc. AMIA Symp. 1942597X. 2015, 1927–1936.

Jiang, B., Deng, C., Yi, H., Hu, Z., Zhou, G., Zheng, Y., Huang, S., Guo, X., Wang, D., Song, Y., Zhao, L., Wang, Z., Sun, P., Zhang, Y., Zhang, D., Li, J., Xu, J., Zhu, X., Gai, K., 2019. XDL: An industrial deep learning framework for high-dimensional sparse data. In: Proceedings of the ACM SIGKDD International Conference on Knowledge Discovery and Data Mining. Association for Computing Machinery, China, pp. 1–9. doi:10.1145/3326937.3341255.

Johnson, A.E.W., Pollard, T.J., Shen, L., Lehman, L.-W.H., Feng, M., Ghassemi, M., Moody, B., Szolovits, P., Celi, L.A., Mark, R.G., 2016. MIMIC-III, a freely accessible critical care database. Sci. Data. 2052-4463. 3 (1). doi:10.1038/sdata.2016.35.

Johnson, J.M., Khoshgoftaar, T.M., 2022. Encoding high-dimensional procedure codes for healthcare fraud detection. SN Comput. Sci. 26618907. 3 (5). Available from: https://www.springer.com/journal/42979. doi:10.1007/s42979-022-01252-4.

Jones, I., Cocker, F., Jose, M., Charleston, M., Neil, A.L., 2023. Methods of analysing patterns of multimorbidity using network analysis: a scoping review. J. Public Health. 16132238. 31 (8), 1217–1223. Available from: https://www.springer.com/journal/10389. doi:10.1007/s10389-021-01685-w.

Kansal, A., Gao, M., Balu, S., Nichols, M., Corey, K., Kashyap, S., Sendak, M., 2021. Impact of diagnosis code grouping method on clinical prediction model performance: a multi-site retrospective observational study. Int. J. Med. Inform. 13865056. 151, 104466. doi:10.1016/j.ijmedinf.2021.104466.

Kanter, J.M., Veeramachaneni, K., 2015. Deep feature synthesis: towards automating data science endeavors. In: Proceedings of the 2015 IEEE International Conference on Data Science and Advanced Analytics, DSAA 2015. Institute of Electrical and Electronics Engineers Inc., United States. pp. 1–10. doi:10.1109/DSAA.2015.7344858.

Kaufman, S., Rosset, S., Perlich, C., 2011. Leakage in data mining: formulation, detection, and avoidance. In: Proceedings of the ACM SIGKDD International Conference on Knowledge Discovery and Data Mining. Association for Computing Machinery, Israel, pp. 556–563. doi:10.1145/2020408.2020496.

Keogh, E., Mueen, A., 2017. Curse of Dimensionality. Springer Science and Business Media LLC, pp. 314–315. doi:10.1007/978-1-4899-7687-1_192.

Khan, O., Parvez, M., Kumari, P., Parvez, S., Ahmad, S., 2023. The future of pharmacy: how AI is revolutionizing the industry. Intell. Pharm. 2949866X. 1 (1), 32–40. doi:10.1016/j.ipha.2023.04.008.

Kulkarni, P., Smith, L.D., Woeltje, K.F., 2016. Assessing risk of hospital readmissions for improving medical practice. Health Care Manag. Sci. 13869620. 19 (3), 291–299. doi:10.1007/s10729-015-9323-5.

Medicine USNL of UMLS Metathesaurus, 2023. HCPCS (HCPCS - Healthcare Common Procedure Coding System). Source Representation https://www.nlm.nih.gov/research/umls/sourcereleasedocs/current/HCPCS/sourcerepresentation.html.

Moran, P., Klinteberg, B.A.F., Batty, G.D., Vågerö, D., 2009. Brief report: childhood intelligence predicts hospitalization with personality disorder in adulthood: evidence from a population-based study in Sweden. J. Pers. Disord. 0885-579X. 23 (5), 535–540. doi:10.1521/pedi.2009.23.5.535.

Mu, X.M., Wang, W., Jiang, Y.Y., Feng, J., 2020. Patterns of comorbidity in hepatocellular carcinoma: a network perspective. Int. J. Environ. Res. Public Health. 16604601. 17 (9). Available from: https://www.mdpi.com/1660-4601/17/9/3108/pdf. doi:10.3390/ijerph17093108.

Newman, M.E.J., 2006. Modularity and community structure in networks. Proc. Natl. Acad. Sci. U. S. A. 0027-8424. 103 (23), 8577–8582. doi:10.1073/pnas.0601602103.

Organization WH, 2023. WHOCC - ATC/DDD Index https://www.whocc.no/atc_ddd_index/.

Pakbin, A., Rafi, P., Hurley, N., Schulz, W., Harlan Krumholz, M., Bobak Mortazavi, J., 2018. Prediction of ICU readmissions using data at patient discharge. In: Proceedings of the Annual International Conference of the IEEE Engineering in Medicine and Biology Society, EMBS. Institute of Electrical and Electronics Engineers Inc., United States, pp. 4932–4935. doi:10.1109/EMBC.2018.8513181.

Panicacci, S., Donati, M., Fanucci, L., Bellin, I., Profili, F., Francesconi, P., 2018. Population health management exploiting machine learning algorithms to identify high-risk patients. In: Proceedings - IEEE Symposium on Computer-Based Medical Systems. Institute of Electrical and Electronics Engineers Inc, Italy, pp. 298–303. doi:10.1109/CBMS.2018.00059.

Pargent, F., Pfisterer, F., Thomas, J., Bischl, B., 2022. Regularized target encoding outperforms traditional methods in supervised machine learning with high cardinality features. Comput. Stat. 0943-4062. 37 (5), 2671–2692. doi:10.1007/s00180-022-01207-6.

Prell, C., 2012. Social Network Analysis: History, Theory & Methodology. SAGE Publications.

Raghupathi, W., Raghupathi, V., 2014. Big data analytics in healthcare: promise and potential. Health Inf. Sci. Syst. 2047-2501. 2 (1). doi:10.1186/2047-2501-2-3.

Shameer, K., Johnson, K.W., Yahi, A., Miotto, R., Li, L.I., Ricks, D., Jebakaran, J., Kovatch, P., Sengupta, P.P., Gelijns, A., Moskovitz, A., Darrow, B., Reich, D.L., Kasarskis, A., Tatonetti, N.P., Pinney, S., Dudley, J.T., 2017. Predictive modeling of hospital readmission rates using electronic medical record-wide machine learning: a case-study using mount sinai heart failure cohort. In: Pacific Symposium on Biocomputing, World Scientific Publishing Co. Pte Ltd, United States, pp. 276–287. http://psb.stanford.edu/. doi:10.1142/9789813207813_0027.

Tanha, J., Abdi, Y., Samadi, N., Razzaghi, N., Asadpour, M., 2020. Boosting methods for multi-class imbalanced data classification: an experimental review. J. Big Data. 2196-1115. 7 (1). doi:10.1186/s40537-020-00349-y.

Traag, V.A., Waltman, L., van Eck, N.J., 2019. From Louvain to Leiden: guaranteeing well-connected communities. Sci. Rep. 20452322. 9 (1). Available from: www.nature.com/srep/index.html. doi:10.1038/s41598-019-41695-z.

Varnosfaderani, S.M., Forouzanfar, M., 2024. The role of AI in hospitals and clinics: transforming healthcare in the 21st century. Bioengineering. 2306-5354. 11 (4), 337. doi:10.3390/bioengineering11040337.

Wang, H., Cui, Z., Chen, Y., Avidan, M., Abdallah, A.B., Kronzer, A., 2018. Predicting Hospital Readmission via Cost-Sensitive Deep Learning. IEEE/ACM Trans. Comput. Biol. Bioinform. 1545-5963. 15 (6), 1968–1978. doi:10.1109/tcbb.2018.2827029.

Yu, K., Xie, X., 2020. Predicting hospital readmission: a joint ensemble-learning model. IEEE J. Biomed. Health Inform. 21682208. 24 (2), 447–456. Available from: http://ieeexplore.ieee.org/xpl/RecentIssue.jsp?punumber=6221020. doi:10.1109/JBHI.2019.2938995.

Zhang, M., Long Jason, L., 2013. Modules in Networks, Algorithms and Methods. Springer Science and Business Media LLC, pp. 1447–1450. doi:10.1007/978-1-4419-9863-7_557.

Zhao, P., Yoo, I., Naqvi, S.H., 2021. Early prediction of unplanned 30-day hospital readmission: model development and retrospective data analysis. JMIR Med. Inform. 22919694. 9 (3). Available from: https://medinform.jmir.org/2021/3/e16306. doi:10.2196/16306.

Zhou, D., Wang, L., Ding, S., Shen, M., Qiu, H., 2022. Phenotypic disease network analysis to identify comorbidity patterns in hospitalized patients with ischemic heart disease using large-scale administrative data. Healthcare. 2227-9032. 10 (1), 80. doi:10.3390/healthcare10010080.

CHAPTER

27

Artificial intelligence in pharmacotherapy—Methods and approaches

Olaf Rose[a], *Kreshnik Hoti*[b], *Christopher Mosch*[c], *and Michael Bücker*[d]

[a]Department of Pharmaceutical Biology and Clinical Pharmacy, Institute of Pharmacy, Paracelsus Medical University, Salzburg, Austria

[b]University of Pristina, Pristina, Serbia

[c]Pharmaceutical Biology and Clinical Pharmacy, Pharmacotherapy Research Group, Institute of Pharmacy, Paracelsus Medical University, Salzburg, Austria

[d]Münster School of Business - FH Münster, University of Applied Sciences, Münster, Germany

CHAPTER OBJECTIVES

After reading this chapter, the reader should be able to:

- Explain the rationale for using artificial intelligence (AI) in pharmacotherapy, particularly in the context of complex medication regimens and increasing therapeutic knowledge.
- Differentiate between the major categories of AI approaches, including traditional machine learning (ML) models [e.g., decision trees, random forests, artificial neural networks (ANNs)] and transformer-based generative models, such as large language models (LLMs).
- Understand key methods for evaluating AI models in pharmacotherapy, including classification metrics, regression metrics, calibration approaches, and validation strategies.
- Recognize the practical barriers to implementing AI-based clinical decision support systems (CDSS) in pharmacotherapy, such as limited

Contemporary Research Methods in Pharmacy and Health Services - Volume 2
https://doi.org/10.1016/B978-0-443-44607-8.00030-3

datasets, model interpretability, and the integration of patient preferences.
- Describe the concept of hybrid AI systems, including retrieval-augmented generation (RAG) and neuro-symbolic architectures, and explain why these approaches may be particularly suitable for clinical decision support in medication management.
- Critically assess the role of AI in pharmacotherapy, recognizing both its potential benefits and its limitations in safety-critical healthcare environments.

1 Background and rationale for using AI in pharmacotherapy

Contemporary and evidence-based pharmacotherapy is grounded in randomized controlled trials and therapy guidelines wherever possible. General practitioners and pharmacists often feel overwhelmed by the rapid changes in therapeutic standards. Consequently, guideline adherence is limited, even in prevalent diseases such as hypertension, dyslipidemia, coronary heart disease, or heart failure (Hobbs, 2002; Komajda et al., 2003; Vonbank et al., 2013). Furthermore, medication errors are common, with prescribing errors being the most prevalent (Naseralallah et al., 2023). CDSS are software tools designed to directly aid clinicians. They are widely accepted and integrated into current medical and pharmaceutical practice (Sim et al., 2001; Jaspers et al., 2011). To date, AI in the medical field is predominantly engaged in diagnosis or in situations where a large amount of data needs to be analyzed (Das et al., 2018; Hollon et al., 2020; Koh et al., 2022). A software application has been introduced that can guide the correct use and application of devices such as insulin pens (Zhao et al., 2021). In contrast to its application in diagnosis, AI is rarely employed to guide therapy, particularly in the field of pharmacotherapy. While LLMs like ChatGPT, Gemini, and others can provide excellent recommendations when prompted with a patient case and a request for optimizing therapy, there are many valid reasons to keep AI out of therapy decisions. Pharmacotherapy is an extremely sensitive matter, and every mistake can have dramatic and immediate consequences. Additionally, several risks specific to the use of LLMs in clinical contexts must be considered. These include so-called "hallucinations," where models generate fluent but factually incorrect or misleading content (Ji et al., 2023), and the lack of transparency in how recommendations are derived, often referred to as the "black box" problem (Amann et al., 2020). Moreover, biases in training data may lead to unfair or unsafe suggestions, particularly for underrepresented patient groups (Obermeyer et al., 2019). Concerns about patient privacy and the secure handling of health data also remain unresolved, especially in light of legal frameworks such as the GDPR and the challenges in ensuring anonymization in complex language data (Price and Cohen, 2019). Finally, the mere availability of seemingly plausible AI output may increase the risk of overreliance among health professionals, even when those outputs are incorrect (Cabitza et al., 2017).

Furthermore, comprehensive patient data are not always available in a digital format. Even though generative AI can collect such information from analog sources, this particularly applies to patients' complaints and expectations, which are gathered through interactions between the healthcare provider and the patient (McCahon et al., 2022). These personal interactions seem inevitable and valuable for shared decision-making. Even though patients appreciate the aid of AI in collecting data, they primarily prefer decision-making by and with a human (Young et al., 2021; Witkowski et al., 2024; Cavalier et al., 2025; Graham, 2025). Personal preferences and mutual trust cannot easily be replaced (Buchegger et al., 2023). CDSS in pharmacotherapy can be designed as simple input-output software, such as a drug-drug interaction checker. Algorithm-based software with interactive feedback loops is much more helpful, as it can respond to preset personal valuations. Unfortunately, software that merely reconciles lists may face limitations in multimorbid patients with conflicting therapies (Kerliu et al., 2021). A simple example is the prescription of two blood pressure-lowering drugs. While this combination therapy is clearly indicated in most cases, it might cause or contribute to a drug-related problem (DRP) in certain other patients. More information is needed in such cases to draw the right conclusion. A review on AI in pharmacy practice found only one study that employed AI in medication management. AI helped to identify patients and reduce costs but was not utilized in therapy planning (Kessler et al., 2021). In this chapter, we aim to present AI models, discuss barriers to the application of these models in pharmacotherapy within patient care (i.e., the patient clinical context), and explore future approaches.

2 Basic AI models as a tool to inform pharmacotherapy

As the field of pharmacotherapy becomes increasingly data-driven, the application of AI models allows for nuanced analysis of complex clinical and biological datasets. AI models can be distinguished between those handling structured datasets, as they are often available for pharmacotherapy CDSS. This is typically referred to as ML. In contrast, LLM models, such as those used for the recognition of pictures or handwritten text, are based on transformer-based neural networks handling unstructured, sequential data. To distinguish between the two, it can be proposed that traditional ML models, like decision trees, are powerful for structured data and focused tasks, while generative AI leverages deep learning (transformers) to process unstructured data and exhibit more generalized, adaptive behavior. Transformers are deep neural network architectures composed of stacked layers that utilize multihead self-attention mechanisms to compute contextualized representations of input sequences in parallel, thereby enabling the modeling of long-range dependencies without recurrence and achieving state-of-the-art performance across a variety of sequence modeling tasks.

2.1 Machine learning

Among the foundational models in this space are decision trees, random forests, and ANNs. These models differ in complexity, interpretability, and predictive power, each offering unique value in pharmacotherapy research and practice.

2.1.1 Decision trees

A decision tree is a supervised learning model used for classification or regression. It splits the input space into regions based on feature values through a recursive binary partitioning process. The resulting structure is a tree with nodes (decision points) and leaves (outcomes).

The tree is built using algorithms such as Classification and Regression Trees, optimizing a splitting criterion like Gini impurity (for classification) and mean squared error (MSE) (for regression).

The decision tree shows high interpretability, requires little data preprocessing, and is well-suited for rule-based modeling. Even though it seems very simple, a decision tree offers many advantages in CDSS pharmacotherapy modeling, which is rule-based in most cases. However, a decision tree faces some limitations, as it tends to overfit, especially with noisy or high-dimensional data, and it demonstrates poor performance on very complex datasets.

Pharmacotherapy example

A decision tree can be used to stratify patients for anticoagulant therapy:

- IF age > 75 AND HAS-BLED score ≥ 3, THEN consider reduced-dose Direct Oral Anticoagulant (DOAC).
  If such rules apply, the decision tree leads to 100% performance.

2.1.2 Random forests

A random forest is an ensemble of decision trees built using bootstrap aggregation (bagging) and random feature selection. Each tree is trained on a bootstrapped subset of the data, and final predictions are made via majority voting (for classification) or averaging (for regression).

Randomness is introduced by sampling with replacement for each tree (bootstrap) and a random subset of features considered at each node (decorrelation). This results in low bias and low variance when tuned properly. Strengths of random forests include high predictive accuracy on structured or tabular data, robustness to overfitting, and the ability to handle nonlinear interactions and variable importance estimation. However, random forests are less interpretable than single trees and exhibit slower inference times with large forests.

Pharmacotherapy example

A random forest could be trained on electronic health record data (age, Body Mass Index (BMI), renal function, medication history) to predict the 30-day risk of drug-induced prolongation of the QT interval (QT prolongation):

- Features: age, sex, estimated Glomerular Filtration Rate (eGFR), loop diuretics, macrolide use.
- Output: binary classification (high-risk vs. low-risk)

The model would not only yield predictions but also indicate which features most influenced the risk.

2.1.3 *Artificial neural networks*

ANNs are inspired by the structure of biological neural networks. They consist of layers of interconnected "neurons" (units), each performing a weighted sum of inputs followed by a nonlinear activation function (e.g., rectified linear unit (ReLU), which is a simple activation function used in neural networks that outputs the input value if it is positive and zero otherwise, or sigmoid).

Neural networks often include multiple hidden layers (deep learning), which increases their capacity to model complex patterns. They show excellent performance on large, high-dimensional datasets, can model complex, nonlinear interactions, and are applicable to structured, unstructured, and time-series data (e.g., notes, lab time-series data). Neural networks exhibit low interpretability ("black box"), are prone to overfitting without regularization, and require large training datasets (Fig. 27.1).

Pharmacotherapy example

ANNs can be used for dose prediction models in chemotherapy drugs or immunosuppressants:

- Inputs: Weight, age, genotype (e.g., CYP3A5), liver function
- Output: Optimal starting dose of tacrolimus

Such models can learn intricate relationships between patient factors and pharmacokinetics that are not captured by conventional dosing formulas.

In summary, there is no single perfect underlying model for all data, but the right approach must be chosen with regard to the data characteristics (Table 27.1). For explainable decision support, decision trees or simpler random forests are preferred. For high-dimensional data (e.g., imaging), ANNs show better performance. Decision trees are suitable for most pharmacotherapy tasks, as the data tends to be less complex and the number of cases is limited.

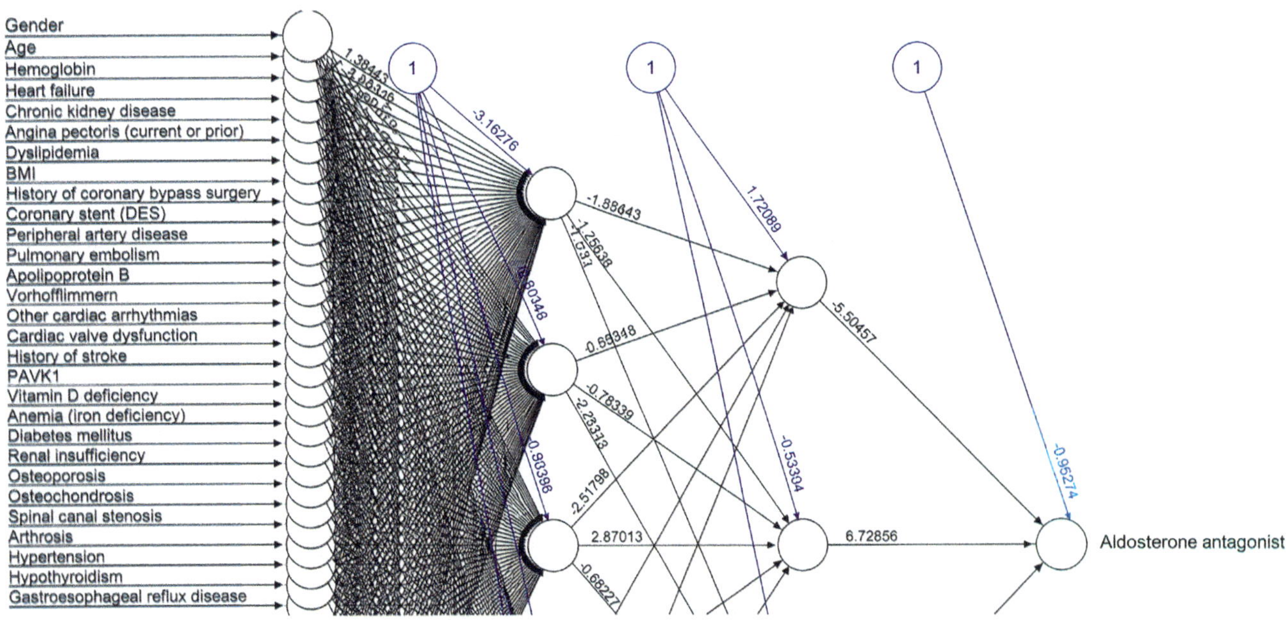

FIG. 27.1 An artificial neural network for decision-making regarding mineralocorticoid-receptor blockers, progressing from the diagnoses (left, in German) to the decision-making process of adding an aldosterone antagonist to the medication regimen of a patient.

TABLE 27.1 A comparison of the three basic AI models and their characteristics.

Model	Data complexity	Interpretability	Typical input types	Example use case
Decision tree	Low-moderate	High	Structured/tabular	Rule-based decision support (e.g., dose adjustment)
Random forest	Moderate	Moderate	Structured/tabular	Risk prediction (e.g., adverse drug events)
Neural network	High	Low	Tabular, time series, text	Natural language processing on clinical notes

2.2 Deep learning

2.2.1 *Overview of the transformer architecture*

Transformers are deep neural architectures designed for sequence modeling tasks. Unlike recurrent or convolutional networks, they rely entirely on self-attention mechanisms to compute relationships between sequence elements. This enables the modeling of long-range dependencies in parallel.

2.2.2 *Scaled dot-product attention*

The core component is the scaled dot-product attention. Given an input matrix $X \in R^{n \times d}$, the attention mechanism is defined as:

$$\text{Attention}(Q, K, V) = \text{softmax}\left(\frac{(QK^{T})}{\sqrt{d_k}}\right)v$$

where:

- $Q = XW^Q$, $K = XW^K$ and $V = XW^V$ are the query, key, and value matrices.
- $W^Q, W^K, W^V \in R^{d \times dk}$ are learnable projection matrices.

$\sqrt{\{d_k\}}$ is a scaling factor to prevent gradient vanishing or explosion.

2.2.3 *Multihead attention*

Instead of applying attention once, the transformer applies it in multiple parallel heads, each with its own learned projections:

$$\text{MultiHead}(Q, K, V) = \text{Concat}(\text{head}_1, \ldots, \text{head}_h)W^O$$

This allows the model to jointly attend to information from different representational subspaces.

2.2.4 *Feedforward network*

Each layer also includes a position-wise feedforward network (FFN) applied independently to each token:

$$FFN(x) = ReLU(xW_1 + b_1)W_2 + b_2$$

2.2.5 *Layer composition and normalization*

Each transformer layer includes:

- A multi-head self-attention block
- A feedforward block
- Residual connections and layer normalization: LayerNorm(x + Sublayer(x))

These architectural choices support stable training and deep stacking.

2.2.6 *Positional encoding*

Because transformers lack recurrence, they inject positional information through positional encodings:

$$\text{PE}_{(\text{pos},2i)} = \sin\left(\frac{\text{pos}}{10000^{2i/d}}\right), \text{PE}_{(\text{pos},2i+1)} = \cos\left(\frac{\text{pos}}{10000^{2i/d}}\right)$$

These are added to the input embeddings, X, before the first layer.

2.2.7 Training strategy

Transformers are trained using variants of stochastic gradient descent, often with the Adam optimizer, label smoothing, and a warm-up learning rate schedule. Depending on the application, the architecture may be encoder-only (e.g., BERT), decoder-only (e.g., GPT), or encoder–decoder (e.g., T5).

3 ML model evaluation and validation in pharmacotherapy applications

Developing an ML model for pharmacotherapy tasks (e.g., risk prediction, dose adjustment, adverse event detection) requires not only model selection but also rigorous evaluation using appropriate statistical methods. The clinical utility of a model hinges on its accuracy, calibration, and generalizability.

3.1 Data splitting and validation strategies

To avoid overfitting and to assess generalization performance, models are validated on unseen data using one or more of the following strategies:

- Train/test split
- The dataset is divided into two portions (e.g., 80% training, 20% testing)
- Simple but can be unstable with small datasets
- K-Fold Cross-Validation
- The data is divided into *k* subsets (folds). Each fold is used once as a test set, while the remaining *k-1* folds are used for training
- Provides a robust estimation of model performance
- Typical values: $k = 5$ or 10
- Nested Cross-Validation
- Combines model selection (inner loop) with model assessment (outer loop).
- Useful for avoiding data leakage during hyperparameter tuning
- Bootstrapping
- Repeatedly resamples the data with replacement and estimates performance over many iterations
- Useful for estimating confidence intervals of performance metrics

3.2 Classification metrics

In pharmacotherapy, many tasks are classification problems (e.g., predicting adverse drug reactions, therapy success/failure). The most relevant metrics include true positives and true negatives, as shown in the confusion matrix (Tables 27.2 and 27.3). Table 27.2 lists the possible options, while Table 27.3 provides the formulas and interpretations associated with these options. These are important metrics within pharmacotherapy and pharmacy practice, as noted in the example below.

Example

: A model predicting bleeding risk after NOAC initiation should aim for high sensitivity (to catch all high-risk patients) while balancing precision (to avoid unnecessary therapy withholding).

TABLE 27.2 Confusion matrix.

	Actually positive (1)	**Actually negative (0)**
Predicted positive (1)	True positives (TPs)	False positives (FPs)
Predicted negative (0)	False negatives (FNs)	True negatives (TNs)

TABLE 27.3 Most relevant metrics in AI

Metric	Formula	Interpretation
Accuracy	$\frac{TP+TN}{TP+TN+FP+FN}$	Overall correctness
Sensitivity (Recall)	$\frac{TP}{TP+FN}$	True positive rate (detects actual positives).
Specificity	$\frac{TN}{TN+FP}$	True negative rate
Precision (PPV)	$\frac{TP}{TP+FP}$	How many predicted positives are correct?
F1 Score	$\frac{2 \cdot \text{Precision} \cdot \text{Recall}}{\text{Precision} + \text{Recall}}$	Balance between precision and recall
AUC-ROC	Area under the receiver operating characteristic curve $AUC = \int_0^1 \text{TPR}(\text{FPR})\, d(\text{FPR})$	Discrimination ability of the model
AUC-PR	Area under the precision-recall curve $PRAUC = \int_0^1 \text{Precision}(\text{Recall})\, d(\text{Recall})$	More useful than ROC when classes are imbalanced.

FN, false negative; *FP*, false positive; *PR*, precision-recall; *TN*, true negative; *TP*, true positive.

3.3 Calibration metrics

3.3.1 *Calibration and its importance in pharmacotherapy risk prediction*

When developing or applying predictive models in pharmacotherapy, such as estimating a patient's risk of adverse drug reactions or treatment failure, two critical aspects of model performance must be considered: discrimination and calibration. While discrimination reflects how well the model separates patients with different outcomes (e.g., ranking highest risk to lowest), calibration ensures that the predicted probabilities actually correspond to real-world outcomes.

Calibration curve/reliability plot

- Definition: A calibration curve (also called a reliability plot) visually compares predicted probabilities with observed event rates, grouping patients into bins based on their predicted risk.
- How it works: For example, if a group of patients receives predictions in the 10%–20% risk range for an adverse drug event, the actual event rate in this group should ideally match the predicted average. Each point on the plot represents a bin's mean predicted probability against the observed proportion experiencing the outcome.
- Perfect calibration: Points falling on the diagonal 45° line indicate perfect calibration—the model's predictions match reality. Points above or below this line highlight overestimation or underestimation, which can mislead therapy decisions.

Practical application in pharmacotherapy: Suppose a clinical decision tool predicts the chances of bleeding in patients starting oral anticoagulants. If the model assigns a 30% risk to a certain subgroup, but in reality, 40 out of 100 such patients experience bleeding, the model underestimates the risk—a miscalibration with potential patient safety implications.

Brier score

- Definition: The Brier Score quantitatively assesses calibration by computing the mean squared difference between each patient's predicted probability and their actual outcome (where "outcome" is 1 if the event occurs and 0 if it does not).

  Formula: $\text{Brier} - \frac{1}{N}\sum_{i=1}^{N}(f_i - y_i)^2$

where pip_ipi is the predicted probability and yiy_iyi is the true outcome.

- Interpretation: Lower scores are better. The score ranges from 0 (perfect prediction) to 1 (worst). For rare events, a model that always predicts "no event" can still achieve a deceptively low Brier Score, so both discrimination and calibration should be reviewed.

3.3.2 *Pharmacotherapy case example*

In selecting antithrombotic therapy, a clinician may rely on a model to estimate bleeding or thrombotic risk. An accurately calibrated model ensures that, for patients assigned a 20% risk, about 20 out of 100 actually experience the event. This alignment supports safer, more personalized treatment choices—ensuring neither overtreatment nor undertreatment.

3.3.3 *Why calibration matters in clinical practice*

- Clinical decision-making: Poor calibration can lead to undertreatment or overtreatment. For example, underestimating bleeding risk might prompt the unnecessary prescription of anticoagulants, increasing harm to patients.
- Patient counseling: Accurately calibrated risks help clinicians communicate expected outcomes, thereby improving shared decision-making.
- Regulatory and local context: In places like North Rhine-Westphalia (NRW), models aiding pharmacotherapy must be regularly calibrated to local populations to ensure their continued relevance and safety.

By incorporating tools such as calibration curves and the Brier Score, clinicians can better judge whether a risk model's probabilities are trustworthy for guiding therapeutic decisions in pharmacotherapy. This can be a useful resource for many healthcare professionals, notably pharmacists.

3.4 Regression metrics

Prediction tasks in clinical and pharmacotherapeutic contexts often require the estimation of continuous variables rather than simple categorical outcomes. For example, clinicians may need models that predict a patient's exact blood concentration of a drug, the required dose for optimal therapeutic effect, or a lab value such as creatinine clearance. In these cases, the model's output isn't just about sorting patients into "high-risk" or "low-risk" categories but providing precise numerical values that can directly inform medical decisions.

Such continuous predictions are central in scenarios like:

- Determining personalized medication dosages (e.g., warfarin, insulin).
- Forecasting serum drug levels to avoid toxicity or subtherapeutic dosing.
- Estimating kidney function (e.g., glomerular filtration rate) or other lab values relevant to therapy adjustments.

Therefore, it is essential to use regression metrics, such as mean absolute error (MAE), MSE, root mean squared error (RMSE), and the coefficient of determination (R^2), to systematically assess model accuracy, error magnitude, and how well predictions match observed clinical data. These metrics help clinicians and pharmacists understand not only how often a model's predictions are close to reality but also the extent and clinical relevance of any errors made. Ultimately, applying appropriate regression metrics ensures model outputs are reliable, actionable, and safe for guiding patient care in real-world settings. Table 27.4 provides an overview of regression metrics typically employed in clinical pharmacy questions.

Example

An ANN trained to predict warfarin dose based on genotype, age, and INR should be evaluated using MAE and R^2.

3.5 Other key concepts

Model interpretability

- Permutation feature importance
- Shapley Additive Explanations? (SHAP) values → explain predictions at the patient-level
- Local Interpretable Model-agnostic Explanations? (LIME) → interpretable local approximations

TABLE 27.4 Core regression metrics for evaluating predictive model accuracy in pharmacotherapy.

Metric	Formula	Description
Mean absolute error (MAE)	$MAE = \frac{1}{n}\sum_{i=1}^{n}\lvert y_i - \hat{y}_i \rvert$	The residual shows how much the prediction differs from the actual value and is used to assess the model's quality.
Mean absolute percentage error (MAPE)	$MAPE = \frac{100\%}{n}\sum \left\lvert \frac{y - \hat{y}}{y} \right\rvert$	
Mean squared error (MSE)	$MSE = \frac{1}{n}\sum_{i=1}^{n}(y_i - \hat{y}_i)^2$	The MSE measures the average squared difference between actual and predicted values in a dataset. It is used to assess how well a model predicts outcomes; a lower MSE indicates better model accuracy.
Root MSE (RMSE)	$RMSE = \sqrt{MSE}$	The RMSE measures the average distance between predicted and actual values, giving higher weight to large errors.
Coefficient of determination (R^2)	$R^2 = 1 - \frac{SS_{res}}{SS_{tot}}$	R^2 measures how well a model explains the variation in the actual data. It ranges from 0 to 1.

n, number of observations; SS_res, residual sum of squares; SS_tot, total sum of squares; *y_i*, actual value (true value); *ŷ_i*, predicted value.

TABLE 27.5 Common AI tasks and corresponding evaluation metrics.

Task type	Metrics used	Key consideration
Classification	Accuracy, AUC, Precision, Recall, F1	Measures how well classes are predicted. It is important to balance sensitivity (recall) and specificity (precision), especially with imbalanced data or rare events (e.g., adverse drug reactions).
Probability estimation	Brier Score, Calibration Curve	Evaluates how well predicted probabilities reflect true outcome likelihoods, which is essential for risk stratification and decision support tools.
Regression	MAE, RMSE, R^2	Quantifies errors in predicting continuous values. Lower errors indicate better performance, R^2 R^2 shows explained variance, which is important for tasks like dose prediction.

Class imbalance handling

- Oversampling (e.g., Synthetic Minority Over-sampling Technique, SMOTE), Undersampling
- Class weighting
- Ensemble methods with balanced bagging

External validation

- Models must be tested on independent datasets to ensure generalizability beyond the development cohort

Once a model has been developed and a strategy for external validation is in place, its performance must be quantified using specific metrics. The selection of an appropriate evaluation metric is a crucial decision that is determined by the goals of the ML task. For example, the criteria for success in a classification task (e.g., identifying spam emails) are different from those in a probability estimation task (e.g., predicting a patient's risk of disease). This distinction is critical because the chosen metric directly influences how a model's performance is interpreted and whether it is deemed successful for its intended purpose. Table 27.5 provides a guide to common task types in AI, their associated evaluation metrics, and the key considerations that should inform this selection process.

Metrics by model type

Example application: NOAC bleeding risk prediction

- Model: Random Forest
- Inputs: Age, renal function, concurrent medications, prior GI bleed
- Outcome: Major bleeding event within 30 days
- Metrics:
- AUC: 0.84 (discrimination)
- Brier Score: 0.11 (calibration)
- Precision: 0.46, Recall: 0.72
- External validation: Performed on an independent hospital registry

3.6 Generative AI

Generative AI refers to a class of AI systems designed to create new content. These systems learn patterns from training data and use that knowledge to generate original outputs that resemble the data they were trained on. Typical tasks performed by generative AI include writing coherent text, creating realistic images, composing music, writing computer code, and generating videos. The word "generative" signifies the model's ability to generate or produce novel data—often creative or free-form content—rather than just analyzing or categorizing existing data.

3.7 Nongenerative AI

Nongenerative AI, by contrast, refers to models that do not create new content. Instead, they are designed to analyze input data, classify or label data, make predictions, detect anomalies, recommend options, and make decisions based on learned patterns. These models are often referred to as discriminative models because they are trained to distinguish between different categories or outcomes. An example of a nongenerative AI model can be a decision tree that splits data based on features to make decisions (e.g., "Does this patient have diabetes?") or a logistic regression with a statistical model for binary outcomes (e.g., "yes/no" predictions).

3.8 Language models

Many modern generative models are called language models because they were originally designed to predict the next word in a sequence—a core task in natural language processing. Over time, these models have evolved to become foundation models, capable of handling not only text but also images, audio, and more. Still, the core mechanism of predicting and generating sequences remains central—which is why the name "language model" persists. LLMs, trained on vast collections of data, have achieved remarkable results in natural language processing. However, they may sometimes generate hallucinations—outputs that are factually incorrect, misleading, or even nonsensical, often presented as if they were accurate. Unlike factual errors stemming from simple data mistakes, LLM hallucinations arise because these models generate text by predicting statistically likely word sequences rather than verifying information or consulting external sources. This can lead to fabricated details, source conflation, and unsubstantiated claims, especially in contexts with ambiguous prompts or insufficient training data. In critical applications such as AI-based CDSS for pharmacotherapy, hallucinations present a serious limitation, as inaccurate or fabricated recommendations can directly impact patient safety and treatment outcomes. Therefore, it is essential to rigorously validate LLM outputs and incorporate safeguards, such as human review or external fact-checking, when using these systems for high-stakes decision-making.

4 Barriers to AI models in pharmacotherapy: Results of a feasibility study

A study by Bücker et al. applied different AI models to a data set drug classes, diagnoses, and patients' demographic data for various individuals with cardiovascular diseases (Bücker et al., 2024). Decision trees were built based on the approach of Breiman et al. (2017). R software, version 4.2.3 (R Foundation for Statistical Computing, Vienna, Austria), along with the package tidymodels (R package version 0.1.0), was used for calculations and modeling. All codes and data are published at https://github.com/mchlbckr/paper_ai_pharmacotherapy/tree/main. To avoid overfitting, bootstrapping was employed. This was applied to an initial split of 74% of the data, with simultaneous optimization of hyperparameters (complexity parameter, tree depth, minimal number of cases per node). Based on the AUC, the best decision tree was chosen. The remaining 26% of the data was used to test predictive performance on the holdout dataset. Decision trees were generated for eight frequently used cardiovascular drug classes, namely ACE-inhibitors/angiotensin receptor blockers (ACEI/ARB), thiazide diuretics, beta-blockers (BB), dihydropyridine calcium channel-blockers (DHP-CCB), mineralocorticoid receptor-blockers (MRA), loop diuretics, isosorbide mono- or di-nitrate (nitrates, ISMN/ISDN), and inhaled nitroglycerin (Bücker et al., 2024). A decision tree for loop diuretics is displayed in Fig. 27.2. The probability for a decision and the affected percentage of patients are shown. The probability for patients with heart failure to take a loop diuretic was 82%. The model identifies patients with renal failure as a second indication.

Accuracy of predictions on the test data set was >50% for all drug classes, except for DHP-CCB, where the numbers decreased from an accuracy of 59% with training data to 38% with testing data, indicating that there is still overfitting involved in the model used. Results for AUC and accuracy on both training and test data sets for all eight drug classes are displayed in Table 27.6.

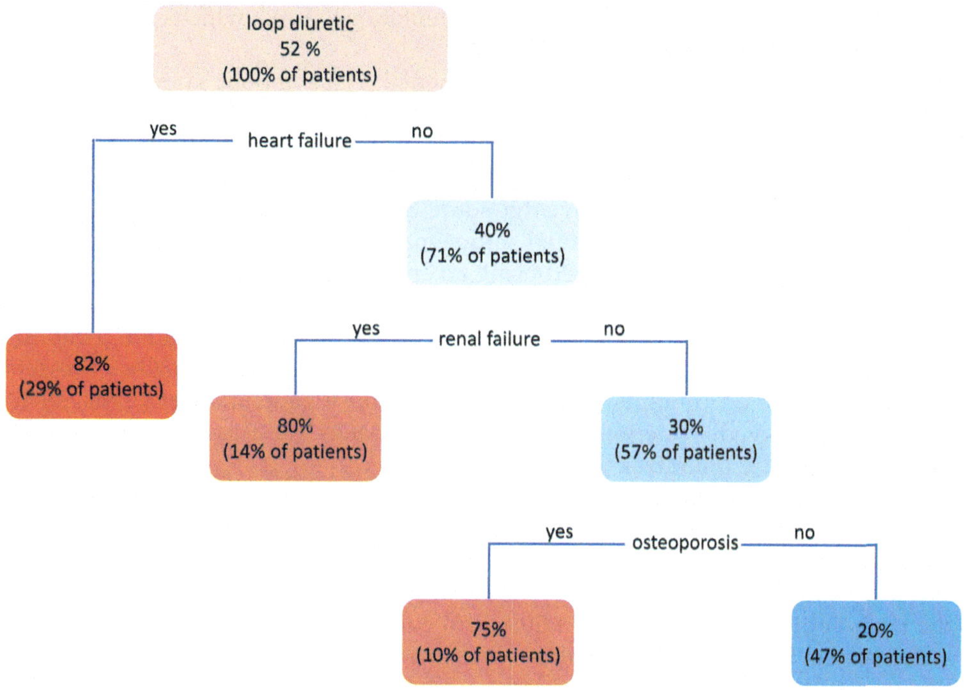

FIG. 27.2 Decision tree for loop diuretics in the feasibility study by Bücker et al. (2024).

TABLE 27.6 AI results on accuracy for eight specific drugs.

Variable	AUC training (%)	ACC training (%)	AUC testing (%)	ACC testing (%)
Nitroglycerin	99	99	100	100
MRA	86	88	100	100
ISMN/ISDN	68	85	50	81
Loop diuretics	66	64	70	65
Beta-blocker	64	80	50	65
Thiazide diuretics	57	76	56	69
ACEI/ARB	55	97	NA	100
DHP-CCB	52	59	31	38

ACC, accuracy; *ACEI*, ACE-inhibitor; *ARB*, angiotensin receptor blocker; *AUC*, area under the curve; *DHP-CCB*, dihydropyridine calcium channel blocker; *MRA*, mineralocorticoid receptor antagonist; *NA*, not available.

5 Hybrid AI

As shown previously in the feasibility study, the complexity of pharmacotherapeutic decision-making necessitates AI systems that combine probabilistic reasoning with deterministic rule enforcement (Bücker et al., 2024). Pure ML models, while excelling at pattern recognition and natural language processing, are prone to hallucinations and lack the interpretability required for clinical applications. In domains such as pharmacotherapy—where safety, transparency, and regulatory compliance are critical—purely data-driven ML models or solely rule-based systems often fall short. ML models, especially LLMs, offer remarkable flexibility and generalization. Rule-based systems, by contrast, ensure transparency and enforce domain constraints but are brittle and lack adaptability. Hybrid AI approaches seek to reconcile these limitations by integrating statistical learning with symbolic reasoning, thereby enabling systems that are both adaptive and trustworthy.

Hybrid AI architectures combine the contextual understanding and generative capabilities of LLMs with structured, knowledge-based reasoning components such as ontologies, knowledge graphs, and explicit rule sets. This integration—often referred to as neuro-symbolic AI—enables reasoning under uncertainty while maintaining verifiable logical consistency. A particularly impactful implementation is RAG, which enhances generative responses by grounding them in curated, authoritative sources.

The architecture typically encompasses three core components: (1) a symbolic knowledge base containing structured domain expertise, (2) an integration layer that orchestrates information flow between these subsystems, and (3) a neural component for natural language understanding and generation. This configuration enables reasoning under uncertainty while maintaining transparent logical traces. The process initiates with document preprocessing, for instance, using LangChain, where clinical knowledge sources—including evidence-based guidelines, medication ontologies, and regulatory bulletins—are segmented into semantically coherent chunks. These chunks, typically ranging from 200 to 1000 tokens, are then vectorized using an embedding model such as OpenAI's text-embedding-ada-002. The vectorized chunks are then indexed using tools like LlamaIndex within specialized databases optimized for similarity search, such as Pinecone. Queries undergo the same vectorization, enabling the retrieval of semantically relevant knowledge fragments using similarity-based retrieval strategies. The retrieved context is integrated into carefully engineered prompts that guide the response generation of LLMs, such as GPT-4, while maintaining adherence to retrieved evidence. Leveraging techniques such as chain-of-thought prompting and dynamic few-shot learning further optimizes the model's output.

Within pharmacotherapy, hybrid AI confers three key benefits: Traceable guideline compliance rules can be encoded in the knowledge graph and are surfaced alongside each recommendation, facilitating audits and clinician trust. Rapid evidence uptake, such as new drug safety alerts or dosing updates, can be indexed by the retrieval engine without retraining the LLM. For context-aware reasoning, the LLM interprets narrative discharge summaries, while the symbolic layer applies rules, e.g., dose-adjustment rules for renal impairment or drug-gene interactions. This setup allows the system to deliver fluent, natural interactions while grounding its responses in authoritative, structured knowledge, resulting in fewer hallucinations.

Ong et al. evaluated a RAG-based LLM CDSS across 61 simulated prescribing error scenarios in 23 complex vignettes spanning 12 clinical specialties. Their findings demonstrate that RAG-augmented LLMs significantly outperform LLMs alone in detecting DRPs. Specifically, the best-performing hybrid model achieved an accuracy of 42.6%, compared to 29.5% for standalone GPT-4. When deployed in a copilot configuration—where junior pharmacists reviewed cases with the support of RAG-LLM recommendations—accuracy increased further to 54.1%, with gains observed across DRP categories such as adverse drug reactions, drug-drug interactions, and therapeutic duplications. The study confirms that RAG-LLM systems can process complex medication profiles and highlight clinically significant prescribing risks missed by either humans or AI alone. This hybrid approach enables both adaptive natural language generation and verifiable, document-grounded output, which is crucial for auditability and clinician trust. Although the study did not directly compare against commercial rule-based CDSS or quantify clinical acceptance rates, it illustrates the feasibility and promise of neuro-symbolic methods for safe, scalable medication review.

Despite their demonstrated advantages, hybrid systems retain certain vulnerabilities that ongoing research seeks to address. Retrieval failures, stemming from inadequate chunk segmentation or embedding quality, can propagate errors throughout the reasoning chain. Similarly, knowledge base staleness poses risks when clinical evidence evolves rapidly.

In domains such as pharmacotherapy, neither pure machine-learning models nor rule-based systems alone deliver the necessary performance. Pharmacotherapy demands decision support systems that are reliable, trustworthy, and interpretable, surpassing the inherent limitations of purely neural or symbolic approaches. By integrating the adaptive capabilities of LLMs with the reliability and interpretability of structured knowledge systems, hybrid architectures could achieve the critical balance of flexibility, safety, and transparency required for clinical implementation. The empirical evidence—studies such as Ong et al.—demonstrates substantial improvements in accuracy and safety, positioning hybrid AI as a possible foundational technology for next-generation healthcare AI systems.

6 Discussion

The study by Bücker et al. provided an initial approach to the use of AI in decision-making within pharmacotherapy (Bücker et al., 2024). With an accuracy of 100% for three out of eight drugs, the results indicate a certain degree of reliability in the models. However, one would expect higher quality before considering its use as a CDSS. More interestingly, the following barriers and potential solutions for AI use in pharmacotherapy were identified:

6.1 Modeling

Due to the limited data, a decision tree was chosen instead of other ML models, such as random forests, boosted trees, or a neural network. Another argument for using a decision tree was the traceability of results. Results showed high accuracy for most drugs. Overfitting can be assumed for DHP-CCB, as the results were significantly better for training data than for testing data. The AUC for testing of ACEI/ARB was difficult to interpret, as all patients in the testing group received these drugs.

Results can also help answer a few general questions about the employment of AI in a highly sensitive field, such as pharmacotherapy. Each potential mistake could potentially be life-threatening.

How this barrier can be addressed: AI models in pharmacotherapy need larger sets of data, which can be sourced from registries.

6.2 Sampling

It is obvious that it is difficult to generate a high number of patients with pharmacotherapy data, which previously has been optimized by specialists. The definition of specialists is unclear, and in pharmacotherapy, there are preferences of patients and prescribers, which are ambiguous. Furthermore, the sample needs to be representative of the setting in which the model is intended to be employed. In the case of the typical cardiovascular patient in a pharmacy or clinic, this would indicate that healthy patients and patients with a typical indication would need to be added to the database.

How this barrier can be addressed: a larger sample with data from healthy individuals needs to be collected, which must be representative of the setting.

6.3 Laboratory data and vital signs

In the mentioned feasibility study, laboratory data and vital signs were available for most patients but were not helpful (Bücker et al., 2024). As blood pressure is lowered by the drugs in use, this medicated blood pressure is of little validity for decision-making. The model would need the native blood pressure to interpret the effects of antihypertensive drugs, which is not available in most cases in clinical practice. Hence, it might even interpret antihypertensives as counteracting, as most patients with high blood pressure are taking these drugs despite still having high blood pressure. The same problem applies to laboratory data. Whereas all additional patient information theoretically would be beneficial for the model, this question remains unsolved for now.

How this barrier can be addressed: A combination of the information provided by an LLM can add rules, such as how much a certain dose of an antihypertensive drug can lower blood pressure. LLMs can thus help interpret laboratory values.

6.4 Novel therapies and drug alerts

As AI models generate decisions based on existing data and probability, it would take a long time before new drug regimens are more likely to be adopted than older ones. This delay would keep patients from benefiting from the latest research. An example is the switch from triple to quadruple therapy with MRA, BB, ACEI, and, nowadays, additional Sodium-Glucose Cotransporter 2 inhibitors (SGLT-2) inhibitors in heart failure. This combination would not be recommended unless more than 85% of patients have it documented in their records. A rapid response is also required in sudden alerts regarding drug safety.

This barrier can be addressed: A decision tree provides the opportunity to simply manually overwrite the numbers. Hence, an SGLT-2 inhibitor can easily be set to a 100% probability in cases where this seems to be always indicated. Combining static content in a hybrid AI model with information from the LLM can also help address this issue, facilitating faster adoption of clinical research or, conversely, the generation of alerts.

6.5 Patient preferences

According to recent studies, including patients' preferences and shared decision-making is rarely implemented in clinical practice, even though it is clearly recommended by all guidelines (Fleming et al., 2023). It is widely believed that patient preferences can only be assessed and translated by human healthcare providers.

How this barrier can be addressed: As time to consult a physician or pharmacist is sometimes very limited, patients might even feel better if they can talk to an avatar and communicate about their disease state without pressure (Hong et al., 2022). This contrasts with most physicians' and pharmacists' expectations that such sensitive situations can only be handled through human interactions. However, results of such an AI-based conversation need to be included in the pharmacotherapy CDSS if all facets of prescribing are to be digitalized. Another approach can be specific prompting, which incorporates patient preferences in a translational way.

6.6 Limited data

A further insight of this study is that it is difficult to produce many optimized patient treatment plans, which are surely needed to train an AI system. If trained using routine care data, AI-based pharmacotherapy models would only suggest average drug regimens. One approach to create better data could involve expert panels. Unfortunately, such panels are very time-consuming and cannot produce large quantities either (Meslin et al., 2018). To maximize the information available, these specialists would need to be permanently updated in all medical fields and must also be familiar with the patient, the perspectives, and the setting.

How this barrier can be addressed: A combination with an LLM can incorporate data from guidelines, which represent expert consensus. Guidelines can also be part of RUGs in a hybrid AI system.

6.7 Cutoff

In the mentioned study by Bücker et al., an accuracy of 100% was achieved by only 3 out of 8 drugs (Bücker et al., 2024). On the other hand, it can be assumed that an accuracy of >50% from optimized data was better than the current status quo in therapeutics. However, given the potential harm of a wrong therapeutic decision, responsibility must remain on the physicians' or pharmacists' side, and a CDSS would be regarded as a clinical aid with a remaining inaccuracy, as is true for any drug-drug interaction checker.

How this barrier can be addressed: Any CDSS, regardless of whether it is AI-based or not, should be seen as a tool rather than a solution. It might help the practitioner in their daily work, but results should be evaluated critically.

7 Conclusion

AI models can be built on several basic concepts. For structured data, decision trees, random forests, and ANNs are frequently utilized. Generative AI for unstructured data, in contrast, is based on transformer-based neural networks. The right model needs to be selected with regard to the underlying data and the desired outcomes. In pharmacotherapy, AI models based on the simple information of patients' diagnoses have shown remarkably high accuracy for some of the analyzed drugs. This can be a useful tool for healthcare professionals to aid in pharmacotherapy analyses and decision-making. To increase the robustness of future AI models, the underlying data set, however, should be large, representative of the setting, and provide options for updating. Included pharmacotherapy regimens must be calibrated to a higher level than standard care, and they must evolve with new recommendations and therapeutic standards. A hybrid approach, combining defined data with LLMs, can be a promising future approach.

8 Questions for future discussion

1. To what extent should AI systems be allowed to influence pharmacotherapy decisions in clinical practice? Should AI remain purely advisory, or could certain decisions eventually be automated?
2. How can the explainability and transparency of AI models be ensured, especially when neural networks or LLMs are used in clinical decision support?
3. What level of predictive accuracy is required before an AI system can be safely implemented in pharmacotherapy decision support? Should thresholds differ depending on the clinical context or the drug risk profile?
4. How can patient preferences and shared decision-making be integrated into AI-based medication management systems?

5. What governance frameworks are needed to ensure that AI models remain updated with new clinical evidence and drug safety alerts?
6. How can healthcare systems obtain sufficiently large and representative datasets to train reliable pharmacotherapy AI models?

9 Application exercise

Case scenario: AI-supported pharmacotherapy decision
A 78-year-old male patient presents with the following clinical characteristics:

- Diagnosis: heart failure with reduced ejection fraction (HFrEF).
- Comorbidities: hypertension, chronic kidney disease, Stage 3
- Current medications:

- ACE inhibitor
- beta-blocker
- loop diuretic
- Laboratory findings:
- eGFR: 42 mL/min
- potassium: 4.6 mmol/L
- Blood pressure: 132/78 mmHg

A clinical decision support system, using a ML model combined with guideline-based rules, evaluates whether additional therapy should be recommended.

10 Tasks

1. Identify which type of AI model could best support this decision, considering interpretability and the type of available data.
2. Explain how a hybrid AI system might process this patient case, including:
   - structured patient data
   - guideline recommendations
   - Probabilistic risk prediction.
3. Discuss potential limitations of relying on AI recommendations in this scenario, including issues related to data availability, model accuracy, and patient-specific factors.
4. Propose how the clinician should integrate AI recommendations with clinical judgment and patient preferences.

AI Disclosure

During the preparation of this work, the author(s) used Wordvice in order to improve readability and language. After using this tool/service, the author(s) reviewed and edited the content as needed and take(s) full responsibility for the content of the publication.

References

Amann, J., Blasimme, A., Vayena, E., Frey, D., Madai, V.I., 2020. Explainability for artificial intelligence in healthcare: a multidisciplinary perspective. BMC Med. Inform. Decis. Mak. 1472-6947. 20 (1). doi:10.1186/s12911-020-01332-6.

Breiman, L., Friedman, J.H., Olshen, R.A., Stone, C.J., 2017. Classification and Regression Trees. CRC Press, United States, pp. 1–358. Available from http://www.tandfebooks.com/doi/book/10.1201/9781315139470. doi:10.1201/9781315139470.

Buchegger, S., Iglseder, B., Alzner, R., Kogler, M., Rose, O., Kutschar, P., Krutter, S., Dückelmann, C., Flamm, M., Pachmayr, J., 2023. Patient perspectives on, and effects of, medication management in geriatric fallers (the EMMA study): protocol for a mixed-methods pre-post study. BMJ Open. 2044-6055. 13 (2), e066666. doi:10.1136/bmjopen-2022-066666.

Bücker, M., Hoti, K., Rose, O., 2024. Artificial intelligence to assist decision-making on pharmacotherapy: a feasibility study. Explor. Res. Clin. Soc. Pharm. 26672766. 15, 100491. doi:10.1016/j.rcsop.2024.100491.

Cabitza, F., Rasoini, R., Gensini, G.F., 2017. Unintended consequences of machine learning in medicine. JAMA. 15383598. 318 (6), 517–518. Available from: http://jamanetwork.com/journals/jama/data/journals/jama/936418/jama_cabitza_2017_vp_170094.pdf. doi:10.1001/jama.2017.7797.

Cavalier, J.S., Goldstein, B.A., Ravitsky, V., Bélisle-Pipon, J.-C., Bedoya, A., Maddocks, J., Klotman, S., Roman, M., Sperling, J., Chun, X., Poon, E.G., Chowdhury, A., 2025. Ethics in patient preferences for artificial intelligence–drafted responses to electronic messages. JAMA Netw. Open. 2574-3805. 8 (3), e250449. doi:10.1001/jamanetworkopen.2025.0449.

Das, N., Topalovic, M., Janssens, W., 2018. Artificial intelligence in diagnosis of obstructive lung disease: current status and future potential. Curr. Opin. Pulm. Med. 15316971. 24 (2), 117–123. Available from: https://www.journals.lww.com/co-pulmonarymedicine/pages/default.aspx. doi:10.1097/MCP.0000000000000459.

Fleming, V., Prasad, A., Connie, G., Crawford, S., Meraj, S., Hough, C.L., Bernard, L., Carson, S.S., Steingrub, J., White, D.B., Muehlschlegel, S., 2023. Prevalence and predictors of shared decision-making in goals-of-care clinician-family meetings for critically ill neurologic patients: a multi-center mixed-methods study. Crit. Care. 1364-8535. 27 (1). doi:10.1186/s13054-023-04693-2.

Graham, C.M., 2025. Artificial intelligence vs human clinicians: a comparative analysis of complex medical query handling across the USA and Australia. J. Health Organ. Manag. 14777266. Available from: http://www.emeraldinsight.com/info/journals/jhom/jhom.jsp. doi:10.1108/JHOM-02-2025-0100.

Hobbs, F.R., 2002. Acceptance of guideline recommendations and perceived implementation of coronary heart disease prevention among primary care physicians in five European countries: the Reassessing European Attitudes about Cardiovascular Treatment (REACT) survey. Fam. Pract. 14602229. 19 (6), 596–604. doi:10.1093/fampra/19.6.596.

Hollon, T.C., Pandian, B., Adapa, A.R., Urias, E., Save, A.V., Khalsa, S.S.S., Eichberg, D.G., D'Amico, R.S., Farooq, Z.U., Lewis, S., Petridis, P.D., Marie, T., Shah, A.H., Garton, H.J.L., Maher, C.O., Heth, J.A., McKean, E.L., Sullivan, S.E., Hervey-Jumper, S.L., Patil, P.G., Thompson, B.G., Sagher, O., McKhann, G.M., Komotar, R.J., Ivan, M.E., Snuderl, M., Otten, M.L., Johnson, T.D., Sisti, M.B., Bruce, J.N., Muraszko, K.M., Trautman, J., Freudiger, C.W., Canoll, P., Lee, H., Camelo-Piragua, S., Orringer, D.A., 2020. Near real-time intraoperative brain tumor diagnosis using stimulated Raman histology and deep neural networks. Nat. Med. 1546170X. 26 (1), 52–58. Available from: http://www.nature.com/nm/index.html. doi:10.1038/s41591-019-0715-9.

Hong, G., Smith, M., Lin, S., 2022. The AI will see you now: feasibility and acceptability of a conversational AI medical interviewing system. JMIR Form. Res. 2561-326X. 6 (6), e37028. doi:10.2196/37028.

Jaspers, M.W.M., Smeulers, M., Vermeulen, H., Peute, L.W., 2011. Effects of clinical decision-support systems on practitioner performance and patient outcomes: a synthesis of high-quality systematic review findings. J. Am. Med. Inform. Assoc. 1067-5027. 18 (3), 327–334. doi:10.1136/amiajnl-2011-000094.

Ji, Z., Lee, N., Frieske, R., Tiezheng, Y., Dan, S., Yan, X., Ishii, E., Bang, Y.J., Madotto, A., Fung, P., 2023. Survey of hallucination in natural language generation. ACM Comput. Surv. 0360-0300. 55 (12), 1–38. doi:10.1145/3571730.

Kerliu, L., Citaku, D., Rudhani, I., Hughes, J.D., Rose, O., Hoti, K., 2021. Exploring instruments used to evaluate potentially inappropriate medication use in hospitalised elderly patients in Kosovo. Eur. J. Hosp. Pharm. 2047-9956. 28 (4), 223–228. doi:10.1136/ejhpharm-2019-001904.

Kessler, S., Desai, M., McConnell, W., Jai, E.M., Mebine, P., Nguyen, J., Kiroyan, C., Dennis, H., Schweber, E.V., Schweber, L.V., 2021. Economic and utilization outcomes of medication management at a large Medicaid plan with disease management pharmacists using a novel artificial intelligence platform from 2018 to 2019: a retrospective observational study using regression methods. J. Manag. Care Spec. Pharm. 2376-0540. 27 (9), 1186–1196. doi:10.18553/jmcp.2021.21036.

Koh, D.M., Papanikolaou, N., Bick, U., Illing, R., Kahn, C.E., Kalpathi-Cramer, J., Matos, C., Martí-Bonmatí, L., Miles, A., Mun, S.K., Napel, S., Rockall, A., Sala, E., Strickland, N., Prior, F., 2022. Artificial intelligence and machine learning in cancer imaging. Commun. Med. 2730664X. 2 (1). Available from: https://www.nature.com/commsmed/. doi:10.1038/s43856-022-00199-0.

Komajda, M., Follath, F., Swedberg, K., Cleland, J., Aguilar, J.C., Cohen-Solal, A., Dietz, R., Gavazzi, A., Van Gilst, W.H., Hobbs, R., Korewicki, J., Madeira, H.C., Moiseyev, V.S., Preda, I., Widimsky, J., Freemantle, N., Eastaugh, J., Mason, J., 2003. The EuroHeart Failure survey programme—a survey on the quality of care among patients with heart failure in Europe. Part 2: treatment. Eur. Heart J. 24 (5), 464–474. doi:10.1016/S0195-668X(02)00700-5.

McCahon, D., Duncan, P., Payne, R., Horwood, J., 2022. Patient perceptions and experiences of medication review: qualitative study in general practice. BMC Prim. Care. 2731-4553. 23 (1). doi:10.1186/s12875-022-01903-8.

Meslin, S.M.M., Zheng, W.Y., Day, R.O., Tay, E.M.Y., Baysari, M.T., 2018. Evaluation of clinical relevance of drug-drug interaction alerts prior to implementation. Appl. Clin. Inform. 18690327. 9 (4), 849–855. Available from: https://www.thieme-connect.com/products/ejournals/journal/10.1055/s-00035026. doi:10.1055/s-0038-1676039.

Naseralallah, L., Stewart, D., Price, M., Paudyal, V., 2023. Prevalence, contributing factors, and interventions to reduce medication errors in outpatient and ambulatory settings: a systematic review. Int. J. Clin. Pharm. 2210-7703. 45 (6), 1359–1377. doi:10.1007/s11096-023-01626-5.

Obermeyer, Z., Powers, B., Vogeli, C., Mullainathan, S., 2019. Dissecting racial bias in an algorithm used to manage the health of populations. Science. 0036-8075. 366 (6464), 447–453. doi:10.1126/science.aax2342.

Price, W.N., Cohen, I.G., 2019. Privacy in the age of medical big data. Nat. Med. 1546170X. 25 (1), 37–43. Available from: http://www.nature.com/nm/index.html. doi:10.1038/s41591-018-0272-7.

Sim, I., Gorman, P., Greenes, R.A., Haynes, R.B., Kaplan, B., Lehmann, H., Tang, P.C., 2001. Clinical decision support systems for the practice of evidence-based medicine. J. Am. Med. Inform. Assoc. 1067-5027. 8 (6), 527–534. doi:10.1136/jamia.2001.0080527.

Vonbank, A., Saely, C.H., Rein, P., Sturn, D., Drexel, H., 2013. Current cholesterol guidelines and clinical reality: a comparison of two cohorts of coronary artery disease patients. Swiss Med. Wkly. 14243997. 143. Available from: http://www.smw.ch/scripts/stream_pdf.php?doi=smw-2013-13828. doi:10.4414/smw.2013.13828.

Witkowski, K., Dougherty, R.B., Neely, S.R., 2024. Public perceptions of artificial intelligence in healthcare: ethical concerns and opportunities for patient-centered care. BMC Med. Ethics. 1472-6939. 25 (1). doi:10.1186/s12910-024-01066-4.

Young, A.T., Amara, D., Bhattacharya, A., Wei, M.L., 2021. Patient and general public attitudes towards clinical artificial intelligence: a mixed methods systematic review. Lancet Digit. Health. 25897500. 3 (9), e599. Available from: https://www.sciencedirect.com/journal/the-lancet-digital-health. doi:10.1016/S2589-7500(21)00132-1.

Zhao, M., Hoti, K., Wang, H., Raghu, A., Katabi, D., 2021. Assessment of medication self-administration using artificial intelligence. Nat. Med. 1078-8956. 27 (4), 727–735. doi:10.1038/s41591-021-01273-1.

CHAPTER

28

Healthcare data integration using machine learning: A case study evaluation with health information-seeking behavior databases

Ardalan Mirzaei, Parisa Aslani, and Carl Richard Schneider

Faculty of Medicine and Health, School of Pharmacy, The University of Sydney, Sydney, NSW, Australia

CHAPTER OBJECTIVES

- To explain the principles of machine learning (ML) and their relevance to healthcare data integration.
- To describe the challenges associated with integrating heterogeneous healthcare datasets.
- To present a taxonomy-guided framework for harmonizing variable definitions across datasets.
- To evaluate ML models for automating schema mapping and improving reproducibility.
- To compare different database integration methods and assess their applicability in pharmacy and healthcare settings.
- To explore ethical considerations in data integration, including privacy, equity, and governance.
- To demonstrate the potential applications of ML-based integration in clinical, public health, and research contexts.

1 Introduction

ML has emerged as a pivotal technology across various sectors, particularly in the healthcare industry. Its origins date back to the mid-20th century, when researchers began developing algorithms that could enable computers to learn from data and make decisions without being explicitly programmed. At its core, ML involves the dynamic interaction between data and algorithms, allowing systems to detect patterns, make predictions, and refine their

Contemporary Research Methods in Pharmacy and Health Services - Volume 2
https://doi.org/10.1016/B978-0-443-44607-8.00025-X

performance over time. This capability has positioned ML as a powerful tool for automating complex tasks and extracting insights from large, diverse datasets (Beam and Kohane, 2018).

Initially, ML relied on rule-based systems designed to perform narrowly defined tasks. However, the field underwent a transformation in the 1990s with the introduction of statistical and probabilistic models, which enabled algorithms to generalize from data and adapt to new scenarios. The rapid expansion of data-generating technologies, such as electronic health records (EHR), wearable devices, and genomic sequencing, combined with advances in computational power, has further accelerated the development of sophisticated models (Sarker, 2021). These modern algorithms are capable of capturing detailed relationships within data, enabling more accurate predictions and deeper analytical capabilities across domains.

Healthcare data is often fragmented and inconsistently recorded across multiple systems and settings, resulting in challenges in linking datasets for comprehensive analysis. This fragmentation hinders the ability to coordinate care, identify population-level patterns, and conduct longitudinal studies. Database integration is the process of harmonizing disparate datasets into a unified, consistent schema. The process is crucial for enhancing data accessibility, reducing redundancy, and improving the quality of healthcare delivery (de la Torre Díez et al., 2016; Janssen et al., 2017; Oliveira, 2019; Stanford Medicine, 2017; Wang, 2019).

The challenge in database integration lies in mapping fields between datasets that differ in structure, terminology, and population focus. Manual mapping is time-consuming and prone to errors, especially when dealing with large-scale datasets (Goodhue et al., 1992; Sherman, 2015). Traditional approaches, such as string matching, offer limited scalability and accuracy, particularly when field names vary in length or semantics (Doan et al., 2012; Hakak et al., 2019).

Achieving semantic consistency across datasets is also challenging due to inconsistent variable naming and structural heterogeneity. To address this, a taxonomy-based approach offers a structured solution by categorizing variables into predefined conceptual domains. This method involves developing a classification system that encompasses key thematic areas such as sociodemographic attributes, clinical indicators, and behavioral factors, and then using it to guide the mapping of dataset fields. By applying this taxonomy, researchers can systematically align disparate variables to a unified schema, facilitating cross-dataset comparisons and longitudinal analyses (Cheatham and Pesquita, 2017).

This taxonomy-driven process is further enhanced through an ontology-guided framework, which leverages semantic relationships between concepts to improve mapping accuracy (Cheatham and Pesquita, 2017; Liyanage et al., 2015). Ontologies provide a formal representation of domain knowledge, enabling the interpretation of free-text field descriptions and their alignment with standardized categories. When combined with ML techniques, this framework enables scalable and automated classification of variables, thereby reducing manual effort and enhancing reproducibility (Bertaux et al., 2024). The integration of datasets using this approach supports more robust data harmonization, enabling richer insights and more comprehensive analyses across diverse healthcare data sources.

ML models, particularly those designed for text classification, can automate the mapping of field descriptions to taxonomy categories (Ikonomakis et al., 2005). For example, logistic regression (LR), random forest classifiers (RFCs), and neural networks can be trained to recognize patterns in field labels and assign them to appropriate schema elements. These models have been successfully applied in EHRs to highlight relevant patient information and support clinical decision-making (King et al., 2019).

2 Methods

2.1 Machine learning background

This section presents a structured methodology for integrating diverse healthcare databases through ML. The strategy focuses on aligning variable definitions across datasets to support cohesive analysis of health information-seeking behavior (HISB) and other patient-level data. The integration workflow comprises three main phases: acquiring and preparing data, mapping schemas using ML-driven text classification, and evaluating model performance.

Statistical learning provides a theoretical and practical framework for understanding how data can be used to infer relationships between inputs (features) and outputs (responses). At its core, it involves constructing models that approximate an unknown function mapping inputs to outputs, often under conditions of uncertainty and noise. ML uses techniques common to statistical learning to develop models that learn from data, improving their predictive accuracy by identifying patterns and structures that generalize beyond the training set. The learning process is

TABLE 28.1 Common machine learning terminology and its definitions.

Term	Definition	Analogy	Healthcare example
Supervised learning	A machine learning approach where models are trained on labeled data, with each input paired with a known output. The goal is to learn a mapping from inputs to outputs for prediction or classification tasks.	Teaching a pet with examples: you show it what to do, and it learns to follow your lead.	For instance, training a model with patient data and outcomes to predict future health statuses.
Unsupervised learning	A method where models learn patterns from unlabeled data. The algorithm explores the structure of the data without predefined categories or outcomes.	Letting a child explore a room alone, they group toys by shape or color without being told how to do so.	Similarly, the algorithm identifies hidden patterns or clusters in health-related data.
Classification	A supervised learning task where the goal is to assign inputs to predefined categories or classes.	Sorting a mixed bag of fruits into apples, oranges, and bananas.	In healthcare, it involves sorting patients into diagnostic categories, such as diabetic or hypertensive.
Regression	A supervised learning technique is used to predict continuous numerical values based on input features.	Predicting someone's height based on their age.	In medicine, it could involve estimating blood pressure based on age, weight, and lifestyle factors.
Clustering	An unsupervised learning method that groups data points based on similarity without predefined labels.	Sorting marbles into groups by color without knowing the names of the colors.	In healthcare, it helps to group patients with similar symptoms or risk profiles.
Feature Engineering	The process of selecting, transforming, or creating relevant input variables (features) improves model performance.	Choosing the best ingredients for a recipe.	In healthcare ML, selecting the right patient or clinical features helps the model understand the data better and make more accurate predictions.

typically categorized into two categories: the first is supervised learning, where the output is known and guides the model, and the second is unsupervised learning, which seeks to uncover latent structures without labeled outcomes (Hastie et al., 2009) (see Table 28.1).

A central challenge in statistical learning is managing the tradeoff between bias and variance. Simple models may underfit the data, failing to capture important patterns (high bias), while overly complex models may overfit, capturing noise rather than signal (high variance). The goal is to find a model that balances these forces to minimize prediction error on unseen data. Choices influence this balance in model complexity, loss functions, and estimation techniques. Statistical learning also emphasizes model assessment and selection, using tools such as cross-validation to estimate generalization error and guide the selection of appropriate algorithms.

The advent of deep learning, a subset of ML, has further fueled progress in the field. Deep learning models, such as neural networks, draw inspiration from the human brain's neural structure and are capable of learning intricate representations from raw data, often outperforming traditional algorithms in complex tasks like image recognition and natural language processing. Deep learning is particularly effective for complex tasks such as medical image analysis, natural language processing of clinical notes, and genomics data analysis. convolutional neural networks and recurrent neural networks (RNNs) are examples of deep learning architectures.

Model evaluation in ML is a critical step that assesses how well a trained model performs on unseen data. It involves applying statistical metrics, such as accuracy, precision, recall, F1-score, and the area under the receiver operating characteristic (ROC) curve, to quantify predictive performance. These metrics help determine whether the model generalizes beyond its training data or suffers from issues such as overfitting or underfitting. Evaluation often includes techniques like cross-validation, which partitions the data into subsets to test the model's robustness across different samples. In addition to quantitative measures, qualitative validation, such as expert review or domain-specific relevance checks, can provide deeper insights into the reliability of the model. Effective evaluation ensures that the model is not only statistically sound but also practically useful in real-world applications (Zollanvari, 2023).

2.2 Methods of database integration

Database integration is a foundational process in data management, enabling the consolidation of disparate data sources into a unified structure for analysis, decision-making, and interoperability. This section outlines six principal methods of database integration, detailing their mechanisms and associated risks.

2.2.1 *Manual integration*

Manual integration involves human-led efforts to reconcile and merge data from multiple sources. This method is typically employed in small-scale or highly specialized contexts where automated tools are unavailable or impractical. Practitioners manually inspect schema structures, interpret field meanings, and align data formats using spreadsheets, custom scripts, or direct database queries.

While manual integration allows for nuanced interpretation and domain-specific adjustments, it is inherently labor-intensive and prone to human error. The lack of standardization and reproducibility poses significant risks, particularly in regulated domains such as healthcare and finance. Moreover, manual processes do not scale well with increasing data volume or complexity, limiting their utility in modern data ecosystems (Doan et al., 2012).

2.2.2 *Extract, transform, load*

Extract, transform, load (ETL) is a structured and widely adopted method for integrating data into centralized repositories, such as data warehouses. The process consists of three stages: extracting data from source systems, transforming it into a standardized format, and loading it into a target system. ETL tools often support batch processing, scheduling, and error handling, making them suitable for enterprise-scale integration (Janssen et al., 2017).

Despite its robustness, ETL pipelines are susceptible to schema drift, which is a change in source data structures that can disrupt the integration process. In addition, ETL is typically not real-time, introducing latency that may be unsuitable for time-sensitive applications. Poorly designed transformation logic can also result in semantic inconsistencies or data loss (Janssen et al., 2017).

2.2.3 *Schema matching*

Schema matching is the process of identifying and aligning corresponding fields across different databases. This method is essential for semantic integration, ensuring that similar concepts are consistently represented. Matching can be performed manually, through rule-based systems, or semiautomatically using heuristics and similarity measures (Hakak et al., 2019).

The primary challenge in schema matching lies in semantic ambiguity. Fields with similar names may represent different concepts, while identical concepts may be labeled differently. Without domain knowledge or contextual metadata, mismatches can lead to erroneous data merging and compromised analytical validity (Hakak et al., 2019).

2.2.4 *Data federation*

Data federation enables unified access to multiple data sources without physically merging them. It creates a virtual layer that allows users to query distributed databases as if they were a single system. Middleware components translate and route queries to the appropriate sources, aggregating results in real-time (de la Torre Díez et al., 2016; Oliveira, 2019).

While data federation preserves data locality and supports dynamic querying, it introduces performance challenges. Complex queries across large datasets can result in latency and resource bottlenecks. Moreover, federated systems depend on the availability and responsiveness of underlying sources and require robust access control mechanisms to ensure data security (de la Torre Díez et al., 2016; Oliveira, 2019).

2.2.5 *Middleware-based integration*

Middleware-based integration employs intermediary software to facilitate communication and data exchange between heterogeneous systems. Middleware solutions, such as message brokers, application programming interface (API) gateways, and enterprise service buses, can translate data formats, manage transactions, and ensure reliable delivery (Wang, 2019; Goodhue et al., 1992). These solutions act as a layer between different systems, facilitating seamless interactions.

This approach supports real-time integration and asynchronous communication, making it suitable for dynamic and distributed environments. However, middleware introduces architectural complexity and potential points of failure. Misconfiguration or incompatibility between systems can lead to data corruption or loss. Continuous monitoring and maintenance are essential to ensure system integrity (Wang, 2019; Goodhue et al., 1992).

2.2.6 *Ontology-based integration*

Ontology-based integration leverages formal representations of domain knowledge to align data across systems. Ontologies define concepts, relationships, and constraints, enabling semantic interoperability and consistent interpretation of data elements. This method is particularly effective in domains with established vocabularies, such as biomedical research (Goldberg and Levy, 2014; Martínez-García and Hernández-Lemus, 2022).

The development and maintenance of ontologies require significant expertise and resources. Misalignment between ontology definitions and real-world data can result in semantic errors. In addition, integrating new data sources may necessitate extensive reconfiguration of the ontology framework (Goldberg and Levy, 2014; Martínez-García and Hernández-Lemus, 2022).

2.3 Examples applied to pharmacy

Each approach offers unique advantages and challenges when consolidating data from various health sources. The following table (Table 28.2) illustrates practical examples of how these methods can be applied within the pharmacy domain, helping to understand their real-world relevance and potential use cases.

TABLE 28.2 Examples of different integration methods and possible applications in pharmacy.

Method	Description	Example
Manual integration	Data from different sources is combined manually using human judgment to align fields, formats, and meanings.	A pharmacist researcher wants to combine two small datasets: • One is from a local hospital listing patient prescriptions. • Another example from a clinical trial lists adverse drug reactions (ADRs). They manually match drug names and patient IDs using spreadsheets, ensuring that "acetaminophen" and "paracetamol" are treated as the same drug.
Extract, transform, load	Data is pulled from source systems, cleaned, and standardized, then loaded into a central database for analysis.	A pharmacy chain integrates data from multiple branches into a central data warehouse: • *Extract*: Pull daily sales and inventory data from each branch's point-of-sale (POS) system. • *Transform*: Standardize drug codes to match WHO ATC classification (Anatomical Therapeutic Chemical (ATC) classification, 2021). • *Load*: Store in a centralized database for analytics on stock levels and demand forecasting.
Schema matching	Corresponding fields across databases are identified and aligned to ensure that similar concepts share a consistent structure and meaning.	Two pharmaceutical databases need to be merged: • One uses the field name 'Drug_Name', while another uses 'Medication'. • Both have dosage fields, but one uses "Dose (mg)" and the other "Strength". Schema matching ensures these fields are correctly aligned before integration.
Data federation	A virtual layer provides unified access to multiple databases, allowing users to query them as if they were a single system without moving the data.	A clinical pharmacist queries multiple sources in real-time: • Hospital electronic health record for patient medication history. • National Drug Database for Contraindications. Instead of merging data physically, a federated system allows a single query to retrieve relevant information from both sources dynamically.
Middleware-based integration	Intermediary software enables different systems to exchange data reliably by translating formats and managing communication.	A pharmacy system integrates with an insurance provider's application programming interface (API): • Middleware translates prescription data into the insurer's format. • It handles secure message exchange and transaction logging. This enables real-time claim approvals when a prescription is dispensed.
Ontology-based integration	Domain ontologies provide standardized concepts and relationships to semantically align data elements across diverse sources.	A research team integrates pharmacogenomics data with clinical drug response data using RxNorm (Medicine NLo, 2023) and SNOMED CT (Benson and Grieve, 2021) ontologies: • Ontologies ensure that "warfarin", and its brand variations are consistently interpreted across datasets to explore drug-gene interactions.

2.4 Ethical considerations

Healthcare data integration offers immense potential for delivering better clinical care and improving population health, enabling the generation of data insights and the utilization of generative artificial intelligence (AI). However, it is important to consider how integration can be performed ethically. It can be argued that the ethical integration of healthcare data requires a dual focus: protecting individual autonomy and privacy while also addressing systemic equity concerns (Caplan and Koopman, 2025). These two concepts are expanded on below:

Individual Privacy and Autonomy: Privacy and consent emerge as the most critical ethical challenges in healthcare data integration. Traditional informed consent models falter when data are aggregated and repurposed beyond their original intent. Individuals may consent to data sharing within the constraints of their primary healthcare provider but remain unaware that their information may be integrated with external databases or used for secondary research applications. This challenge is compounded by the technical complexity of data integration processes, making it difficult for individuals to fully understand how their information will be utilized, stored, and potentially shared across organizational boundaries. A survey of patients in Germany revealed a broad willingness to permit the secondary use of their health data, provided that equivalent safeguards are in place regarding data security and privacy (Köngeter et al., 2022). The concept of "meta consent" has emerged as a potential solution, allowing individuals to specify their preferences regarding different types of data use, from specific consent for particular applications to broader consent for research purposes (Ploug and Holm, 2016). Although patients prefer a meta or broad-based consent process, they still would like the opportunity for periodic reconsent (Köngeter et al., 2022). However, even with the ideal implementation of a consent framework that allows for the secondary use of data, the integration of legacy systems and existing data repositories remains problematic.

Systemic Equity and Justice: A key structural consideration when integrating datasets is the risk of amplifying health disparities if certain populations are underrepresented or if data quality varies by demographic group. Marginalized communities may experience fragmented data records, resulting in biased analytics and unequal access to benefits derived from data integration. This is particularly concerning when data integration may result in an increased risk of marginalization through the integration of sensitive or protected information (Iloanusi and Chun, 2024), such as sexual orientation or residency status.

2.4.1 Ethical and governance considerations in healthcare data integration

Existing regulatory frameworks and ethical guidelines provide an essential foundation for healthcare data integration, but they remain insufficient for addressing the scale and complexity of contemporary data-sharing initiatives. Major regulations, such as the Health Insurance Portability and Accountability Act in the United States and the General Data Protection Regulation in Europe, establish baseline protections for data security, privacy, and patient rights (Edemekong et al., 2024; Intersoft Consulting, 2025). However, these frameworks were largely designed around traditional, bounded healthcare relationships and do not fully anticipate large-scale, cross-organizational data integration or secondary data use. As a result, important regulatory and governance gaps persist.

In response, professional bodies and international organizations have begun to develop more context-specific guidance. The Australian Medical Association's Data Governance Position Statement, for example, emphasizes patient-centered governance and requires that data-sharing initiatives demonstrate clear and tangible value in improving healthcare systems (AMA Position Statement on Data Governance and Patient Privacy, 2023). Similarly, the World Health Organization's health data principles frame health data as a public good while underscoring the importance of safeguarding individual rights, community trust, and social license (WHO data principles, 2025). Together, these initiatives highlight a shift toward governance models that balance public benefit with ethical stewardship.

Healthcare organizations implementing data integration initiatives should, therefore, adopt comprehensive ethical frameworks that extend beyond regulatory compliance alone. Such frameworks must address individual-level concerns, such as privacy, consent, and data security, alongside structural considerations, including equity, justice, and the fair distribution of benefits. Robust governance mechanisms, supported by continuous stakeholder engagement across the data lifecycle, are essential to ensuring that integrated data systems remain socially legitimate and ethically grounded.

The ethical considerations mentioned above are closely aligned with broader principles of responsible data governance. Effective governance ensures that data collection, integration, and modeling practices uphold standards of data quality, integrity, and legitimate access, consistent with the European Union's emphasis on strong privacy protections and data stewardship. In addition, all data integration and AI-supported analytical activities should be guided by a clearly articulated societal and environmental purpose, ensuring that data use advances public well-being, equity, and sustainability. As such, the EU's Guidelines for Trustworthy AI emphasize transparency, including clear communication of system capabilities, data provenance, and limitations, as well as mechanisms that support explainability and traceability. Equally critical is accountability, which may be operationalized via robust human oversight, auditability, and risk management mechanisms to ensure responsible use of integrated datasets and machine-learning models. Embedding these principles throughout the data integration pipeline strengthens trust, enhances ethical compliance, and aligns healthcare data integration initiatives with internationally recognized standards for responsible and socially beneficial AI.

Disclosure: All data used in the following example is publicly available and de-identified. Ethical considerations include transparency in model design, fairness in classification across demographic groups, and reproducibility of results.

3 Application scenario

In the context of HISB, integration becomes particularly complex. HISB data, which captures how individuals seek information about health, illness, and wellness, is often embedded within broader surveys and lacks consistent labeling (Lambert and Loiselle, 2007; Mirzaei et al., 2021). To address this, a taxonomy was developed to classify HISB-related fields, including sociodemographic, informational, health, and affective domains (Goldberg and Levy, 2014; Mirzaei et al., 2021). This taxonomy serves as an ontology-guided framework for mapping free-text field descriptions to standardized concepts, enabling semantic alignment across datasets.

In the context of HISB data integration, ML models can classify variables across multiple datasets, enabling the construction of unified databases for large-scale analysis. Tools such as PhenDisco in genomics research demonstrate the feasibility of using ML for semantic integration, retrieving phenotype information from heterogeneous sources (Doan et al., 2012). While most prior work has focused on patient-level record linkage, our approach emphasizes field-level mapping—aligning variable definitions across datasets to build harmonized research resources.

Neural networks, in particular, show promise for this task; however, their performance depends on the volume and consistency of the training data. When applied to HISB datasets, ML models can achieve high classification accuracy, significantly reducing the manual effort required for integration. This methodological innovation facilitates the creation of large, longitudinal datasets that provide deeper insights into health information behaviors and their impact on health outcomes.

For this scenario, we will work on data integration similar to the HISB case study (Mirzaei et al., 2022). The process will follow these steps:

1. Data acquisition and preprocessing
2. Taxonomy-guided schema mapping
3. Building a training set
4. ML models
5. Model evaluation

The original case study utilized Python 3 for modeling, but any programming software with ML capabilities will be suitable (e.g., R, Julia). For this application scenario, the focus will be on using the health information national trends survey (HINTS) (Nelson et al., 2004) (hints.cancer.gov) data solely. The boxes provide process steps that you can follow yourself.

3.1 Data acquisition and preprocessing

Healthcare datasets often originate from diverse sources, such as national health surveys, EHRs, and patient-reported outcomes. These datasets typically vary in structure, terminology, and granularity. To facilitate integration, each dataset is first parsed to extract metadata, specifically variable names and field descriptions. Parsing, in this context, involves taking a sentence or a string and breaking it into its syntactic components.

What to collect from each cycle (Box 28.1):

- Variable name (e.g., *HC9SeekCancerInfo*),
- Short label/question text (e.g., "Have you ever looked for cancer information?")

For each variable's name and label/question, standardize the text encoding to UTF-8 and avoid heavy cleaning to preserve semantics for the short strings. This includes standardizing character encoding, replacing symbols (e.g., "#" with "number"), and retaining punctuation to preserve semantic cues (Mirzaei et al., 2022).

Minimal preprocessing is applied to preserve the natural language structure of field labels, which are used as input features for ML models.

3.2 Taxonomy-guided schema mapping

A domain-specific taxonomy is employed to guide the classification of variables into consistent categories. For HISB datasets, this includes fields related to sociodemographics, information sources, health status, and affective responses (Mirzaei et al., 2021). The taxonomy serves as an ontology, enabling semantic alignment across datasets (Goldberg and Levy, 2014).

This condensed schema (Box 28.2) is consistent with HISB frameworks and prior taxonomy work that grouped predictors/variables across studies—see the systematic literature review and taxonomy in HISB (Mirzaei et al., 2021).

Each field label is treated as a text input for classification. The task is framed as a multiclass classification problem, where the goal is to assign each variable to one of the predefined taxonomy categories. This approach allows for scalable schema mapping with minimal manual intervention.

3.3 Building a training set

Keep an annotation spreadsheet (Box 28.3) in Excel, Google Sheets, or a similar platform (variable → label → taxonomy class) to serve as ground truth and for interrater checks (simple percent agreement). This approach is consistent with ontology-guided, expert-reviewed mapping practices (e.g., phenotype metadata standardization).

BOX 28.1

Data acquisition step

Go to HINTS Data (hints.cancer.gov) and download one or more cycles [e.g., HINTS 5, Cycle 4 (2020), and HINTS 6 (2022)]. You'll find data files (SAS/SPSS/Stata), methodology reports, and an interactive merging tool.

Retrieve survey instruments (codebooks and questionnaires) for those cycles. You need the variable names and field descriptions/question text for ML input.

BOX 28.2

Building a taxonomy

Use a domain-specific HISB taxonomy to guide classification.

A practical four-bin version is:

- *Sociodemographic* (e.g., *age, sex, education*)
- *Informational* (e.g., *source, search, trust, access*)
- *Health* (e.g., *condition, status, behaviors*)
- *Affective* (e.g., *worry, confidence, risk perception*)

Keep your bins small to start; you can later split informational categories (e.g., source types, search behaviors) as your training data grows.

BOX 28.3

Building a training set

Retrieve one to three HINTS cycles and begin hand-labeling ~200–400 variables into the four taxonomy bins. This mirrors "field-level mapping" rather than patient-level linkage and is feasible at a small scale.

BOX 28.4

Feature engineering

Use TF-IDF, a technique for assigning importance values to words, on the concatenation of the variable name and label/question text. This provides a robust baseline for short text classification, pairing well with linear models.

BOX 28.5

Reporting

Report your 's performance and compare how well your ML models supported your task. It may require going back and tuning your ML models to improve their performance.

3.4 Machine learning models

Several ML algorithms are evaluated for their effectiveness in schema mapping:

- **LR:** A baseline model known for its interpretability and efficiency in text classification tasks (Ikonomakis et al., 2005).
- **RFC:** An ensemble method that handles nonlinear relationships and performs well with imbalanced data (Kowsari et al., 2019).
- **Fully connected neural networks (FCNNs):** Deep learning models capable of capturing complex semantic patterns in field descriptions (Gul et al., 2012).
- **Long short-term memory networks:** RNNs that account for word order and context, particularly useful for structured field labels (Chen et al., 2025).

Models are trained using labeled datasets derived from prior manual classification efforts. Tokenization and embedding techniques (Box 28.4) are applied to convert text into numerical representations that are suitable for model input.

3.5 Model evaluation

Model performance (Box 28.5) is assessed using standard classification metrics, including precision, recall, F1-score, and accuracy. The evaluation is undertaken on the test dataset (or sometimes the validation dataset). Cross-validation is employed to ensure generalizability, and ablation studies are conducted to evaluate the impact of individual datasets on model performance (Mirzaei et al., 2022).

In addition to quantitative metrics, qualitative validation is performed by comparing predicted classifications against expert-reviewed mappings. This dual approach ensures both statistical robustness and domain relevance.

4 Discussion

The integration of heterogeneous databases using ML represents a significant advancement in data-driven research and operational analytics across healthcare, biomedical sciences, and public health domains. The application scenario demonstrates that ML-based schema mapping can effectively address the challenges of semantic inconsistency, structural heterogeneity, and scalability in database integration.

4.1 Key findings and contributions

The chapter and the application scenario presented a framework for integrating heterogeneous healthcare datasets using ML, with a focus on harmonizing variable definitions across sources. This framework was grounded in statistical learning principles and employed supervised and unsupervised methods to model relationships between variables. Taxonomy-guided schema mapping enabled the consistent classification of variables, which was particularly useful in public health and pharmaceutical research, where terminology varies widely.

The chapter also outlined six principal methods of database integration: manual integration, ETL, schema matching, data federation, middleware-based integration, and ontology-based integration, each with distinct applications. Manual integration was suitable for small-scale research, while ETL was ideal for centralizing data from multiple pharmacy branches. Schema matching helped reconcile inconsistently labeled fields, and data federation allowed real-time querying across distributed systems. Middleware-based integration facilitated secure communication between pharmacy systems and insurers, enabling the real-time processing of claims. Ontology-based integration supported semantic alignment in research settings, such as pharmacogenomics. Together, these methods provided a flexible toolkit for addressing the challenges of data fragmentation, enabling more effective use of healthcare and pharmacy data in both operational and research contexts.

In the application scenario, we worked with ML models, particularly LR, RFC, and FCNNs, which were trained to classify and align variable definitions across disparate datasets with high accuracy. These models outperformed traditional rule-based or string-matching approaches, which often failed to capture semantic nuances and contextual relationships between field labels (Doan et al., 2012; Hakak et al., 2019).

The use of ML for schema alignment enables automated, scalable integration of databases, reducing the reliance on manual curation and domain-specific expertise. This is particularly valuable in contexts where datasets are large, frequently updated, or originate from multiple institutions with varying data standards. The integration process facilitates cross-dataset analyses, supports longitudinal research, and enhances the utility of secondary data sources.

4.2 Methodological implications

The success of ML-based integration depends on several factors. First, the quality and consistency of training data are critical. Models trained on well-labeled datasets with representative examples of variable types consistently outperform those trained on sparse or noisy data. Second, the choice of model architecture needs to strike a balance between complexity and interpretability. While deep learning models offer flexibility and abstraction, simpler models, such as LR and RFC, often provide sufficient performance with greater transparency and lower computational costs (Kowsari et al., 2019).

Embedding techniques such as GloVe and word2vec further enhanced model performance by capturing semantic relationships between terms, enabling more accurate classification of field labels (Goldberg and Levy, 2014). However, these techniques required careful preprocessing and tuning to avoid overfitting and ensure generalizability.

4.3 Challenges and limitations

Despite the advantages of ML-based integration, several challenges remain. One major limitation is the "black box" nature of deep learning models, which can obscure the rationale behind classification decisions. This lack of interpretability might hinder adoption in regulated environments or clinical settings where transparency is essential (Buhrmester et al., 2019).

Another challenge was the propagation of bias. If training datasets contained biased or incomplete representations of certain populations or concepts, the resulting models could reinforce these biases during integration. Addressing this required the incorporation of fairness-aware ML techniques and ongoing validation across diverse datasets.

In addition, integration across international or multilingual datasets introduces linguistic and cultural variability that existing models might not have adequately captured. Future work should explore multilingual embeddings and culturally adaptive taxonomies to improve global applicability.

4.4 Applications and future directions

The implications of this work extend beyond the healthcare sector. ML-based database integration can be applied to domains such as genomics, environmental health, epidemiology, and social sciences, where data fragmentation can be a persistent barrier to synthesis and discovery. For example, integrating genomic and clinical data could support precision medicine initiatives, while harmonizing public health surveillance data might improve outbreak detection and response.

Future research should explore hybrid approaches that combine ML with rule-based systems, leveraging domain knowledge to guide model predictions. Transfer learning and federated learning may also enable integration across institutions without sharing raw data, preserving privacy while enhancing collaboration.

Ultimately, the development of standardized evaluation frameworks and open-source tools for ML-based integration will be crucial in promoting reproducibility, transparency, and widespread adoption.

5 Conclusions

This chapter has outlined a methodological framework for integrating heterogeneous healthcare datasets using ML. By leveraging taxonomy-guided schema mapping, text classification models, and a suite of integration techniques, the approach addresses key challenges in semantic alignment, scalability, and automation. The methods discussed not only reduce manual effort and improve reproducibility but also enable the construction of unified databases that support longitudinal research and operational analytics.

The potential applications of these methods span clinical decision support, public health surveillance, pharmacy informatics, and precision medicine. As healthcare data continues to grow in volume and complexity, ML provides a scalable solution for harmonizing diverse data sources. Future work should focus on enhancing model interpretability, addressing bias, and developing open-source tools to facilitate broader adoption. Lastly, the integration of data through intelligent systems holds promise for enhancing healthcare delivery, improving research efficiency, and advancing patient outcomes.

6 Questions for further discussion

- How can ML models be adapted to handle multilingual healthcare datasets while preserving semantic accuracy?
- What strategies can be employed to ensure fairness and reduce bias in ML-based data integration, especially for underrepresented populations?
- In what ways can ontology-based integration be scaled for use in real-time clinical decision support systems?
- How might federated learning frameworks be used to integrate sensitive healthcare data across institutions without compromising privacy?
- What are the ethical implications of automating schema mapping in healthcare, and how can transparency be maintained?
- How can pharmacy informatics benefit from real-time data federation, and what infrastructure is needed to support it?
- What role should professional organizations play in standardizing taxonomies and integration protocols across healthcare domains?
- How can ML-based integration methods be validated across different healthcare systems with varying data quality and standards?

7 Further scenarios

7.1 Manual integration of medication adherence data

You are a pharmacy researcher conducting a small-scale study on medication adherence among patients with hypertension in either a community or hospital setting. You have access to two datasets:

- Dataset A: Pharmacy dispensing records showing refill dates and quantities
- Dataset B: Patient self-reported adherence surveys, collected during clinic visits

Task: Manually integrate these datasets using spreadsheet tools. Your goal is to:

- Identify matching patient IDs across both datasets
- Standardize medication names and formats
- Create a unified table that links dispensing patterns with self-reported adherence

Challenges and outcomes: The datasets use inconsistent naming conventions and formats. You must reconcile these differences and produce a clean, integrated dataset suitable for basic analysis.

The final outcome should be a harmonized dataset that can be used to explore correlations between refill behavior and self-reported adherence. From here, you would conduct further statistical analysis.

7.2 ML-based integration of pharmacovigilance data

You are part of a research team investigating adverse drug reactions (ADRs) using national pharmacovigilance reports and EHRs. Each source uses different terminology and structures for drug names, symptoms, and patient demographics.

Task: Use ML to automate schema mapping and integrate the datasets. You will:

- Extract variable names and descriptions from both sources
- Apply a taxonomy to classify variables (e.g., drug, symptom, demographic)
- Train a text classification model (e.g., LR or neural network) to assign variables to taxonomy bins
- Evaluate model performance using metrics such as precision and F1-score

Challenges and outcomes: A challenge with this task is to ensure semantic consistency across datasets while minimizing manual effort. Upon completion, you would expect to have an integrated dataset that supports large-scale analysis of ADR patterns across populations and drug classes.

AI disclosure

During the preparation of this work, the author(s) used Microsoft CoPilot and Grammarly to support drafting, editing, and refining content, ensuring language harmonization and the condensation of concept paragraphs. After using these tools/services, the author(s) reviewed and edited the content as needed and take(s) full responsibility for the content of the publication.

References

AMA Position Statement on Data Governance and Patient Privacy, 2023. [press release].

Anatomical therapeutic chemical (ATC) classification (2021).

Beam, A.L., Kohane, I.S., 2018. Big data and machine learning in health care. JAMA. 0098-7484. 319 (13), 1317. doi:10.1001/jama.2017.18391.

Benson, Grieve, G., 2021. SNOMED CT. In: Principles of Health Interoperability: FHIR, HL7 and SNOMED CT. Springer Cham, p. 293–324. https://link.springer.com/book/10.1007/978-3-030-56883-2.

Bertaux, A., Ghidalia, S., Narsis, O.L., Nicolle, C., 2024. Combining machine learning and ontology: a systematic literature review. arXiv. 2331-8422. Available from: https://arxiv.org. doi:10.48550/arXiv.2401.07744.

Buhrmester, V., Münch, D., Arens, M., 2019. Analysis of explainers of black box deep neural networks for computer vision: a survey. arXiv. 2331-8422. Available from: https://arxiv.org. doi:10.48550/arxiv.1911.12116.

Caplan, A.B., Koopman, C., 2025. The ethics of data interoperability: mapping problems and strategies in biomedical data and beyond. Big Data Soc. 2053-9517. 12 (2). Available from: https://journals.sagepub.com/home/BDS. doi:10.1177/20539517251352815.

Cheatham, M., Pesquita, C., 2017. Semantic data integration. In: Handbook of Big Data Technologies. Springer International Publishing, United States, pp. 263–305. Available from: http://www.springer.com/in/book/9783319493398. doi:10.1007/978-3-319-49340-4_8.

Chen, Y.M., Hsiao, T.H., Lin, C.H., Fann, Y.C., 2025. Unlocking precision medicine: clinical applications of integrating health records, genetics, and immunology through artificial intelligence. J. Biomed. Sci. 1423-0127. 32 (1). Available from: https://jbiomedsci.biomedcentral.com. doi:10.1186/S12929-024-01110-W.

de la Torre Díez, I., Cosgaya, H.M., Garcia-Zapirain, B., López-Coronado, M., 2016. Big data in health: a literature review from the year 2005. J. Med. Syst. 1573-689X. 40 (9). Available from: www.wkap.nl/journalhome.htm/0148-5598. doi:10.1007/s10916-016-0565-7.

Doan, A., Halevy, A., Ives, Z., 2012. 1—Introduction. In: Doan, A., Halevy, A. (Eds.), Principles of Data Integration. Morgan Kaufmann Publishers Inc, San Francisco. 978-0-12-416044-6, pp. 1–19.

Edemekong, P., Annamaraju, P., Afzal, M., Haydel, M., 2024. Health insurance portability and accountability act (HIPAA) compliance. In: StatPearls. https://www.ncbi.nlm.nih.gov/books/NBK500019/.

Goldberg, Y., Levy, O., 2014. word2vec Explained: deriving Mikolov et al.'s negative-sampling word-embedding method.

Goodhue, D.L., Wybo, M.D., Kirsch, L.J., 1992. The impact of data integration on the costs and benefits of information systems. MIS Q. 0276-7783. 16 (3), 293. doi:10.2307/249530.

Gul, O., Al-Qutayri, M., Vu, Q.H., Yeun, C.Y. 2012 Data integration of electronic health records using artificial neural networks.In: International Conference for Internet Technology and Secured Transactions, ICITST 2012. United Arab Emirates, 313–317.

Hakak, S.I., Kamsin, A., Shivakumara, P., Gilkar, G.A., Khan, W.Z., Imran, M., 2019. Exact string matching algorithms: survey, issues, and future research directions. IEEE Access. 2169-3536. 7, 69614–69637. Available from: http://ieeexplore.ieee.org/xpl/RecentIssue.jsp?punumber=6287639. doi:10.1109/ACCESS.2019.2914071.

Hastie, Tibshirani, Friedman, J., 2009. The elements of statistical learning.

Ikonomakis, M., Kotsiantis, S., Tampakas, V., 2005. Text classification using machine learning techniques. WSEAS Trans. Comput. 4 (8), 966–974.

Iloanusi, N.J., Chun, S.A. 2024 AI impact on health equity for marginalized, racial, and ethnic minorities. In: ACM International Conference Proceeding Series. 9798400709883. Association for Computing Machinery, United States. 841–848. http://portal.acm.org/. doi:10.1145/3657054.3657152.

Intersoft Consulting, 2025. General data protection regulation (GDPR). Available from: https://gdpr-info.eu/.

Janssen, M., van der Voort, H., Wahyudi, A., 2017. Factors influencing big data decision-making quality. J. Bus. Res. 0148-2963. 70, 338–345. doi:10.1016/j.jbusres.2016.08.007.

King, A.J., Cooper, G.F., Clermont, G., Hochheiser, H., Hauskrecht, M., Sittig, D.F., Visweswaran, S., 2019. Using machine learning to selectively highlight patient information. J. Biomed. Inform. 1532-0464. 100. Available from: http://www.elsevier.com/inca/publications/store/6/2/2/8/5/7/index.htt. doi:10.1016/j.jbi.2019.103327.

Köngeter, A., Schickhardt, C., Jungkunz, M., Bergbold, S., Mehlis, K., Winkler, E.C., 2022. Patients' willingness to provide their clinical data for research purposes and acceptance of different consent models: findings from a representative survey of patients with cancer. J. Med. Internet Res. 1438-8871. 24 (8), e37665. doi:10.2196/37665.

Kowsari, K., Meimandi, K.J., Heidarysafa, M., Mendu, S., Barnes, L., Brown, D., 2019. Text classification algorithms: a survey. Information. 2078-2489. 10 (4), 150. doi:10.3390/info10040150.

Lambert, S.D., Loiselle, C.G., 2007. Health information-seeking behavior. Qual. Health Res. 1552-7557. 17 (8), 1006–1019. doi:10.1177/1049732307305199.

Liyanage, H., Krause, P., De Lusignan, S., 2015. Using ontologies to improve semantic interoperability in health data. J. Innov. Health Inform. 2058-4563. 22 (2), 309–315. doi:10.14236/jhi.v22i2.159.

Martínez-García, M., Hernández-Lemus, E., 2022. Data integration challenges for machine learning in precision medicine. Front. Med. 2296-858X. 8. doi:10.3389/fmed.2021.784455.

Medicine NLo, 2023. RxNorm overview.

Mirzaei, A., Aslani, P., Luca, E.J., Schneider, C.R., 2021. Predictors of health information–seeking behavior: systematic literature review and network analysis. J. Med. Internet Res. 1438-8871. 23 (7), e21680. doi:10.2196/21680.

Mirzaei, A., Aslani, P., Schneider, C.R., 2022. Healthcare data integration using machine learning: a case study evaluation with health information-seeking behavior databases. Res. Soc. Adm. Pharm. 1551-7411. 18 (12), 4144–4149. Available from: http://www.journals.elsevierhealth.com/periodicals/rsap. doi:10.1016/j.sapharm.2022.08.001.

Nelson, D., Kreps, G., Hesse, B., Croyle, R., Willis, G., Arora, N., Barbara Rimer, K.V.V., Weinstein, N., Alden, S., 2004. The health information national trends survey (HINTS): development, design, and dissemination. J. Health Commun. 1081-0730. 9 (5), 443–460. doi:10.1080/10810730490504233.

Oliveira, A.L., 2019. Biotechnology, big data and artificial intelligence. Biotechnol. J. 1860-7314. 14 (8). Available from: http://onlinelibrary.wiley.com/journal/10.1002/(ISSN)1860-7314. doi:10.1002/biot.201800613.

Ploug, T., Holm, S., 2016. Meta consent—a flexible solution to the problem of secondary use of health data. Bioethics. 0269-9702. 30 (9), 721–732. doi:10.1111/bioe.12286.

Sarker, I.H., 2021. Machine learning: algorithms, real-World applications and research directions. SN Comput. Sci. 2661-8907. 2 (3). Available from: https://www.springer.com/journal/42979. doi:10.1007/s42979-021-00592-x.

Sherman, R., 2015. Data integration processes. In: Business Intelligence Guidebook, pp. 301–333. doi:10.1016/b978-0-12-411461-6.00012-5.

Stanford Medicine, 2017. Health trends report. Harnessing the power of data in health.

Wang, Z., 2019. Data integration of electronic medical record under administrative decentralization of medical insurance and healthcare in China: a case study. Isr. J. Health Policy Res. 2045-4015. 8 (1). doi:10.1186/s13584-019-0293-9.

WHO data principles, 2025. Available from: https://www.who.int/data/principles.

Zollanvari, A., 2023. Model Evaluation and Selection. Springer Science and Business Media LLC, pp. 237–281. doi:10.1007/978-3-031-33342-2_9.

CHAPTER

29

Creating digital practice support tools with generative artificial intelligence

Reginald Amin Yakob[a], Adeola Bamgboje-Ayodele[b], Jack C. Collins[a], and Parisa Aslani[a]

[a]Faculty of Medicine and Health, School of Pharmacy, The University of Sydney, Camperdown, NSW, Australia
[b]Discipline of Design, School of Architecture, Design and Planning, The University of Sydney, Camperdown, NSW, Australia

CHAPTER OBJECTIVES

- This chapter acknowledges the current influence of artificial intelligence (AI) on healthcare practice, such as supporting clinical decision-making and documentation (Tierney et al., 2024; Haberl et al., 2025; Kutbi, 2024). With the rapid advancements in AI, particularly in its capacity to generate contextually relevant outputs, and using ChatGPT as a representative example of generative AI based on a large language model (LLM), this chapter focuses on how healthcare professionals (HCPs) may leverage generative AI to create digital practice support (DPS) tools. The objectives are to:
- Provide an overview of LLM-based AI used in healthcare.
- Describe the specific knowledge and skills that HCPs may need to work with LLMs effectively.
- Describe different methods HCPs can use when interacting with LLMs.
- Guide readers through the iterative prompting method, explaining each step and demonstrating how repeated refinement results in the desired DPS tool.
- Describe an example of using iterative prompting with ChatGPT to create a DPS tool that advises on drug crushability, including its functionality testing, tool outcomes, and the process of employing an alternative approach.
- Discuss the considerations related to HCPs' use of LLMs for creating DPS tools within the context of an AI-integrated healthcare ecosystem.

Contemporary Research Methods in Pharmacy and Health Services - Volume 2
https://doi.org/10.1016/B978-0-443-44607-8.00027-3

1 Introduction

We are currently in an era of AI, marked by growing expectations about the transformative impact of AI on our everyday work and lives (Mucci, 2024; Jindal et al., 2024; Azaria et al., 2024; Altman, 2023). Much like the computer revolution that reshaped essential sectors such as education, health, and the global economy, the advent of AI is poised to bring about similar far-reaching changes (Mucci, 2024; Altman, 2023; Haigh, 2024).

Generative AI, for instance, represents a type of AI technology that uses deep artificial neural networks to learn and recognize patterns from large datasets and generate contextually relevant outputs such as text, code, or images; in contrast, nongenerative AI classifies, predicts, or makes decisions based on inputs, with actions constrained to specific tasks such as forecasting clinical outcomes (Mucci, 2024; Hasan et al., 2025). In this field, LLMs are a subset of generative AI models trained on vast volumes of data, enabling them to engage in context-rich conversations with users (Azaria et al., 2024; Annepaka and Pakray, 2025).

In clinical practice, generative AI technologies are increasingly used as ambient, real-time transcription tools to facilitate clinical documentation of visits and communication between HCPs and patients (Tierney et al., 2024). In medical imaging, generative AI has been used to create synthetic medical images from real-world data, yielding images with reportedly high validity and quality, which may be useful for increasing the diversity of training data for other AI models (Haberl et al., 2025; Kutbi, 2024).

Beyond imaging, generative AI is also making significant strides in pharmacy practice research (Morath et al., 2024; Albogami et al., 2024; Al-Dujaili et al., 2023). However, unlike traditional resources whose outputs are deterministic (i.e., they produce the same result every time), LLMs can generate different outputs for the same query, leading to variations in accuracy and reproducibility (Morath et al., 2024; Albogami et al., 2024; Al-Dujaili et al., 2023; van Nuland et al., 2024a). These characteristics present both opportunities and challenges for HCPs, as technology plays a central role in practice, raising an important question: how will LLMs support HCPs in engaging in technological innovation?

Here, the conversational ability of LLMs, coupled with their broad scope of information and task-handling capacity, offers strong support, especially for complex undertakings such as creating DPS tools. Previously, such tasks would have required extensive human training, effort, and time (Feldman and Anderson, 2024). For instance, ChatGPT has been utilized by pharmacists to create DPS tools that serve as prototypes for collaborative innovation within practice (Yakob et al., 2025). In this chapter, when we mention generative AI, we primarily refer to LLM-based AI. Most importantly, we use ChatGPT as a representative example due to its popularity (Ryazanov et al., 2025).

For many HCPs, the gap between their health expertise and digital competence may hinder their ability to create DPS tools. Supporting HCPs through training has been suggested as a way to improve their use of technology in practice (Silva et al., 2022; Martini et al., 2024). In the interim, LLMs, particularly general models (e.g., ChatGPT), enable HCPs, even those in resource-constrained settings, to experiment with creating DPS tools.

When HCPs combine their domain expertise with digital literacy and leverage LLMs for tool prototyping, this may enhance their confidence and facilitate collaboration with technology experts. In this way, AI is not only enhancing individual practice but also fostering a culture of innovation within the broader healthcare ecosystem.

1.1 Digital competence required for creating DPS tools with LLMs

A HCP's level of digital competency is likely to influence the complexity of DPS tools they can create with an LLM. For instance, the European Union's (EU) digital competency framework includes listed competency areas: *1. Information search, evaluation, and management; 2. Communication and collaboration; 3. Content creation; 4. Safety, wellbeing, and responsible use; and 5. Problem identification and solving* (European Commission, 2025). Notably, the competency area of content creation encompasses knowledge and skills related to the creative use of digital technologies, whereas safety, well-being, and responsible use encompass awareness of applicable regulations, such as the EU AI Act (European Commission, 2025; European Union, 2024). These competencies also align with key AI skills recommended by the International Pharmaceutical Federation (FIP) to enable pharmacists to incorporate AI into their practice more effectively and harness its full potential (International Pharmaceutical Federation, 2025).

These recommended competencies are adapted from the FIP AI Toolkit:

- **An understanding of AI's generative capabilities and limitations:** In the context of HCPs creating DPS tools with LLMs, this competency relates to the HCP's knowledge that AI can actually provide the software for a tool, such as in the form of code, as this chapter presents. This knowledge may not be apparent to HCPs who lack exposure to using LLMs for this purpose and to LLM limitations, such as usage quotas. Some LLM providers may set usage limits depending on whether the version is paid or free. For example, as of August 2025, ChatGPT-5 allows free users up to 10 messages every five hours with the standard model, after which usage shifts to a lighter mini-model (OpenAI Help Center, 2025). Full LLM capabilities and limitations are often available from the specific LLM provider.

- **Data literacy:** The ability of HCPs to interpret and evaluate data outputs from AI tools such as LLMs is essential for accurate and safe practice when using AI. In creating DPS tools with LLMs, HCPs may apply data literacy to test and evaluate the outputs of the DPS tools. This may be as simple as testing whether your intended data is returned by the DPS tool you create, and we will see an example of this in the application scenario. Although HCPs may not have the requisite programming knowledge to evaluate an LLM-provided code appropriately, this can serve as a basis for collaboration with technical experts, especially beyond idea prototyping and before DPS tool implementation or dissemination (Feldman and Anderson, 2024).
- **Ethical and legal considerations of AI use:** HCPs should be familiar with the ethical and regulatory guidelines governing the use of AI technologies (Jindal et al., 2024; Therapeutic Goods Administration, 2024). Within the context of applying LLMs for DPS tools, for example, HCPs should be aware of ethical issues, such as obtaining organizational or owner consent before creating DPS tools on nonpersonally-owned computers (e.g., shared clinical or organizational workstations, where information may be retained or organizational policies may affect storage and information access), avoiding the use of restricted or biased information, and complying with regulations such as privacy laws surrounding the creation of DPS tools that collect personal information. Ethical and regulatory issues concerning the creation of DPS tools with LLMs will be further elaborated in Discussion Section 4.
- **Critical thinking and decision-making:** This competency relates to HCPs taking responsibility for their use of AI, with the ultimate decision-making remaining with the HCP. HCPs are trained experts in their domain, and their critical thinking can be applied to testing or validating the outputs of the DPS tool. HCPs need to make an informed decision about whether to use or discard the DPS tool's outputs and take responsibility for their use of AI.
- **Communication skills:** This competency relates to HCPs' ability to communicate AI-generated information to patients and other stakeholders. This competency also covers the ability to translate complex AI data into simple, usable advice for patients and stakeholders transparently and justifiably. In the context of HCP use of LLMs for DPS tools, effective communication will be required, particularly when DPS tools are created collaboratively among a team and for the intended user. Disclosure of how the DPS tool was created and its intended function is necessary to obtain stakeholders' informed consent.
- **Continuous learning and adaptability:** This relates to HCPs' ongoing education on the evolving influence of AI technologies. HCPs' continuous learning and adaptability to AI technologies ensure they apply AI more effectively to facilitate their own practice and improve healthcare services. In the context of HCPs using LLMs for DPS tools, an example is leveraging an LLM to create a webpage that communicates and promotes the unique aspects of a practice to the public, thereby improving information accessibility, as presented in the application exercise at the end of this chapter.
- **Collaborative skills for interdisciplinary teams:** This competency relates to collaboration between HCPs and experts in other domains, such as Internet technology (IT), data scientists, and programmers, as well as between HCP groups. As previously noted under data literacy, collaboration with a technical expert is essential to developing a final DPS tool beyond a prototype, as HCPs may lack the knowledge to evaluate the generated code or improve it directly. Similarly, HCP groups may collaborate with IT experts to create a DPS tool that performs functions aligned with their combined needs, followed by testing and validation beyond the prototype stage.
- **Patient-centered care:** HCPs have a responsibility to place patients at the center of care provision activities (American Society of Health-System Pharmacists, 2020; Guthrey and Taylor, 2024). The application of AI within healthcare must ultimately improve healthcare service provision as a tenet of patient-centered care. In the context of using LLMs to create DPS tools, an example is using an LLM to build a health service webpage that disseminates health information, thereby supporting service provision by making important information, such as healthcare location details, publicly accessible.
- **Innovation and creativity:** HCPs have an opportunity to find innovative and creative ways to apply AI. AI presents opportunities for trained HCPs to adapt the technology to their practices (Jindal et al., 2024; International Pharmaceutical Federation, 2025). This requires an innovative, creative mindset that may encompass developing adaptable workflows and enabling an HCP workforce capable of implementing AI to

improve their specific domains of care (Jindal et al., 2024). When HCPs use AI to create a DPS tool, they may develop competence through experience. LLMs can support HCPs' creativity in this process by translating their ideas into prototypical DPS tools.

The relevance of specific competencies can vary across stages of the DPS tool-creation process. For example, understanding AI's generative capabilities and limitations is essential in the early stages of DPS tool creation, as HCPs may need to determine the type of code required before using an LLM like ChatGPT to generate code for the DPS tool. For instance, they might ask ChatGPT for Python code to create a DPS tool or for a webpage; in that case, Hypertext Markup Language (HTML) code may be required. The appropriate code type is often recommended by the LLM, depending on the user's description of the DPS tool and its function.

The competencies related to patient-centered care (example use case: applying AI responsibly to support aspects of providing patient care), collaborative skills for interdisciplinary teams, and data literacy (example use case: testing and reviewing the DPS tool's accuracy and reliability), as well as continuous learning and adaptability (example use case: responsible experimentation with LLMs within domain-specific practices), are equally important with reference to the example use cases. Similarly, the competency related to innovation and creativity is relevant to HCPs' imagination regarding which particular tool to create to support their practice.

Competency in critical thinking and decision-making is necessary for writing prompts for the LLM to create the DPS tool, as well as for the HCP to correctly follow the guidelines provided by the LLM to acquire and subsequently test the DPS tool. The competency *"ethical and legal considerations of AI use"* influences how HCPs finalize the DPS tool prototype and how they intend to use it, including considerations for personal or public use and responsibility for proper testing, validation, and compliance with any regulatory requirements specific to the DPS tool and its function. For example, DPS tools such as rule-based drug calculators may function by coded rules or formulas and may not qualify as AI systems; however, the professional use of AI by HCPs (besides personal use) may be covered by regulations such as the EU AI Act, where HCPs deploying AI systems in their professional capacity take responsibility for their use of the AI system and must ensure they have an appropriate level of AI literacy in accordance with the Act (European Union, 2024). An appropriate level of AI literacy includes understanding the key ethical requirements for deploying trustworthy AI, specifically: human agency and oversight; privacy and data governance; avoiding unfair bias in AI outputs; safety and technical robustness; transparency; societal and environmental well-being; and accountability (European Commission, 2019). Lastly, communication skills are essential for seeking perspectives and information, such as from stakeholders and regulatory experts, that are relevant to the DPS tool's creation process and intended use.

As mentioned earlier, LLMs must be prompted to create the DPS tool. We will now explore methods of prompting LLMs and determine the best approach for HCPs to create DPS tool prototypes with LLMs.

2 Methods of prompting LLMs

Prompting is the method used to query an LLM to generate the desired output (OpenAI Developers, 2025). Prompt engineering involves crafting prompts that produce LLM results that meet the user's needs (Gao, 2023). There are several established methods for prompting LLMs, including zero-shot, few-shot, role-play, and iterative prompting, which are explained below. LLM prompting methods, their main use cases, and practical examples for each are also summarized in Table 29.1.

Zero-shot prompting: This approach uses a direct query to the model without prior examples or context (International Pharmaceutical Federation, 2025; OpenAI Help Center, 2025). Zero-shot prompts work well for exploring initial ideas, brainstorming, or seeking alternative perspectives. Because the results depend on the LLM's pretraining and reasoning abilities, zero-shot prompts often yield more variable, less targeted outputs (Giray, 2023).

Few-shot prompting: Here, the model receives a limited number of examples or contextual background information (Gao, 2023). Providing examples helps guide the LLM toward more preferred responses. This approach is useful for clarifying concepts, mapping ideas, or troubleshooting problems because it allows users some control over the output.

Role-play prompting: This method asks the model to take on a specific role or character (International Pharmaceutical Federation, 2025). By adopting a defined persona, the LLM tailors its responses in structure, style, depth, and length to match the intended role (OpenAI Developers, 2025; Gao, 2023). Users may initiate role-play through system prompts or directly at the LLM interface. For instance, in clinical practice research, prompts like "act as a clinical pharmacist" or "act as an herbalist" have been shown to improve LLM performance in providing domain-specific answers (Munir et al., 2024; Poonprasartporn et al., 2023).

TABLE 29.1 Methods of prompting large language models, with illustrative use cases and examples.

Prompt	Use Cases	Example
Zero-shot prompt	*Initial idea exploration *Brainstorming ideas *Broad learning	*A new patient has been diagnosed with Type 2 diabetes mellitus. Should I recommend gliclazide?*
Few-shot prompt	*Rule-based and/or informed guidance *Mapping and/or refining concepts *Troubleshooting problems	Preemptive prompt: *Our pharmacy's imprest diabetes drug stock includes semaglutide, metformin, acarbose, dapagliflozin, empagliflozin, and insulin. We keep other drugs from multiple classes; however, we prefer avoiding prescribing sulfonylureas as we are also a weight loss and exercise clinic. Please consider this information for any questions regarding diabetes management drugs and regimens at our clinic.* *A new patient is diagnosed with Type 2 diabetes mellitus. Should I recommend gliclazide?*
Role-play	*Prompt automation *Function restriction *System framing *Model character/persona	*You are a clinical pharmacist, and your role is to provide accurate counseling bullet points for all incoming patient inquiries.* *"Act as a herbal therapy expert and answer the following consumer questions ... "*
Iterative prompts	Creating specific projects and/or resources *Modifying projects, resources, and design* Exploring code effects and targeted learning	Prompt 1: *I need a resource on my computer for calculating drug and volume doses. How should I go about it?* Prompt 2: *Change the color of the resource to blue and make the output units in mL,* etc., i.e., *multiple prompts.*

Iterative prompting: This technique involves an ongoing dialog with the LLM, starting from an initial query and refining outputs through multiple rounds of feedback (Azaria et al., 2024). Iterative prompting is especially important when creating a DPS tool, as a single prompt rarely yields the desired final prototype. By providing feedback and requesting adjustments, users can gradually steer the LLM toward a satisfactory outcome. This process supports exploratory thinking and creative problem-solving (Azaria et al., 2024).

2.1 Focus on the iterative prompting method

Since the interactive nature of iterative prompting enables the achievement of a targeted objective, HCPs may engage in iterative dialog with LLMs to generate DPS tool prototypes. A conceptual flow diagram of a typical iterative prompting process with LLMs is shown in Figure 29.1.

2.1.1 Stages of an iterative prompting method for digital practice support tool creation with ChatGPT

The compositional stages of an iterative prompting method include:

Planning

The planning stage involves imagining, envisioning, and determining which DPS tools or resources are required to support a specific task. It can include several decisions, such as:

- The functions the DPS tool must perform to adequately support the intended task(s).
- The DPS tool's interface requirements and appearance (i.e., user interface design).
- Ease of use, such as the option to choose between automated suggestions and manual entries. For example, a drug crushability advice DPS tool might offer users the option to let the system autocomplete drug names or allow them to enter the names manually to capture entry data.
- The device or platform on which the DPS tool operates, such as a phone, computer, or online platform.
- Type of LLM to use—availability and performance often influence the selection of an LLM. For instance, some LLMs are multimodal, handling text, images, videos, and audio, while others may handle text only (Annepaka and Pakray, 2025).

The planning stage can also provide an opportunity for collaboration among HCPs and key stakeholders, including end users, administrators, and IT specialists. During this phase, participants may codesign and define project goals, identify user needs, and outline essential features for the DPS tool prototype, ensuring that diverse perspectives shape the final tool prototype.

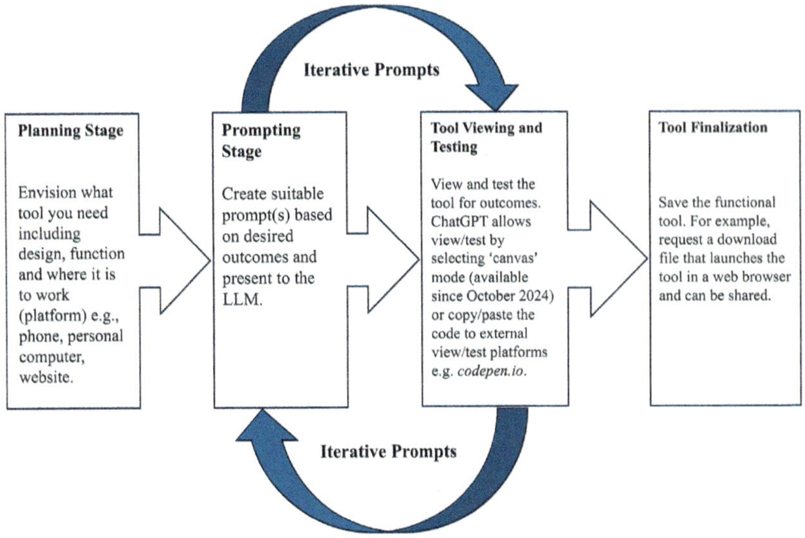

FIG. 29.1 An iterative prompting process for creating digital practice support tools with ChatGPT. This figure illustrates the iterative prompting method as a flow diagram consisting of the planning, prompting, DPS tool viewing/testing, and DPS tool finalization stages. The diagram cycles between the prompting and tool viewing/testing stages until a satisfactory tool outcome is achieved.

Prompting (initial and iterative)

This involves creating an appropriate initial prompt for engaging the LLM. For example, to create a DPS tool that solves complex problems, the LLM might first be given the problem and then involved in a guided dialog to create a tool based on the solved problem, i.e., for handling similar future queries (Yakob et al., 2025). The DPS tool is reviewed, tested, and refined with additional prompts based on the initial results or responses. This cycle of prompting, reviewing, testing, and re-prompting continues until a functional and satisfactory tool is achieved.

Viewing and testing

This stage confirms that the LLM has produced the intended DPS tool, such as by generating code or a downloadable file, and that the DPS tool works as expected. Some LLMs offer built-in viewing and testing features, such as ChatGPT's *'Canvas'* mode or *'Artifact'* within the Claude LLM (OpenAI, 2024; Claude Help Center, 2026). Alternatively, the generated DPS tool code can be saved to a compatible device, such as a computer, or uploaded to external platforms, such as codepen.io, for viewing and testing.

In addition, in a collaborative team, designating separate groups for creating and testing the DPS tool can enhance methodological rigor and minimize potential bias in tool evaluation. In such cases, the following steps are suggested:

- ***DPS tool design group***: This team is responsible for planning and creating the DPS tool using appropriate prompts.
- ***DPS tool evaluation group:*** A separate group, "blinded" to the DPS tool creation details (meaning they have no prior knowledge of how the tool was made), evaluates its functionality and usability. This approach helps ensure unbiased, informative feedback.
- ***Iterative improvement:*** Based on the testers' feedback, the DPS tool is refined and improved by the creating group.
- ***Final confirmation***: A final round of testing ensures that the DPS tool meets functionality and usability expectations before it is finalized as a prototype.

Finalization

This stage involves saving the satisfactory DPS tool to the target device or platform for use. Practical steps might include "copying", "pasting", and "saving" the code in an appropriate file format, or requesting the LLM to generate a downloadable file, such as an HTML document that can be opened directly in a web browser. In many cases, the LLM may also provide device-specific guidance for saving and finalizing the DPS tool.

Beyond saving and finalizing the DPS tool, HCPs should also consider several practical factors when using LLMs to create the DPS tool. These include LLM availability and capabilities (e.g., ChatGPT's *'Canvas'* or Claude's *'Artifacts'* mode for viewing code outputs), user knowledge and experience, location-specific resources, and relevant regulatory and ethical requirements. It is important to note that the iterative approach described here is appropriate for HCPs' exploration and prototyping of innovative tool concepts; however, progression beyond this stage requires collaboration with technological, legal, and regulatory experts to ensure that such tools are validated and refined in accordance with their intended purpose and scope. These factors will be further discussed in Section 4.

2.2 Application scenario of the iterative prompting method

Of the prompting strategies outlined in Table 29.1, iterative prompting is particularly advantageous for HCPs without formal programming training because it enables incremental refinement and exploration of ideas without requiring technical expertise (Azaria et al., 2024; Feldman and Anderson, 2024). This approach allows users to interactively develop and improve tool prototypes, making it accessible and practical for HCPs focused on practice innovation.

An application of iterative prompting to create a DPS tool that advises on drug crushability is demonstrated using ChatGPT.

2.2.1 Tool selection for creation with ChatGPT

A drug crushability tool was chosen for this practice scenario because pharmacists often need to address questions about crushing drugs or alternative dosing for elderly, pediatric, palliative, or community settings where swallowing difficulties exist (Cornish, 2005; Fodil et al., 2017).

A drug-crushability tool can provide quick guidance on crushing solid drug formulations. More importantly, the reference resource used by the created tool can be customized to include personalized or location-specific information, such as uncommon drug names, differences in crushability across brands of the same generic medicine, and other details unique to healthcare workers who intend to use the digital tool. See Table 29.2 for an example project template relevant to this application scenario. Specific stages within the template are illustrated in Figures 29.2–29.5.

Figure 29.2 shows an Excel spreadsheet containing drug-crushability advice requested from ChatGPT, using Prompt 1 in the project template (Table 29.2).

Figure 29.3 shows ChatGPT's provided options for Prompt 3 in the project template (Table 29.2).

Figure 29.4 shows ChatGPT's response to the image request using Prompt 4 in the project template (Table 29.2).

Figure 29.5 shows ChatGPT's response to an autosuggest function requested with Prompt 6 in the project template (Table 29.2).

Medication	Crushing Advice	Medication2	Crushing Advice2	Medication3	Crushing Advice3
Acetaminophen ER	Do Not Crush	Famotidine	Crush	Naproxen	Crush
Acetaminophen IR	Crush	Fentanyl buccal	Do Not Crush	Nifedipine XL	Do Not Crush
Alendronate	Do Not Crush	Ferrous sulfate	Crush	Nitroglycerin SL	Do Not Crush
Allopurinol	Crush	Fluoxetine	Do Not Crush	Olanzapine	Crush
Alprazolam XR	Do Not Crush	Folic acid	Crush	Omeprazole DR	Do Not Crush
Amiodarone	Crush	Furosemide	Crush	Ondansetron ODT	Do Not Crush
Amlodipine	Crush	Gabapentin	Crush	Oxycodone CR	Do Not Crush
Amoxicillin	Crush and mask taste	Glipizide XL	Do Not Crush	Pantoprazole DR	Do Not Crush
Apixaban	Crush	Glyburide	Crush	Paracetamol ER	Do Not Crush
Aspirin EC	Do Not Crush	Haloperidol	Crush	Paracetamol IR	Crush
Atorvastatin	Crush	Heparin	Do Not Crush	Potassium chloride ER	Do Not Crush
Bisoprolol	Crush	Hydralazine	Crush	Prednisolone	Crush
Calcium carbonate	Crush	Hydrochlorothiazide	Crush	Prednisone	Crush
Canagliflozin	Crush	Hydrocortisone	Crush	Propranolol XR	Do Not Crush
Carbamazepine XR	Do Not Crush	Ibuprofen	Do Not Crush	Propylthiouracil	Crush
Carvedilol	Crush	Insulin	Do Not Crush	Quetiapine XR	Do Not Crush
Celecoxib	Do Not Crush	Isotretinoin	Do Not Crush	Ranitidine	Crush
Celecoxib	Do Not Crush	Lamotrigine	Crush	Risedronate	Do Not Crush
Citalopram	Crush	Levetiracetam	Crush	Risperidone ODT	Do Not Crush
Clonidine	Crush	Levothyroxine	Crush	Rivaroxaban	Crush
Clopidogrel	Crush	Liraglutide	Do Not Crush	Sertraline	Crush
Codeine	Crush	Lisinopril	Crush	Simvastatin	Crush
Colchicine	Crush	Lithium	Crush	Sitagliptin	Crush
Cyanocobalamin	Crush	Loperamide	Crush	Sotalol	Crush
Dabigatran	Do Not Crush	Loratadine	Crush	Spironolactone	Crush
Diazepam	Do Not Crush	Lorazepam	Crush	Tacrolimus XL	Do Not Crush
Diclofenac EC	Do Not Crush	Losartan	Crush	Topiramate	Crush
Digoxin	Crush	Magnesium oxide	Crush	Tramadol ER	Do Not Crush
Diltiazem XR	Do Not Crush	Meloxicam	Crush	Tramadol IR	Crush
Donepezil XR	Do Not Crush	Metformin IR	Crush	Valproate	Crush
Duloxetine	Do Not Crush	Metformin XR	Do Not Crush	Venlafaxine XR	Do Not Crush
Empagliflozin	Crush	Methotrexate	Do Not Crush	Verapamil SR	Do Not Crush
Enoxaparin	Do Not Crush	Methylphenidate XR	Do Not Crush	Vitamin D tablet	Crush
Erythromycin EC	Do Not Crush	Metoclopramide	Crush	Warfarin	Crush
Escitalopram	Crush	Morphine SR	Do Not Crush	Zolpidem	Crush

FIG. 29.2 Excel spreadsheet of drug crushability advice created with ChatGPT, serving as an editable reference for the tool. This was requested from Prompt 1 in the project template (Table 29.2). The Excel spreadsheet contains a list of drugs and their "crush" or "do not crush" advice. This Excel sheet was generated by the LLM as the reference resource for the drug crushability advice tool.

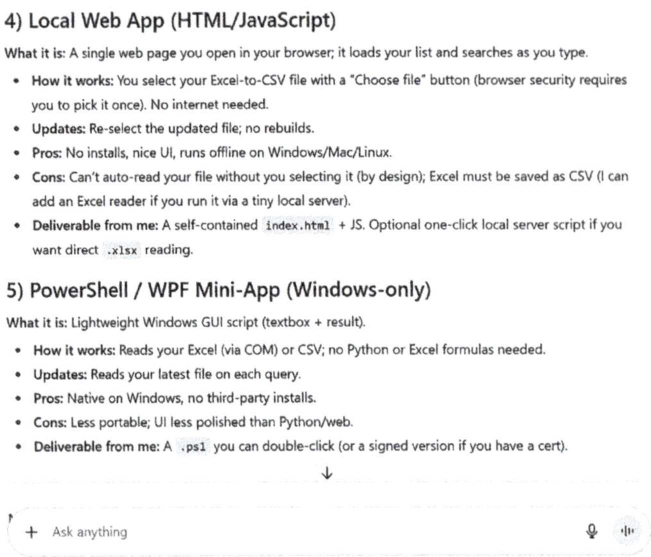

4) Local Web App (HTML/JavaScript)

What it is: A single web page you open in your browser; it loads your list and searches as you type.

- **How it works:** You select your Excel-to-CSV file with a "Choose file" button (browser security requires you to pick it once). No internet needed.
- **Updates:** Re-select the updated file; no rebuilds.
- **Pros:** No installs, nice UI, runs offline on Windows/Mac/Linux.
- **Cons:** Can't auto-read your file without you selecting it (by design); Excel must be saved as CSV (I can add an Excel reader if you run it via a tiny local server).
- **Deliverable from me:** A self-contained `index.html` + JS. Optional one-click local server script if you want direct `.xlsx` reading.

5) PowerShell / WPF Mini-App (Windows-only)

What it is: Lightweight Windows GUI script (textbox + result).

- **How it works:** Reads your Excel (via COM) or CSV; no Python or Excel formulas needed.
- **Updates:** Reads your latest file on each query.
- **Pros:** Native on Windows, no third-party installs.
- **Cons:** Less portable; UI less polished than Python/web.
- **Deliverable from me:** A `.ps1` you can double-click (or a signed version if you have a cert).

+ Ask anything

FIG. 29.3 ChatGPT's response options for Prompt 3 within the project template (Table 29.2). ChatGPT provided options for creating the described tool, including either a web application or a Windows application.

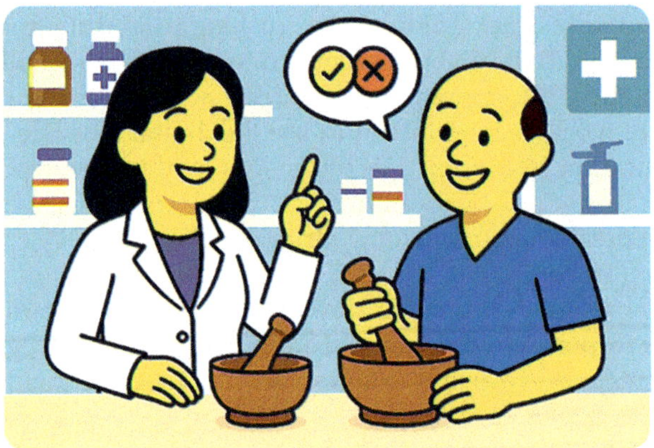

FIG. 29.4 ChatGPT's output response to Prompt 4 in the project template (Table 29.2). A cartoon image was generated by ChatGPT to serve as the background for the created tool.

2.2.2 *Tool overview*

The final drug crushability advice tool, which resulted from using the prompts within the project template, is presented in Fig. 29.6.

A weblink and QR code are provided for accessing the tool for online viewing and testing in Fig. 29.7.

2.2.3 *Tool preliminary functionality test*

The DPS tool's intended function was to provide "crush", "do not crush", or "Drug not found—contact pharmacist" advice when a drug name was entered. This advice is based on the Excel reference resource presented in Fig. 29.2.

Drugs are selected from the Excel reference resource to test whether the tool provides each drug's associated advice as outlined in the Excel reference resource presented in Fig. 29.2.

The DPS tool is accessed via the webpage at https://reginaldy.github.io/crushornotautocomplete/ .

For example, querying the DPS tool by entering *"Amoxicillin"* into the search bar displays the associated advice: "CRUSH AND MASK TASTE". This advice is consistent with the information provided in the Excel reference resource for the *"Amoxicillin"* entry.

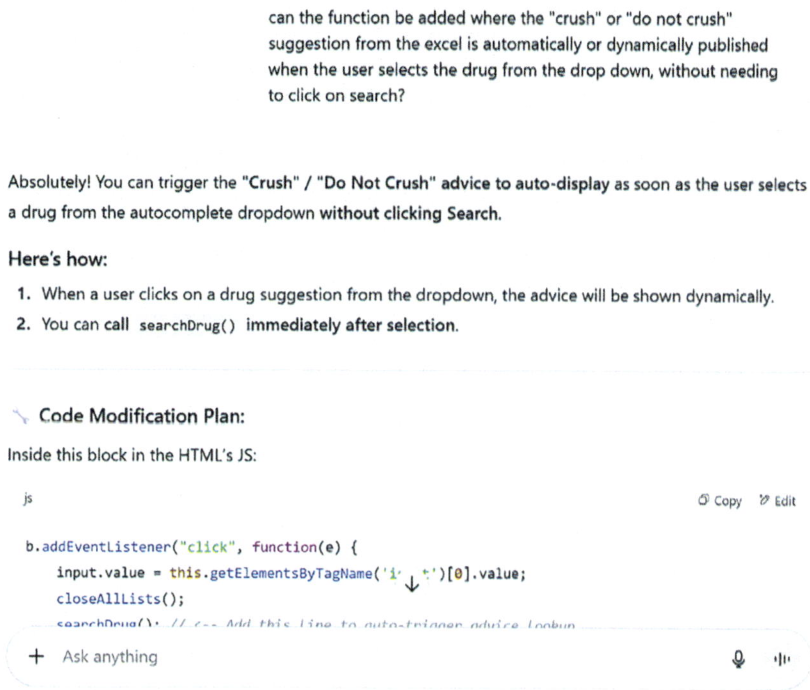

FIG. 29.5 ChatGPT's output response to Prompt 6 within the project template (Table29.2). The output from ChatGPT for an iterative request to add an autosuggest function to the created tool.

TABLE 29.2 Project template: using ChatGPT for creating a drug crushability tool.

Clinician: pharmacist	Task: Creating a digital crushability tool with ChatGPT Date: 10th August 2025 LLM used: ChatGPT-5 duration: two hours
Planning stage	• My pharmacy assistants, patients, interns, and aged care homes, which we service, often request information about which tablets can be crushed and which cannot be crushed. • I need an inventory of the common drugs, including all those within our imprest, with crushability or "do not crush" advice. • I would like this tool to report "crush" or "do not crush" advice when the drug name is entered. • The tool must work on our desktop computer in the pharmacy or through a webpage. • I will use ChatGPT (https://chatgpt.com/) as I have free access, and it can generate code. Note: Although it is not required, creating an account and logging in allows you to save your prompts and work history, revisit previous sessions, and manage your projects.
Prompting Stage	• Prompt 1: "I would like to create an Excel file on my computer desktop and then create a tool with an interface that reports from the file on my desktop. The tool's interface is for inputting the name of a drug. When a drug is typed into the interface, information on whether it is "crush" or "do not crush" is returned based on the type of drug input. The information should come from my list of drugs, which I will subsequently provide as an Excel spreadsheet on my desktop. Please provide me with an Excel list of 100 drugs and their crush or do not crush advice for me to edit and use as a reference resource for the tool." (See Fig. 29.2 for the generated Excel spreadsheet.) • Prompt 2: "I have attached an Excel spreadsheet of drugs and their 'crush' or 'do not crush' advice. I want a tool that works on my computer and reports from this Excel spreadsheet. When I type the name of a drug into the tool, it should provide the corresponding crushability advice. I will often change or update the drugs in the Excel spreadsheet. When a drug is not listed, the tool should state 'Drug not Found—Contact Pharmacist' in red. Please provide the available options you can offer for such a tool." NB: The Excel spreadsheet was generated from ChatGPT using Prompt 1. • Prompt 3: "I choose option 4—local web app. Since it will work on my local computer, it will be easy for me to upload it to our website in the future." (See Fig. 29.3 for ChatGPT's provided options for creating a local web app.)
Tool viewing and testing	• The tool was reviewed and tested by running the code on ChatGPT's *"Canvas"*. • *Optional test* • Download the HTML code to the desktop and open it with a web app (e.g., Google Chrome, Mozilla Firefox, or Internet Explorer).

Continued

TABLE 29.2 Project template: using ChatGPT for creating a drug crushability tool—cont'd

Clinician: pharmacist	**Task: Creating a digital crushability tool with ChatGPT Date: 10th August 2025 LLM used: ChatGPT-5 duration: two hours**
Iterative prompts	• Prompt 4: Provide a cartoon image of a pharmacist in a white coat instructing an assistant about whether to crush or not crush tablets. The assistant is wearing a blue coat. Both characters have smiley faces and are depicted in a pharmacy setting with a crushing mortar and pestle. The pharmacist is female, and the assistant is male. (See Fig. 29.4 for ChatGPT's response). • Prompt 5: How do I use this image as the background of the tool page? • Prompt 6: Can a function be added where the "crush" or "do not crush" suggestion from the Excel file is automatically or dynamically published when the user selects the drug from the drop-down menu, without needing to click on search? (See Fig. 29.5 for ChatGPT's output response.) • **Optional** (Tool upload to webpage) • Prompt 7: I have uploaded the tool code to a webpage. Here is a weblink to the spreadsheet (i.e., *enter the spreadsheet web address).* Make the tool load the reference resource automatically so users can begin searching from the webpage without needing to upload a spreadsheet. Add the text "A reference resource has been uploaded for illustrative purposes only—Do not use in clinical practice! Begin search." in red color beneath the search bar. (See Fig. 29.6 for the tool outcome from this prompt.)
Tool finalization	• Download the HTML code to your desktop and open it with a web app (Google Chrome, Mozilla Firefox, or Internet Explorer). • Upload the Excel drug information worksheet and use the tool.

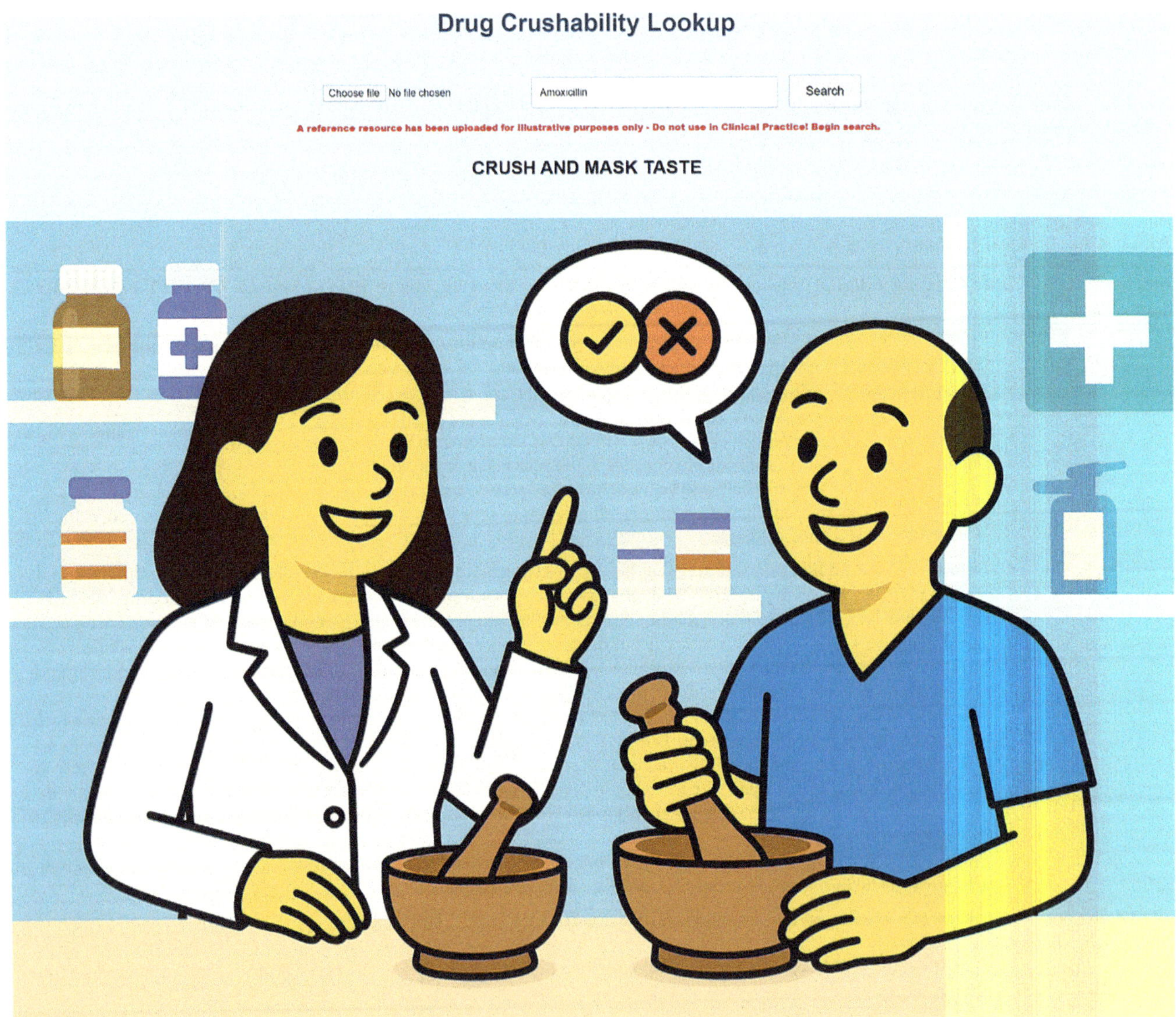

FIG. 29.6 A web-based prototype drug crushability advice tool created using iterative prompting with ChatGPT. The finalized web-based tool prototype features a cartoon image as the background and text entry fields for drug names to provide crushability advice.

FIG. 29.7 A QR code to access the drug crushability advice tool prototype. A scannable barcode provides access to the drug crushability advice tool prototype, along with a Weblink to access the tool prototype: https://reginaldy.github.io/crushornotautocomplete/.

TABLE 29.3 Functionality assessment of the drug crushability advice tool.

Tool	Intended function	Test and reference answer	Tool result	Pass/Fail
Drug crushability lookup	1. Provide a "crush", "do not crush", or "Drug not found—contact pharmacist" advice upon entry of a drug name based on the reference resource. The tool's background is rendered with the generated image, i.e. (Prompt 1 to 5)	1. Amoxicillin—"CRUSH AND MASK TASTE" Acetaminophen ER—"DO NOT CRUSH" Acetaminophen IR—"CRUSH" Pregabalin—"Drug Not Found—Contact Pharmacist" (i.e., written in red as per "Prompt 2"). Tool background = generated image.	1. Amoxicillin—"CRUSH AND MASK TASTE" Acetaminophen ER—"DO NOT CRUSH" Acetaminophen IR—"CRUSH" Pregabalin—"Drug Not Found—Contact Pharmacist" written in red. Observed background = generated image.	Pass
	2. Autosuggest drug names from a dropdown list as they are entered, i.e., as per Prompt 6.	2. Begin drug name entry and confirm. e.g. "ibupro … "—autosuggests "Ibuprofen" as per the reference resource.	2. Autosuggested "Ibuprofen" as per the reference resource.	Pass
	3. If the drug is on the list, provide crush advice immediately without clicking the search button, i.e., as per Prompt 6.	3. Select a suggested drug name, e.g., isotretinoin, and confirm the advice—"DO NOT CRUSH". Enter a different drug, e.g., amlodipine, and confirm the immediate change of advice to "CRUSH".	3. Entering "isotretinoin" displayed "DO NOT CRUSH" without pressing the search button. A subsequent search for "amlodipine" immediately changed the advice to "CRUSH".	Pass

Similarly, for extended-release (ER) *"acetaminophen ER"*, the returned advice is "DO NOT CRUSH" and for immediate-release (IR) *"acetaminophen IR"*, the returned advice is "CRUSH". The returned advice outputs are concordant with the associated entry for each drug in the Excel reference resource presented in Fig. 29.2.

If a drug is not listed in the Excel reference resource (e.g., *pregabalin*), the DPS tool returns "Drug Not Found—Contact Pharmacist". This advice is concordant with Prompt 2 in the project template (Table 29.2).

The DPS tool's outputs are, therefore, concordant with the information within our Excel reference resource, which is presented in Fig. 29.2. The tool reliably returns each drug's associated advice within the Excel reference resource presented in Fig. 29.2.

A summary functional test of the DPS tool is presented in Table 29.3.

2.2.4 Beyond creation: Tool validation and collaboration

Beyond DPS tool creation (prototyping), DPS tools intended for production use or dissemination to other users (e.g., on a commercial basis) would typically be required to meet performance, safety, and legal or regulatory requirements beyond the methods demonstrated in this chapter. A thorough validation of a DPS tool may, for example, include reliability testing that ensures the tool gives consistent answers each time and can be performed using sample data, e.g., testing the tool with problems for which it has been created to solve (Syed et al., 2024). For reliability, test-retest (sequential testing) has been used in studies to assess the consistency of technology outputs in healthcare (Al-Dujaili et al., 2023; van Nuland et al., 2024a, 2024b).

Users' acceptance and intention to use a digital tool may also be assessed using validated measures such as the Technology Acceptance Model or the Unified Theory of Acceptance and Use of Technology (Ifinedo, 2012; Venkatesh et al., 2003). In addition, the System Usability Scale is a validated measure that can be used in healthcare to assess a digital tool's user-friendliness and user satisfaction (Syed et al., 2024; Dowding et al., 2019).

In addition, studies evaluating the accuracy of digital tools in healthcare have relied on expert user scoring, consensus agreements, and comparisons of outputs with standard reference sources (Albogami et al., 2024; Poonprasartporn et al., 2023; van Nuland et al., 2024b).

Although this chapter reports a preliminary functional test of the DPS tool prototype, readers interested in further validating the tools they have created may consider the methods suggested here. Progression beyond early, unlicensed prototypes would require appropriate collaboration with technical (e.g., software developers) and regulatory or legal expertise [e.g., intellectual property (IP) specialists]. Since the primary goal of this chapter is to demonstrate the iterative prompting method by which HCPs can use LLMs to create a functional DPS tool, the examples presented here are illustrative prototypes and are not provided for clinical use. Responsibilities of HCPs, along with ethical and regulatory considerations related to the use of LLMs for DPS tool creation, are discussed in Section 4.

2.2.5 Alternative tool creation approach enabled by ChatGPT: Executable applications

Although an HTML approach was selected for webpage accessibility, ChatGPT proposed other methods for creating the DPS tool, such as an executable application that displays data from a reference drug-crushability spreadsheet on the desktop. The guidelines provided by ChatGPT for creating the DPS tool required running a local command prompt, installing relevant software (Python), and ultimately installing the DPS tool outcome as an executable application. As such, it was slightly more technical and required system administrator permissions to install executable application files, which may not be permissible when implemented on public or institutional computers for security reasons. Nonetheless, the resulting desktop DPS tool, following ChatGPT's guidance, is shown in Fig. 29.8.

The prompts provided to ChatGPT for creating the local desktop DPS tool are shown in Fig. 29.9 and were as follows: Initial prompt: "I want to create a tool that works on my computer, with an interface for inputting the name of a drug. When a drug is typed into the interface, information on whether 'appropriate to crush' or 'do not crush' is returned based on the type of drug input. The information should come from my list of drugs, which I have attached as an Excel sheet. I want to be able to update the Excel sheet often with new information; as such, a standalone tool that reports from my Excel file is preferred. I want to download this tool onto my computer, and it reports from my Excel file, which is on my computer. Can you create and provide me with this tool?" Iterative prompt: "Provide this as a desktop button with autocomplete from the Excel file uploaded, and without the need to operate through Python each time."

In response to the initial prompt, ChatGPT provided the tool code along with implementation guidelines. Since the code was based on Python, the guidance was to install the Python program using the computer system's command prompt; doing so allowed the tool to appear on the computer through the system's command prompt terminal.

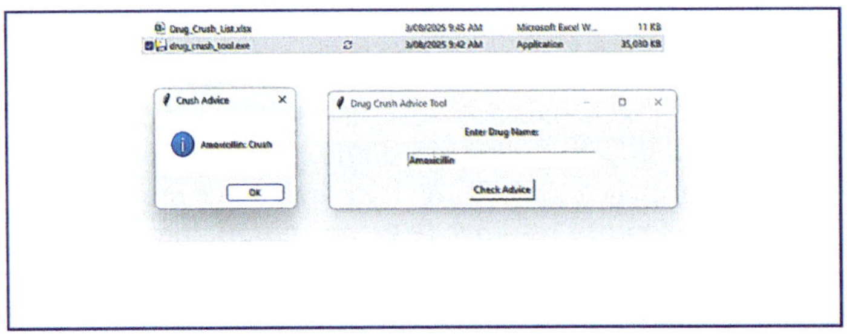

FIG. 29.8 An executable desktop application for drug crushability advice, created using iterative prompting with ChatGPT. An executable Windows desktop application for drug crushability advice was also created using iterative prompts with ChatGPT.

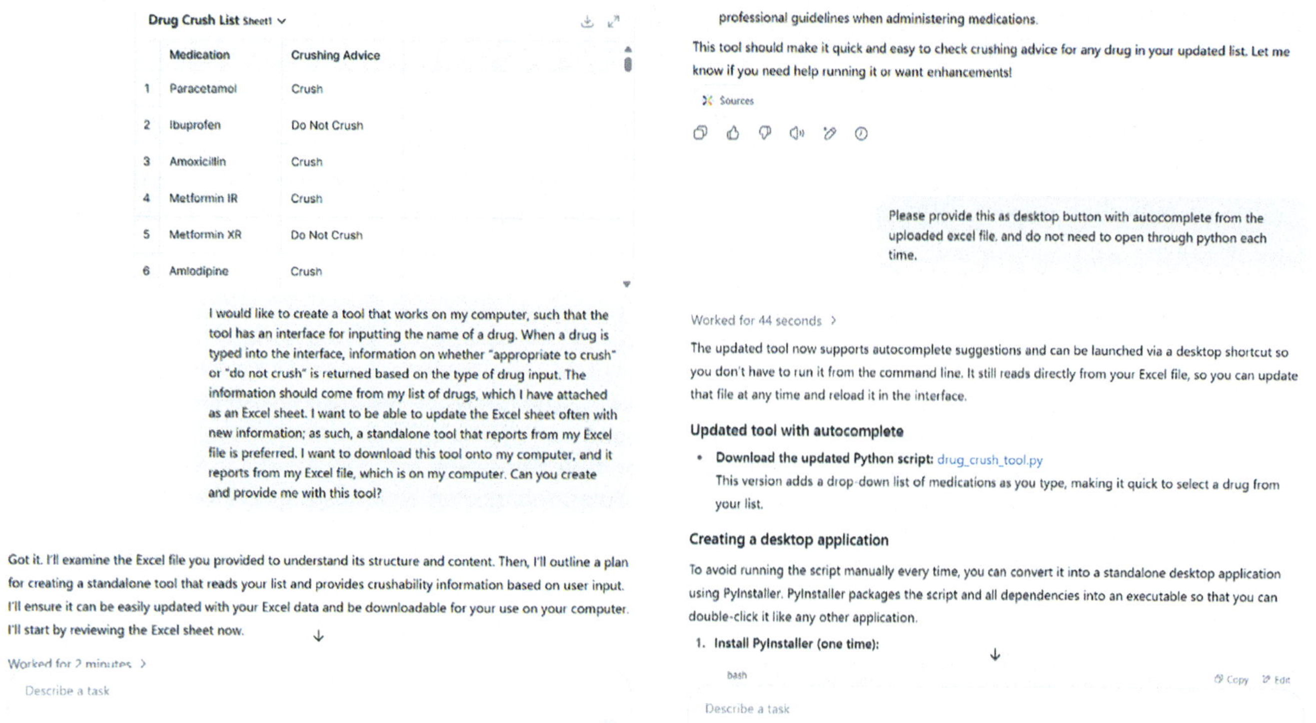

FIG. 29.9 Prompts and ChatGPT guidance for creating an executable drug-crushability advice tool. Prompts were provided to ChatGPT to develop an executable desktop application for a drug-crushability advice tool.

In response to the iterative prompt,ChatGPT provided an updated tool code with guidelines on how to install a free program, PyInstaller, on the computer, allowing the tool to be created as an executable application installed on the computer desktop, as seen in Fig. 29.8.

Choosing either the HTML or the executable application approach presented unique considerations, as outlined below:

2.2.6 Pros and cons of tool creation approaches: HTML versus executable applications

HTML approach

Pros:

- The process for creating the DPS tool is simpler because external programming tools, such as Python, are not required.
- Easy and safer to implement, as it does not require installing the created DPS tool on the computer and can be opened in the computer's web browser.
- The HTML code can be hosted on an online web page for wider accessibility.
- If hosted online, the HTML-based DPS tool can be updated centrally, allowing access to the most recent version immediately without requiring local reinstallation or manual updates.
- If saved to a computer instead of being hosted online, the HTML-based DPS tool and reference resources can be used without internet connectivity, thereby avoiding online data transmission and reducing the risk of information exposure.

Cons:

- A standard web browser is typically required to open and use the HTML-based DPS tool.
- The HTML-based DPS tool's performance and functionality may be constrained by local browser capabilities or specifications.
- If the reference resource is not incorporated into the code, it may need to be re-uploaded whenever the browser session restarts. In contrast, embedding the reference resource within the code can complicate

updates, such as when new drug names are introduced, requiring code modifications. This can potentially increase code size and affect performance.
- Saving and using the tool on a local computer reduces the risk of online information exposure and security risks; however, hosting the tool on a website requires consideration of web security, maintenance, web updates, host platform performance, and appropriate web IT and cybersecurity expertise.
- If an HTML-based tool is hosted online, the source code may be visible and potentially copied by others, raising intellectual property (IP) considerations that may require legal expertise regarding appropriate IP protections.

Executable application approach

Pros:

- Because the DPS tool is installed on the local computer where the reference resource is also stored, there is no need to re-upload the reference resource to use the DPS tool.
- The DPS tool can be accessed locally without the need for a web browser.
- When the DPS tool is saved and installed on a local computer, reliance on web hosting services and platform updates is avoided, reducing the risk of exposing source code or sensitive information online.
- Executable applications often provide performance advantages over HTML-based applications, as they run directly on local hardware without relying on web browser functionality.
- Updates to the DPS tool outputs can be implemented locally by adding or modifying information in the reference resource, whereas updates to the tool's design or behavior can be applied by redesigning the interface through iterative reprompting of the LLM for changes.

Cons:

- Installing a programming language such as Python and implementing the executable DPS tool-creation process may be more challenging for HCPs compared to an HTML-based DPS tool.
- Executable applications cannot be installed on computers without an administrator user's permission.
- Before installing an application on a local computer, executable files should be obtained from trusted sources and inspected for malicious code; consulting IT professionals may help assess their trustworthiness.
- DPS tools created on one platform may not work when transferred to another platform due to differences in operating systems, system architectures, or security restrictions affecting performance.

3 Discussion of AI in healthcare, its uses, and considerations

AI has made tasks previously considered difficult much easier (Feldman and Anderson, 2024; Yakob et al., 2025; Gao, 2023). LLMs generate coherent text and respond to diverse queries, enabling nonexperts to create digital tools (Feldman and Anderson, 2024; Gao, 2023). This chapter explores iterative prompting as a method for HCPs to leverage commonly available LLMs to create DPS tools. In today's rapidly evolving AI landscape, it is essential for clinical education programs to incorporate training on the applications and implications of healthcare AI, preparing personnel, such as HCPs, to benefit from and navigate AI's societal influence, as well as the legal and ethical frameworks that govern its use (Silva et al., 2022; Martini et al., 2024).

Public interest in LLMs surged with the release of ChatGPT-3.5 in 2022 (Annepaka and Pakray, 2025; Leiter et al., 2024; Ryazanov et al., 2025). Advancements continue with multimodal models like ChatGPT-5, which also interpret audiovisual content (OpenAI Help Center, 2025). With models from providers such as Anthropic, Microsoft, and Meta, AI is heralded as a new technological frontier (Mucci, 2024; Annepaka and Pakray, 2025; Haberl et al., 2025; The White House, 2025).

A more obvious benefit is the reduction of skills gaps, especially between digital needs and the means to meet them. This trend, often referred to as the democratization of technology, is evident when individuals use AI to create digital tool prototypes without formal coding or programming skills (World Economic Forum, 2023; Shukla, 2019; Costa et al., 2024). These prototypes can serve as initial practice support tools and facilitate collaboration with technology experts to develop more advanced and validated tools. Since the tool's underlying logic or formulas are derived from natural language dialog (iterative prompts) between the HCP and the LLM, the HCP's functional requirements for the DPS tool are represented in the generated code. This transparency may support auditability by IT experts and facilitate prototyping, interdisciplinary collaboration, stakeholder involvement, and HCP competency building.

To this end, this chapter includes an outcome-oriented application scenario in which an LLM was prompted to create a functional DPS tool. In the scenario, iterative prompting was used with ChatGPT to obtain a reference resource and a drug crushability advice tool that reports information from the reference resource. As explored in the application scenario section, ChatGPT offered multiple pathway options to develop the tool, including an HTML option, which was primarily chosen to make the tool accessible on a webpage.

An alternative approach provided by ChatGPT was also followed to create a local desktop application. This method required executing local command-line prompts and installing the tool as a desktop application. In contrast, the HTML approach was available for download from ChatGPT and could be run directly on a desktop or uploaded to a webpage. While the application scenario emphasizes the HTML method, guidance and results for the alternative approach were also presented. The HTML approach is considered safer and more straightforward on devices because it eliminates the need to use system command lines or install executables, which often require administrator permissions.

Specific to the application scenario presented in this chapter, iterative prompts were used to provide a background user interface of cartooned characters, request drug autosuggest features, and initially generate a list of 100 common drugs and their crushability advice, which served as a reference resource for the tool—all within no more than two hours from planning to tool completion, as shown in the project template. With increasing HCPs' knowledge and advancements in LLMs, it is expected that DPS tool creation will evolve from simple ones, as illustrated here, to more complex ones, and also in a shorter timeframe, to achieve a functional tool prototype.

3.1 Factors influencing HCP use of generative AI for creating DPS tools

Ultimately, HCPs' use of generative AI technologies, such as LLMs, for DPS tool creation, as described in this chapter, is influenced by individual factors, including creativity, clinical knowledge, experience, and specific needs. The ability to effectively prompt an LLM for particular DPS tools may be enhanced by qualities such as self-efficacy, creativity, and collaboration. For instance, self-efficacy may encourage HCPs to confidently experiment with new prompting strategies and refine their approaches based on outcomes. Creativity fosters interactive solutions and innovative applications when working with LLMs. Collaboration, such as through joint workshops among HCPs, the technology industry, and regulatory agencies, ensures that diverse perspectives inform the project and ultimately lead to more practice-oriented tools.

LLM outputs, performance characteristics, and user requirements vary across providers such as Llama by Meta AI, Claude by Anthropic, and Copilot by Microsoft, and prompting an LLM to achieve a desired outcome is often considered both an art and a science (OpenAI Developers, 2025). It is essential for users to investigate and choose an appropriate LLM type and provider. While advanced LLMs have generally demonstrated greater consistency on tasks than less advanced models (Bazzari and Bazzari, 2024; Al-Ashwal et al., 2023) the goal of tool creation is outcome-focused: the LLM should be engaged in dialog to produce a tool that performs its intended task.

3.2 Ethical and regulatory considerations of HCP use of generative AI for creating DPS tools

Not surprisingly, the novelty and widespread adoption of AI, along with its rapid evolution, pose challenges to established regulations across key sectors, including education, healthcare, and society as a whole (Azaria et al., 2024). These regulatory authorities must find ways to balance regulating AI development and use with the need to avoid restrictions that could hinder technological progress (Therapeutic Goods Administration, 2024; The White House, 2025; Davtyan, 2025). The popular commentary, "AI will not replace you; you will be replaced by someone who uses AI," captures this dilemma (Harvard Business Review, 2023; Siu, 2024). For HCPs, leveraging LLMs to create DPS tools may reduce barriers to participation in digital innovation (Yakob et al., 2025). When such applications yield cost savings, they may also contribute to a broader goal of making healthcare resources affordable, especially for underresourced settings. Furthermore, a reduction in technological acquisition costs, such as through LLMs, may facilitate innovative collaborations that promote work efficiency (World Economic Forum, 2023; DevelopmentAid, 2023).

Despite their benefits, AI technologies must be used ethically (Azaria et al., 2024; Bazzari and Bazzari, 2024). Ethical considerations with respect to the creation of DPS tools include avoiding the use of copyrighted information in tool creation without appropriate permissions, avoiding privacy violations such as failing to seek administrator consent for tool creation on nonpersonal devices, and avoiding the use of patients' personal data in tool creation. In addition, it is important to avoid the use of biased information, such as culturally insensitive or inappropriate language prompts used with LLMs, and to exercise human professional oversight over the accuracy of LLMs' output. The EU AI Act, for example, governs the use of AI in professional contexts beyond personal use and requires AI deployers to possess an appropriate level of AI literacy, including an understanding of the requirements for meeting the definition of trustworthy AI (i.e., human agency and oversight, technical robustness and safety, privacy and data governance, transparency, diversity, nondiscrimination and fairness, societal and environmental well-being, and accountability) (European Commission, 2019; European Union, 2024). Article 3, point (1), in the EU AI Act defines an AI system as *"a machine-based system designed to operate with varying levels of autonomy and that may exhibit adaptiveness after deployment, and that, for explicit or implicit objectives, infers, from the input it receives, how to generate outputs such as predictions, content, recommendations, or decisions that can influence physical or virtual environments"* (European Union, 2024). DPS tools created with generative AI, however, may fall under medical device regulations based on their function, complexity, and risk level. Regulatory bodies such as the United States Food and Drug Administration and the Australian Therapeutic Goods Administration do not currently classify simple digital tools, for example, as medical devices and do not require stricter regulations if they support or enhance, rather than replace, HCPs' capacity or decision-making (Therapeutic Goods Administration, 2021; Food and Drug Administration, 2026). However, it is always prudent to seek direct clarification from the relevant authorities in your specific setting regarding the tool itself and its intended purpose. For example, when a tool is designed to collect patient information, privacy and data protection laws typically apply (Therapeutic Goods Administration, 2024). If a tool is created for commercial purposes, one should expect that commercial and consumer laws would apply. For these purposes, HCPs should consult legal and local regulatory authorities for specific guidance.

In summary, iterative prompting enables HCPs to leverage LLMs to create DPS tools that can serve as prototypes for subsequent innovative collaborations with the technology sector. In resource-limited settings, following DPS tool validation and regulatory guidance, such tools may support service provision by offering customization, such as location-specific drug names and processes, while potentially facilitating tasks. The potential of advanced LLMs to bridge technological gaps underscores the importance of integrating AI education into healthcare training. Given the rapidly evolving AI landscape and its growing influence in healthcare, a deeper understanding of AI and its purposeful application, as highlighted in this chapter, may encourage HCPs to remain engaged with technological advancements and foster confidence to contribute to an AI-integrated healthcare ecosystem.

3.3 Dos and don'ts when creating DPS tools with LLMs

Dos

- Utilize advanced LLMs, as they typically provide greater accuracy and may require less detailed prompting to accomplish tasks. Free users can benefit from available "thinking models" by crafting effective initial prompts. If access is later limited to a lower-performing model, the initial results generated by the "thinking model" can be further refined using the lower-performing model.
- Craft effective initial prompts with sufficient details, such as button designs and autosuggest features. This can reduce the number of subsequent iterative prompts required to complete the task.
- For free users, be aware of message limits that cap the number of requests you can make within a given period. If possible, combine prompts into single queries.
- Before using the LLM, ensure it is configured with the desired or required data privacy settings, such as preventing the use of information entered for model training by accessing the model settings option.

Don'ts

- When creating digital tools with LLMs, avoid using LLM tokens (usage quotas) for nontool-related or diversionary chats.
- Do not create DPS tools on nonpersonal computers without administrative permission, especially if they involve system command prompts or installing executable files, as doing so may violate system policies and acceptable use guidelines.

- Avoid entering personal or proprietary information, such as names and passwords, or organizationally sensitive material into general-purpose LLMs (e.g., ChatGPT), as it could violate data privacy laws. For creative tasks that require such input, consult a technology expert and a legal advisor.
- Be aware that, unless explicitly excluded by the LLM provider or via model settings such as "opt-out", data entered into LLMs may be used to train the LLM model. Therefore, make an informed choice about the data you enter into LLMs or the model's current settings before using it.

4 Conclusion

This chapter presented iterative prompting as a method HCPs can use with LLMs to create DPS tools. It included a practice scenario that demonstrated the creation of a drug crushability tool by engaging an LLM (ChatGPT-5) with iterative prompts. Preliminary testing indicated that the tool achieved its target functionality of advising on the crushability of various drugs using a reference resource. The chapter described digital competencies that could help HCPs use LLMs effectively, particularly for creating DPS tools. Key HCP competencies identified include innovation and creativity, continuous learning and adaptability, critical thinking, and decision-making, all of which are vital for HCPs' use of LLMs in DPS tool creation. Furthermore, interdisciplinary collaboration, effective communication, and consideration of regulatory requirements are important throughout the tool creation process, as such collaboration helps ensure that the tool is reliable, compliant with relevant legal requirements, validated, and capable of progressing beyond a prototype. Different LLMs vary in their strengths, limitations, and user requirements, which may influence the DPS tool creation process. This variability underscores the importance of users making an informed choice when selecting an appropriate LLM to leverage for DPS tool creation. Furthermore, incorporating AI training into HCP education may help maximize AI's potential and foster ongoing innovation in healthcare practice.

5 Questions for further discussion

1. How might the stages of iterative prompting be adapted when developing a DPS tool for different clinical settings and teams?
2. How could the performance differences and access restrictions between advanced and standard LLMs influence your approach to creating DPS tools?
3. You are planning to develop a digital tool that provides simplified information about drugs for patients with diabetes. Describe the components, duties, and functions of a multidisciplinary team in contributing toward this endeavor.
4. What harms could arise if HCPs rely too heavily on LLM-suggested guidance without responsible human oversight?
5. How can institutions support and enable HCP innovation and experimentation with LLMs for DPS tool creation while still protecting computer system security?
6. As AI becomes integrated into daily life and healthcare, what are the risks of a disconnect between educational systems and real-world AI influences?
7. What are the potential implications and considerations for HCPs using LLMs for creating DPS tools in underresourced settings?

See the application exercise in Section 7. For further reading and ideas for tool creation, refer to the publication: "Harnessing ChatGPT for digital tools in pharmacy practice" (Yakob et al., 2025).

6 Application exercise

This application exercise involves disseminating health service information by creating a health website using ChatGPT. The end goal is to create a webpage similar to the example shown in Fig. 29.10. Using the supplied project template in Table 29.4, complete the sections based on the iterative prompting method, and use the completed template as a guide to creating the webpage.

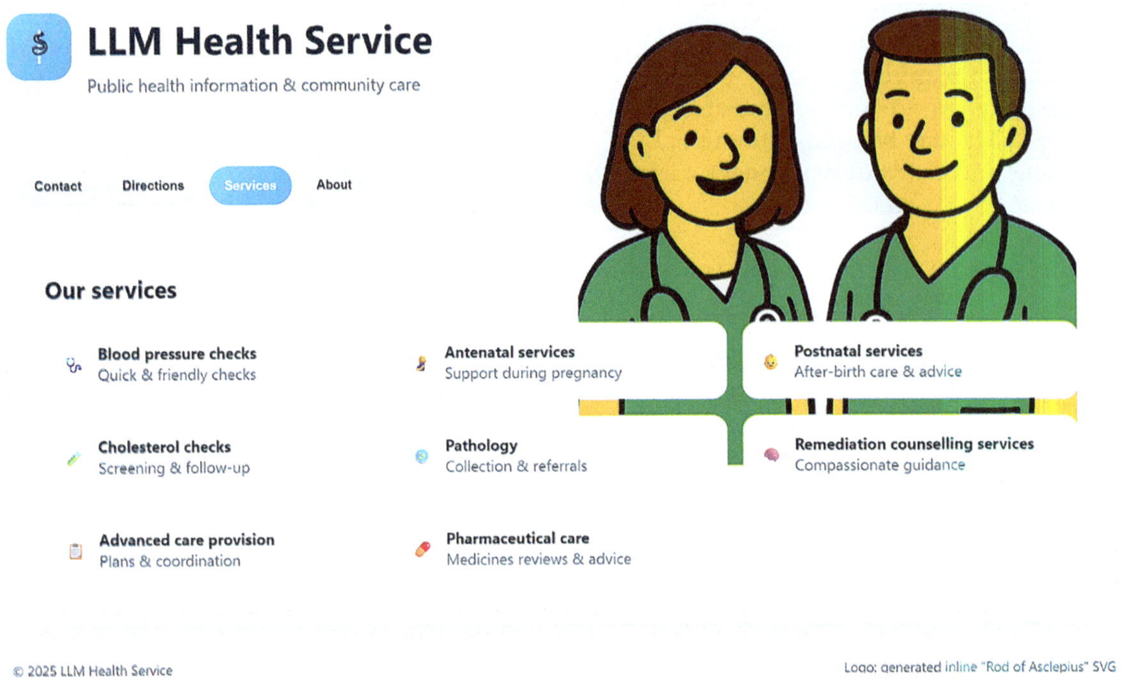

FIG. 29.10 Example outcome of the project template guide: A health services webpage created with ChatGPT LLM. Application exercise outcome: A medical website page providing public information on health and medical services, created with ChatGPT using an iterative prompting method.

TABLE 29.4 Project template guide: using ChatGPT to create a health services Webpage.

Clinician	Task: .... Date: .... LLM used: ....Duration: ....
Planning stage	• What do you want to create? (Health service webpage) • Why do you want to create this tool? • What is the tool's purpose? What do you want it to do? • How do you want it to do it? E.g., how should the results be presented? • Where would you like the tool to be created? E.g., on a desktop computer, a web page, or a mobile device. • What LLM do you have access to, and what are your accessible limits, e.g., the number of prompts per hour? • Is this an individual or team project? What are each team member's roles, e.g., prompting, testing, and reviewing? • Have you created an LLM user account to save your work?
Prompting stage	• Create an initial prompt that includes a description of the tool, its purpose, function, and the platform it operates on. Add a query for the LLM to provide information about other options to acquire the tool if you are unsure. • Consider the options provided by the LLM in relation to the required needs and functions of the tool, the team's skill level, the capacity to implement the guidance, and any computer user restrictions. • Choose a suggested option and follow the guidance from the LLM step-by-step. You may ask for clarification on specific stages from the LLM if unsure.
Tool viewing and testing	• Download to view or view the tool within the LLM interface, if possible (e.g., ChatGPT Canvas). • Check that the tool matches the prompts presented to the LLM. • Test the tool based on its intended functions. • If necessary, perform accuracy, reliability, and usability testing with a collaborative team.
Iterative prompts	• Provide further prompts for the LLM to correct the tool. • Query the LLM with any problems discovered while operating the tool or following the guidelines. • Request for modifications, corrections, designs, and additional functions to be incorporated into the tool. • View and test the tool after each change implemented by the LLM.
Tool finalization	• Request the code to be generated in a ready-to-use, downloadable format.

Pearl/Practice advice

Most available LLMs permit free use, though typically with limits on the number of prompts within a given period. As of August 2025, for example, ChatGPT-5 allows free users up to 10 messages every five hours with the standard model, after which usage shifts to a lighter mini-model. Its advanced "thinking model," designed for more complex tasks, provides free users with one prompt per day (OpenAI Help Center, 2025). *For HCPs seeking to create DPS tools with ChatGPT, it may be advantageous to consolidate prompts, including preplanned iterations, into a single comprehensive initial request directed to the high-end thinking model. Subsequent refinements can then be carried out with the step-down model, allowing for iterative improvement while remaining within usage constraints.*

References

Al-Ashwal, F.Y., Zawiah, M., Gharaibeh, L., Abu-Farha, R., Bitar, A.N., 2023. Evaluating the sensitivity, specificity, and accuracy of ChatGPT-3.5, ChatGPT-4, Bing AI, and Bard against conventional drug-drug interactions clinical tools. Drug, Healthc. Patient Saf. 1179-1365. 15, 137–147. doi:10.2147/dhps.s425858.

Al-Dujaili, Z., Omari, S., Pillai, J., Faraj, A.A., 2023. Assessing the accuracy and consistency of ChatGPT in clinical pharmacy management: a preliminary analysis with clinical pharmacy experts worldwide. Res. Social Adm. Pharm. 1551-7411. 19 (12), 1590–1594. doi:10.1016/j.sapharm.2023.08.012.

Albogami, Y., Alfakhri, A., Alaqil, A., Alkoraishi, A., Alshammari, H., Elsharawy, Y., Alhammad, A., Abdulaziz Alhossan, 2024. Safety and quality of AI chatbots for drug-related inquiries: a real-world comparison with licensed pharmacists. Digit Health. 2055-2076. 10. doi:10.1177/20552076241253523.

Altman, S., 2023. Planning for AGI and beyond, OpenAI. https://openai.com/index/planning-for-agi-and-beyond/. (Accessed 21 October 2025).

American Society of Health-System Pharmacists, 2020. ASHP practice advancement initiative, 2030: new recommendations for advancing pharmacy practice in health systems. Am. J. Health Syst. Pharm. 1079-2082. 77 (2), 113–121. doi:10.1093/ajhp/zxz271.

Annepaka, Y., Pakray, P., 2025. Large language models: a survey of their development, capabilities, and applications. Knowl. Inf. Syst. 0219-1377. 67 (3), 2967–3022. doi:10.1007/s10115-024-02310-4.

Azaria, A., Azoulay, R., Reches, S., 2024. ChatGPT is a remarkable tool—for experts. Data Intell. 2641-435X. 6 (1), 240–296. doi:10.1162/dint_a_00235.

Bazzari, F.H., Bazzari, A.H., 2024. Utilizing ChatGPT in telepharmacy. Cureus. 2168-8184. 16 (1). doi:10.7759/cureus.52365.

Claude Help Center, 2026. What are artifacts and how do I use them?. https://support.claude.com/en/articles/9487310-what-are-artifacts-and-how-do-i-use-them. (Accessed 8 July 2025).

Cornish, P., 2005. "Avoid the crush": hazards of medication administration in patients with dysphagia or a feeding tube. Can. Med. Assoc. J. 0820-3946. 172 (7), 871–872. doi:10.1503/cmaj.050176.

Costa, C.J., Aparicio, M., Aparicio, S., Aparicio, J.T., 2024. The democratization of artificial intelligence: theoretical framework. Appl. Sci. 2076-3417. 14 (18), 8236. doi:10.3390/app14188236.

Davtyan, T., 2025. The U.S. Approach to AI regulation: federal laws, policies, and strategies explained. J. Law, Technol. Internet. 1949-6451. 16 (2). Available from: https://scholarlycommons.law.case.edu/jolti/vol16/iss2/2.

DevelopmentAid, 2023 AI will not replace you, but someone who uses it might | opinion. https://www.developmentaid.org/news-stream/post/165338/ai-will-not-replace-you. 7 31 2025 8 22.

Dowding, D., Merrill, J.A., Barrón, Y., Onorato, N., Jonas, K., Russell, D., 2019. Usability evaluation of a dashboard for home care nurses. CIN Comput. Inform. Nurs. 1538-9774. 37 (1), 11–19. Available from: http://www.cinjournal.com. doi:10.1097/CIN.0000000000000484.

European Commission, 2019. Ethics guidelines for trustworthy AI. https://digital-strategy.ec.europa.eu/en/library/ethics-guidelines-trustworthy-ai. (Accessed 5 Febuary 2026).

European Commission, 2025. DigComp 3.0. https://joint-research-centre.ec.europa.eu/projects-and-activities/education-and-training/digital-transformation-education/digital-competence-framework-citizens-digcomp/digcomp-framework_en. (Accessed 21 October 2025).

European Union, 2024. Artificial Intelligence Act. Official Journal of the European Union. https://eur-lex.europa.eu/eli/reg/2024/1689/oj. (Accessed 21 October 2025).

Feldman, M.Q., Anderson, C.J., 2024. Non-expert programmers in the generative AI future. In: ACM International Conference Proceeding Series. 9798400710179. Association for Computing Machinery, United States. http://portal.acm.org/. doi:10.1145/3663384.3663393. 6 25 2024/06/25.

Fodil, M., Nghiem, D., Colas, M., Bourry, S., Poisson-Salomon, A.-S., Rezigue, H., Trivalle, C., 2017. Assessment of clinical practices for crushing medication in geriatric units. J. Nutr., Health Aging. 1279-7707. 21 (8), 904–908. doi:10.1007/s12603-017-0886-3.

Food and Drug Administration, 2026. Clinical Decision Support Software Guidance for Industry and Food and Drug Administration Staff. https://www.fda.gov/regulatory-information/search-fda-guidance-documents/clinical-decision-support-software. (Accessed 5 June 2026).

Gao, A., Prompt engineering for large language models. (2023), Available from: https://papers.ssrn.com/sol3/papers.cfm?abstract_id=4504303.

Giray, L., 2023. Prompt engineering with ChatGPT: a guide for academic writers. Ann. Biomed. Eng. 0090-6964. 51 (12), 2629–2633. doi:10.1007/s10439-023-03272-4.

Guthrey, Taylor, S., PHARMACISTS IN 2030. (2024), Available from: https://www.psa.org.au/advocacy/working-for-our-profession/pharmacists_in_2030/.

Haberl, D., Ning, J., Kluge, K., Kumpf, K., Josef, Y., Jiang, Z., Constantino, C., Monaci, A., Starace, M., Haug, A.R., Calabretta, R., Camoni, L., Bertagna, F., Mascherbauer, K., Hofer, F., Albano, D., Sciagra, R., Oliveira, F., Costa, D., Nitsche, C., Hacker, M., Spielvogel, C.P., 2025. Generative artificial intelligence enables the generation of bone scintigraphy images and improves generalization of deep learning models in data-constrained environments. Eur. J. Nucl. Med. Mol. Imaging. 1619-7070. 52 (7), 2355–2368. doi:10.1007/s00259-025-07091-8.

Haigh, T., 2024. Between the booms: AI in winter. Commun. ACM. 0001-0782. 67 (11), 18–23. doi:10.1145/3688379.

Harvard Business Review, 2023. AI Won't Replace Humans—but Humans With AI Will Replace Humans Without AI. https://hbr.org/2023/08/ai-wont-replace-humans-but-humans-with-ai-will-replace-humans-without-ai. (Accessed 8 May 2025).

Hasan, S.S., Woo, J.J., Cote, M.P., Ramkumar, P.N., 2025. Generative versus nongenerative artificial intelligence. Arthroscopy. 0749-8063. 41 (3), 545–546. Available from: https://www.sciencedirect.com/science/article/pii/S0749806324010181. doi:10.1016/j.arthro.2024.12.001.

Ifinedo, P. 2012 Technology acceptance by health professionals in Canada: an analysis with a modified UTAUT model. In: Proceedings of the Annual Hawaii International Conference on System Sciences. IEEE Computer Society, Canada, pp. 2937–2946. doi:10.1109/HICSS.2012.556 15301605

International Pharmaceutical Federation, 2025. An Artificial Intelligence Toolkit for Pharmacy: An Introduction and Resource Guide for Pharmacists, International Pharmaceutical Federation, The Hague.

Jindal, J.A., Lungren, M.P., Shah, N.H., 2024. Ensuring useful adoption of generative artificial intelligence in healthcare. J. Am. Med. Inform. Assoc. 1527-974X. 31 (6), 1441–1444. Available from: http://jamia.oxfordjournals.org/content/22/e1. doi:10.1093/jamia/ocae043.

Kutbi, M., 2024. Artificial intelligence-based applications for bone fracture detection using medical images: a systematic review. Diagnostics. 2075-4418. 14 (17), 1879. doi:10.3390/diagnostics14171879.

Leiter, C., Zhang, R., Chen, Y., Belouadi, J., Larionov, D., Fresen, V., Eger, S., 2024. ChatGPT: a meta-analysis after 2.5 months. Mach. Learn. Appl. 2666-8270. 16, 100541. doi:10.1016/j.mlwa.2024.100541.

Martini, N., Sajtos, L., Idio, L., Kaur, M., Sweeney, N., Zhang, C., Scahill, S., 2024. The future of pharmacy work: how pharmacists are adapting to and preparing for technology infusion. Explor. Res. Clin. Soc. Pharm. 2667-2766. 15, 100472. doi:10.1016/j.rcsop.2024.100472.

Morath, B., Chiriac, U., Jaszkowski, E., Deiß, C., Nürnberg, H., Hörth, K., Hoppe-Tichy, T., Green, K., 2024. Performance and risks of ChatGPT used in drug information: an exploratory real-world analysis. Eur. J. Hosp. Pharm. 2047-9956. 31 (6), 491–497. doi:10.1136/ejhpharm-2023-003750.

Mucci, T., 2024. The History of Artificial Intelligence | IBM. The history of artificial intelligence. IBM. https://www.ibm.com/think/topics/history-of-artificial-intelligence. (Accessed 21 October 2025).

Munir, F., Gehres, A., Wai, D., Song, L., 2024. Evaluation of ChatGPT as a tool for answering clinical questions in pharmacy practice. J. Pharm. Pract. 0897-1900. 37 (6), 1303–1310. doi:10.1177/08971900241256731.

OpenAI Developers, 2025. GPT-5 prompting guide. https://cookbook.openai.com/examples/gpt-5/gpt-5_prompting_guide. (Accessed 8 July 2025).

OpenAI Help Center, 2025. GPT-5 in ChatGPT. https://help.openai.com/en/articles/11909943-gpt-5-in-chatgpt. (Accessed 8 July 2025).

OpenAI, 2024. Introducing Canvas: a new way of working with ChatGPT to write and code. 10 3 2024.

Poonprasartporn, A., Uttaranakorn, P., Chuaybamroong, R., 2023. Comparing the accuracy and referencing of ChatGPT's responses to herbal medicine queries: a zero-shot versus roleplay prompting approach. Thai J. Pharm. Sci. 3027-7922. 47 (4). doi:10.56808/3027-7922.2838.

Ryazanov, I., Öhman, C., Björklund, J., 2025. How ChatGPT changed the media's narratives on AI: a semi-automated narrative analysis through frame semantics. Minds Mach. 1572-8641. 35 (1). doi:10.1007/s11023-024-09705-w.

Shukla, M. 2019. The Democratization of Technology https://www.forbes.com/councils/forbestechcouncil/2019/11/07/the-democratization-of-technology/. 11 7 2025 8 22.

Silva, R.D.O.S., de Araújo, D.C.S.A., Dos Santos Menezes, P.W., Neves, E.R.Z., de Lyra, D.P., 2022. Digital pharmacists: the new wave in pharmacy practice and education. Int. J. Clin. Pharm. 2210-7711. 44 (3), 775–780. Available from: http://springerlink.metapress.com/content/2210-7703/. doi:10.1007/s11096-021-01365-5.

Siu, E., 2024. AI may not replace you, but someone who uses it can — here's the No. 1 skill you need to stay relevant. CNBC, https://www.cnbcafrica.com/2024/ai-may-not-replace-you-but-someone-who-uses-it-can-heres-the-no-1-skill-you-need-to-stay-relevant/. (Accessed 5 December 2025).

Syed, J., Ramesh, M., Kumar, T.M.P., Patil, V., Chalasani, S.H., 2024. Dose 4 you: dose division calculator—A tool to reduce calculation errors. Hosp. Pharm. 1945-1253. 59 (2), 223–227. Available from: https://journals.sagepub.com/home/HPX. doi:10.1177/00185787231207757.

The White House, 2025. https://www.whitehouse.gov/articles/2025/07/white-house-unveils-americas-ai-action-plan/. 7 23 2025 8 21.

Therapeutic Goods Administration, 2021. Is my software regulated?. https://www.tga.gov.au/products/medical-devices/software-and-artificial-intelligence-ai/manufacturing/artificial-intelligence-ai-and-medical-device-software-regulation/my-software-regulated. (Accessed 30 August 2025).

Therapeutic Goods Administration, 2024. Consultation on clarifying and strengthening the regulation of artificial intelligence. https://www.tga.gov.au/resources/consultation/consultation-clarifying-and-strengthening-regulation-artificial-intelligence-ai. 10 20 2025 9 18 (Accessed 20 October 2025).

Tierney, A.A., Gayre, G., Hoberman, B., Mattern, B., Ballesca, M., Kipnis, P., Liu, V., Lee, K., 2024. Ambient artificial intelligence scribes to alleviate the burden of clinical documentation. NEJM Catal. 2642-0007. 5 (3). doi:10.1056/cat.23.0404.

van Nuland, M., Erdogan, A., Açar, C., Contrucci, R., Hilbrants, S., Maanach, L., Egberts, T., van der Linden, P.D., 2024b. Performance of ChatGPT on factual knowledge questions regarding clinical pharmacy. J. Clin. Pharmacol. 0091-2700. 64 (9), 1095–1100. doi:10.1002/jcph.2443.

van Nuland, M., Lobbezoo, A.-F.H., van de Garde, E.M.W., Herbrink, M., van Heijl, I., Bognàr, T., Houwen, J.P.A., Dekens, M., Wannet, D., Egberts, T., van der Linden, P.D., 2024a. Assessing accuracy of ChatGPT in response to questions from day to day pharmaceutical care in hospitals. Explor. Res. Clin. Soc. Pharm. 2667-2766. 15, 100464. doi:10.1016/j.rcsop.2024.100464.

Venkatesh, V., Morris, M.G., Davis, G.B., Davis, F.D., 2003. User acceptance of information technology: toward a unified view. MIS Q. 0276-7783. 27 (3), 425–478. Available from: http://misq.org/misq/downloads/. doi:10.2307/30036540.

World Economic Forum, 2023. https://www.weforum.org/stories/2023/01/here-s-why-democratize-access-technology-davos2023/. 1 9 2025 8 22.

Yakob, R.A., Bamgboje-Ayodele, A., Collins, J.C., Aslani, P., 2025. Harnessing ChatGPT for digital tools in pharmacy practice. Res. Social Adm. Pharm. 1551-7411. 21 (11), 943–950. Available from: https://www.sciencedirect.com/science/journal/15517411. doi:10.1016/j.sapharm.2025.06.106.

CHAPTER

30

Preventing, identifying, and managing fraudulent participants in research

Carole Bandiera[a], Donna Thomas[b], Jack C. Collins[a], Kate Lowrie[c], Sabuj Kanti Mistry[d], Mark F. Harris[e], and Parisa Aslani[a]

[a]Sydney Pharmacy School, Faculty of Medicine and Health, University of Sydney, Sydney, NSW, Australia
[b]Sydney School of Health Sciences, Faculty of Medicine and Health, University of Sydney, Sydney, NSW, Australia
[c]Research Integrity and Ethics Administration, University of Sydney, Sydney, NSW, Australia
[d]School of Population Health, University of New South Wales, Sydney, NSW, Australia
[e]International Centre for Future Health Systems, University of New South Wales, Sydney, NSW, Australia

CHAPTER OBJECTIVES

- To explore strategies to minimize the inclusion of fraudulent participants and prevent bots in online research studies (prevention)
- To understand how to identify fraudulent participants and detect bots in online research (identification)
- To understand how to manage the inclusion of fraudulent participants and bots in online research (management)

1 Introduction

Data integrity and quality are prerequisites for trustworthy research. Incorrect or biased data can mislead researchers, clinicians, and practitioners and may ultimately result in ineffective interventions. Generating evidence-based data in pharmacy practice informs clinical decisions and public health policies. The reliability of data collected directly impacts the validity of the findings, the evidence, and, in turn, the recommendations made to researchers, healthcare professionals, policymakers, and the population. There is an ethical imperative and a core responsibility for researchers, clinicians, and practitioners to rigorously ensure the quality and accuracy of the data they collect.

Research conducted online has been growing since the Coronavirus (COVID-19) pandemic, primarily because face-to-face contact was reduced for all research purposes, and participants were advised not to visit health centers and pharmacies to avoid infection and contamination (Keen et al., 2022; Kobakhidze et al., 2021). This shift in data collection from face-to-face to online, in both quantitative and qualitative studies, has been rapid and essential to ensure the continuation of research during the pandemic. Beyond the practicalities necessitating a move to online

Contemporary Research Methods in Pharmacy and Health Services - Volume 2
https://doi.org/10.1016/B978-0-443-44607-8.00029-7

data collection, collecting data online offers numerous advantages: it provides greater accessibility to studies for participants in remote and rural areas or those with mobility difficulties, and it expands the geographic area for recruitment, enabling a more diverse population to be included. It is also time-efficient, as neither researchers nor participants need to travel to the study site for data collection. Consequently, resources and costs can be kept low (Keen et al., 2022; Darko et al., 2022). However, online research poses challenges, such as verifying the authenticity and eligibility of participants recruited online (Jones et al., 2021). Fraudulent or imposter participants are defined as individuals who take part in research inappropriately or under false pretenses, provide false information, or have unethical intentions for participating (Jones et al., 2021).

Experiences of scamming in online research have been increasingly reported since 2023, including fraud in recruitment, participation, and responses provided, both in online qualitative (Sharma et al., 2024; Mistry et al., 2024; Sefcik et al., 2023; Pullen Sansfaçon et al., 2024; Ridge et al., 2023; Andrew et al., 2024; Kumarasamy et al., 2024; Bandiera et al., 2025) and quantitative studies, such as online clinical or intervention trials (Davies et al., 2024; Glazer et al., 2021) or online surveys (Salinas, 2023; Chung et al., 2019; Lawrence et al., 2023; Levi et al., 2022; Pozzar et al., 2020; Comachio et al., 2025; Mozaffarian et al., 2025). For example, in a Canadian study, imposter participants were interviewed online as part of a qualitative study recruiting young people who detransitioned after a gender transition (Pullen Sansfaçon et al., 2024). During the second wave of recruitment, the study poster was shared on the social media platforms TikTok and Twitter, and specified a reimbursement of canadian dollars (CAD) 30. Researchers became suspicious about imposter participants taking part, as participants systematically refused to turn their cameras on, and some information shared by participants seemed erroneous (Pullen Sansfaçon et al., 2024). Other similar experiences have occurred in Australia, such as in an online qualitative study recruiting families of Australian children with neurodevelopmental disorders (Sharma et al., 2024) and in a study recruiting primary caregivers of preschool-aged children (Andrew et al., 2024). Similar issues have also been reported in the United States, where caregivers for individuals with a diagnosis of Alzheimer's disease were recruited online (Sefcik et al., 2023). A scoping review included 23 studies that described the identification of fraudulent responses with online recruitment and reported that 18 of the studies (78%) experienced fraudulent responses (Comachio et al., 2025). Among the included studies, 3% to 94% of participants were excluded from the research because of fraudulent or suspicious responses (Comachio et al., 2025).

In pharmacy practice research, reports of scamming or fraudulent participation are limited in the literature. To our knowledge, only one article reported that fraudulent participants were interviewed as part of a research study in pharmacy practice (Bandiera et al., 2025). Although it is possible that other studies are yet to be published, this remains an underexplored issue, as the current litterature in pharmacy practice research has not reported suspected fraudulent participation or failed to recognize the involvement of fraudulent participants.

It is important to note that fraud does not only exist in healthcare research but also in research across other disciplines, where, similarly, authors are discussing strategies to identify and prevent fraud as well as the implications of such actions. For example, a recent publication on fraudulent research in the social sciences noted that focusing on methods to identify fraudulent participants may inadvertently exclude genuine participants from marginalized communities. The authors also emphasized the need for reflection on current epistemologies in social science research, including reflecting on what defines "authenticity" in research, challenging historic notions of researchers as gatekeepers of knowledge, and acknowledging the structural power imbalances that exist between researchers and those being researched (Merchant et al., 2025). Another study reported the methods used to identify and prevent suspected bots and fraudulent responses in online surveys within education research (Schles and Deheck, 2025). In this study, 75.4% of the responses received across the surveys were removed due to fraud. The authors noted that many responses were removed because the research team suspected the surveys were completed by bots. Although they were unable to confirm that bots were used, they observed that the responses were not valid human responses (Schles and Deheck, 2025).

Such fraud, if not identified, raises ethical concerns and poses challenges to research integrity and data quality, impacting the validity of research findings. There is a lack of awareness and guidance on how to prevent and identify scams in online qualitative and quantitative research, as well as on the management of fraud once it has been detected. Importantly, as technology and artificial intelligence (AI) are increasingly used by people in parallel with the rapid evolution of AI technologies, strategies to reduce the risk of fraud need to be regularly reviewed and updated. A research team recently published the Prevent FRaudulent Online STudy participation (P-FROST) recommendations, which provide a standardized approach to preventing, identifying, and managing scams in online qualitative research (Mistry et al., 2024). Recommendations are provided at different levels, such as study set-up (e.g., involving experienced qualitative researchers, including methods to prevent fraud in the study design), reimbursement (e.g., carefully considering the need to advertise incentives, posting local vouchers), recruitment (e.g., in person or in closed groups), data collection (e.g., screening questions to verify participant eligibility and identity, requiring participants to have their cameras turned on), data analysis (e.g., identifying suspicious responses, managing fraudulent participants' data following team consensus), reporting fraud, and supporting research teams. No additional recommendations are made regarding fraud in quantitative studies, such as online surveys.

In this chapter, we discuss potential fraudulent participation in both online qualitative and quantitative studies and aim to present strategies to minimize the inclusion of fraudulent participants in online research (prevention), understand how to identify fraudulent participants in online research (identification), and manage inclusion of fraudulent participants in online research (management).

2 Case studies

This section presents several case studies drawn from the lived experiences of fraud in the authors' qualitative and quantitative research studies.

2.1 Scam in a qualitative study

The authors conducted a qualitative study to describe how community health workers (CHWs) and pharmacists work together and to identify the barriers and facilitators to this collaborative practice from the perspectives of pharmacists and CHWs (Bandiera et al., 2026). Participants were eligible if they had been working in health services for at least six months in Australia or New Zealand, spoke English, and did not require an interpreter.

The 30-minute semi-structured interviews were conducted either face-to-face or online via Zoom (Zoom Communications, Inc.) or Microsoft Teams videoconferencing, were audio-recorded, transcribed verbatim, and thematically analyzed. All participants were reimbursed with a physical or electronic gift voucher for a local grocery store (Australian dollars (AUD) 100/New Zealand dollars (NZD) 120 for pharmacists and AUD 75/NZD 90 for CHWs), either given in person right after the interview or sent by email immediately after the interview (Bandiera et al., 2026).

CHWs and pharmacists were recruited in two phases. Firstly, the study was promoted to closed groups, i.e., researchers' professional networks and through professional pharmaceutical associations' newsletters. Secondly, the study flyer was promoted online via the researchers' LinkedIn (LinkedIn Corporation) accounts, a social media platform for professional networking (Bandiera et al., 2026). The scamming occurred during this second phase of recruitment, where some participants pretended to be pharmacists or CHWs.

Within five days of advertising on LinkedIn, the investigator received more than 10 emails with a similar structure and content from people interested in participating in the study, identifying themselves as pharmacists or CHWs. After ensuring that the participants had signed the consent form, all the interviews were planned to be conducted online. After three interviews were conducted, the investigator realized that the three participants were impostors. Indeed, several emails from potential participants were received in a short period of time; the emails had similar content and address structures, the participants showed a specific interest in the reimbursement, their cameras were switched off during the entire interview, and there were inconsistencies in their responses to questions (Bandiera et al., 2025). When the investigator asked for the participants' healthcare professional registration numbers, they were unable to provide them. Subsequently, the investigator did not hear from the fraudulent participants again and did not receive emails from other potential participants interested in participating (Bandiera et al., 2025).

This experience resulted in a significant waste of time for the researchers (including interview preparation, ordering electronic gift vouchers, preparing materials, conducting interviews, and data management), a waste of research funds, and, as highlighted in the literature, an emotional impact, including stress, for the research team (Mistry et al., 2024; Pullen Sansfaçon et al., 2024; Kumarasamy et al., 2024).

2.2 Scam in a quantitative study

The authors conducted an online questionnaire study to understand how caregivers of children with a specific type of speech impairment, Childhood Apraxia of Speech (CAS), engaged with speech-language pathology services (Thomas, 2026). They were interested in understanding the caregivers' experiences with the diagnostic process for their children and the type of speech-language therapy service delivery they received. Participants were eligible if they were caregivers of a child under 18 years of age who had been diagnosed with CAS and could read and write English sufficiently to complete the survey.

An online questionnaire hosted on Qualtrics (Provo, UT) (Qualtrics, 2025) was selected for data collection. The questionnaire utilized all of the Qualtrics Fraud Detection features (Qualtrics, 2025). Participants were offered a United States dollars (USD) 15 Starbucks e-gift voucher for their participation. If they wished to claim the voucher, they followed a link in the survey to provide their name and email address. This process ensured that their questionnaire responses remained anonymous. The coffee company vouchers were sent in monthly batches during data collection.

Participants were recruited in two phases. Phase one recruitment was for caregivers whose children (aged 3 years, 6 months to 7 years, 11 months) had recently completed the treatment study for CAS. These caregivers were provided with information about the questionnaire by their speech-language therapist during the final follow-up session of their treatment study. Phase two recruitment was for all caregivers who had a child (< 18 years) diagnosed with CAS. During phase two, the study was advertised online via social media, LinkedIn, and the researchers' professional networks.

During the first month of phase two of recruitment, there was a large increase in responses, rising from approximately six per month in phase one to 450. Although this was initially encouraging for the investigators, a closer inspection of the data revealed inconsistencies, such as hundreds of responses within a two-hour period, the submission of up to 40 identical questionnaires, and a discrepancy between the number of coffee vouchers requested and surveys completed. These response patterns were consistent with what occurs when an internet bot—short for robot—completes a questionnaire (King-Nyberg et al., 2023; Chen et al., 2023). A bot is a software application that performs an automated task (script) over the internet. When completing a questionnaire, a bot mimics human behavior by combining the content of the questionnaire with large language models to produce plausible answers (Feng et al., 2024). Once the suspected bot attacks were identified, data collection was paused while additional questions were added to facilitate differentiation between genuine and bot responses (Chen et al., 2023; Griffin et al., 2022; King-Nyberg et al., 2023). When recruitment was reopened, there were intermittent periods during which significant numbers of responses were received in a short time, but the volume was less than during the first bot attack.

As an example of the sophistication of the bots, we provide this example of an email exchange (Appendix). During phase two data collection, the investigator received an email purporting to be from a caregiver interested in participating in the study. There were several 'red flags' indicating that the email may not have been from a genuine caregiver. The email subject line was the URL for the questionnaire, the email address consisted of a series of random letters '@ google.com' with no correlation to the person's name, the investigator was not addressed by name, and there was an unusual focus on the voucher. The bot, however, responded to all questions asked by the investigator and even provided information from the questionnaire that was not requested, such as giving the capital city of their state when asked where they were from. One final suspicion was raised due to the time the emails were sent—3:14 a.m. local time.

To differentiate between fraudulent and genuine responses, the research team developed guidelines to evaluate the responses based on previous research (e.g., Chen et al., 2023; Griffin et al., 2022; King-Nyberg et al., 2023; Pinzón et al., 2024). These guidelines provided information on how to interpret Qualtrics metrics (e.g., Fraud Detection), survey completion time, internal consistency, and the plausibility of open-ended responses. Each survey response was manually and independently reviewed by two members of the research team using these guidelines. This process was very time-consuming, and during it, the investigators noted that over the four months the survey was open for phase two recruitment, the bot responses became increasingly sophisticated and harder to differentiate from genuine human responses. There was good agreement between the two raters, who made a categorical decision regarding each questionnaire as 'genuine', 'bot', or 'incomplete' (< 10% complete), with agreement achieved for 692 responses (96%). Discrepancies were resolved via team discussion. There were 161 valid responses from the initial 721 (22%) survey responses.

3 Recommendations and strategies

We provide indicators and strategies to prevent, identify, and manage the inclusion of fraudulent participants in online research, based on the experiences of fraud identified by the authors in their qualitative and quantitative studies, as well as evidence from the literature. Researchers also need to consider that imposter participants can respond to surveys, not just participate in interviews. It is important to balance the risk of including fraudulent participants and verifying authenticity with privacy and ethical considerations (see Sections 5.4 and 5.5). By the nature of online research, fraudulent participants may reside anywhere in the world, and researchers should be alert to signs indicating that participants may not reside in the expected setting.

3.1 Contact details of fraudulent participants

Researchers should be suspicious of multiple emails with a similar email address structure and content received from potential participants within a short period of time following the online promotion of the study (King-Nyberg et al., 2023; Sharma et al., 2024; Pullen Sansfaçon et al., 2024). Notably, the names of the interested individuals may be common or similar to one another.

Another suspicious behavior that researchers should be cautious of is when participants ask the investigator to promote the study to their "colleagues" through email addresses that they send via the online chat, with all email addresses having the same address structure as mentioned above. In addition, suspicious email activity, based on the location and time and focused on the compensation, should raise alarm bells for the researchers (Pinzón et al., 2024) (see example in Appendix).

In the case of a limited number of suspicious email activities, we suggest that researchers carefully verify the identity of potential participants one by one. If the number of emails is too large to respond to each individually, we recommend replying with a message indicating that the participant's identity will be thoroughly verified before recruitment in order to deter fraud.

It should be noted that if the email addresses were part of a questionnaire, this may involve deleting all of the participants' responses. For questionnaire studies, it might be useful to have a two-step process where people interested in the study complete a more detailed screening process, possibly by phone, prior to being allocated a unique identifier.

In studies recruiting professionals, participants should be encouraged to correspond through their professional email addresses, accompanied by a professional signature. When email addresses are not collected, we recommend that contact details be obtained to reduce fraud. We suggest collecting the home or work postal address of participants in addition to other demographic data. However, such information should be used solely to verify participant identity and stored separately from participants' responses to limit access to their personal data.

3.2 Focused interest in the reimbursement

We recommend informing potential participants about the level of reimbursement through the participant information statement, reminding them that payment will only be sent after rigorous data and proof-of-identity checking (Jones et al., 2021; Mistry et al., 2024; Davies et al., 2024; Glazer et al., 2021), and providing reimbursement with physical or electronic vouchers to be used in local stores only, rather than international vouchers, to deter international impostors.

Researchers should be suspicious when participants show a special interest in the reimbursement or ask to exchange the local gift card for an international voucher (Sharma et al., 2024; Pullen Sansfaçon et al., 2024; Andrew et al., 2024). For example, when a participant asks whether it is possible to obtain an electronic voucher that can be used internationally (e.g., a prepaid debit card rather than a voucher for a local store) even before the interview has started. In this scenario, we advise researchers to remind the participant that the voucher is intended for the local context and that no other voucher or incentive can be provided.

Other researchers have recommended sending a nontransferable e-voucher by mail (Davies et al., 2024; Glazer et al., 2021; Pellicano et al., 2024) or texting the voucher to a mobile phone (Pellicano et al., 2024). In some contexts, reducing reimbursement or proposing reimbursement in the form of an entry to a gift card draw (i.e., participants aren't guaranteed reimbursement) may help deter fraud without negatively impacting the recruitment of genuine participants. In addition, where possible, we suggest that the level or existence of reimbursement not be included in the study flyer, after consultation with the relevant ethics office. Details about reimbursement can be provided once potential participants contact investigators for participation and their identities have been verified.

3.3 Anonymity

Although research has historically prioritized participant anonymity, this needs to be balanced with the need to ensure the integrity of the data. Decreasing anonymity may increase data integrity. For example, if participants in questionnaires upload copies of documents to confirm their eligibility, researchers can be more confident in the data provided, even though this decreases the participants' anonymity. Similarly, in qualitative interviews, if researchers request the participant to turn their camera on, it decreases the participant's anonymity but also reduces the risk of including a fraudulent participant.

Researchers should consider the possibility of fraudulent participation if the camera remains turned off during the entire interview. Unless the participant is using a blurred or virtual background in their video-call software, researchers should also assess whether the surroundings of the participant during the interview align with what they would reasonably expect, such as indicators of the time of day, the country of residence, or the participant's place of work. Where appropriate, the researcher may kindly request the participant to temporarily disable their blurred or virtual background to assist in verifying their identity.

Some researchers suggest the use of cameras as a prerequisite for participation in online interviews, at least for a short period—for instance, right before or at the start of the interview (Sefcik et al., 2023; Ridge et al., 2023; Andrew et al., 2024; Kumarasamy et al., 2024; Pellicano et al., 2024). We recommend requiring participants to switch their cameras on during interviews so that researchers can observe participants' body language when answering questions, detect the presence of a second screen or use of a smartwatch, and determine whether participants are using resources such as AI to answer questions (Sharma et al., 2024; Sefcik et al., 2023). In addition, if participants use an AI-based language tool, researchers can assess how they utilize it. We recommend that the requirement to have the camera turned on during the interview be explicitly stated in the participant information statement and consent form. Where video is captured as part of the online interview, it is important to address any privacy concerns and ensure that appropriate data management procedures are in place. Researchers should consider whether any visual data is necessary for analysis or whether it can be erased immediately to mitigate privacy concerns, retaining only the audio recordings for analysis.

3.4 Language skills of fraudulent participants

Indicators of potential research fraud include: (1) the participant struggles to speak the language of the research setting, (2) it is difficult to understand the participant throughout the interview, (3) the participant's understanding of the questions is limited, and the researcher needs to repeat the questions multiple times.

However, when it comes to including participants from diverse linguistic backgrounds, it is worthwhile to consider the participants' language skills with sensitivity so as not to profile or unintentionally exclude those who have limited proficiency in the language of the interview. Furthermore, it is important to differentiate between poor language skills (as might occur due to cognitive difficulties or neurological issues) and difficulty with understanding and using the language of the interview.

Researchers recommend setting up a prestudy verification process, such as a preinterview with the participant for qualitative studies, either over the phone or online with the camera switched on. For a questionnaire, this might involve an email to the study team followed by a phone call. This process would allow researchers to check the eligibility criteria and verify the participant's identity (Sharma et al., 2024; Sefcik et al., 2023; Davies et al., 2024; Pellicano et al., 2024), as well as ensure the validity of the participant's phone number and the host country of the phone number. In addition, it would provide an opportunity to assess the participant's proficiency in the language of the interview or questionnaire before conducting the study, and to match the demographic data filled out online by the participant or the data declared during the interview with the information provided during the preinterview (Sharma et al., 2024; Sefcik et al., 2023; Ridge et al., 2023). Researchers should also consider any language requirements as part of the study's eligibility criteria and determine whether an interpreter may be needed, where appropriate.

3.5 Quality of responses to interview questions

Fraud can be identified in a qualitative study when: (1) the conversation does not flow naturally, (2) there are delays in answering each question (which may indicate the use of AI to answer the questions), (3) suspicious responses are provided regarding eligibility to participate, (4) participants provide short, vague, and very general responses, do not respond directly to the questions, or provide responses not relevant to the study topic, (5) inaccurate responses to questions are provided (e.g., participants state that they heard about the study through social media, whereas the study was not promoted on that specific social media platform), (6) no experiences are reported that are applicable to being a member of the population of interest (e.g., a pharmacist), (7) participants do not report their personal experiences as part of answering the questions, and (8) the sound quality is poor.

We recommend adapting the interview guide by adding screening questions and questions that allow participants to report on their personal experiences in order to give researchers the opportunity to detect fraudulent participants early in the interview. During the interview, we recommend ensuring that terms used for medical conditions or health services, as relevant, are consistent with those used within the participant's geographic area.

3.6 Proving the authenticity of meeting the study inclusion criteria

When recruiting healthcare professionals, their registration number, membership certificate from a professional organization or similar credentials should be verified prior to conducting the interview (e.g., through the local agency responsible for registering healthcare professionals). If the participant is a healthcare professional but is not formally registered with a professional body (e.g., a CHW), we suggest that participants provide a confirmation of their work status from their institution or employer. For consumers or patients, it may be helpful to ask them to provide evidence that they have the condition under investigation. This could involve providing the name and organization of a healthcare professional who can verify the condition or uploading reports that confirm their diagnoses. While this approach may not be appropriate in all circumstances and could potentially infringe upon patient confidentiality, it may nonetheless warrant consideration. It is important to note that fraudulent diagnosis data may be provided by imposters, and the systematic collection of proof of diagnosis could deter genuine participants from participating. Researchers may decide whether proof of diagnosis should be required for all participants or only for those suspected of fraudulent participation. Some authors suggest adding the inclusion criteria to the consent form, requiring participants to confirm the criteria before signing the document, which may dissuade imposters from participating (Andrew et al., 2024).

Asking the participant to provide identification (e.g., driver's license) might be another way of verifying the participant's identity (Glazer et al., 2021). However, anonymity may be important in certain qualitative studies to encourage honest and legitimate responses; therefore, using multi-factor identification may be an alternative option, although it could deter some participants from taking part. Alternatively, researchers could use separate anonymized forms to check eligibility criteria or conduct interviews via phone calls, where the researcher contacts the participant directly. In addition, if the study's eligibility criteria limit the inclusion of participants to certain countries, researchers should consider selecting the corresponding option in the Zoom (Zoom Communications, Inc.) application settings to prevent individuals from joining from other countries (Sharma et al., 2024).

Fraud may be identified when participants are screened against eligibility criteria. For example, participants may immediately disconnect from the interview and cease all communication when they are asked questions related to eligibility. Communication from similar email addresses may also decrease, potentially indicating that all communication was coming from the same fraudulent individual or syndicate.

3.7 Prevent, detect, and manage bots in online surveys

As noted by King-Nyberg et al. (2023), there is a fine line between the responses provided by humans and bots. The longer a questionnaire remains open, the more sophisticated the bot responses become, and the harder they are to distinguish from human responses. Although there are some strategies that reduce the likelihood of bots, there is no single screening technique that accurately distinguishes between humans and bots. Instead, it is important to consider multiple metrics to arrive at a holistic impression of the responses. Some general strategies are listed below:

Prevention:

- Enable fraud detection features in the survey platform (e.g., prevent ballot-box stuffing in Qualtrics)
- Consider using personalized survey links rather than public links. Personalized links can be provided once the participant has passed verification checks, such as an email exchange with the research team or uploading verification details like reports, healthcare provider numbers, or healthcare registration numbers
- Avoid using incentives; however, if incentives are to be used, follow these guidelines: i) consider using entries into a draw rather than a fixed reimbursement, so that participants are not guaranteed an incentive, ii) add information to the study indicating that incentives are provided only after a strict verification process has been completed, iii) do not advertise the incentive alongside the study information on social media, iv) avoid using high-value incentives, and v) use some open-ended questions within the questionnaire, which must be completed in order to progress through it

Detection:

- Review the fraud detection metrics within the survey platform and scrutinize responses that are flagged by the platform. It is important to note that most survey platforms do not report details of how each metric is computed, possibly to prevent this information from being accessed by those who write automated scripts
- Monitor responses for duplicate surveys in which the answers to all questions are identical
- Check the time taken to complete the survey. The time required for a human to complete the survey should be determined through pilot testing. If a questionnaire response is faster than this, it may indicate the presence of a bot (Comachio et al., 2025)
- Review the responses to open-ended questions to ensure they make sense and are internally consistent. For example, check that the unit of measurement (ounces, grams, kilometers) matches the stated country of residence, and that the words used for a condition are appropriate (e.g., in speech pathology, 'assignment' is not a synonym for 'homework')
- Be skeptical about receiving a large number of responses within a short time frame

Management:

- Regularly review survey responses
- Keep the survey open for the shortest time possible
- If fraud is detected, close the survey, increase the security, and change the link

- Remove fraudulent responses prior to data analysis
- Report the number of fraudulent responses in the results
- Report the strategies used for bot prevention, detection, and management

4 Ongoing considerations to prevent and identify fraudulent participants in research

4.1 Minimizing fraud when screening and recruiting participants

Prevention measures should be implemented during the screening phase to identify fraudulent participants before recruiting them and to secure the online recruitment process. For instance, we recommend promoting the study within closed networks or social media groups. Potential participants matching the eligibility criteria could be targeted via small group communities, e.g., in closed Facebook groups or other social media platforms that restrict membership rather than using public profiles and communication channels (Andrew et al., 2024; Kumarasamy et al., 2024).

In addition, the use of market research companies to recruit participants can be an option to facilitate the recruitment process and obtain data. However, no report has been conducted on how strict these companies are when recruiting their panels and how they verify that the data are not only self-reported but also carefully checked to ensure that participants are not fraudulent. Given the limited information available about the procedures used by these companies, their use should be approached with caution. We recommend that researchers discuss this matter with individual market research companies and, if needed, implement additional checks to ensure the validity of the identification and eligibility of potential participants before recruiting them.

Finally, it is worth considering that, while this chapter focuses on online research, fraud can also occur when participants are met face-to-face (e.g., in interviews). Researchers should apply the principles outlined in this chapter to all research settings and designs to mitigate the risk of fraudulent participants.

4.2 Motivations behind fraudulent activities

A study evaluated the association between reimbursement and participant deception about research eligibility and concluded that reimbursement was associated with fraudulent participants compared to the control condition (Fernandez Lynch et al., 2019). Interestingly, higher reimbursements were not associated with increased rates of fraud (Fernandez Lynch et al., 2019). Even though the most common reason behind fraudulent activities in research might be financial gain, reimbursement may not be the only reason for scammers to commit fraud. Imposter participants may participate out of curiosity or might want to corrupt research data (Pullen Sansfaçon et al., 2024; Bauermeister et al., 2012). Other reasons may include political orientation or a desire to show opposition to certain sensitive issues. Other layers of scamming need to be considered: for instance, even if participants are eligible to participate, they may deliberately lie for the reasons cited above.

4.3 Use of AI while conducting qualitative studies

With the growing use of AI globally, participants may use it to answer questions or generate content during interviews. Indeed, there is already a proliferation of fraudulent activity where AI has been used in online surveys (Pinzón et al., 2024). Researchers will need to remain aware of rapidly evolving AI capabilities that could allow impostors to commit fraud (e.g., including AI-generated voice, photo or video (Clark and Lewandowsky, 2026)).

However, AI may be useful when used by participants or researchers for the translation of questions and responses or to improve understandability and communication, particularly in studies involving participants from culturally and linguistically diverse backgrounds. In such contexts, we recommend that participants discuss the use of AI with the researchers. During an interview, we suggest that any use of AI for language purposes be simultaneously visible to both the interviewer and interviewee, e.g., via screen share.

We recommend that the participant information statement be adapted accordingly, and the participant consent form could include a paragraph such as:

"We are interested in your personal knowledge and experiences, so we kindly ask that you do not use generative artificial intelligence (AI) tools to help you respond to the questions we will ask you. However, AI-based language tools may be used by participants who do not speak the dominant language of the research setting to facilitate translation, understanding, and communication. If you choose to use such tools, we kindly ask that you discuss this with the researcher before the interview starts and ensure that any AI-based language tool is used in real time and shared with the interviewer, e.g., *via screen share."*

4.4 Tension between privacy and data integrity

The prevention of fraud in research raises ethical concerns, as there is tension between privacy, identity checks, and the integrity of data. Ethics committees and the research community will need to work collaboratively with the wider community to find a new threshold they are comfortable with to balance the loss of confidentiality against data integrity. Decisions may need to be made on a case-by-case basis, considering the potential extent and impact of fraudulent activity on the research. Currently, ethics committees and the ethical standards and frameworks to which they must adhere may not sufficiently focus on fraud as a potential issue when reviewing ethics applications. Researchers should explicitly state in study protocols how they will prevent and address fraud if experienced (Sharma et al., 2024). Ethics committees should take action to require researchers to have protocols for fraud detection and should revise the participant information statements and participant consent forms accordingly to limit fraud. There is a need to develop ethics committee members' understanding of measures that can be taken to reduce the risk of fraudulent participation in research so they can effectively assess the potential for fraud in research studies.

4.5 Raising awareness of fraud and fraudulent participants among the research community: Roles of researchers, ethics committees, and institutions

After fraud is detected, researchers should report their experiences to the relevant ethics committee(s). To improve transparency, researchers should include their experiences in the dissemination of the research, detailing the methods used to prevent and detect fraud, the proportion of fraudulent participants excluded, if any, and explaining the actions taken to manage fraudulent participants (Mistry et al., 2024; Pellicano et al., 2024; Teitcher et al., 2015).

Specifically, researchers should report (1) how they prevented fraudulent participants from taking part in their study, (2) how they ensured that participants were not fraudulent, (3) if fraudulent participants took part, the number of participants involved, (4) what actions were implemented to deal with fraudulent data, and (5) how they prevented fraud from happening again. We encourage journal editors to require this information before publishing online qualitative study articles and suggest that reporting checklists be developed or revised to incorporate considerations relating to fraud. We also recommend that funding bodies scrutinize the methods of studies to ensure that strategies are in place to minimize and detect fraudulent participants.

Importantly, awareness about fraud in research should also be raised within the research community, such as at research conferences. Researchers can be upskilled through workshops on scam prevention and the key elements of detecting impostor participants.

More research should be conducted on the extent of fraud in research, e.g., a study that examines the number of fraudulent participants and the correlation with incentives provided in the context of a pharmacy practice study. However, this needs to go hand in hand with transparent reporting of fraud in research.

Universities and research institutions are called upon to develop guidance and support training initiatives on how to safeguard online research activities and prevent further occurrences of scamming. Guidance and training initiatives should be developed to educate early-career and student researchers, as well as staff researchers, on fraud in research.

Furthermore, guidelines need to be developed on how to manage fraudulent data if fraud is suspected or confirmed. Researchers may need to seek advice from local ethics committees, for example, on declining reimbursement to a fraudulent participant. We advise keeping all information and participant data collected as justification of fraud and disregarding them for the data analysis. Retention of data, even in cases of fraud, can be useful, such as when there is a complaint about a fraudulent participant not receiving reimbursement. In this scenario, it is important to show the ethics committee that the person was not eligible and to validate suspicions that the data was fake or fraudulent.

Finally, it should be acknowledged that all of these additional measures to prevent, detect, and manage fraud may have other unintended consequences. Firstly, these measures increase the potential burden on researchers, which could be addressed by implementing more automated and streamlined systems for data collection and reporting. Secondly, they may adversely affect the recruitment of participants who might be reluctant to provide identification or complete extra steps due to time constraints and concerns about their personal information being collected—and potentially hacked in the cloud. Thirdly, they may result in some genuine data being excluded from analysis, for example, if participants have poor language skills or misinterpret questions. These issues need to be carefully considered by researchers, ethics committees, and guideline developers.

5 Conclusions

Fraudulent participation in online qualitative and quantitative research represents a threat to data integrity. Based on the authors' experiences, this chapter reports how impostors have participated in online interviews and bots have generated responses in online surveys. While fraudulent participants may be detected by their suspicious contact details, inconsistent responses, a focused interest in the reimbursement, or refusal to appear on camera, researchers can prevent fraud by promoting the study to a closed network, carefully verifying participant identity, using fraud-detection tools in the survey platform, personalized links, or open-ended questions within the questionnaire. Ethics committees and research communities should work collaboratively to determine the balance between participant privacy and data verification processes. Research protocols, participant information statements, and consent forms will need to be revised to prevent future occurrences of fraud. Researchers will need to reinforce and constantly adapt their fraud prevention strategies, especially with the growing capacities of AI in generating responses, voices, and videos. Universities and research institutions have a key role to play in developing guidance and training and raising awareness of fraud in online research within the research community.

6 Questions for further discussion

- How can researchers balance the need to verify participant identity and eligibility with the ethical imperative to protect participant privacy and avoid excluding genuine, marginalized participants?
- What are the trade-offs between requiring cameras to be turned on during qualitative interviews and maintaining participant anonymity, particularly in sensitive research topics?
- How might the increasing sophistication of AI-generated text, voice, and video (as noted in Section 4.3) change the strategies researchers need to use to detect fraudulent participants over the next five years?
- What responsibilities do ethics committees have in requiring researchers to proactively plan for and report on fraud prevention, identification, and management in their protocols?
- How should researchers decide whether to report suspected fraudulent participation in their published research findings, and what are the implications of not doing so for the broader research community?
- In what ways might reimbursement structures (e.g., vouchers vs. cash, local vs. international) unintentionally influence the risk of fraudulent participation, and how should this be weighed against the goal of fairly compensating genuine participants?

7 Application exercise/scenario

7.1 Scenario 1 (qualitative study)

You are planning a qualitative study to explore pharmacists' strategies for conducting medication reviews with migrants. You are planning to recruit both pharmacists and migrants to conduct separate online interviews. You will advertise the study online to reach more participants.

- Provide five recommendations to incorporate into the protocol to prevent the inclusion of fraudulent participants.
- Provide two statements to be included in the participant information statement and consent form to deter fraudulent participants from taking part.

7.2 Scenario 2 (quantitative study)

You are planning a survey to explore pharmacists' roles in supporting medication adherence in children with asthma. You intend to distribute an online survey to both pharmacists and parents of children with asthma.

- Provide five recommendations to incorporate into the protocol to prevent the inclusion of fraudulent participants.
- Provide two statements to be included in the participant information statement and consent form to discourage fraudulent participants from taking part.

Appendix: Example of an email exchange between a researcher and a bot

Email 1
From: (bot)
To: (researcher)
Hello
I am taking part in this research survey. Is it still valid? I am eligible. I want to get this 15 Starbucks gift card.
Waiting for your reply.

Email 2
From: (researcher)
To: (bot)
Hi XX,
Great to hear from you. Yes, we are interested in hearing from caregivers of children with CAS.
The insights that caregivers provide about their experiences with assessment and treatment will help future families with CAS. Unfortunately, we have experienced some difficulties with computers (rather than humans) completing the survey. We have worked with some colleagues to identify the different characteristics of humans and robots. To help inform our efforts in this regard, could you please advise: (1) the age of your child with CAS, and (2) how you heard about the survey?
We sincerely thank you for your interest in the study.
Kind regards
The CAS Family Questionnaire team

Email 3
From: (bot)
To: (researcher)
Thank you for your response.
Thank you for reaching out! I appreciate the opportunity to contribute to this important study.
(1) My child with CAS is 8 years old.
(2) I learned about the survey through a Facebook post by XX, which you can find here: [Facebook link].
Thank you for your efforts in ensuring valuable insights from caregivers. I look forward to seeing the positive impact of this research!
I shared this survey with some friends who qualify and have completed it. I promised them it was a paid survey, and this is what I committed to them. Will they receive compensation?
Best regards,
XX

Email 4
From: (researcher)
To: (bot)
Hi XX,
We sincerely appreciate your time and effort of all caregivers of children with CAS. Where are you located? We're so keen to hear from people from around the globe.
XX

Email 5
From: (bot)
To: (researcher)
I am located in the United States, specifically in Nevada. The capital of my state is Carson City.

AI disclosure

During the preparation of this work, the author(s) used ChatGPT and Microsoft Copilot to correct spelling mistakes and to improve the flow of some sentences. After using these tools/services, the author(s) reviewed and edited the content as needed and take(s) full responsibility for the content of the publication.

References

Andrew, L., Gizzarelli, E., Estai, M., Wallace, R., 2024. Participant misrepresentation in online focus groups: red flags and proactive measures. Ethics Hum. Res. 2578-2363. 46 (1), 37–42. Available from: https://onlinelibrary.wiley.com/journal/25782363. doi:10.1002/eahr.500198.

Bandiera, C., Darwood, M., Mistry, S.K., Harris, E., Harris, M.F., Aslani, P., 2026. Interprofessional collaboration between community health workers and pharmacists. Health Expect. 1369-6513. 29 (1), e70538. Available from: https://www.ncbi.nlm.nih.gov/pmc/articles/PMC12815246. doi:10.1111/hex.70538.

Bandiera, C., Lowrie, K., Thomas, D., Mistry, S.K., Harris, E., Harris, M.F., Aslani, P., 2025. I have been scammed in my qualitative research. Res. Integr. Peer Rev. 2058-8615. 10 (1). doi:10.1186/s41073-025-00179-7.

Bauermeister, Pingel, Zimmerman, Couper, Carballo-Diéguez, Strecher, 2012. Data quality in web-based HIV/AIDS research: handling invalid and suspicious data. Field Methods 24 (3), 272–291.

Chen, A.T., Komi, M., Bessler, S., Mikles, S.P., Zhang, Y., 2023. Integrating statistical and visual analytic methods for bot identification of health-related survey data. J. Biomed. Inform. 1532-0464. 144. Available from: http://www.elsevier.com/inca/publications/store/6/2/2/8/5/7/index.htt. doi:10.1016/j.jbi.2023.104439.

Chung, S.Y., Hacker, E.D., Rawl, S., Ellis, R., Bakas, T., Jones, J., Welch, J., 2019. Using Facebook in recruiting kidney transplant recipients for a REDCap study. West. J. Nurs. Res. 1552-8456. 41 (12), 1790–1812. Available from: http://www.sagepub.com/ejournals. doi:10.1177/0193945919832600.

Clark, S., Lewandowsky, S., 2026. The continued influence of AI-generated deepfake videos despite transparency warnings. Commun. Psychol. 2731-9121. 4 (1), 13. Available from: https://doi.org/10.1038/s44271-025-00381-9. doi:10.1038/s44271-025-00381-9.

Comachio, J., Poulsen, A., Bamgboje-Ayodele, A., Tan, A., Ayre, J., Raeside, R., Roy, R., O'hagan, E., 2025. Identifying and counteracting fraudulent responses in online recruitment for health research: a scoping review. BMJ Evid. Based Med. 2515-4478. 30 (3), 173–182. Available from: http://ebm.bmj.com/. doi:10.1136/bmjebm-2024-113170.

Darko, E.M., Kleib, M., Olson, J., 2022. Social media use for research participant recruitment: integrative literature review. J. Med. Internet Res. 1438-8871. 24 (8), e38015. doi:10.2196/38015.

Davies, M.R., Monssen, D., Sharpe, H., Allen, K.L., Simms, B., Goldsmith, K.A., Byford, S., Lawrence, V., Schmidt, U., 2024. Management of fraudulent participants in online research: practical recommendations from a randomized controlled feasibility trial. Int. J. Eat. Disord. 1098-108X. 57 (6), 1311–1321. Available from: http://onlinelibrary.wiley.com/journal/10.1002/(ISSN)1098-108X. doi:10.1002/eat.24085.

Feng, S., Wan, H., Wang, N., Tan, Z., Luo, M., Tsvetkov, Y., 2024. What does the bot say? Opportunities and risks of large language models in social media bot detection. arXiv. 2331-8422. Available from: https://arxiv.org. doi:10.48550/arXiv.2402.00371.

Fernandez Lynch, H., Joffe, S., Thirumurthy, H., Xie, D., Largent, E.A., 2019. Association between financial incentives and participant deception about study eligibility. JAMA Netw. Open. 2574-3805. 2 (1), e187355. doi:10.1001/jamanetworkopen.2018.7355.

Glazer, J.V., MacDonnell, K., Frederick, C., Ingersoll, K., Ritterband, L.M., Liar!, L., 2021. Identifying eligibility fraud by applicants in digital health research. Internet Interv. 2214-7829. 25. Available from: http://www.journals.elsevier.com/internet-interventions/. doi:10.1016/j.invent.2021.100401.

Griffin, M., Martino, R.J., LoSchiavo, C., Comer-Carruthers, C., Krause, K.D., Stults, C.B., Halkitis, P.N., 2022. Ensuring survey research data integrity in the era of internet bots. Qual. Quant. 1573-7845. 56 (4), 2841–2852. Available from: https://link.springer.com/journal/11135. doi:10.1007/s11135-021-01252-1.

Jones, A., Caes, L., Rugg, T., Noel, M., Bateman, S., Jordan, A., 2021. Challenging issues of integrity and identity of participants in non-synchronous online qualitative methods. Methods Psychol. 2590-2601. 5, 100072. doi:10.1016/j.metip.2021.100072.

Keen, S., Lomeli-Rodriguez, M., Joffe, H., 2022. From challenge to opportunity: virtual qualitative research during COVID-19 and beyond. Int. J. Qual. Methods. 1609-4069. 21. Available from: https://journals.sagepub.com/home/IJQ. doi:10.1177/16094069221105075.

King-Nyberg, B., Thomson, E.F., Morris-Reade, J., Borgen, R., Taylor, C., 2023. The bot toolbox an accidental case study on how to eliminate bots from your online survey. J. Soc. Thought 7 (1). Available from: https://ojs.lib.uwo.ca/index.php/jst/article/view/14331.

Kobakhidze, M.N., Hui, J., Chui, J., González, A., 2021. Research disruptions, new opportunities: re-imagining qualitative interview study during the COVID-19 pandemic. Int. J. Qual. Methods. 1609-4069. 20. Available from: http://ijq.sagepub.com/content/by/year. doi:10.1177/16094069211051576.

Kumarasamy, V., Goodfellow, N., Ferron, E.M., Wright, A.L., 2024. Evaluating the problem of fraudulent participants in health care research: multimethod pilot study. JMIR Form. Res. 2561-326X. 8. Available from: https://formative.jmir.org/2024/1/e55798. doi:10.2196/51530.

Lawrence, P.R., Osborne, M.C., Sharma, D., Spratling, R., Calamaro, C.J., 2023. Methodological challenge: addressing bots in online research. J. Pediatr. Health Care. 0891-5245. 37 (3), 328–332. Available from: http://www.sciencedirect.com/science/journal/08915245. doi:10.1016/j.pedhc.2022.12.006.

Levi, R., Ridberg, R., Akers, M., Seligman, H., 2022. Survey fraud and the integrity of web-based survey research. Am. J. Health Promot. 2168-6602. 36 (1), 18–20. Available from: https://journals.sagepub.com/home/AHP. doi:10.1177/08901171211037531.

Merchant, A.A., Atherton, S., García-Iglesias, J., 2025. Imposter participants: a call for social science intervention. Sociol. Res. Online. 1360-7804. Available from: https://journals.sagepub.com/home/sro. doi:10.1177/13607804251340013.

Mistry, K., Merrick, S., Cabecinha, M., Daniels, S., Ragan, J., Epstein, M., Lever, L., Venables, Z.C., Levell, N.J., 2024. Fraudulent participation in online qualitative studies: practical recommendations on an emerging phenomenon. Qual. Health Res. 1552-7557. Available from: https://journals.sagepub.com/home/QHR. doi:10.1177/10497323241288181.

Mozaffarian, R.S., Norris, J.M., Kenney, E.L., 2025. Managing sophisticated fraud in online research. JAMA Netw. Open. 2574-3805. 8 (2), e2460168. Available from: https://jamanetwork.com/journals/jamanetworkopen. doi:10.1001/jamanetworkopen.2024.60168.

Pellicano, E., Adams, D., Crane, L., Hollingue, C., Allen, C., Almendinger, K., Botha, M., Haar, T., Kapp, S.K., Wheeley, E., 2024. Letter to the editor: a possible threat to data integrity for online qualitative autism research. Autism. 1461-7005. 28 (3), 786–792. Available from: https://journals.sagepub.com/home/AUT. doi:10.1177/13623613231174543.

Pinzón, N., Koundinya, V., Galt, R.E., Dowling, W.O.R., Baukloh, M., Taku-Forchu, N.C., Schohr, T., Roche, L.M., Ikendi, S., Cooper, M., Parker, L.E., Pathak, T.B., 2024. AI-powered fraud and the erosion of online survey integrity: an analysis of 31 fraud detection strategies. Front. Res. Metr. Anal. 2504-0537. 9. Available from: https://www.frontiersin.org/journals/research-metrics-and-analytics/about. doi:10.3389/frma.2024.1432774.

Pozzar, R., Hammer, M.J., Underhill-Blazey, M., Wright, A.A., Tulsky, J.A., Hong, F., Gundersen, D.A., Berry, D.L., 2020. Threats of bots and other bad actors to data quality following research participant recruitment through social media: cross-sectional questionnaire. J. Med. Internet Res. 1438-8871. 22 (10). Available from: http://www.jmir.org/2020/10/e23021/. doi:10.2196/23021.

Pullen Sansfaçon, A., Gravel, E., Gelly, M.A., 2024. Dealing with scam in online qualitative research: strategies and ethical considerations. Int. J. Qual. Methods. 1609-4069. 23. Available from: https://journals.sagepub.com/home/IJQ. doi:10.1177/16094069231224610.

Qualtrics, 2025. Fraud Detection. https://www.qualtrics.com/support/survey-platform/survey-module/survey-checker/fraud-detection/

Qualtrics, 2025. Qualtrics website. https://www.qualtrics.com./

Ridge, D., Bullock, L., Causer, H., Fisher, T., Hider, S., Kingstone, T., Gray, L., Riley, R., Smyth, N., Silverwood, V., Spiers, J., Southam, J., 2023. Imposter participants' in online qualitative research, a new and increasing threat to data integrity?. Health Expect. 1369-7625. 26 (3), 941–944. Available from: http://onlinelibrary.wiley.com/journal/10.1111/(ISSN)1369-7625. doi:10.1111/hex.13724.

Salinas, M.R., 2023. Are your participants real? Dealing with fraud in recruiting older adults online. West. J. Nurs. Res. 1552-8456. 45 (1), 93–99. Available from: https://journals.sagepub.com/home/WJN. doi:10.1177/01939459221098468.

Schles, R.A., Deheck, C.M.K., 2025. Identifying and mitigating the influence of invalid responses in online surveys: a longitudinal case study. Qual. Quant. 1573-7845. Available from: https://www.springer.com/journal/11135. doi:10.1007/s11135-025-02333-1.

Sefcik, J.S., Hathaway, Z., DiMaria-Ghalili, R.A., 2023. When snowball sampling leads to an avalanche of fraudulent participants in qualitative research. Int. J. Older People Nurs. 1748-3743. 18 (6). Available from: http://onlinelibrary.wiley.com/journal/10.1111/(ISSN)1748-3743. doi:10.1111/opn.12572.

Sharma, P., McPhail, S.M., Kularatna, S., Senanayake, S., Abell, B., 2024. Navigating the challenges of imposter participants in online qualitative research: lessons learned from a paediatric health services study. BMC Health Serv. Res. 1472-6963. 24 (1). Available from: https://bmchealthservres.biomedcentral.com/. doi:10.1186/s12913-024-11166-x.

Teitcher, J.E.F., Bockting, W.O., Bauermeister, J.A., Hoefer, C.J., Miner, M.H., Klitzman, R.L., 2015. Detecting, preventing, and responding to "fraudsters" in internet research: ethics and tradeoffs. J. L. Med. Ethics. 1748-720X. 43 (1), 116–133. Available from: http://lme.sagepub.com/. doi:10.1111/jlme.12200.

Thomas, D.C. et al., 2026. Caregivers' Experiences of Assessment and Treatment for Their Child With Childhood Apraxia of Speech: An International Questionnaire Study. Am J Speech Lang Pathol 35 (2), 743–762. doi:10.1044/2025_AJSLP-25-00358.

Thomas, D.C., Gomez, M., Muis, A., Trezise, N., Williamson, E., Choo, J.X.M., Case, J., Murray, E., Grigos, M.I., Iuzzini-Seigel, J., Velleman, S.L. (n.d.) Caregivers' Experiences of Assessment and Treatment for their Child with CAS: an International Questionnaire Study. Submitted.

Index

Note: Page numbers followed by *f* indicate figures, *b* indicate boxes, *t* indicate tables.

Q

R

S

T

U

V

W

Z

Printed and bound by CPI Group (UK) Ltd, Croydon, CR0 4YY
14/09/2026
02216388-0008